DICTIONARY OF
Optometry and Vision Science

Content Strategist: Russell Gabbedy
Content Development Specialist: Sharon Nash
Project Manager: Julie Taylor
Design: Brian Salisbury
Illustration Manager: Karen Giacomucci
Marketing Manager: Claire McKenzie

EIGHTH EDITION

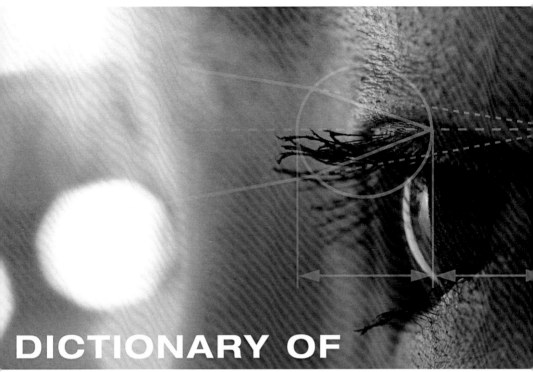

DICTIONARY OF
Optometry and Vision Science

MICHEL MILLODOT
OD, PhD, DOSc(Hon), FAAO, FCOptom
Honorary Professor, School of Optometry and Vision Sciences, Cardiff University, UK;
Professor Emeritus, The Hong Kong Polytechnic University, Hong Kong, China

For additional online content, visit ExpertConsult.com

ELSEVIER

ELSEVIER

First edition 1986
Second edition 1990
Third edition 1993
Reprinted 1994, 1995
Fourth edition 1997
Reprinted 1998
Fifth edition 2000
Reprinted 2001, 2002
Sixth edition 2004
Reprinted 2005, 2006
Seventh edition 2009

Notices

Knowledge and best practice in this field are constantly changing. As new research and experience broaden our understanding, changes in research methods, professional practices, or medical treatment may become necessary.

Practitioners and researchers must always rely on their own experience and knowledge in evaluating and using any information, methods, compounds, or experiments described herein. In using such information or methods they should be mindful of their own safety and the safety of others, including parties for whom they have a professional responsibility.

With respect to any drug or pharmaceutical products identified, readers are advised to check the most current information provided (i) on procedures featured or (ii) by the manufacturer of each product to be administered, to verify the recommended dose or formula, the method and duration of administration, and contraindications. It is the responsibility of practitioners, relying on their own experience and knowledge of their patients, to make diagnoses, to determine dosages and the best treatment for each individual patient, and to take all appropriate safety precautions.

To the fullest extent of the law, neither the Publisher nor the authors, contributors, or editors, assume any liability for any injury and/or damage to persons or property as a matter of products liability, negligence or otherwise, or from any use or operation of any methods, products, instructions, or ideas contained in the material herein.

ISBN: 978-0-7020-7222-2
E-ISBN: 978-0-7020-7223-9
Inkling ISBN: 978-0-7020-7224-6

ELSEVIER your source for books, journals and multimedia in the health sciences

www.elsevierhealth.com

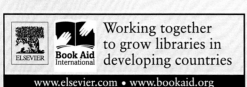

Working together to grow libraries in developing countries

www.elsevier.com • www.bookaid.org

The publisher's policy is to use paper manufactured from sustainable forests

Contents

Preface to the eighth edition

The continued acceptance of the *Dictionary of Optometry and Vision Science* has been very gratifying. It has now become a recommended text in most optometry courses around the world. For this new edition, I have felt compelled to carry out an exhaustive revision of all the existing definitions, to expand many to include more relevant and up-to-date information and to improve the clarity wherever this was deemed necessary. Some obsolete terms were also deleted. The education and practice of optometry has changed in the last few years as optometrists in many countries (e.g. UK, U.S., Canada, Australia) have become legally entitled to use therapeutic drugs for the treatment of eye diseases. They have thus become more involved in the management and co-management of some eye diseases, in addition to the traditional fields of optometric practice, and it became imperative to reflect these changes in the dictionary. Therefore in this edition there are more than 400 new terms relating to ocular pathology, ocular pharmacology, ocular anatomy, optometric techniques, physiology and psychology of vision, contact lenses, optics ocular genetics, research methodology and neuroimaging techniques.

The aim of the *Dictionary of Optometry and Vision Science* remains to serve as a repository of all common terms used in this discipline and as a source of information for clinicians, students and researchers in optometry, ophthalmology, orthoptics, dispensing optics and vision science, as well as others searching for an answer to their query regarding visual anomalies, eye diseases, systemic diseases and syndromes with ocular manifestations, anatomy, physiology and optics of the eye, and the phenomenon of vision.

A dictionary defines words, unlike an encyclopaedia, which describes subjects, albeit to various degrees of comprehensiveness. Thus the entries are relatively concise, although the foremost aim has been to provide the most relevant information in each definition. Thus a given disease will consist of a description of the condition including its aetiology, its main signs, symptoms and a brief note about its treatment. An anatomical structure is described in terms of its morphology and function. Busy practitioners and students would thus be spared the need to search through various sources for the desired information. Within each definition, technical words are often used by necessity; however, all these words are defined elsewhere in the dictionary.

New illustrations have been added and several older ones have been modified to improve their presentation. They enhance the understanding of the definitions and in many cases additional information is provided with the illustrations. The dictionary also contains many tables. They not only summarize some of the written text but also frequently supplement the definitions. They appear with related terms throughout the text and not in appendices, as is sometimes done in some dictionaries.

Overall the text now contains about 12% more material than in the last edition.

The dictionary now includes more than 5600 terms, 90 tables and 253 illustrations and I hope that this new edition represents the most up-to-date and informative compilation of optometric and vision science terms available, yet in a new, approachable and affordable format.

I would like to thank the staff of Elsevier, especially Russell Gabbedy, Sharon Nash and Julie Taylor, for their continuous support and help in the preparation of this new edition.

Michel Millodot
mmillodot@gmail.com

About the dictionary

Entries are listed alphabetically. This is easy when the entry consists of a single word. However, in optometry and vision science, a great number of terms are compounds made up of more than one word. In almost all instances, compound entries made up of one or more adjectives appear under the noun (e.g. crystalline lens capsule and confocal scanning laser ophthalmoscope appear at capsule and ophthalmoscope, respectively). There are exceptions to this rule, especially eponymous terms in which the noun is almost the only one listed (e.g. Mallett fixation disparity unit, Krukenberg spindle, Landolt ring, Necker cube, Scheimpflug photography, Wilbrand's knee appear at the name of the individual; but Graves' disease, Marfan's syndrome or the duochrome test in which there are many entries with that noun appear in the list at disease, syndrome and test, respectively). Also when the noun is almost the only one listed while the adjective forms part of a long list of entries (e.g. corneal stroma and retinal pigment epithelium), they are placed in the list of the words (corneal and retinal, respectively). A few entries are placed under the most important word (e.g. back optic zone radius and resting potential of the eye are placed at optic and potential, respectively). *In any case, compound terms are listed under the alternative entry and cross-referred to where they are defined, if applicable.*

Many entries have **subentries**, in bold letters, on subjects that are related to the main entry. In many instances, they are defined there rather than repeating the definition elsewhere. The entries often end with the common **synonyms** *(Syn.)* and sometimes with a *Note*. Synonyms are very common in the vocabulary of optometry. I have, however, retained the most common synonyms. They also vary from country to country. For example, stimulus deprivation amblyopia is the preferred term in the UK, whereas image degradation amblyopia is favoured in the U.S. Some synonyms also appear within a definition and are then given in brackets.

Cross-references (See) accompany many entries as they help the reader obtain additional information that is either directly or indirectly linked to them and to continue in the path of learning. Cross-references as main entries merely refer to another entry where it is more conveniently defined or it may be a synonym or a subentry of an entry defined elsewhere.

The names of medicinal *drugs* are given using the Recommended International Nonproprietary Name (rINN), which are those used in the British National Formulary.

Abbreviations and *symbols* are assembled in a table at the beginning of the dictionary. They have become very fashionable in the last few years, perhaps because of the widespread use of personal computers. Not all those which exist are listed here; it has been necessary to try to distinguish between those that seem ephemeral and those that are destined to endure. And there is the added complication of existing differences between common usage in different countries.

Prefixes and *suffixes* are frequently used in the formation of words. Thus a list of prefixes and suffixes employed in this dictionary appears at the beginning of the dictionary. It was also felt that the **linguistic origin** of some of the most common terms used in the language of this discipline may be of interest. This is also given at the beginning of the dictionary.

British spelling has been used throughout this dictionary. However, because American spelling (e.g. esthesiometer, edema) differs from British spelling, both terms are listed, but the definition is placed with the British spelling (e.g. aesthesiometer, oedema).

Abbreviations, acronyms and symbols

Å	ångström unit = 0.1 nm		BP	blood pressure
A	ocular accommodation		BPR	back peripheral radius
AACG	acute angle-closure glaucoma		BPZD	back peripheral zone diameter
AAU	acute anterior uveitis		BRAO	branch retinal artery occlusion
AC	anterior chamber			(see retinal artery)
AC/A	accommodative convergence/		BRVO	branch retinal vein occlusion (see
	accommodation ratio			retinal vein)
acc	accommodation		BSV	binocular single vision
ACG	angle-closure glaucoma		BU	base-up (prism)
ACh	acetylcholine		BUT	break-up time
ACIOL	anterior chamber intraocular lens		BV	binocular vision
ACT	alternating cover test		BVP	back vertex power
add	addition for near vision		BVS	best vision sphere
AFD	afferent pupillary defect		C/D	cup-disc ratio
AFPP	apparent frontoparallel plane		CAB	cellulose acetate butyrate
AIDS	acquired immunodeficiency		CACG	chronic angle-closure glaucoma
	syndrome		CAG	closed-angle glaucoma
AION	anterior ischaemic optic		CAT	computerized axial tomography
	neuropathy		cc	chief complaint; concave; cum
AKC	atopic keratoconjunctivitis			corrections (with correction)
AMD	age-related macular degeneration		CCTV	closed-circuit television
amp acc	amplitude of accommodation		cd	candela
ANS	autonomic nervous system		CD	centration distance
AOSLO	adaptive optics scanning laser		CDT	corneal damage threshold
	ophthalmoscope		CF	counting fingers
ARC	abnormal retinal correspondence		CFF	critical fusion frequency
ARM	age-related maculopathy		CFT	corneal epithelial fragility threshold
ARMD	age-related macular degeneration		CHED	congenital hereditary endothelial
As	spectacle accommodation			dystrophy
Ast	astigmatism		CHRPE	congenital hypertrophy of the
ATP	adenosine triphosphate			retinal pigment epithelium
A–V	arteriole–venule crossing		CIE	Commission Internationale de
BAT	Brightness Acuity Tester			l'Eclairage
BC	base curve; back central radius		CISS	convergence insufficiency
BCOD	back central optic diameter			symptom survey
BCOR	back central optic radius		CL	contact lens
BCVA	best corrected visual acuity		CLAPC	contact lens-associated papillary
BD	base-down (prism)			conjunctivitis
BDR	background diabetic retinopathy		CLARE	contact lens acute red eye
BE	both eyes		CLPC	contact lens papillary conjunctivitis
BI	base-in (prism)		CMO	cystoid macular oedema
BIO	binocular indirect ophthalmoscope		CMV	cytomegalovirus
BO	base-out (prism)		CNS	central nervous system
BOZD	back optic zone diameter		CNV	choroidal neovascularization
BOZR	back optic zone radius		COR	critical oxygen requirement

CORVIST	cortical vision screening test	EOP	equivalent oxygen pressure (see oxygen pressure)
CP	centration point		
cpd	cycle per degree	ER	enlargement ratio
CPEO	chronic progressive external ophthalmoplegia	ERG	electroretinogram
		ERP	early receptor potential
CR-39	Columbia Resin 39	eso	esophoria
CRAO	central retinal artery occlusion	ESOP	esophoria
CRVO	central retinal vein occlusion	esoT	esotropia
CSCR	central serous chorioretinopathy	ET	esotropia at distance
CSF	contrast sensitivity function	ET′	esotropia at near
CSLO	confocal scanning laser ophthalmoscope	EVD	equivalent viewing distance
		EVES	electronic vision enhancement system
CSR	central serous retinopathy		
CT	cover test; computed tomography	EVP	equivalent viewing power
CTT	corneal touch threshold	EW	extended wear contact lens
CV	colour vision	exo	exophoria
CVS	computer vision syndrome	exoT	exotropia
cx	convex	f'	second focal length
CXL	corneal collagen cross-linking	f	first focal length
cyl	cylindrical power	F	focal power; refractive power; surface power; vergence power
D	dioptre; optical density		
DALK	deep anterior lamellar keratoplasty	FAAO	Fellow of the American Academy of Optometry
dB	decibel		
DBL	distance between lenses	FB	foreign body
DBR	distance between rims	fc	footcandle
DC	dioptric cylindrical power	FCOptom	Fellow of the College of Optometrists
DCLP	Diploma in Contact Lens Practice		
DDST	Denver Developmental Screening Test	FDA	Food and Drug Administration (U.S.)
dec	decentration	FDP	frequency doubling perimetry
DEM	developmental eye movement test	F_e	equivalent power; power of the eye
DFP	diisopropyl fluorophosphate		
Dk	oxygen permeability	FES	floppy eyelid syndrome
Dk/t	oxygen transmissibility	FFA	fundus fluorescein angiography
DNA	deoxyribonucleic acid	fL	footlambert
DOrth	Diploma in Orthoptics	FM100	Farnsworth–Munsell 100 Hue test
DOS	Doctor of Ocular Science; Doctor of Optometric Science	fMRI	functional magnetic resonance imaging
DPA	diagnostic pharmaceutical agent	FOH	familial ocular history
DR	diabetic retinopathy	FOZD	front optic zone diameter
DS	dioptric spherical power	FRCOphth	Fellow of the Royal College of Ophthalmologists
DSAEK	Descemet's stripping automated endothelial keratoplasty		
		FRCS	Fellow of the Royal College of Surgeons
DSEK	Descemet's stripping endothelial keratoplasty		
		F'_v	back vertex power
DV	distance vision	F_v	front vertex power
DVD	dissociated vertical deviation	FVP	front vertex power
DVP	distance visual point	FXS	fragile X syndrome
Dx	diagnosis	GH	general health
E	esophoria at distance; illumination	GP	gas permeable contact lens
E′	esophoria at near	GPC	giant papillary conjunctivitis
ECCE	extracapsular cataract extraction (see cataract extraction)	GPCL	gas permeable contact lens
		GPL	gas permeable lens
EDTA	ethylenediamine tetraacetic acid	H	hypermetropia; hyperopia
EF	eccentric fixation	h	object height
EMG	electromyogram	h'	image height
EOG	electrooculogram	HA	headache

HARC	harmonious abnormal retinal correspondence	LVA	low vision aid
		lx	lux
HEMA	hydroxyethyl methacrylate	M	myopia; magnification
HGP	hard gas permeable contact lens	ma	metre angle
HHV	human herpesvirus	MAR	minimum angle of resolution
HIC	Humphriss immediate contrast test	MBCO	Member of the British College of Optometrists
HIV	human immunodeficiency virus	mfERG	multifocal electroretinogram
HM	hand movements	MGD	meibomian gland dysfunction
HRR	Hardy, Rand and Rittler colour vision test	MPD	monocular pupillary distance
		MR	medial rectus
HSV	herpes simplex virus	mRGC	melanopsin retinal ganglion cell
Hx	patient's history	MRI	magnetic resonance imaging
Hz	hertz	MS	multiple sclerosis
I	luminous intensity	MTF	modulation transfer function
ICCE	intracapsular cataract extraction	n	index of refraction
ICE	iridocorneal endothelial syndrome	NAD	nothing abnormal discovered
INO	internuclear ophthalmoplegia	NCD	near centration distance
IO	inferior oblique	NCT	Non-Contact Tonometer
IOL	intraocular lens	ND	neutral density filter
IOP	intraocular pressure	NGF	nerve growth factor
IOT	interocular transfer	NIBUT	non-invasive break-up time test
IPD	interpupillary distance	NLP	no light perception
IR	inferior rectus; infrared	nm	nanometre
ISO	International Organization for Standardization	NPC	near point of convergence
		NPS	nearpoint stress
J	Jaeger test type	NRA	negative relative accommodation
jnd	just noticeable difference	NRC	normal retinal correspondence
K	centre corneal curvature of longest radius as measured with a keratometer; ocular refraction; spectacle refraction; degree kelvin	NSAID	non-steroidal antiinflammatory drug
		NTG	normal-tension glaucoma
		NV	near vision
KC	keratoconus	NVP	near visual point
KCS	keratoconjunctivitis sicca	OCA	Ophthalmological Congress Amsterdam notation
KP	keratic precipitates		
L	lambert; left; luminance; vergence	Occ	occupation
l	object distance	OCG	oculogyric crisis
l'	image distance	OCT	optical coherence tomography
L/R	left hyperphoria	OD	Doctor of Optometry; oculus dexter; overall diameter
LASEK	laser assisted epithelial keratomileusis		
		ODM	ophthalmodynamometer
LASER	light amplification by stimulated emission of radiation	OH	ocular history
		OKN	optokinetic nystagmus
LASIK	laser in situ keratomileusis or laser assisted intrastromal keratoplasty	ONH	optic nerve head
		OPD	optic zone diameter
LCA	longitudinal chromatic aberration	OS	oculus sinister; overall size
LE	left eye	OU	oculus uterque
LGB	lateral geniculate body (see geniculate body)	PAL	progressive addition lens
		PAM	Potential Acuity Meter
LGN	lateral geniculate nucleus	PCCR	posterior central curve radius
lm	lumen	PCI	partial coherence interferometry
LOCS	lens opacity classification system	PCIOL	posterior chamber intraocular lens
LP	light perception	PD	interpupillary distance; prism dioptre
LR	lateral rectus; light reaction		
LRI	limbal relaxing incision	PDR	proliferative diabetic retinopathy
LRK	laser refractive keratoplasty	PDS	pigment dispersion syndrome
LTG	low tension glaucoma	PDT	photodynamic therapy

PEK	photoelectric keratoscope; punctate epithelial keratitis	**SLK**	superior limbic keratoconjunctivitis
pERG	pattern electroretinogram	**SLO**	scanning laser ophthalmoscope
PERRLA	pupils equal, round and reactive to light and accommodation	**SLP**	scanning laser polarimetry
		SM	spectacle magnification
PET	positron emission tomography	**SMD**	senile macular degeneration
pH	hydrogen ion concentration	**SO**	superior oblique
ph	pinhole	**SOP**	esophoria
PK	penetrating keratoplasty	**SOT**	esotropia
PHPV	persistent hyperplastic primary vitreous	**sph**	spherical power
		SPK	superficial punctate keratitis
PL	preferential looking	**SR**	superior rectus
PMMA	polymethyl methacrylate	**SV**	single vision
PNS	peripheral nervous system	**SWAP**	short wavelength automated perimetry
POAG	primary open-angle glaucoma		
POH	past ocular history	**TA**	tonic accommodation
POHS	presumed ocular histoplasmosis syndrome	**TABO**	Technischer Auschuss für Brillenoptik
PPV	pars plana vitrectomy	**TBUT**	tear break-up time
PRA	positive relative accommodation	**TCA**	transverse chromatic aberration
PRK	photorefractive keratectomy	**TD**	total diameter
PSF	point-spread function	**TIB**	Turville Infinity Balance test
PSP	progressive supranuclear palsy	**TNO**	Technisch Natuurwetenschappelijk Onderzoek
PVD	posterior vitreous detachment		
Px	patient	t_o	geometrical centre thickness (contact lens)
PXF	pseudoexfoliation		
PXS	pseudoexfoliation syndrome	**TPA**	therapeutic pharmaceutical agent
r	radius of curvature of a surface	**TRIC**	trachoma inclusion conjunctivitis (see conjunctivitis, adult inclusion)
R	right		
R/L	right hyperphoria	**TVAS**	Test of Visual Analysis Skills
RAPD	relative afferent pupillary defect (see pupil, Marcus Gunn)	**Tx**	treatment
		UV	ultraviolet
RCT	randomized controlled trial; randomized clinical trial	**UVR**	ultraviolet radiation
		V	Abbè's number; constringence; vision; V-value
RD	retinal detachment		
RDS	random-dot stereogram	**V1**	visual area 1
RE	right eye	**VA**	visual acuity
REM	rapid eye movements	**VDT**	video display terminal
ret	retinoscopy	**VDU**	visual display unit
RGC	retinal ganglion cell	**VECP**	visual evoked cortical potential
RGP	rigid gas permeable contact lens	**VEGF**	vascular endothelial growth factor
RK	radial keratotomy		
RNA	ribonucleic acid	**VEP**	visual evoked potential
RNFL	retinal nerve fibre layer	**VER**	visual evoked response
ROP	retinopathy of prematurity	**VF**	visual field
ROS	reactive oxygen species	**VKC**	vernal keratoconjunctivitis
RP	retinitis pigmentosa	**VKH**	Vogt–Koyanagi–Harada syndrome
RPE	retinal pigment epithelium	**VSRT**	Visual Skills for Reading Test
RSM	relative spectacle magnification	**VZV**	varicella-zoster virus
R_x	prescription	**WD**	working distance
S	spherical power	**WHO**	World Health Organization
SBV	single binocular vision	**WT**	wearing time
SCL	soft contact lens	**X**	exophoria at distance
SEAL	superior epithelial arcuate lesion (see staining, fluorescein)	**X′**	exophoria at near
		x-axis	transverse axis
SiH	silicone hydrogel	**XOP**	exophoria
SITA	Swedish Interactive Thresholding Algorithm	**XOT**	exotropia
		XT	exotropia at distance

XT′	exotropia at near	θ	angle theta
YAG	yttrium-aluminium-garnet	κ	angle kappa
y-axis	anteroposterior axis	λ	angle lambda; wavelength
z-axis	vertical axis	ν	frequency of light
α	angle alpha	ρ	reflection factor
Δ	prism dioptre	ω	angle omega
η	stereoscopic visual acuity	∞	infinity (6 m (or 20 ft) or more)

Common prefixes and suffixes

prefix	meaning	example
a-	not, without	aniridia (without an iris)
ab-	away from	abduct (turning away from midline)
ad-	to, towards	adduct (turning towards the midline)
alb-	white	albinism (hypopigmentation of eye, skin and hair)
ambi-	both	ambiocular (use either eye separately)
ana-	up, towards, apart	anatomy (to cut apart)
angi-, angio-	blood or lymph vessels	angioscotoma (scotoma due to blood vessels)
aniso-	unequal, dissimilar	anisophoria (variation in the amount of heterophoria)
anti-	against, opposed	antimetropia (opposite refraction in each eye)
bi-	twice, double	bifocal (two foci)
blephar-, blepharo-	eyelid	blepharitis (inflammation of the eyelids)
chrom-	colour	chromatic (pertaining to colour)
contra-	opposed, against	contralateral (opposite side)
cry-, cryo-	cold	cryotherapy (use of cold to treat retinal detachment)
cyano-	blue	cyanophobia (aversion to blue)
cycl-, cyclo-	circle	cycloduction (rotation of an eye)
dacry-, dacryo-	tears	dacryocystitis (inflammation of the lacrimal sac)
de-	separation, reversal	degeneration (worsening), deterioration
dextro-	right	dextroduction (rotation of an eye to the right)
deuter-, deutero-	two, second	deuteranopia (vision of two primary colours)
di-	two, apart	distichiasis (two rows of eyelashes)
dis-	apart, reversal, to separate	dispersion (separation of monochromatic components)
dys-	bad, difficult	dyslexia (difficulty with reading)
end-, endo-	within, inner	endothelium (the inner corneal layer)
epi-	upon, beside	episclera (upon the sclera)
erythr-, erythro-	red	erythrolabe (red cone pigment)
exo-	from, out of, outside	exophthalmos (eye protruding out of the orbit)
extra-	outside of, beyond the scope of	extraocular (outside the eye)
gonio-	angle	gonioscopy (measurement of the anterior chamber angle)
haema-	blood	haematoma (tumour containing blood)
hemi-	half	hemianopia (loss of vision in half of visual field)
hetero-	different, other	heterochromia (different coloured eyes)
hyper-	above, excessive	hyperaesthesia (above normal sensitivity)
hypo-	under, deficient, below	hypopyon (pus at the bottom of the anterior chamber)
infra-	below, under	infraduction (rotation of an eye downward)
inter-	between, among	interocular (between the eyes)
intra-	within, inside	intraocular (within the eye)
irid-, irido-	iris	iridoplegia (paralysis affecting the iris)
iso-	equal	isocoria (pupils of equal sizes)
kerat-, kerato-	cornea	keratoconus (bulging of the cornea)
kin-, kine-	movement	kinetic (pertaining to movement)

prefix	meaning	example
leuk-, leuko-	white, colourless	leukocoria (a white reflex within the pupil)
macro-	large, long	macropsia (large visual object)
meg-, mega-	large, oversize	megalophthalmos (abnormally large eye)
melan-, melano-	black	melanoma (a brown or black mass)
micro-	small, one millionth (1/1 000 000 or 10^{-6})	microphthalmia (very small eyeball) micrometre (one millionth of a metre)
milli-	one thousandth (1/1000 or 10^{-3})	millisecond (one thousandth of) a second
mono-	one, single	monocular (pertaining to one eye)
multi-	many	multifocal (many foci)
nano-	one-billionth (10^{-9})	nanometre (one billionth of a metre)
neur-, neuri-, neuro-	nerve, nervous system	neuropathy (disorder of nerves or the nervous system)
ocul-	eye	ocular (pertaining to the eye)
ophthalm-	relate to eye	ophthalmia (inflammation of the eye)
ortho-	straight, correct, right	orthophoria (straight eyes)
pan-	all	panoramic vision (vision in all directions)
para-	beside, beyond, near, wrong	paraxial (near the axis)
peri-	around, near	perimetry (measurement of visual field 'around the centre')
phaco-	crystalline lens	phacoemulsification (a method of cataract removal)
phot-, photo-	light	photophobia (fear of light)
poly-	many	polyopia (many visual images)
post-	after, behind	postlenticular (behind the lens)
presby-	old	presbyopia (old eye)
pro-	before, in front of, in place of, forward	prophylaxis (prevention of a disease); projector (presentation of an image forward)
pseudo-	false	pseudoglaucoma (false glaucoma)
re-	again, backward	reflex (respond backward)
retro-	backward, behind	retrobulbar (behind the eye)
scot-, scoto-	darkness, shadow	scotoma (a dark area of the visual field)
sub-	under, below	subconjunctival haemorrhage (rupture of blood vessels beneath the conjunctiva)
supra-	above	supraversion (both eyes rotate upward)
sym-, syn-	together, with	symblepharon (adhesion of the bulbar and palpebral conjunctiva)
tele-	distant, far off	telescope (to view distant objects)
tono-	pressure, tension	tonometer (to measure intraocular pressure)
trans-	through, across	transmission (passage through)
tri-	three	trichromatic (three colours)
ultra-	beyond, extreme	ultraviolet (beyond the violet)
uni-	one	uniocular (one eye)
xanth-, xantho-	yellow	xanthelasma (yellow plaque on the eyelid)
xero-	dry	xerophthalmia (dryness of the cornea and conjunctiva)

suffix	meaning	example
-aemia	referring to blood	hyperaemia (excessive accumulation of blood)
-al	pertaining to, relating to	deuteranomal (pertaining to deuteranomaly)
-ase	enzyme	acetylcholinesterase (an enzyme which hydrolyses acetylcholine)
-asis	condition, process	mydriasis (condition of an eye with a large pupil)
-ation	a resulting state or thing	illumination (resulting in a brighter object)
-cele	protrusion	descemetocele (bulging of Descemet's membrane)

suffix	meaning	example
-ectomy	excision of	iridectomy (excision of the iris)
-gram	recording	electrooculogram (recording of eye movements)
-ia	state or condition	amblyopia (condition of reduced visual acuity)
-ic	pertaining to, relating to	chromatic (pertaining to colour)
-ism	condition, action	achromatism (being totally colour blind)
-ist	person or agent	optometrist
-itis	inflammation	conjunctivitis (inflammation of the conjunctiva)
-lysis	separating, dissolution	iridodialysis (disinsertion of the iris from the ciliary body)
-malacia	softening	keratomalacia (an abnormally soft cornea)
-meter	measures	photometer (measures light)
-metry	process of measuring	keratometry (process of measuring the cornea)
-ogist	person or agent	ophthalmologist
-ology	science, study of, knowledge of	physiology (study of living organisms)
-oma	tumour	retinoblastoma (tumour of the retina)
-opia	condition or defect	polyopia (many visual images)
-opsia	condition or defect	chromatopsia (objects appear falsely coloured)
-osis	condition, process	madarosis (loss of the eyelashes); proptosis (abnormal protrusion of one eye)
-otomy	cutting, incision, division	iridotomy (creating an opening in the iris)
-oxia	oxygen	hypoxia (state of decreased oxygen)
-pathy	disease	keratopathy (disease of the cornea)
-pexy	fixation	retinopexy (re-attaching the sensory retina to the pigment epithelium)
-phobia	abnormal fear or intolerance	photophobia (abnormal fear or intolerance to light)
-plasty	surgical intervention or repair	keratoplasty (corneal transplant)
-plegia	paralysis	ophthalmoplegia (paralysis of some ocular muscle/s)
-rrhaphy	suturing in place	tarsorrhaphy (suturing the eyelids)
-scope	instrument for examining	ophthalmoscope (examining inside the eye)
-scopy	act of examining	retinoscopy (process of measuring refraction)
-spasm	muscle contraction	blepharospasm (sudden contraction of the orbicularis muscle)
-tic	pertaining to	anaesthetic (pertaining to anaesthesia)
-tion	state or condition	perception (recognizing a percept)
-tropia	to turn	exotropia (eye turning outward)
-trophy	nutrition, growth	hypertrophy (excessive growth of an organ)

Linguistic origin of common terms (G. Greek; L. Latin)

aberration	L. *aberratio,* a distorted state
accommodation	L. *accommodatio*, adjustment
adaptation	L. *adaptatio*, process of adapting
amblyopia	G. *amblys*, dull + *ops*, eye + *ia*, a condition
ametropia	G. *ametros*, irregular + *ops*, eye + *ia*, a condition
anaesthesia	G. *an,* without + *aesthesis,* sensation
aniseikonia	G. anisos, unequal + *eikon,* image + *ia,* a condition
anisocoria	G. *anisos,* unequal + *kore,* pupil
anisotropic	G. *anisos,* unequal + *tropos,* turn + ic
anopsia	G. *an,* without + *opsis,* vision + *ia,* a condition
aphakia	G. *a*, without + *phakos*, lens
artery	L. *arteria*, elastic vessel
asthenopia	G. *astheneia*, weakness + *ops*, eye + *ia*, a condition
astigmatism	G. *a,* without + *stigma*, point
blindness	Anglo Saxon *blind*
blepharitis	G. *blepharon,* eyelid + *itis,* inflammation
blepharorrhaphy	G. *blepharon,* eyelid + *rhaphe,* suture
cataract	L. *cataracta* or G. *katarrhaktes*, a waterfall
chiasma	G. *chiasma,* two crossing lines
chromatism	G. *chroma,* colour
chromatophobia	G. *chroma,* colour + *phobos,* fear + *ia,* a condition
conjunctiva	L. *conjunctivus,* connecting
conjunctivitis	L. *conjunctivus* + G. *itis,* inflammation
cornea	L. *corneus,* horn-like
cryopexy	G. *kryos,* cold + *pexis,* fixing in place
dacryocele	G. *dakryon,* tear + *kele,* swelling
dacryocyst	G. *dakryon,* tear + *kystis,* sac
dacryoma	G. *dakryon,* tear + *oma,* tumour
dextroversion	L. *dexter,* right + *versio,* turning
deuteranopia	G. *deuteros*, second + *a*, without + *ops*, eye + *ia*, a condition
diplocoria	G. *diploos*, double + *kore*, pupil + *ia*, a condition
diplopia	G. *diploos*, double + *ops*, eye + *ia*, a condition
dyslexia	G. *dys*, bad + *lexis,* word + *ia,* a condition
emmetropia	G. *emmetros*, proportioned + *ops*, eye + *ia*, a condition
endothelium	G. *endon,* within + *thele,* nipple
epithelium	G. *epi,* upon + *thele,* nipple
eye	Anglo Saxon *éage*
fovea	L. a pit
fusion	L. *fusio,* a pouring
haematoma	G. *haima*, blood + *oma,* tumour
hemeralopia	G. *hemera*, day + *alaos*, obscure + *ops*, eye + *ia*, a condition

heterophoria	G. *heteros*, different + *phora*, movement + *ia*, a condition
hemianopsia	G. *hemi*, half + *an*, without + *opsia*, seeing
hordeolum	L. *hordeolus*, a stye
humour	L. *umor*, a liquid
hypermetropia	G. *hyper*, above + *metron*, measure + *ops*, eye + *ia*, a condition
illusion	L. *illusio*, mock
iridology	G. *irid*, rainbow + *logos*, study
iridoplegia	G. *irid*, rainbow + *plege*, stroke
isotropic	G. *isos*, equal + *tropos*, turn + ic
keratitis	G. *keras*, horn + *itis*, inflammation
keratoconus	G. *keras*, horn + *konos*, cone
keratoplasty	G. *keras*, horn + *plasso*, to form
lens	L. *lentil*
luxation	L. *luxation*, dislocation
macropsia	G. *makros*, large + *opsia*, seeing
macula	L. a spot
macula lutea	L. a spot + *luteus*, yellow
megalocornea	G. *megas*, big + L. *corneus*, horny
melanoma	G. *melan*, black + *oma*, tumour
microaneurysm	G. *mikros*, small + *aneurusma*, dilatation
microscope	G. *mikros*, small + *skopeo*, to examine
miosis	G. *meiosis*, diminution
mitosis	G. *mitos*, thread + *osis*, a process
monochromat	G. *monos*, single + *chroma*, colour
myopathy	G. *myos*, muscle + *pathos*, suffering
myopia	G. *myo*, to close + *ops*, eye + *ia*, a condition
nekrosis	G. *nekrosis*, death
neuropathy	G. *neuron*, nerve + *pathos*, suffering
nyctalopia	G. *nyx*, night + *alaos*, obscure + *ops*, eye + *ia*, a condition
nystagmus	G. *nystagmos*, a nodding
ophthalmic	G. *ophthalmos*, eyeball
ophthalmoscope	G. *ophthalmos*, eyeball + *skopeo*, to examine
optics	G. *optikos*, of sight
optometry	G. *optikos*, of sight + *metron*, measure
orthophoria	G. *orthos*, straight + *phora*, movement + *ia*, a condition
orthoptics	G. *orthos*, straight + *optikos*, of sight
penumbra	L. *paene*, almost + *umbra*, shadow
perimeter	G. *peri*, around + *metron*, measure
periscope	G. *peri*, around + *skopeo*, to examine
phakometer	G. *phakos*, lens + *metron*, measure
photophobia	G. *photos*, light + *phobos*, fear
presbyopia	G. *presbys*, old man + *ops*, eye + *ia*, a condition
ptosis	G. *ptosis*, falling
pupil	L. *pupilla*, little doll
reflection	L. *reflexus*, bent back
reflex	L. *reflecto*, to bend back
refraction	L. *refraction*, breaking up
retina	L. *rete*, a net
sclera	G. *skleros*, hard
sclerectomy	G. *skleros*, hard + *ektome*, excision
sclerotomy	G. *skleros*, hard + *tome*, incision
scotoma	G. *skotos*, darkness + *oma*, tumour
stereopsis	G. *stereos*, solid + *opsis*, vision
strabismus	G. *strabismos*, a squint
synapse	G. *sunapsias*, connection
syndrome	G. *syn*, together + *dromos*, running
synechia	G. *sunekheia*, continuity

telescope	G. *tele,* far off + *skopeo,* to examine
tonometer	G. *tonos,* tension + *metron,* measure
tritanopia	G. *tritos*, third + *a*, without + *ops*, eye + *ia*, a condition
ultrasonography	L. *ultra,* beyond + *sonus,* sound + G. *grapho,* to write
uvea	L. *uva*, grape
vision	L. *visio*, seeing

Greek alphabet

letter name	lower case	upper case
alpha	α	A
beta	β	B
gamma	γ	Γ
delta	δ	Δ
epsilon	ε	E
zeta	ζ	Z
eta	η	H
theta	θ	Θ
iota	ι	I
kappa	κ	K
lambda	λ	Λ
mu	μ	M
nu	ν	N
xi	ξ	Ξ
omicron	ο	O
pi	π	Π
rho	ρ	P
sigma	σ or ς	Σ
tau	τ	T
upsilon	υ	Y
phi	φ	Φ
chi	χ	X
psi	ψ	Ψ
omega	ω	Ω

Acknowledgements

Many textbooks, journals and dictionaries were used as sources for the writing of this *Dictionary of Optometry and Vision Science*. However, the following represent the primary references to which I am indebted:

D M Albert and F A Jakobiec, *Principles and Practice of Ophthalmology*, W B Saunders Co.; J F Amos, *Diagnosis and Management in Vision Care*, Butterworth-Heinemann; J D Bartlett and S D Jaanus, *Clinical Ocular Pharmacology*, Butterworth-Heinemann; W J Benjamin, *Borish's Clinical Refraction*, W B Saunders company; J Birch, *Diagnosis of Defective Color Vision*, Butterworth-Heinemann; B Bowling, *Kanski's Clinical Ophthalmology*, Elsevier; A J Bron, R C Tripathi and B J Tripathi, *Wolff's Anatomy of the Eye and Orbit*, Chapman and Hall Medical; S E Caloroso and M W Rouse, *Clinical Management of Strabismus*, Butterworth-Heinemann; J Cronly-Dillon, *Vision and Visual Dysfunction*, 16 volumes, Macmillan Press; H Davson, *The Eye*, vols. 1–4, Academic Press; A K O Denniston and P I Murray, *Oxford Handbook of Ophthalmology*, Oxford University Press; C Dickinson, *Low Vision; Principles and Practice*, Butterworth-Heinemann; W A Douthwaite *Contact Lens Optics and Lens Design*, Butterworth-Heinemann; N Efron, *Contact lens Practice*, Butterworth-Heinemann; N Efron, *Contact Lens Complications*, Butterworth-Heinemann; D B Elliott, *Primary Eye Care*, Butterworth-Heinemann; J B Eskridge, J F Amos and J D Bartlett, *Clinical Procedures in Optometry*, J B Lippincott Company; D L Easty and J M Sparrow, *Oxford Textbook of Ophthalmology*, Oxford Medical Publications; B J W Evans, *Pickwell's Binocular Vision Anomalies*, Butterworth-Heinemann; T E Fannin and T Grosvenor, *Clinical Optics*, Butterworth-Heinemann; I Fatt and B A Weissman, *Physiology of the Eye*, Butterworth-Heinemann; E E Faye, *Clinical Low Vision*, Little Brown and Company; M H Freeman, *Optics*, Butterworth-Heinemann; B S Fine and M Yanoff, *Ocular Histology,* Harper and Row Publishers; K Gegenfurtner and L T Sharpe, *Color Vision, From Genes to Perception*, Cambridge University Press; R G Gilman, *Behavioral Optometry,* Paradox Publishing; J R Griffin and J D Grisham, *Binocular Anomalies*, Butterworth-Heinemann; T P Grosvenor, *Primary Care Optometry*, Butterworth-Heinemann; T P Grosvenor and M C Flom, *Refractive Anomalies: Research and Clinical Applications*, Butterworth-Heinemann; W M Hart, *Adler's Physiology of the Eye*, Mosby Year Book; D B Henson, *Optometric Instrumentation*, Butterworth-Heinemann; D B Henson, *Visual Fields*, Butterworth-Heinemann; M J Hogan, J A Alvarado and J E Weddell, *Histology of the Human Eye*, W B Saunders Co.; G Hopkins and R Pearson, *O'Connor Davies' Ophthalmic Drugs*, Butterworth-Heinemann; M Jalie, *The Principles of Ophthalmic Lenses*, The Association of Dispensing Opticians; J J Kanski, *Clinical Ophthalmology*, Butterworth-Heinemann; S J Leat, R H Shute and C A Westall, *Assessing Children's Vision*, Butterworth-Heinemann; D D Michaels, *Visual Optics and Refraction*, The C V Mosby Co.; F W Newell, *Ophthalmology*, The C V Mosby Co.; G K von Noorden, *Binocular Vision and Ocular Motility*, The C V Mosby Co.; H Obstfeld, *Optics in Vision*, Butterworths; C W Oyster, *The Human Eye, Structure and Function*, Sinauer Associates Inc.; S E Palmer, *Vision Science*, The MIT Press; D Pavan-Langston, *Manual of Ocular Diagnosis and Therapy*, Little, Brown and Company; A J Phillips and L Speedwell, *Contact Lenses*, Butterworth-Heinemann; R B Rabbetts, *Bennett and Rabbetts' Clinical Visual Optics*, Butterworth-Heinemann; H E Records, *Physiology of the Human Eye and Visual System*, Harper and Row, Publishers; M Rosenfield and N Logan, *Optometry*, Butterworth-Heinemann; R P Rutstein and K M Daum, *Anomalies of Binocular Vision*, The C V Mosby Co.; S H Schwartz, *Visual Perception*, Appleton and Lange; R S Snell and M A Lemp, *Clinical Anatomy of the Eye*, Blackwell Scientific Publications; W Tasman et al, *Duane's Clinical Ophthalmology*, 6 volumes, Lippincott Williams and Wilkins; D Vaughan, T Asbury and P Riordan-Eva, *General Ophthalmology*, Appleton and Lange; H J Wyatt, *Manual of Visual Anatomy and Physiology*, Professional Press Books; M Yanoff and J S Duker, *Ophthalmology*, Mosby.

I am most grateful to the following professional colleagues who have read some of the manuscript of this and earlier editions for their comments, suggestions and corrections: Professor Brian Brown, Professor Wolfgang Drexler, Mr. Richard Earlam, Professor Jez Guggenheim, Dr. Daniel M Laby, Mrs. Susan Millodot, Mr. Len Morrison, Professor Rachel North, Mr. Henri Obstfeld, Dr. Ron Ofri, Ms. Dinah Paritzky, Mr. Ron Rabbetts, Professor Gordon Ruskell, Mr. Jonathan Shapiro, Professor Avi Solomon, Dr. Howard Solomons, Dr. Yu Chun Pong and Ms. Anne Marie Taylor.

Michel Millodot, 2016

Figure credits

Fig. A19 Kandel ER, Schwartz JH, Jessell TM. *Principles of Neural Science*. 4th edn. New York: McGraw-Hill; 2000; **Fig. B3** Kanski J. *Clinical Ophthalmology*. 5th edn. Edinburgh: Butterworth-Heinemann; 2003; **Fig. C5** Kanski J. *Clinical Ophthalmology*. 6th edn. Edinburgh: Butterworth-Heinemann; 2007; **Fig. C14** Kanski J. *Clinical Ophthalmology*. 5th edn. Edinburgh: Butterworth-Heinemann; 2003; **Fig. C19** Kanski J. *Clinical Ophthalmology*. 6th edn. Edinburgh: Butterworth-Heinemann; 2007; **Fig. D11** Kanski J. *Clinical Ophthalmology*. 6th edn. Edinburgh: Butterworth-Heinemann; 2007; **Fig. D12** Bowling B. *Kanski's Clinical Ophthalmology*. 8th edn. Elsevier; 2016; **Fig. E4** Kanski J. *Clinical Ophthalmology*. 5th edn. Edinburgh: Butterworth-Heinemann; 2003; **Fig. E7** Kanski J. *Clinical Ophthalmology*. 5th edn. Edinburgh: Butterworth-Heinemann; 2003; **Fig. E9** Millodot M. *What do you know about vision*. Montreal: Aquila Communications; 1976; **Fig. G4** Kanski J. *Clinical Ophthalmology*. 6th edn. Edinburgh: Butterworth-Heinemann; 2007; **Fig. H6** Bowling B. *Kanski's Clinical Ophthalmology*. 8th edn. Elsevier; 2016; **Fig. H7** Bowling B. *Kanski's Clinical Ophthalmology*. 8th edn. Elsevier; 2016; **Fig. I6** Colman AM. *A Dictionary of Psychology*. New York: Oxford University Press; 2003; **Fig. I16** Millodot M, Hendler K, Péer J. Iris melanoma: a case report and review. *Ophthal Physiol Opt* 2006; 26: 120–126; **Fig. K1** Bowling B. *Kanski's Clinical Ophthalmology*. 8th edn. Elsevier; 2016; **Fig. L19** Bowling B. *Kanski's Clinical Ophthalmology*. 8th edn. Elsevier; 2016; **Fig. M7** Millodot M, Hendler K, Péer J. Iris Melanoma: a case report and review. *Ophthal Physiol Opt* 2006; 26: 120–126; **Fig. M9** Kanski J. *Clinical Ophthalmology*. 6th edn. Edinburgh: Butterworth-Heinemann; 2007; **Fig. M12** Pritchard RM. Stabilized images on the retina. Scientific American, June 1961; **Fig. M14** Millodot M. *What do you know about vision?* Montreal: Aquila Communications; 1976; **Fig. N3** Kanski J. *Clinical Ophthalmology*. 6th edn. Edinburgh: Butterworth-Heinemann; 2007; **Fig. N4** Huber A. *Eye signs and symptoms in brain tumours*. 3rd edn. St Louis: Mosby; 1976; **Fig. P2** Bowling B. *Kanski's Clinical Ophthalmology*. 8th edn. Elsevier; 2016; **Fig. P12** Kanski J. *Clinical Ophthalmology*. 5th edn. Edinburgh: Butterworth-Heinemann; 2003; **Fig. P23** Kanski J. *Clinical Ophthalmology*. 5th edn. Edinburgh: Butterworth-Heinemann; 2003; **Fig. P24** Kanski J. *Clinical Ophthalmology*. 6th edn. Edinburgh: Butterworth-Heinemann; 2007; **Fig. P25** Atchison, Smith G. *Optics of the Human Eye*. Edinburgh: Butterworth-Heinemann; 2000; **Fig. R10** Bowling B. *Kanski's Clinical Ophthalmology*. 8th edn. Elsevier; 2016; **Fig. R12** Kanski J. *Clinical Ophthalmology*. 6th edn. Edinburgh: Butterworth-Heinemann; 2007; **Fig. S11** Kanski J. *Clinical Ophthalmology*. 6th edn. Edinburgh: Butterworth-Heinemann; 2007; **Fig. S15** Bowling B. *Kanski's Clinical Ophthalmology*. 8th edn. Elsevier; 2016; **Fig. T9** Kanski J. *Clinical Ophthalmology*. 6th edn. Edinburgh: Butterworth-Heinemann; 2007; **Fig. T22** Kanski J. Clinical Ophthalmology. 5th edn. Edinburgh; 2003; **Fig. U3** Bowling B. *Kanski's Clinical Ophthalmology*. 8th edn. Elsevier; 2016.

List of tables

A

Aarskog's syndrome *See* syndrome, Aarskog's.

abathic distance *See* plane, apparent frontoparallel.

Abbé's condenser *See* condenser, Abbé's.

Abbé's condition *See* sine condition.

Abbé's number *See* constringence.

Abbé's refractometer *See* refractometer.

abducens muscle *See* muscle, lateral rectus.

abducens nerve *See* nerve, abducens.

abducens nerve palsy *See* paralysis of the sixth nerve.

abduct To turn away from the midline, as when the eye rotates outward.

abduction Outward rotation of an eye; that is, away from the midline.
See duction; syndrome, Duane's.

abductors Extraocular muscles that move the eye outward, such as the lateral rectus, the inferior oblique and the superior oblique.

aberrant regeneration *See* regeneration, aberrant.

aberration An optical defect in which the rays from a point object do not form a perfect point after passing through an optical system (Table A1).
See astigmatism, oblique; curvature of field; distortion; lens, best-form.

axial chromatic a. *See* aberration, longitudinal chromatic.

coma a. A component of the wavefront aberrations in which the image is elevated on one side and depressed on the other side, relative to the reference (or ideal) wavefront.

hexafoil a. A component of the wavefront aberrations in which there are six areas where the emerging wavefront is elevated and six areas where it is depressed with six distinct axes and with different curvatures relative to the reference wavefront.

higher-order a. Term referring to the wavefront aberrations above the 2nd order which include coma, hexafoil, pentafoil, quadrafoil, secondary astigmatism, secondary spherical aberration and trefoil. *See* Table A1.

lateral chromatic a. *See* aberration, transverse chromatic.

longitudinal chromatic a. Defect of an optical system (eye, lens, prism, etc.) due to the unequal refraction of different wavelengths (dispersion) which results in an extended image along the optical axis. In the eye, blue rays are focused in front of the retina (by about 1 D) and red rays slightly behind the retina (0.25–0.5 D) when relaxed. When the eye is accommodated for a near target, blue rays tend to be focused near the retina and red rays are focused behind the retina (1 D) because of a lag of accommodation, usually occurring when viewing near targets (Fig. A1). *Syn*. axial chromatic aberration.
See chromoretinoscopy; chromostereopsis; constringence; dispersion; doublet; lens, achromatizing; pigment, macular; test, duochrome.

lower-order a. Term referring to the wavefront aberrations' order 0 to 2nd. They include astigmatism, defocus (hyperopia, myopia), piston and tilt. *See* Table A1.

monochromatic a. Defect of an optical system (eye, lens, prism, etc.) occurring for a single wavelength of light. Classically, they were the five Seidel aberrations: spherical aberration, coma, curvature of field, oblique astigmatism and distortion. The mathematical description of these aberrations was based on the assumption that the optics of the system is rotationally symmetrical, which is the case in most lenses and optical systems, but not in the eye. The monochromatic aberrations of the eye are nowadays part of the wavefront aberrations, which have replaced the older approach to aberrations.
See aberration, wavefront.

pentafoil a. A component of the wavefront aberrations in which there are five areas where the emerging wavefront is elevated and five areas where it is depressed with five distinct axes and with different curvatures relative to the reference wavefront.

prism a. Effects caused by a prism on refracted light, in addition to the expected change in direction of light. These effects include different magnifications, curvature of field and chromatic aberration.

piston a A lower-order wavefront aberration. It appears as a symmetrical, circular deviation of the emerging wavefront.

quadrafoil a. A component of the wavefront aberrations in which there are four areas where the emerging wavefront is elevated and four areas where it is depressed with four distinct axes and with different curvatures relative to the reference wavefront. *Syn*. tetrafoil aberration.

Seidel a. *See* aberration, monochromatic.

spherical a. Defect of an optical system due to a variation in the focusing between peripheral and paraxial rays. The larger the pupil size, the greater the difference in focusing between the two rays. In the gaussian theory, the focus of the optical system is attributed to the paraxial rays. The distance, in dioptres, between the focus of the paraxial rays and the peripheral rays represents the amount of **longitudinal spherical aberration** of the system. When the peripheral rays are refracted more than the paraxial rays, the aberration is said to be **positive** or **undercorrected**. When the peripheral rays are refracted less than the paraxial rays, the aberration is said to be **negative** or **overcorrected**. This relates to optical systems or lenses, which are rotationally

Table A1	**Aberrations of the eye**	
A	Chromatic aberrations: longitudinal and transverse	
B	Monochromatic aberrations: wavefront aberrations	

Lower-order

Order	Zernike polynomial	Name
0	Z_0^0	Piston
1st	Z_1^{-1}	Vertical tilt
1st	Z_1^1	Horizontal tilt
2nd	Z_2^{-2}	Oblique astigmatism
2nd	Z_2^0	Defocus
2nd	Z_2^2	With/against the rule astigmatism

Higher-order

Order	Zernike polynomial	Name
3rd	Z_3^{-3}	Oblique trefoil
3rd	Z_3^{-1}	Vertical coma
3rd	Z_3^1	Horizontal coma
3rd	Z_3^3	Horizontal trefoil
4th	Z_4^{-4}	Oblique quadrafoil
4th	Z_4^{-2}	Oblique secondary astigmatism
4th	Z_4^0	Spherical aberration
4th	$Z4^2$	With/against the rule secondary astigmatism
4th	Z_4^4	Quadrafoil
5th	Z_5^{-5}	Pentafoil
5th	Z_5^{-3}	Horizontal trefoil
5th	Z_5^{-1}	Secondary vertical coma
5th	Z_5^1	Secondary horizontal coma
5th	Z_5^3	Oblique trefoil
5th	Z_5^5	Pentafoil
6th	Z_6^{-6}	Hexafoil
6th	Z_6^{-4}	Quadrafoil
6th	Z_6^{-2}	Secondary oblique astigmatism
6th	Z_6^0	Secondary spherical aberration
6th	Z_6^2	Secondary vertical astigmatism
6th	Z_6^4	Quadrafoil
6th	Z_6^6	Hexafoil

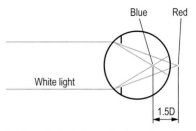

Fig. A1 Longitudinal chromatic aberration of the eye.

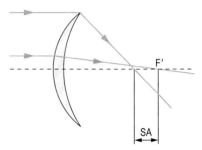

Fig. A2 Spherical aberration of a lens in one meridian. Two parallel rays coming from infinity are focused, one at F′, the secondary focal point corresponding to paraxial rays and the other peripheral ray in front or behind F′, depending on the type of spherical aberration. It is positive in this illustration (SA, longitudinal spherical aberration).

symmetrical about the axis. This is not the case in the eye and thus this aberration forms part of the higher-order wavefront aberrations of the eye. The amount of this aberration in the eye varies with accommodation. (Fig. A2).
See caustic; lens, aplanatic; theory, gaussian.
tetrafoil a. *See* aberration, quadrafoil.
tilt a. A component of the wavefront aberrations in which one part of the emerging wavefront is elevated and the rest depressed relative to the reference wavefront.
transverse chromatic a. Defect of an optical system (eye, lens, prism, etc.) in which the size of the image of a point object is extended at right angle to the optical axis by a coloured fringe, due to the unequal refraction of different wavelengths (dispersion). *Syn.* chromatic difference of magnification; lateral chromatic aberration. *See* dispersion; doublet.
trefoil a. A component of the wavefront aberrations in which there are three areas where the emerging wavefront is elevated and three areas where it is depressed with three distinct axes and with different curvatures relative to the reference wavefront.
wavefront a. The amount of deviation found between an output wavefront emanating from an optical system and a conceptualized ideal (reference) wavefront. The wavefront is perpendicular to the direction of the incident light. The measurement of this aberration can be done subjectively or objectively (e.g. with an aberrometer based on the **Hartmann–Shack principle**). A narrow beam of light is projected onto the retina and reflected from a point source, usually the fovea, and emerges from the eye through the lens and cornea. The emerging wavefront, typically distorted, passes through an array of several hundred microlenses, which

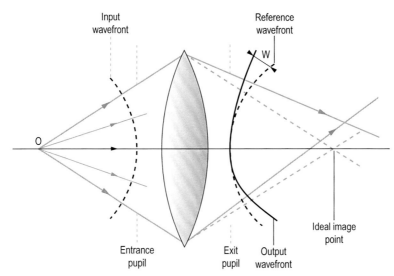

Fig. A3 An input spherical wavefront of light is centred on object O. After emerging from a lens affected by monochromatic aberration, it is no longer spherical and the image-forming rays do not meet in the single ideal image point (the paraxial image). The wavefront aberration W is the distance between the ideal reference wavefront and the actual output wavefront at various distances from the optical axis.

subdivides it into several hundred beams, which are then focused onto a detector. Deviations of the images from their reference positions are used to calculate the shape of the wavefront aberration function of the eye. The wavefront is usually quantified by the sum of Zernike polynomials in which each polynomial corresponds to a different lower-order or higher-order aberration (Table A1). The aberrations are very small, measured in units of micrometres, and given as the root mean square (RMS), a measure of the variance of the wavefront error within the pupil. Qualitative assessment of the shape of the wavefront can be made from a colour-coded map. Typical results show that spherical aberration and coma are the most important components (Fig. A3 and Table A1). *Syn.* wavefront error.
See **aberrometry.**

aberrometer *See* **optometer.**

aberrometry The measurement of aberrations. The term is mainly associated with the measurement of wavefront aberrations of optical systems, such as the eye, the eye with a spectacle correction, with contact lenses (in vitro or in situ), intraocular lenses (in vitro or in situ), corneal refractive surgery, cataract, etc.

aberroscope Instrument for observing aberration. Such an instrument was designed by Tscherning to measure his own spherical aberration. It consists of a planoconvex lens with a grid made up of squares ruled on its plane surface.

abetalipoproteinaemia *See* syndrome, Bassen–Kornzweig.

ablatio retinae *See* **retinal detachment.**

ablation A procedure in which a tissue or body part is removed or destroyed by surgery, radiation or photocoagulation. *Example:* LASIK.
See **photoablation.**

ablepharon *See* **ablephary.**

ablephary Congenital absence, complete or partial, of the eyelids. *Syn.* ablepharon.

ablepsia *See* **blindness.**

ablepsy *See* **blindness.**

Abney's law; phenomenon *See* under the nouns.

abnormal (anomalous) retinal correspondence *See* retinal correspondence, abnormal.

abrasion, corneal *See* corneal abrasion.

abrasive Granular substance used in lens grinding, such as corundum (aluminium oxide), carborundum, etc.
See **roughing; smoothing; surfacing.**

abscess An accumulation of pus located in infected tissue.

absorbance *See* density, optical; transmittance.

absorption Transformation of radiant energy into a different form of energy, usually heat, as it passes through a medium. Light that is absorbed is neither transmitted nor reflected. It may, however, be re-emitted as light of another wavelength as, for example, ultraviolet radiation is converted into visible radiation on absorption by a luminescent material. A substance that absorbs all radiations is called a black body.
See **density, optical; fluorescence.**

absorptive lens *See* lens, absorptive.

AC/A ratio Ratio of the accommodative convergence AC (in prism dioptres) to the stimulus to accommodation A (in dioptres). It is represented by the amount of convergence elicited per dioptre of accommodation. The most common method of determining this ratio is by the **gradient method** (or **gradient test**) in which the heterophoria at near is measured after changing the accommodation with a spherical lens (usually +1.00 D or −1.00 D) placed in front of the two eyes. It is expressed as

$$AC/A = (\alpha - \alpha')/F$$

where α is the phoria at near, and α' is the phoria at the same distance but through a lens of power F. The deviation is measured in prism dioptres, with + for esodeviation and − for exodeviation. *Example*: If the initial phoria is 4 Δ exo and 8 Δ exo when a lens of +1.00 D is placed in front of the eyes, the AC/A ratio is equal to

$$[-4-(-8)]/1 = 4\Delta/D$$

The average AC/A ratio is about 4 in young adults and tends to decline slightly with age. The gradient is not affected by proximal convergence, as the target distance and size are relatively constant. The full gradient test is based on measurements of heterophoria with several lens power in 1.00 D steps and plotting a graph of lens power against induced phoria. The **modified gradient test** is based on heterophoria measured at only two points, with at least a 2.00 D lens difference.
Another method of determining the AC/A ratio (often called the heterophoria method) compares the phoria measured at distance and at near. It is expressed as

$$AC/A = PD + ((N-D)/K)$$

where PD is the interpupillary distance in cm, N the deviation at near, D the deviation at distance and K the near fixation distance in dioptres. *Example*: A patient has a PD of 70 mm, a distance phoria of 4 Δ eso and a near phoria of 8 Δ exo at 33.3 cm from the eyes, the AC/A ratio is equal to

$$7.0 + ([-8-(+4)]/3) = 3\Delta/D$$

See convergence, accommodative; convergence, proximal; dioptre; prism.

acanthamoeba　keratitis *See* keratitis, acanthamoeba.

acanthocytosis *See* syndrome, Bassen–Kornzweig.

acanthosis nigricans A rare skin disorder presenting numerous superficial, pigmented papillomatous growths on various parts of the body. Ocular manifestations are primarily papillomatous lesions of the lid margins, which may be so extensive as to cause punctal occlusion, as well as papillary conjunctivitis. *Syn.* keratosis nigricans.

accessory lacrimal glands *See* glands, accessory lacrimal; gland, of Krause; gland, of Wolfring.

accommodation Adjustment of the dioptric power of the eye. It is generally involuntary and made to see objects clearly at any distance. In man (and primates), this adjustment is brought about by a change in the shape of the crystalline lens. In some animals, this adjustment occurs either as a result of an anteroposterior movement of the crystalline lens or of an alteration in the curvature of the cornea.
See aniso-accommodation; muscle, ciliary; reflex, accommodative; theory, Fincham's; theory, Helmholtz's of accommodation.
amplitude of a. The maximum amount of accommodation A that the eye can exert. It is expressed in dioptres, as the difference between the far point and the near point measured with respect either to the spectacle plane or the corneal apex or some other reference point. Thus,

$$A = K - B$$

where B is the near point vergence and K is the far point vergence. A is always positive. In the emmetropic eye, A = −B, because the far point is at infinity and K = 0. So, if the near point of an emmetrope is at 25 cm from the spectacle plane, the amplitude of accommodation is equal to − [−1/ (25×10^{-2})] = 4 D. The amplitude of accommodation declines from about 14 D at age 10 to about 0.5 D at age 60 (although the measured value is usually slightly higher due to the depth of focus of the eye) (Table A2).
See method, minus lens; method, push-up.
astigmatic a. Postulated unequal accommodation along different meridians of the eye attributed

Table A2 Mean amplitude of accommodation as a function of age, in Caucasians (the plane of reference is the spectacle plane)

Age (years)	Duane (N = 2000 subjects, push-up method)	Turner (N = 500 subjects, push-out method)
10	13.5	13.0
15	12.5	10.6
20	11.5	9.5
25	10.5	7.9
30	8.9	6.6
35	7.3	5.75
40	5.9	4.4
45	3.7	2.5
50	2.0	1.6
55	1.3	1.1
60	1.2	0.7
65	1.1	0.6
70	1.0	0.6

to a differential action of the ciliary muscle, which would lead to a difference in the curvature of the surfaces of the crystalline lens along different meridians. *Syn.* meridional accommodation.

closed-loop a. Accommodative response to visual stimuli in normal viewing conditions. *See* **accommodation, open-loop.**

components of a. The process of accommodation is assumed to involve four components: reflex, vergence (convergence), proximal and tonic accommodation (also called resting state of accommodation). *See* **accommodation, convergence; accommodation, proximal; accommodation, reflex; accommodation, resting state of.**

consensual a. Accommodation occurring in one eye when the other eye has received the dioptric stimulus.

convergence a. 1. Accommodation induced directly by a change in convergence. **2.** That component of accommodation induced by the binocular disparity of the retinal images. *Syn.* vergence accommodation.

correction induced a. Ocular accommodation induced when changing from spectacles to contact lenses in near vision. Spectacles induce less accommodation in myopes and more accommodation in hyperopes than that exerted by an emmetrope fixating at a given distance. Contact lenses do not induce any different accommodation than that required for a given distance. Consequently, myopes require more accommodation and hyperopes less accommodation when they transfer from spectacles to contact lenses. However, this change in accommodative demand is accompanied by a similar change in convergence, so that a myope transferring to contact lenses accommodates and converges more than with spectacles and the reverse applies for a hyperope. *See* **convergence, correction induced.**

far point of a. Point in space that is conjugate with the retina (more specifically the foveola) when accommodation is relaxed. In emmetropia, the far point is at infinity; in myopia, it is at a finite distance in front of the eye; in hyperopia, it is a virtual point behind the eye (Fig. A4). *Syn.* far point of the eye; punctum remotum. *See* **sphere, far point.**

ill-sustained a. *See* **accommodative insufficiency.**

inert a. *See* **accommodative infacility.**

insufficiency of a. *See* **accommodative insufficiency.**

lag of a. 1. The amount by which the accommodative response of the eye is less than the dioptric stimulus to accommodation (or accommodative demand), as usually occurs when fixating an object at near. It could be due to uncorrected hyperopia or indicate accommodative insufficiency. Absence of an accommodative lag may indicate latent hyperopia. Accommodative lag is considered to be myopigenic. *Syn.* lazy lag of accommodation. **2.** The condition occurring in dynamic retinoscopy

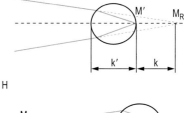

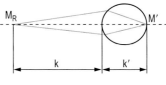

Fig. A4 A hyperopic eye H and a myopic eye M, fixating an object at the far point M_R. k and k′ represent the conjugate object and image distances, respectively, from the reduced eye surface.

in which the neutral point is situated further from the eyes than is the retinoscopic target. *See* **defocus, hyperopic; retinoscopy, dynamic.**

lead of a. The dioptric amount by which the accommodative response of the eye is greater than the dioptric stimulus to accommodation, as occurs when fixating at distance. It only occurs in a few individuals. It can also occur as a result of a spasm of accommodation. *See* **defocus, myopic; retinoscopy, dynamic.**

mechanism of a. Process by which the eye focuses onto an object. It does so by contracting the ciliary muscle which releases the tension on the zonular fibres, allowing the elastic lens capsule to increase its curvature, especially that of the front surface. Along with these changes are an increase in the thickness of the lens, a decrease in its equatorial diameter and a reduction in pupil size. The ciliary muscle is controlled by the parasympathetic system, which is triggered by an out-of-focus retinal image. *See* **accommodation, convergence; accommodation, proximal; accommodative response; muscle, ciliary; reflex, near.**

meridional a. *See* **accommodation, astigmatic.**

microfluctuations of a. Involuntary variations in the contraction of the intraocular muscles responsible for accommodation and resulting in changes of about 0.1–0.5 D with a frequency of 0.5–2.5 Hz.

near point of a. The nearest point in space that is conjugate with the foveola when exerting the maximum accommodative effort. *Syn.* punctum proximum. *See* **method, push-up; rule, near point; sphere, near point; test, Scheiner's.**

negative a. 1. A relaxation of accommodation below the apparent zero level or when shifting from near to distance vision. **2.** *See* **accommodation, relative amplitude of.**

objective a. Accommodation measured without the subject's judgment. This is accomplished by

dynamic retinoscopy, by autorefractors or by visually evoked cortical potentials. The term is sometimes used incorrectly to refer to the amplitude of accommodation without the influence of the depth of focus (e.g. as measured by stigmatoscopy).
See **accommodation, subjective; optometer; potential, visual evoked; retinoscopy, dynamic; stigmatoscopy.**
ocular a. The amplitude of accommodation referred to the front surface of the cornea (Tables A3 and A4). *Symbol:* A.
See **accommodation, spectacle.**
open-loop a. Accommodative response occurring without the usual stimulus to accommodation, such as a blurred retinal image. In these conditions, the accommodative system of the eye tends to return to its position of rest (or tonic accommodation). *Examples:* looking at an empty

field; looking through a very small artificial pupil (0.5 mm or less).
See **accommodation, closed-loop.**
paralysis of a. Total or partial loss of accommodation due to paralysis of the ciliary muscle.
positive a. Normal accommodation that occurs when looking from a distant to a near object.
proximal a. Component of accommodation which is initiated by the awareness of a near object. *Syn.* psychic accommodation.
See **accommodation, components of; accommodation, resting state of.**
psychic a. See **accommodation, proximal.**
range of a. Linear distance between the far point and the near point. Part of the range of accommodation is virtual in the case of the hyperope.
reflex a. An adjustment of the refractive state of the eye stimulated by blur and aimed at reducing

Table A3   Relationship between viewing distance and spectacle and ocular accommodation of a contact lens wearer and of four corrected hyperopes (with thin spectacle lenses). The vertex distance was 14 mm and ocular accommodation was calculated using the formula $A = K - B$. The ocular accommodation exerted by a contact lens wearer is the same for all refractive errors and equal to that of an emmetrope.

Distance from spectacle lens (cm)	Spectacle accom. (D)	Ocular accom. (D) of contact lens wearer	Ocular accom. (D) of hyperopes			
			+2	+4	+6	+8
100	1.00	0.99	1.04	1.11	1.17	1.25
67	1.49	1.46	1.55	1.64	1.74	1.86
50	2.00	1.95	2.06	2.18	2.31	2.46
40	2.50	2.42	2.55	2.71	2.87	3.05
33	3.03	2.91	3.07	3.25	3.45	3.67
25	4.00	3.79	4.00	4.24	4.49	4.77
20	5.00	4.67	4.94	5.22	5.54	5.88
16	6.25	5.75	6.07	6.42	6.80	7.22
14	7.14	6.49	6.86	7.25	7.68	8.14
12	8.33	7.46	7.88	8.32	8.81	9.34
10	10.00	8.77	9.25	9.77	10.34	10.95

Table A4   Relationship between viewing distance and spectacle and ocular accommodation of a contact lens wearer and of five corrected myopes (with thin spectacle lenses). The vertex distance was 14 mm and ocular accommodation was calculated using the formula $A = K - B$. The ocular accommodation exerted by a contact lens wearer is the same for all refractive errors and equal to that of an emmetrope.

Distance from spectacle lens (cm)	Spectacle accom. (D)	Ocular accom. (D) of contact lens wearer	Ocular accom. (D) of myopes				
			−4	−6	−8	−10	−12
100	1.00	0.99	0.89	0.84	0.80	0.76	0.72
67	1.49	1.46	1.31	1.25	1.18	1.13	1.07
50	2.00	1.95	1.75	1.66	1.58	1.50	1.43
40	2.50	2.42	2.17	2.06	1.96	1.87	1.78
33	3.03	2.91	2.61	2.48	2.36	2.25	2.14
25	4.00	3.79	3.41	3.24	3.08	2.93	2.80
20	5.00	4.67	4.21	4.00	3.80	3.62	3.46
16	6.25	5.75	5.18	4.92	4.69	4.47	4.26
14	7.14	6.49	5.85	5.57	5.30	5.05	4.82
12	8.33	7.46	6.73	6.40	6.10	5.82	5.55
10	10.00	8.77	7.92	7.54	7.18	6.85	6.55

blur. It may be initiated when the eye changes fixation from far to near, or it may be induced by convergence. The amount of reflex accommodation rarely exceeds 2 D.

See **accommodation, components of; reflex, near.**

relative amplitude of a. Total amount of accommodation which the eye can exert while the convergence of the eyes is fixed. It can be **positive** (using concave lenses until the image blurs). This is called positive relative accommodation (PRA). It can be **negative** (using convex lenses until the image blurs). This is negative relative accommodation (NRA).

See **zone of clear, single, binocular vision.**

reserve a. *See* **addition, near.**

resting state of a. Passive state of accommodation of the eye in the absence of a visual stimulus, i.e. when the eye is either in complete darkness, or looking at a bright empty field. In this condition, the pre-presbyopic eye is usually focused at an intermediate point (about 80 cm on average, although there are large variations), that is, the emmetropic eye becomes myopic. This is presumably due to a balance between a parasympathetic innervation to the circular fibres of the ciliary muscle and a sympathetic innervation to the longitudinal fibres of the ciliary muscle. Thus, the resting state of accommodation would correspond to a position of equilibrium between the two systems. Accommodation from this state to the near point of accommodation would be the response to parasympathetic stimulation, and accommodation from this state to the far point of accommodation would be the response to sympathetic stimulation. *Syn.* dark accommodation; dark focus (these terms are not strictly synonymous but as they have been found to correlate well, they have been adopted as synonyms); tonic accommodation.

See **hysteresis, accommodative; myopia, night; myopia, space; tonus; vergence, tonic.**

spasm of a. Involuntary contraction of the ciliary muscle producing excess accommodation. It may be constant, intermittent, unilateral or bilateral. Patients typically complain of discomfort, blurred distance vision and sometimes changes in perceived size of objects. If the patient is a low hyperope or emmetrope, it will give rise to **pseudomyopia (false myopia, hypertonic myopia, spurious myopia)**. Diagnosis is facilitated by cycloplegic refraction to rule out latent hyperopia. Although spasm of accommodation can be a separate entity, it is often associated with excessive convergence (esotropia) and miosis; this is referred to as **spasm of the near reflex**. Management includes removal of the primary cause, if possible (e.g. uveitis, or patient taking parasympathomimetic drugs); correction of the underlying refraction, if any; changes in the visual working conditions; positive lenses; accommodative facility exercises and, only rarely, cycloplegics. *Syn.* ciliary spasm.

See **accommodative facility; metamorphopsia.**

spectacle a. The amplitude of accommodation referred to the spectacle plane (Tables A3 and A4). *Symbol*: A_s.

See **accommodation, ocular.**

subjective a. Measurement of the accommodation based on the subject's judgements, such as the push-up or push-out method or the minus lens method.

See **accommodation, objective; method, minus lens; method, push-up.**

tonic a. *See* **accommodation, resting state of.**

vergence a. *See* **accommodation, convergence.**

accommodative Relating to accommodation.

accommodative astigmatism *See* astigmatism, accommodative.

accommodative balance *See* balance, binocular; method, Humphriss; test, balancing; test, Turville infinity.

accommodative convergence *See* convergence, accommodative.

accommodative convergence/accommodation ratio *See* AC/A ratio.

accommodative excess A condition in which the subject exerts more accommodation than required for the visual stimulus or is unable to relax accommodation. It may be due to uncorrected hyperopia, very prolonged near work, emotional problems, spasm of accommodation, uveitis, trigeminal neuralgia, syphilis, meningitis, head trauma or the side effect of some pharmaceutical agent (e.g. a miotic drug). It is usually associated with convergence excess. The subject reports blurred vision at distance, asthenopia and often headaches. Treatment commonly includes plus lenses and facility exercises, besides therapy of the underlying cause. *Syn.* hyperaccommodation. *Note*: Spasm of accommodation is one aspect of the general condition of accommodative excess, although some authors consider this term a synonym.

See accommodation, spasm of; accommodative facility; convergence excess.

accommodative demand *See* accommodation, correction induced; accommodation, lag of.

accommodative esotropia *See* strabismus, accommodative.

accommodative facility Ability of the eye/s to focus on stimuli placed at various distances and in different sequences in a given period of time. Clinically, this is measured either monocularly or binocularly, usually by having the subject fixate a small target alternately through plus and minus lenses, which are interchanged as soon as the target appears clear. The operation is repeated many times and the results are commonly presented in cycles per minute (one cycle indicates that both plus and minus lenses have been cleared). *Syn.* accommodative rock.

See accommodative insufficiency; lens flippers.

accommodative fatigue *See* accommodative insufficiency.

accommodative inertia Difficulty in altering the accommodative response, such that the latency and completion time of the process are delayed. It may occur as a result of prolonged near vision tasks. Orthoptic exercises may help in this condition.

accommodative hysteresis *See* hysteresis, accommodative.

accommodative infacility A condition in which there is a slowness in changing from one level of accommodation to another. Patients may complain of transitory blur. It may be due to diabetes, Graves' disease, measles or the side effects of some drugs. It is commonly associated with asthenopia. Treatment is aimed at the primary cause, but plus lenses and, especially, accommodative facility exercises can be helpful. *Syn.* inert accommodation.

accommodative insufficiency Insufficient amplitude of accommodation that is unequivocally below the appropriate level for the age. It may be due to extreme fatigue, influenza, high stress, systemic medication, ocular inflammation, head trauma, thyroid eye disease or the juvenile form of diabetes mellitus. The condition is often associated with convergence insufficiency, general fatigue, measles, multiple sclerosis, myotonic dystrophy, etc. It is the most common accommodative dysfunction. Patients complain of blurred vision or difficulty in sustaining clear vision at near; this is often accompanied by a frontal headache and even sometimes by pain in the eye. A mild form of accommodative insufficiency is often referred to as **ill-sustained accommodation (accommodative fatigue)** in which the response may be initially normal but cannot be maintained. It is easily discovered with accommodative facility exercises. Ill-sustained accommodation may be a precursor of accommodative insufficiency. Treatment is aimed at the primary cause, but plus lens correction, and in some cases exercises such as accommodative facility training can be helpful. *Syn.* premature presbyopia. *See* convergence insufficiency symptom survey; headache, ocular.

accommodative lag *See* accommodation, lag of.

accommodative reflex *See* accommodation, reflex.

accommodative response The response of the accommodative system when the eye changes fixation from one point in space to another. The reaction time for the accommodative response is about 350–420 ms and the image is suppressed during the process. Clinically, it can be estimated by measuring the accommodative lag or accommodative lead. *See* accommodation, mechanism of; effect, Mandelbaum.

accommodative rock *See* accommodative facility.

acetazolamide *See* carbonic anhydrase inhibitors.

acetone Liquid ketone (dimethyl ketone and propanone) used as a solvent for many organic compounds (e.g. cellulose acetate) and for repairing spectacle frames.

acetylcholine (ACh) A neurotransmitter substance which mediates excitatory properties of all preganglionic autonomic neurons, all parasympathetic postganglionic neurons and a few postganglionic sympathetic neurons. Acetylcholine is synthesized and liberated by the action of the enzyme choline acetyltranferase from the compounds choline and acetyl coenzyme A (acetyl CoA) which occurs in all cholinergic neurons. ACh exists only momentarily after its formation, being hydrolysed by the enzyme **acetylcholinesterase** which is present in the neurons of cholinergic nerves throughout their entire lengths and at neuromuscular junctions. This process is essential for proper muscle function as otherwise the accumulation of ACh would result in continuous stimulation of the muscles, glands and central nervous system. Alternatively, a shortage of ACh has devastating effect (e.g. myasthenia gravis). ACh binds to acetylcholine receptors on skeletal muscle fibres. Sodium enters the muscle fibre membrane, which leads to a depolarization of the membrane and muscle contraction. There are two main types of acetylcholine receptors (cholinergic receptors): (1) **muscarinic receptors,** which are stimulated by muscarine and ACh, belong to a family of G proteins coupled receptors that activate other ionic channels indirectly through a second messenger and thus act on nicotinic receptors. They are found in parasympathetically innervated structures (e.g. the iris and ciliary body); (2) **nicotinic receptors,** which are stimulated by nicotine and ACh, are ligand-gated receptors causing ion channels to open and are situated in striated muscles (e.g. the extraocular muscles). Cholinergic receptors are found in the sympathetic and parasympathetic nervous systems, in the brain and spinal cord. The action of ACh can be either blocked or stimulated by drugs: **Anticholinesterase drugs** (e.g. neostigmine) inhibit acetylcholinesterase and prolong the action of ACh whereas **antimuscarinic drugs** (also referred to as **anticholinergics** or **parasympatholytics**) such as atropine, cyclopentolate, homatropine and tropicamide inhibit the action of ACh at muscarinic receptors. Other drugs mimic the action of ACh. They are known as **parasympathomimetics** (e.g. pilocarpine). *See* cholinergic; cycloplegia; miotics; mydriatic; neurotransmitter; nicotine; synapse; system, autonomic nervous.

acetylcholinesterase An enzyme that degrades and inactivates acetylcholine. This compound is mainly found in neurons and at neuromuscular junctions. Drugs that inhibit this enzyme (e.g. diisopropyl fluorophosphate, physostigmine, edrophonium, echothiophate, DFP) can be used in the diagnosis and possible treatment of myasthenia gravis as well as certain forms of esotropia and glaucoma. *Syn.* specific cholinesterase. *See* anticholinesterase drugs.

acetylcysteine *See* tears, artificial.

achromasia *See* achromatopsia.

achromat *See* lens, achromatic.

achromatic 1. *See* lens, achromatic. **2.** The condition of being totally colour blind.
See achromatopsia; light, white; spectrum, equal energy.

achromatic axis; colour; interval; lens *See* under the nouns.

achromatic light stimulus, specified Any specified illuminant capable of being accepted as white under usual conditions of observation. *Note*: This includes the CIE standard illuminants (CIE).

achromatic prism *See* prism, achromatic.

achromatism 1. The condition of being totally colour blind. *Syn.* achromatopsia. **2.** Absence of colour. **3.** Condition of a lens or an optical system corrected for, or free from, chromatic aberration.
See monochromat.

achromatizing lens *See* lens, achromatizing.

achromatopsia Total colour blindness. The majority of cases are autosomal recessively inherited and caused by a mutation in genes CNGA3, CNGB3 or CNAT2. There are two types of achromatopsia. (1) Complete achromatopsia which results from having only rods and no functional cones (rod monochromat) having photophobia, poor acuity and nystagmus. (2) Incomplete achromatopsia in which there are the same symptoms, but in a diminished form. Patients benefit from dark-tinted lenses. Achromatopsia is non-progressive and very rare: one person in about 35 000 people. A few cases may be acquired resulting from a lesion in cortical area V4 (central achromatopsia). *Syn.* achromasia; achromatic vision; achromatism; acritochromacy; monochromatism.
See colour vision, defective; hemiachromatopsia; monochromat.

achromic Colourless.

acyclovir *See* antiviral agents.

acinar cell *See* cell, acinar.

acidosis An abnormal condition characterized by an increase in acidity and a relative decrease in alkaline content of the blood and body tissues. **Corneal acidosis** occurs as a result of contact lens wear, especially low gas permeable lenses, due to an accumulation of lactic acid and an increase in the concentration of carbon dioxide (hypercapnia), which is associated with a lower pH. This leads to polymegethism and polymorphism of endothelial cells.

acne rosacea A chronic inflammatory disease of the sebaceous glands of the skin of the face. It usually appears in middle-aged individuals. Nearly a third of these patients have blepharoconjunctivitis with staphylococcal infection and a few per cent will develop rosacea keratitis. The patient presents with papules, pustules, erythema, telangiectasia and, in some cases, rhinophyma, as well as facial erythema. Treatment includes lid hygiene with hot compresses, removal of crusts from the lid margins and topical and systemic antibiotics.
See blepharitis, anterior or marginal; keratitis, rosacea.

acorea Absence of the pupil of the eye.

acquired Pertaining to a condition which is contracted after birth and is not hereditary.
See congenital; familial; hereditary.

acquired colour vision deficiency A rare colour vision deficiency that develops equally in males and females of any age, in one eye or asymmetrically. It presents as a blue-yellow and less commonly red-green defect and in many instances there is decreased visual acuity and visual field constriction. It occurs as a result of disease such as glaucoma, diabetic retinopathy, age-related macular degeneration, optic neuritis, drugs or toxic exposure. Ageing may also lead to a blue defect, similar to tritan, due to yellowing of the lens.
See colour, defective; rule, Kollner's; test, colour vision.

Acquired Immune Deficiency Syndrome (AIDS) *See* syndrome, acquired immune deficiency.

acritochromacy *See* achromatopsia.

acrocephalosyndactyly *See* syndrome, Apert's.

actinic Pertaining to the chemical effect of radiant energy (especially ultraviolet) that results from absorption by certain substances. In the eye, the cornea, in particular, but also the lens and retina are most susceptible.
See blindness, eclipse; retinopathy, solar.

actinic keratoconjunctivitis; keratopathy *See* under the nouns.

action, primary Term referring to the greatest effect of an extraocular muscle in the primary position, that is in one plane. The other actions are called the **subsidiary** or **secondary** and **tertiary** actions. The primary action of the inferior rectus is depression; of the superior rectus, elevation; of the inferior oblique, extorsion; and of the superior oblique, intorsion. The medial and lateral recti muscles exert their primary action in the primary position, that is, pure adduction for the medial rectus and pure abduction for the lateral rectus.
See position, primary; Table M6, p. 220; test, forced duction; test, red glass.

action spectrum *See* spectrum, action.

action, tertiary Term referring to the least effect of an extrocular muscle. The tertiary action of the inferior rectus is extorsion; of the superior rectus, intorsion; of the inferior and superior oblique, abduction. The medial and lateral recti muscles are regarded as having only a primary action, at least in the primary position.

active position; transport *See* under the nouns.

acute In health care, pertains to a condition that has an abrupt onset and is severe and usually requires immediate attention. *Example:* acute angle-closure glaucoma.
See chronic.

acuity Term derived from the Latin (*acutus*) meaning acute or sharp: sharpness of vision.

angular visual a. *See* acuity, monotype visual.

central visual a. Visual acuity of the fovea and the macular area. Foveal visual acuity of 6/6 (20/20 or 0.00 logMAR) is considered to be normal. However, it is age-dependent and most young people have acuity better than normal (6/4; 20/14 or −0.18 logMAR), whereas older individuals have normal or less than normal acuity (Table A5).

decimal visual a. Visual acuity expressed as a decimal. The Snellen fraction is reduced, e.g. 6/18 (or 20/60 in feet) = 0.33. If the acuity is given in visual angle, decimal acuity is the reciprocal, e.g. 1/(3 minutes of arc) = 0.33.

dynamic visual a. Capacity to see distinctly moving objects. *Syn*. kinetic visual acuity.

kinetic visual a. *See* acuity, dynamic visual.

letter visual a. **1.** Visual acuity determined with letters on a chart. **2.** Visual acuity determined with single isolated letters.

line visual a. *See* acuity, morphoscopic visual.

logMAR visual a. *See* acuity, visual; chart, logMAR.

minimum separable visual a. *See* acuity, visual.

monotype visual a. Visual acuity determined with single isolated optotypes and therefore uninfluenced by neighbouring contours. *Syn*. acuity, angular visual.

morphoscopic visual a. Visual acuity determined with a group of optotypes such as, for example, a line of letters or Landolt rings. The result may thus be influenced by neighbouring contours. *Syn*. line visual acuity.

See phenomenon, crowding.

near visual a. Capacity for seeing distinctly the details of an object at near. It is specified in various ways: (1) As the angle of resolution (in minutes of arc) at a given near distance. (2) As a Snellen fraction,

either as one that is equivalent to the distance visual acuity (**Snellen equivalent**) or more correctly as one which indicates the actual distance (e.g. 16/32 if the distance is 16 inches). (3) As lines of unrelated words of a Bailey-Lovie Word reading chart in which the progression of each line is logarithmic similar to a distance logMAR chart that uses optotypes. (4) As an arbitrary Jaeger notation (e.g. J6). (5) As **N notation** (using Times Roman typeface) or **Points** (using any typeface), such as N8 at 40 cm (or simply 8-point), where N refers to near and the number to the amount of points (a point is a unit used by printers to specify print size and is equal to 0.35 mm or 1/72 of an inch). Thus, N8 indicates that the overall height is 8/72 inch (or 2.82 mm) or about 4/72 inch (or 1.41 mm) for lower-case letters. (6) As M **Units**. For the usual font styles (e.g. Times Roman, Century) used in newsprint, 8-point print is usually considered to be approximately equal to 1 M Unit, so 1 M = N8, 2 M = N16, etc (Table A6).

See chart, Bailey–Lovie; chart, logMAR; Jaeger test types.

objective visual a. Visual acuity measured without the subject's judgement.

See potential, visual evoked; method, preferential looking; test, optokinetic nystagmus.

peripheral visual a. Visual acuity of the peripheral regions of the retina, outside the macula.

resolution visual a. *See* acuity, visual.

Snellen a. Visual acuity measured with Snellen letters.

static visual a. Acuity determined with stationary test types or test objects.

See acuity, dynamic visual; test type.

stereoscopic visual a. The ability to detect the smallest difference in depth between two objects. It is expressed as the difference η between the two angles subtended at any two objects in the field of view by the base line (or interpupillary distance). This threshold angle η (eta) is given by the approximate relationship, in radians

$$\eta = PD \times \Delta D / d^2$$

where PD is the interpupillary distance, d the test distance of the reference object and ΔD the distance between the two objects. (To convert the result into seconds of arc it should be multiplied by $180/\pi \times 60 \times 60 = 206265$.) The difference between the two angles $u_1 - u_2$ (the difference between the two retinal images) is called **binocular disparity** or **retinal disparity**, and the difference between the two angles β − α is called the **relative binocular parallax** (Fig. A5). Stereoscopic visual acuity is extremely fine, varying between 5 and 15 seconds of arc. It tends to decrease with age and it is positively correlated with Snellen visual acuity. *Example*: Suppose ΔD is equal to 2 mm, d is 827 mm and the PD is 64 mm

$$\eta = \frac{64(2)}{827^2}(206265) = 38 \text{ seconds of arc}$$

Table A5 Average relative visual acuity in the central region of the retina			
Eccentricity (degrees)	Acuity (%)	Snellen fraction (m)	(ft)
0	100	6/6	20/20
0.5	80	6/7.5	20/25
1	66	6/9	20/30
1.5	57	6/11	20/37
2	49	6/12	20/40
2.5	41	6/14.5	20/48
3	39	6/15	20/50
3.5	37	6/16	20/53
4	35	6/17	20/57
4.5	33	6/18	20/60
5	32	6/19	20/63
6	29	6/21	20/70
7	27	6/22	20/73

Table A6 Relationship between several near visual acuity notations

Snellen equivalent in metres (feet)

25 cm	40 cm	Points	M units
6/240 (20/800)	6/144 (20/480)	80	10.0
6/192 (20/640)	6/120 (20/400)	64	8.0
6/144 (20/480)	6/96 (20/320)	48	6.4
6/120 (20/400)	6/72 (20/240)	40	4.8
6/96 (20/320)	6/60 (20/200)	32	4.0
6/72 (20/240)	6/48 (20/160)	24	3.2
6/60 (20/200)	6/36 (20/120)	20	2.4
6/48 (20/160)	6/30 (20/100)	16	2.0
6/36 (20/120)	6/24 (20/80)	12	1.6
6/30 (20/100)	6/18 (20/60)	10	1.2
6/24 (20/80)	6/15 (20/50)	8	1.0
6/18 (20/60)	6/12 (20/40)	6	0.8
6/15 (20/50)	6/9 (20/30)	5	0.6
6/12 (20/40)	6/7.5 (20/25)	4	0.5
6/9 (20/30)	6/6 (20/20)	3	0.4
6/6 (20/20)	6/3.6 (20/12)	2	0.25

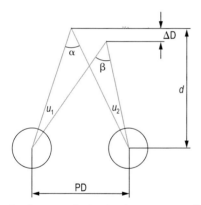

Fig. A5 Stereoscopic visual acuity, $\eta = u_1 - u_2 = \beta - \alpha$

Syn. stereo-acuity; stereo-threshold.
See angle of stereopsis; disparity, retinal; test, Howard–Dolman; test, three needle; vectogram.
Teller a. cards Test cards used to assess the visual acuity of infants. The set consists of 16 rectangular grey cards, each approximately 26 by 56 cm. Fifteen of the cards contain a high-contrast square-wave grating, 12 by 12 cm, each of a given spatial frequency, and located either on the left or the right of a central peephole in the card. The average luminance of the grating is approximately equal to that of the grey background. The spatial frequencies of the gratings range from 0.3 to 38 cpd when viewed from 55 cm. The procedure consists in starting with the card with the lowest spatial frequency (or coarser grating) and proceeding to cards with finer gratings. The observer watches the infant through the central peephole and his or her task is to make a subjective judgment, based on the infant's head and eye movements, of which is the finest grating card that the child can just resolve. The spatial frequency of this last card represents the estimate of the visual acuity. The procedure using these cards is based on the method of preferential looking but it is simpler, quicker and equally reliable.
See cycle per degree; method, preferential looking.
unaided visual a. Visual acuity without any correction. *Syn.* vision; unaided vision.
vernier visual a. The ability to detect the alignment or otherwise, of two lines as in the reading of a vernier scale. This is the finest acuity being of the order of 1–5 seconds of arc depending on the length of the line; the longer the line, the more acute the detection. *Syn.* aligning power.
See hyperacuity.
visual a. (VA) Capacity for seeing distinctly the details of an object. Quantitatively, it is represented in two ways: (1) As the reciprocal of the minimum angle of resolution (in minutes of arc). This is the resolution visual acuity. *Syn.* minimum separable visual acuity. (2) As the $\log_{10}$ of the minimum angle of resolution (logMAR), which is determined using a special logMAR chart. (3) As the Snellen fraction. This is measured using letters or Landolt rings or equivalent objects.
Average clinical visual acuity varies between 6/4 and 6/6 (or 20/15 and 20/20 in feet). Visual acuity varies with the region of the retina (being maximum in the foveola), with general illumination, contrast, colour and type of test, time of exposure, the refractive error of the eye, the patient's age, etc (Tables A6 and A7).
See angle of resolution, minimum; chart, Bailey-Lovie; chart, logMAR; cycle per degree; Glasgow acuity cards; hyperacuity; isoacuity; optotype; sensitivity, contrast; Snellen fraction; test, Cardiff acuity; test, photostress; test, Sheridan–Gardiner; visual efficiency scale; Snell–Sterling.

acyanopsia Inability to recognize blue tints.
See chromatopsia.

Table A7 Relationship between several distance visual acuity notations

Snellen fraction		Min. angle of resolution (min. of arc)	logMAR	Decimal
(m)	(ft)			
6/240	20/800	40.0	1.60	0.025
6/180	20/600	30.0	1.52	0.03
6/150	20/500	25.0	1.40	0.04
6/120	20/400	20.0	1.30	0.05
6/90	20/300	15.0	1.18	0.07
6/60	20/200	10.0	1.0	0.10
6/48	20/160	8.0	0.90	0.125
6/38	20/125	6.3	0.80	0.16
6/30	20/100	5.0	0.70	0.20
6/24	20/80	4.0	0.60	0.25
6/21	20/70	3.5	0.54	0.29
6/18	20/60	3.0	0.48	0.33
6/15	20/50	2.5	0.40	0.40
6/12	20/40	2.0	0.30	0.50
6/9	20/30	1.5	0.17	0.67
6/7.5	20/25	1.25	0.11	0.80
6/6	20/20	1.0	0.00	1.0
6/4.5	20/15	0.75	−0.12	1.33
6/3	20/10	0.5	−0.30	2.0

Adams desaturated D-15 test *See* **test, Farnsworth.**

adaptation 1. Process by which a sensory organ (e.g. the eye) adjusts to its environment (e.g. to luminance, colour or contact lens wear). **2.** The reduction in sensitivity to continuous sensory stimulation. The neurophysiological correlate corresponds to a decrease in the frequency of action potentials fired by a neuron, despite a stimulus of constant magnitude. Visual adaptation is prevented from occurring by the continuous involuntary movements of the eyes.
See **movement, fixation; potential, action; stabilized retinal image.**
chromatic a. Apparent changes in hue and saturation after prolonged exposure to a field of a specific colour.
dark a. Adjustment of the eye (particularly regeneration of visual pigments and dilatation of the pupil), such that, after observation in the dark, the sensitivity to light is greatly increased, i.e. the threshold response to light is decreased. This is a much slower process than light adaptation. Older people usually take longer to adapt to darkness and only reach a higher threshold than young people. It is some 2 log units, i.e. 100 times, higher in an 80-year-old than in a 20-year-old person.
See **adaptometer; hemeralopia; pigment, visual; theory, duplicity.**
light a. Adjustment of the eye (particularly bleaching of visual pigments and constriction of the pupil), such that, after observation of a bright field, the sensitivity to light is diminished, i.e. the threshold of luminance is increased.
See **law, de Vries-Rose; law, Weber's; theory, duplicity.**
prism a. See **adaptation, vergence.**
sensory a. Mechanism by which the visual system adjusts to avoid confusion and diplopia of the perceptual impression due to an abnormal motor condition (e.g. strabismus).
vergence a. A process by which the eyes return to their condition of habitual heterophoria or orthophoria after a heterophoria has been induced by prisms (**prism adaptation**) in front of one or both eyes (as, for example, when lens centration does not coincide with the interpupillary distance), or by spherical lenses, or due to changes in the orbital contents with increasing age. This adaptation process may be related to the phenomenon of orthophorization. People who have symptomatic binocular vision anomalies do not, or only partially, show vergence adaptation to prisms. Vergence adaptation decreases with increasing age.

adaptive optics *See* **optics, adaptive.**

adaptometer An instrument for measuring the variations in threshold of luminance. The most common is that of Goldmann–Weekers.

add *See* **addition, near.**

addition, near (add) The difference in spherical power between the distance and near corrections. A common method of arriving at the power of the addition is to measure the patient's working distance and the amplitude of accommodation. The add is obtained as follows

$$add = (1\,\text{metre}/\text{working distance in metre}) - x(\text{amplitude})$$

where x is the percentage of the total amplitude of accommodation which is to be used: Two-thirds is usually more appropriate for young presbyopes (below about 52 years of age), while one-half is more appropriate for older presbyopes. Thus, this formula allows for a certain amount of the amplitude of accommodation to be left in **reserve** (usually one-third or one-half). It can also be estimated based on age: +1.0 D to +1.25 D for age 45–50 years; +1.5 to +1.75 D for age 50–55 years; +2.0 D to +2.25 D for age 55–60 years; +2.5 D to +3.0 D for older patients. However, these figures may need to be adjusted to take into account the average working distance of the patient. *Syn.* presbyopic addition; reading addition.
See **bracketing; distance, reading; presbyopia; Table R3, p. 305; test at near, cross-cylinder.**

adduct To turn toward the midline.

adduction Rotation of an eye toward the midline (Fig. A6).
See **duction; palsy, third nerve; syndrome, Duane's.**

adductors Extraocular muscles that move the eye inward, such as the medial rectus, the inferior rectus and the superior rectus.
See **muscles, extraocular.**

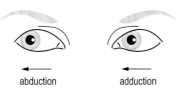

Fig. A6 Abduction of the right eye. Adduction of the left eye. (Although both are drawn on the same figure note that ductions refer to one eye only.)

adenoma A benign tumour consisting of glandular epithelium and some connective tissue.

adenoma, Fuchs' *See* Fuchs' adenoma.

adenoma, pituitary An adenoma of the pituitary gland, which can cause headache, colour vision variations when shown a coloured object across the midline of one eye and a visual field defect, typically asymmetrical bitemporal hemianopia. *See* **gland, pituitary.**

adenopathy *See* lymphadenopathy.

adenovirus A DNA virus, composed of over 40 serotypes. Many serotypes cause ocular infection, including epidemic keratoconjunctivitis caused by serotypes 8, 19 and 37. Other infections include follicular conjunctivitis with or without pseudomembranes and epithelial keratitis. The adenovirus can be identified using, among others, conjunctival swabs for viral antigen. *See* **conjunctivitis, acute.**

adequate stimulus *See* stimulus, adequate.

adherence syndrome *See* syndrome, adherence.

adhesion *See* synechia.

Adie's pupil *See* pupil, Adie's.

Adie's syndrome *See* syndrome, Holmes-Adie.

adipose tissue A type of fatty tissue that is present in large amounts in the orbit. The fat surrounds the orbit and acts as a cushion for the globe. The fat is divided by fibrous septae and is kept posteriorly by Tenon's capsule.

adnexa oculi *See* appendages of the eye.

adrenaline (epinephrine) A hormone of the adrenal medulla which, instilled in the eye, causes a constriction of the conjunctival vessels, dilates the pupil and diminishes the intraocular pressure. *See* **adrenergic receptors; decongestant, ocular; gland, adrenal; naphazoline; neurotransmitter; noradrenaline (norepinephrine).**

adrenergic 1. Relating to a neuron that is activated or capable of releasing adrenaline (epinephrine). **2.** Having an effect similar to adrenaline (epinephrine). **3.** Relating to drugs that mimic the effects of the sympathetic nervous system (sympathomimetic drugs).

adrenergic agonist *See* sympathomimetic drugs.

adrenergic blocking agents *See* sympatholytic drugs.

adrenergic receptors Receptors which are stimulated by catecholamines adrenaline (epinephrine) and noradrenaline (norepinephrine). These receptors belong to a family of G protein coupled receptors and are found in the central nervous system. There are two main types of adrenergic receptors. (1) **α-receptors** of which there are two types; α_1 **receptors** are located in the arterioles, dilator pupillae and Muller palpebral muscles. Stimulation of α_1 **agonists** (e.g. noradrenaline [norepinephrine], phenylephrine) causes mydriasis and lid retraction; α_2 **receptors** are located in the ciliary epithelium. Stimulation of α_2 **agonists** (e.g. apraclonidine, brimonidine) results in a reduction of aqueous secretion and enhancing uveoscleral outflow. (2) **β-receptors** of which there are (at least) two types, β_1 and β_2; β_1 **receptors** are located in the myocardium. Stimulation increases cardiac output. β_2 **receptors** are located in the bronchi and ciliary epithelium. Stimulation causes bronchodilatation and increased aqueous secretion. There are drugs that block the effect of catecholamines on α- or β-adrenergic receptors and are called α- or β-blockers (or sympatholytic drugs or adrenergic receptor agonists). *Example:* The ciliary epithelium contains mainly β_2-receptors, and a β-blocker such as timolol inhibits the secretion of aqueous humour, thus reducing intraocular pressure. *Syn.* adrenoceptor. *See* **alpha-adrenergic agonists; alpha-adrenergic antagonists; beta-blocker; miotics; mydriatic; pathway, uveoscleral; sympatholytic drugs; sympathomimetic drugs; system, autonomic nervous.**

adrenocorticosteroids Compounds created by the adrenal cortex that have distant metabolic effects. There are three types of compounds created by the adrenal cortex: glucocorticoids, mineralocorticoids and androgens. Of these, the glucocorticoids are most important to the visual system due to their antiinflammatory effects. The antiinflammatory effect is thought to be mediated by inhibition of prostaglandin synthesis. *See* **antiinflammatory drug; gland, adrenal; steroid.**

adult inclusion conjunctivitis *See* conjunctivitis, adult inclusion.

advancement A surgical procedure used in strabismus or is some form of ptosis (involutional) in which an extraocular muscle (e.g. rectus or levator palpebrae superioris muscle) is removed from its insertion and repositioned elsewhere on the globe anteriorly to increase its action. *See* **recession.**

aerial image *See* image, aerial.

aerial perspective *See* perspective, aerial.

aerobic Needing oxygen to sustain life. *See* **anaerobic.**

aesthesiometer Instrument for the measurement of tissue sensitivity, especially tactile. The cornea and eyelid margins are the ocular structures measured. There are many types of aesthesiometers. The most common used to be that of **Cochet–Bonnet**

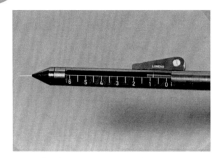

Fig. A7 Cochet–Bonnet aesthesiometer.

(Fig. A7). It consists of a nylon monofilament of constant diameter which, depending upon its length, can exert more or less pressure. The length at which the subject responds to represents the corneal touch threshold. New instruments are non-contact and use a pulse of pressurized air or gas to stimulate the cornea. *Note*: also spelt esthesiometer.
See **corneal fragility; hyperaesthesia, corneal; corneal touch threshold; sensitivity, corneal.**

aetiology The cause or origin of a disease. *Note*: also spelt etiology.
See **diagnosis; epidemiology.**

afferent Carrying nerve impulses from the periphery to the central nervous system.
See **efferent.**

afferent limb, of pupillary pathway Section of the visual pathway originating in the rods and cones of the retina and terminating in the brainstem. The fibres follow the visual pathway, decussating in the optic chiasma, and continuing in the optic tracts. The fibres exit the optic tracts before reaching the lateral geniculate body, and project to the brainstem. After synapsing in the brainstem, the fibres then project to the ipsilateral and contralateral Edinger–Westphal nuclei.
See **reflex, pupil light.**

afferent pupillary defect *See* **pupil, Marcus Gunn.**

aflibercept *See* **anti-VEG drugs.**

afocal Refers to a lens or an optical system with zero focal power, i.e. in which incident rays entering parallel emerge parallel.
See **lens, afocal; lens, aniseikonic.**

after-cataract An opacity in the posterior capsule of the crystalline lens which may have remained or occurred after extracapsular cataract extraction (manual or phacoemulsification). The opacity is caused by migration of lens epithelial cells, which migrate from the anterior surface and form an opaque membrane on the posterior surface of the lens. Treatment is typically with a neodymium-YAG laser to create a central hole in the capsule (**capsulotomy**). *Syn.* secondary cataract.
See **cataract extraction, extracapsular.**

after-effect, motion *See* **after-effect, waterfall.**

after-effect, tilt Observation of a temporary change in the perceived orientation of lines after having adapted to lines tilted in another direction. If, for example, you stare at white and black bars tilted to the left for a minute or so, then look at vertical bars, these will now appear to tilt slightly to the right. This is an example of the adaptation in the visual system of orientation-specific cells, which become fatigued and therefore temporarily less responsive.
See **adaptation; after-effect, waterfall; cell, orientation-specific.**

after-effect, waterfall Observation of a movement in the opposite direction after having looked at a waterfall for some time, when fixating a stationary object. This is an example of phenomena that are used to infer the existence of channels in the visual system. It is suggested that there are two opposed directionally sensitive neural channels (or neurons) which are normally in balance for stationary stimuli, but when the activity of one channel is fatigued by prolonged stimulation, the other one becomes the active one. The waterfall after-effect is a special case of **motion or movement after-effect** (or **motion after-image**). *Syn.* waterfall effect; waterfall illusion.
See **channel; spiral, Plateau's.**

after-image Visual sensation persisting after the original stimulus has been removed. If observed in darkness following stimulation by a high intensity and brief duration light source, seven different after-image phases are frequently noted. The first phase, also called **Hering's after-image**, is a positive after-image, and it is followed by a negative after-image. After a short interval (less than half a second), a second positive after-image, called **Purkinje after-image** or **Bidwell's ghost**, appears, the character of which depends upon the conditions of adaptation, the colour of the stimulus and the retinal region stimulated (best in the periphery). Afterward, a second negative after-image is sometimes observed followed by a third positive after-image, called **Hess after-image**. After a long dark interval, a third negative after-image may appear followed by another long dark interval by a fourth positive after-image. If the light stimulus is of moderate intensity, the last phases will be absent.
See **law, Emmert's; test, after-image; test, after-image transfer.**
complementary a. After-image in which the colour is complementary to the colour of the original stimulus.
Hering's; Hess a. See **after-image.**
homochromatic a. After-image in which the colour appears to be the same as the original stimulus.
motion a. See **after-effect, waterfall; spiral, Plateau's.**
negative a. An after-image in which the light areas of the original stimulus appear dark, the dark areas appear light and the coloured areas appear in a complementary colour.

positive a. After-image that appears to be the same as the original stimulus.
Purkinje a. See after-image.

against movement See movement, against; neutralization; retinoscope.

agnosia Inability to recognize the significance of sensory stimuli (e.g. to recognize colour, faces, shape and the orientation of objects), although the receptors and the sensory pathway are intact. The condition is attributed to bilateral lesions in the association areas of the cortex. If the sense of sight is affected, it is called **visual agnosia** (**perceptual** or **psychic blindness**).
See alexia; apraxia, optical; prosopagnosia.

agonist 1. An agonistic muscle. **2.** A substance (e.g. a drug, hormone or neurotransmitter) that binds with a cell receptor to initiate a physiological response similar to that produced by the natural neurotransmitter or hormone. *Example*: pilocarpine, which mimics the effect of acetylcholine acting on cholinergic receptors.
See antagonist; muscle, agonistic.

agonist drug A drug that combines with the receptor to mimic or enhance the effect of a neurotransmitter.
See neurotransmitter.

agonistic muscle See muscle, agonistic.

agraphia Inability to write, usually as a result of a brain lesion. If the person can write from dictation but not from copying, it is called **visual agraphia**.
See dysgraphia.

Aicardi's syndrome See syndrome, Aicardi's.

AIDS See syndrome, acquired immunodeficiency.

aids, low vision Optical (e.g. loupe) or non-optical (e.g. large numeral telephone) appliances and devices designed to assist the partially sighted patient.
See glass, magnifying; lamp, halogen; lens, telescopic; spectacles, pinhole; typoscope; vision, low.

air-puff tonometer See tonometer, non-contact.

Airy's disc See disc, Airy's.

akinesia Loss or impairment of voluntary movements of the eye and/or the eyelids. It occurs as a temporary muscular paralysis following peribulbar, retrobulbar or sub-Tenon anaesthesia or facial nerve blockage before surgery.
See injection.

akinaesthesia 1. Inability to perceive moving objects. *Example*: As a glass fills up with water, the person cannot see the level moving, but only a succession of fixed images. **2.** Lack or loss of muscular sense.

alacrima Absence of secretion from the lacrimal gland. However, the typical picture is one of reduced tear secretion more correctly termed **hypolacrima**. It may occur as a result of occlusion of the orifices of the lacrimal gland due to trauma, cicatrization, diseases (e.g. trachoma); it may be congenital (e.g. Riley–Day syndrome) or it may be due to a neurogenic cause (secondary to brain damage) or to a systemic disease (e.g. Sjögren's syndrome). Treatment includes artificial tears, bland ointments, sealed scleral contact lenses and, in very severe cases, tarsorrhaphy.
See keratoconjunctivitis sicca.

Alagille's syndrome See syndrome, Alagille's.

albedo retinae Oedema of the retina.

albinism Congenital anomaly due to a defect of melanin production as a result of one of several possible genetic defects. **Oculocutaneous albinism type 1 (OCA1)** is due to a genetic defect in tyrosinase, the enzyme that metabolizes the amino acid tyrosine, which is essential for its conversion to melanin (also called **tyrosinase-negative** albinism). It is an autosomal recessive condition caused by a mutation in the tyrosinase gene TYR on chromosome 11q14, which affects the skin, hair and eyes. The iris is a pale colour, the fundus and the pupil are reddish and the eye transilluminates markedly. There is poor visual acuity, photophobia, nystagmus and strabismus. **Oculocutaneous type 2 (OCA2)** is caused by a mutation of the OCA2 ("P") gene on chromosome 15q resulting in variable amounts of melanin synthesis. The hypopigmentation of the eyes, skin and hair varies from fair to normal (also called **tyrosinase-positive** albinism). It may be associated with the **Hermansky–Pudlak syndrome** in which there is albinism and easy bruising or bleeding and Waardenburg's syndrome. The other type of albinism is **ocular albinism type 1 (OA1)**. It is inherited either as an X-linked or less commonly as an autosomal recessive trait. It affects mainly the eyes and, in most instances, males only and the skin colour is usually normal. Management involves full correction (hyperopia is the most common refractive error), possibly with tinted lenses. Surgery may be required for strabismus.
See fundus, ocular; inheritance; transillumination.

albinoidism A mild form of albinism in which, although there is decreased activity of tyrosinase and hypopigmentation in localized areas, it does not lead to any ocular defects.

Albright's syndrome See syndrome, Albright's.

alcohol See antiseptic.

Alexander's law See law, Alexander's.

alexia Inability to recognize written or printed words due to a lesion in the brain. This is a form of visual agnosia. *Syn.* word blindness.
See agnosia; dyslexia.

Algorithm, Swedish Interactive Thresholding (SITA) A program designed to shorten the time taken to determine the threshold values of each location of the visual field being tested with an automated perimeter. It takes about 3.5 minutes in most patients. Stimulus presentation is altered according to the patient's response time; the quicker the patient responds the faster the rate of presentation and vice versa. Patient's reliability is also taken into account.

aliasing Perceptual phenomenon occurring when the spatial frequency of a visual target is higher than that of the photoreceptor spacing, i.e. there is undersampling. The spatial frequency is then higher than Nyquist frequency.
See **frequency, Nyquist; stroboscope; undersampling.**

aligning power *See* **acuity, vernier visual.**

aligning prism Term recommended to replace the term associated heterophoria.
See **prism, aligning.**

alignment fit *See* **fitted on K.**

alkaptonuria A rare, hereditary, metabolic disorder characterized by dark urine. It is caused by mutation in the homogentisate 1, 2-dioxygenase gene (HGD), which produces an error in the metabolism of the amino acids tyrosine and phenylalanine, which normally break down by oxidation to homogentisic acid. However, in this condition, homogentisic acid is not broken down but stored in tissues, especially cartilage, which it turns bluish-black and is excreted in the urine. Ocular signs are pigmentation of the sclera, most markedly near the insertions of the recti muscles and limbus, and of the cornea and conjunctiva.

all or none law *See* **law, all or none.**

allele *See* **genotype.**

Allen–Thorpe gonioprism *See* **gonioprism.**

allergic reactions *See* **hypersensitivity.**

allergy A state of hypersensitivity induced by re-exposure to a particular antigen (called allergen), usually environmental, such as pollens, foods, microorganisms and drugs resulting in an abnormal immunological response (e.g. hay fever, asthma, urticaria). It typically involves the release of histamine from mast cells in response to an antigen binding to IgE antibodies on the surface of the mast cells. The signs and symptoms in the eye are itching, tearing, hyperaemia and eyelid oedema.
See **conjunctivitis, allergic; hypersensitivity.**

allesthesia, visual A rare disorder in which a visual stimulus located in one half of the visual field is perceived as being located in the other. Occasionally the visual stimulus may be transposed from the lower to the upper quadrant, or vice versa. The condition may occur as a result of damage to the parietal or occipital cortex.

allograft A graft of tissue taken from a donor and implanted in a host of the same species but not of the same genotype (i.e. not in the same person). It is used to replace a diseased or injured tissue. *Example:* a corneal graft performed in a case of severe keratoconus. *Syn.* homograft.
See **keratoplasty; xenograft.**

allometropia Refraction of the eye along any line except the visual axis (or line of sight) therefore representing the refraction of any extrafoveal region. *Example*: if an eye is emmetropic along the visual axis, at 40 degrees of temporal retinal eccentricity the allometropia will be about plano $-2.50 \times 90°$ and at 50 degrees, $+0.50-3.50 \times 90°$.
See **astigmatism, oblique.**

allowance *See* **retinoscope.**

allyl diglycol carbonate *See* **CR-39 material.**

all-trans *See* **rhodopsin.**

alpha-adrenergic agonist An agent that selectively binds and activates alpha-adrenergic receptors. In the eye, it causes mydriasis and reduces the production of aqueous humour. Some are used topically in the treatment of glaucoma, such as apraclonidine and brimonidine tartrate. Other agents include adrenaline (epinephrine) and noradrenaline (norepinephrine).
See **adrenergic receptor; sympathomimetic drugs.**

alpha-adrenergic antagonist An agent that blocks the effect of the catecholamine adrenaline (epinephrine) and noradrenaline (norepinephrine) on adrenergic receptors. It produces miosis and a slight reduction in intraocular pressure. It is used mainly to reverse the mydriatic effect of sympathomimetic drugs (e.g. phenylephrine hydrochloride) or even some antimuscarinic drugs (e.g. tropicamide). Common agents include dapiprazole and moxisylyte (thymoxamine). *Syn.* alpha-blocker.
See **adrenergic receptors; sympatholytic drugs.**

alpha angle *See* **angle, alpha.**

alpha-blocker *See* **alpha-adrenergic antagonist.**

alpha waves Rhythmic oscillation in electrical potential occurring in the cortex of the human brain when awake and at rest. The rate of oscillation is 8–13 Hz. *Syn.* alpha rhythm.
See **potential, resting membrane.**

alphabet patterns *See* **pattern, alphabet.**

Alport's syndrome *See* **syndrome, Alport's.**

alternate cover test *See* **test, cover.**

alternating checkerboard stimulus A type of light stimulus used in performing electrophysiological testing. It is used in the pattern electroretinogram (pERG) and visual evoked potentials. It consists of a checkerboard of black and white squares in which the dark phase of one set of squares coincide with the bright phase of the other set and they alternate at a given rate, but the overall luminance of the screen remains constant.
See **electroretinogram; pattern, checkerboard; potential, visual evoked.**

alternating hypertropia; strabismus *See* under the nouns.

altitudinal hemianopia *See* **hemianopia, altitudinal.**

Alvarez lens *See* **lens, Alvarez.**

amacrine cell *See* **cell, amacrine.**

amaurosis 1. Partial or total loss of sight due to a lesion somewhere in the visual pathway (usually the optic nerve), but not in the eye itself. **2.** Synonym for blindness.
See **pupil, amaurotic.**

amaurosis fugax Transient unilateral loss of vision. The visual loss varies from partial to total blindness and rarely lasts longer than 10 minutes. It is usually caused by a temporary occlusion in the internal carotid artery, which produces an insufficient blood flow to the ophthalmic artery and may lead to closure of the central retinal artery. *Syn.* blackout. *See* **angiography, fluorescein; arteritis, giant cell; blackout; bruit; neuropathy, arteritic anterior ischaemic optic; plaques, Hollenhorst's; retinal artery occlusion.**

amaurosis, Leber's congenital *See* **Leber's congenital amaurosis.**

ambiocularity 1. *See* **dominance, ocular.** 2. In strabismus, the condition in which the patient uses either eye.

ambiguous figure *See* **figure, Blivet; figure, Kanizsa; Necker cube; Schroeder's staircase; vase, Rubin's.**

amblyogenic *See* **amblyopiagenic.**

amblyope Person who has amblyopia.

amblyopia A condition characterized by reduced visual acuity due to a lesion in the eye or in the visual pathway, which hinders the normal development of vision, and which is not correctable by spectacles or contact lenses. The usual clinical criterion is 6/9 (20/30 or 0.17 logMAR) or less in one eye, or a two-line difference or more, on the acuity chart between the two eyes. Amblyopia may occur as a result of: suppression in the deviated eye in strabismus (**strabismic amblyopia;** formerly called **amblyopia ex anopsia,** which amounts to about 20% of all cases); a blurred image in the more ametropic eye in uncorrected anisometropia (**anisometropic amblyopia** which amounts to about 50% of all cases); bilateral blurred images in uncorrected refractive errors (**isoametropic amblyopia**); a blurred image in one of the meridians of high uncorrected astigmatism (**meridional amblyopia**); any of the previous three is also called **refractive amblyopia;** opacities in the ocular media (e.g. congenital cataract, severe ptosis) in infants (**deprivation amblyopia or visual deprivation amblyopia or image degradation amblyopia**) after the lesion has been removed; continuous occlusion of an eye as may occur in occlusion treatment (**occlusion amblyopia**); arsenic, lead or quinine poisoning (**toxic amblyopia**) or the more specific types of toxic amblyopia such as those caused by excessive use of alcohol (**alcohol amblyopia**), methanol (**methanol amblyopia**), quinine (**quinine amblyopia**) or tobacco (**tobacco amblyopia**), although the latter three may actually be due to nutritional deficiencies (**nutritional amblyopia**); psychological origin (**hysterical amblyopia**) or of unknown origin (**idiopathic amblyopia**).

Many of these amblyopias are **functional**, i.e. in which no organic lesion exists as in hysterical, refractive (e.g. meridional amblyopia), isoametropic, strabismic or stimulus deprivation amblyopia. Others are **organic**, i.e. they are due to some pathological (e.g. congenital cataract) or anatomical anomalies (e.g. malorientation of retinal receptors), as nutritional or toxic poisoning or excessive alcohol or tobacco. However, there may be cases in which a functional amblyopia is due in part to some accompanying undetected pathology or structural defects (e.g. a change in retinal fibre layer thickness). Amblyopia occurs in 2–4% of the population. There is usually a reduction in the amplitude of accommodation in amblyopic eyes. Treatment of amblyopia depends on the type. However, the younger the patient is, the more likely that the treatment will be successful. Typically, the principal treatment is occlusion of the fixating eye (or the eye with the best acuity) by patching or blurring with atropine sulfate to force the other eye to take up fixation, after full refractive correction and treatment of the underlying pathology. Other procedures (alternatives or supplemental to patching) include penalization, kicking a ball toward a specific target, playing catch a ball, bar reading, pleoptics (when there is eccentric fixation as well) and any other procedures which require fixation like drawing, duplicating letter sequences on a typewriter, cutting out patterns, etc.
See **cheiroscope; disc, pinhole; fixation, eccentric; Glasgow acuity cards; occlusion treatment; penalization; perceptual learning; period, critical; phenomenon, crowding; pleoptics; suppression; test, bar reading; test, neutral density filter.**
functional a. See amblyopia.
hysterical a. Apparent loss of vision due to a psychological disorder. The patient really believes that he or she cannot see, although this is not supported by physiological impairment. The condition is often characterized by a constricted visual field or tunnel vision.
meridional a. Amblyopia in one of the two principal meridians of an astigmatic eye. The amblyopia usually affects the most defocused meridian and its severity tends to vary with the amount of astigmatism. This amblyopia is of neural origin. Optical correction of the patient as young as possible usually prevents this condition. *Syn.* astigmatic amblyopia.
organic a. See amblyopia.

amblyopiagenic Pertains to factors causing amblyopia, such as anisometropia, strabismus, opacities in the ocular media, etc. *Syn.* amblyogenic.

amblyopic eye nystagmus *See* under the nouns.

amblyoscope, major *See* amblyoscope, Worth.

amblyoscope, Wheatstone Amblyoscope using mirrors to change the angle of convergence or divergence. *Syn.* Wheatstone stereoscope.

amblyoscope, Worth A modified haploscope introduced by Worth, consisting of two angled tubes held in front of the eyes which present a different image to each eye, and which can be turned to any degree of convergence or divergence. Using various images (slides), the instrument can be used to measure the angle of deviation and vergence amplitudes, and to investigate retinal correspondence, fusion, suppression and stereopsis. If the instrument is incorporated into a table, it is called a **major amblyoscope** of which there are various types called **Synoptiscope** or **Synoptophore**.

Ames room *See* room, Ames.

amethocaine hydrochloride *See* tetracaine.

ametrope Person who has ametropia.

ametropia Anomaly of the refractive state of the eye in which, with relaxed accommodation, the image of objects at infinity is not formed on the retina. Thus vision may be blurred. The ametropias are: **astigmatism, hyperopia (hypermetropia)** and **myopia**. The absence of ametropia is called **emmetropia**. Ametropia is thought to develop when there is a failure in the correlation of the optical components that constitute the dioptrics of the eye, thus hindering the emmetropization process. *Syn.* refractive error; error of refraction; refraction (although not strictly correct since this term may also refer to the lack of ametropia). *See* **defocus, hyperopic; defocus, myopic; emmetropization; refraction; refractive error; theory, biological-statistical; theory, emmetropization; theory, nativistic.**

axial a. Ametropia due primarily to an abnormal length of the eye while the refractive power is approximately normal. This is the most common cause of ametropia. (Fig. A8).

refractive a. Ametropia due primarily to an abnormal refractive power of the eye while the length is approximately normal. Refractive ametropias can be attributed to either an abnormal radius of curvature of the surfaces of the cornea or the crystalline lens (**curvature ametropia**), or to an abnormal index of refraction of one or more of the ocular media (**index ametropia**).

amikacin sulfate *See* antibiotic.

amino acids *See* protein.

aminoglycoside Any one of a group of antibiotics composed of amino sugars in glycoside linkage which act by interfering with the synthesis of bacterial proteins. It is used in the treatment of infections caused by Gram-negative bacteria. *Examples*: framycetin, gentamicin, neomycin and tobramycin.

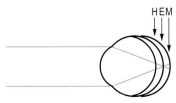

HEM

Fig. A8 Emmetropia E, axial hyperopia H and axial myopia M. In emmetropia, parallel rays are focused on the retina. In hyperopia, the eye is relatively too short and the principal focus is behind the retina. In myopia, the eye is relatively too long and the principal focus is situated in front of the retina.

Ammann's test *See* test, neutral density filter.

amphotericin B *See* antifungal agent.

amplitude of accommodation *See* accommodation, amplitude of.

amplitude of convergence *See* convergence, amplitude of.

ampulla 1. A small dilatation of the canaliculus located near the lacrimal punctum at the junction of the vertical and horizontal portions. There are two ampullae, one in the upper and the other in the lower eyelid. **2.** The dilated sacs of the vortex veins. They are found at the equator with at least one per quadrant and receive blood from the posterior uveal tract. *See* **lacrimal apparatus; vein, vortex.**

Amsler chart; grid *See* chart, Amsler.

amyloidosis A rare condition in which deposits of amyloid are found in various organs and tissues of the body. It can be primary and inherited or secondary to chronic infection or associated with other diseases. In the eye, it can be found in the cornea, vitreous humour, the ocular nerves, blood vessels and in the orbit (**orbital amyloidosis**). The patient may present with abnormal ocular motility, ptosis and proptosis. Management includes treatment of the primary cause and surgical excision of abnormal tissue may be necessary. *See* **dystrophy, lattice.**

anaerobic Ability to sustain life in an atmosphere devoid of oxygen. *See* **aerobic.**

anaesthesia 1. A loss of sensation in a part, or in the whole body, induced by the administration of a drug (an **anaesthetic agent**). **2.** A loss of sensation, usually touch, in a part of the body as a result of some nervous lesion. *Example*: corneal anaesthesia. *Note*: also spelt anesthesia. *See* **injection, peribulbar.**

topical a. Application of a local anaesthetic agent to an area of the skin or mucous membrane (e.g. conjunctiva) to produce anaesthesia. The application may be via direct instillation, soaked swabs, ointments or sprays. *Syn.* surface anaesthesia.

anaesthetic Any substance used to produce a loss of pain sensation either in the whole of the body when unconscious (**general anaesthetic**) or to some part of the body when awake (**local anaesthetic**). *Note*: also spelt anesthetic.

local a's. Chemical agents that prevent the transmission of nerve impulses by binding to the sodium channel and thus blocking the transient rush of sodium ions through the cell membrane. They act locally and without loss of consciousness. They can be either ester-linked (e.g. benoxinate, cocaine, oxybuprocaine hydrochloride [benoxinate], proxymetacaine hydrochloride, and tetracaine hydrochloride) or amide-linked (e.g. bupivacaine, lidocaine hydrochloride and procaine). Ester types are applied mainly topically whereas amide types are usually administered by injection. *See* **injection, peribulbar; potential, receptor.**

anaglyph Stereogram consisting of two superimposed and laterally displaced drawings or photographs of the same scene but taken from two directions and in complementary colours (usually red and green). If the anaglyphs are viewed through filters of the same colour, one to each eye, and induce retinal disparity (of a fixed amount) they give rise to the perception of depth or stereopsis. A set of scenes or targets on the same card, to induce various amounts of retinal disparity can be used to detect and train fusion and stereopsis (e.g. Tranaglyphs). *See* colour, complementary; disparity, retinal; fusion, sensory; perception, depth; stereogram, random-dot; stereopsis.

analgesic A remedy or agent that relieves pain.

analyser 1. Polarizing device used to determine the plane of vibration of a beam of polarized light. *Examples*: Nicol prism, polaroid sheet, tourmaline crystal. **2.** In a polariscope, the second of the two polarizing elements, the first being the polarizer. *See* light, polarized.

analyser, Friedmann visual field Instrument designed to examine the central visual field. The instrument has been discontinued. *See* perimeter, automated.

Analyser, Humphrey Vision Subjective refractometer using continuously variable-power lenses developed by Alvarez. The instrument has been discontinued. *See* lens, Alvarez; optometer.

analysis of variance *See* Student's t-test.

anaphoria *See* hypertropia, alternating.

anastigmatic lens *See* lens, anastigmatic.

anastomosis A natural communication between two blood vessels or other tubular structures. *Example*: The long posterior ciliary artery divides into two branches as it enters the posterior part of the ciliary muscle, and at its anterior end these branches anastomose with each other and with the anterior ciliary arteries to form the major arterial circle of the iris. *See* arterial circle of the iris, major.

anatomical position of rest *See* position of rest, anatomical.

anatropia *See* hypertropia, alternating.

Andersen–Warburg syndrome *See* disease, Norrie's.

anesthesia *See* anaesthesia.

aneuploidy *See* chromosome.

aneurysm A localized dilatation of the walls of a blood vessel, usually an artery, as a result of infection, injury or degeneration. It is filled with fluid or clotted blood. Aneurysms occur in diabetic retinopathy, and retinal vein occlusion leading to haemorrhages and oedema.

angiogenesis The formation of new blood vessels in the body. In ophthalmology, the term neovascularization is generally used. *See* VEGF.

angiogenic Pertains to factors causing the formation of new blood vessels. *See* anti-VEGF drugs; neovascularization, choroidal.

angiogram The photographic image obtained in fluorescein angiography.

angiography, fundus fluorescein A technique aimed at observing the choroidal and retinal vessels of the eye by using photography following the intravenous injection of sodium fluorescein, a dye that is excited by blue radiations. It is a useful technique, which facilitates the diagnosis of various retinal (e.g. diabetic retinopathy, retinal artery occlusion, retinal vein occlusion, age-related maculopathy) and choroidal (e.g. tumour of the choroid) disorders. Those of the choroid are more difficult to observe, but better resolution of the choroidal circulation is made possible by injecting indocyanine green, a dye that is excited by infrared radiations. The technique of angiography may also be applied to observe the iris vessels and detect iris disorders. *See* choroidal flush; indocyanine green; fluorescence; retinopathy, diabetic.

angioid streaks Degeneration of Bruch's membrane characterized by brown or reddish lines or streaks in the fundus of the eye. Patients may occasionally be aware of some visual impairment in the visual field depending on the location of the streaks. The membrane is very fragile and liable to rupture in the case of ocular trauma, which may lead to macular haemorrhage and visual loss. Angioid streaks are often found in association with pseudoxanthoma elasticum, Ehlers–Danlos syndrome, Paget's disease or sickle-cell anaemia. *See* neovascularization, choroidal; pseudoxanthoma elasticum.

angioma Tumour of the blood vessels.

angiomatosis retinae *See* disease, von Hippel's.

angioscotoma A scotoma produced by the shadow cast by the retinal blood vessels. It looks like the branches of a tree extending from the blind spot. It is seen only in special conditions of illumination as when illuminating the fundus of the eye by gently moving a penlight over the closed eyelid, when illuminating the fundus through the sclera or when plotting the visual field. This phenomenon is sometimes used as a test to predict gross macular function in a patient with dense cataract where visualization of the fundus is impossible, although better results are obtained with the blue field entoptoscope. *Syn.* Purkinje figures; Purkinje shadows; Purkinje tree. *See* image, entoptic.

angle 1. The figure formed by two intersecting lines or planes at one point. **2.** The direction from which an object is viewed. **3.** The form produced by a change in direction of a line or plane.

a. alpha Angle between the visual axis and the optical axis formed at the first nodal point of the eye. The visual axis usually lies nasal to the optical axis on the plane of the cornea (**positive** angle

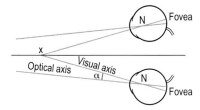

Fig. A9 Angle alpha.

alpha). It is, on average, equal to about 5° in the adult eye. If it lies temporal to the optical axis, the angle is denoted **negative** (Fig. A9). *Symbol*: a.
See **angle lambda.**
a. of altitude 1. Angle through which the eyes have turned up or down from the primary position by a rotation about the transverse axis (x-axis). **2.** The angle between the plane of regard and the subjective horizontal plane. *Syn.* angle of elevation.
a. of anomaly Angle between the line of visual direction of the fovea and the line of visual direction of the abnormal corresponding point of the same deviated eye. It is usually represented by the difference between the objective and subjective angles of deviation in abnormal retinal correspondence.
See **line of direction; retinal correspondence, abnormal.**
a. of the anterior chamber Angle at the periphery of the anterior chamber formed by the root of the iris, the front surface of the ciliary body and the trabecular meshwork. *Syn.* angle of filtration; drainage angle; iridocorneal angle.
See **gonioscope; method, van Herick, Shaffer and Schwartz; method, Smith's; test, shadow.**
apical a. *See* **angle, prism.**
a. of azimuth The angle through which the eyes have turned right or left from the primary position by a rotation about the vertical axis.
Brewster's a. *See* **angle of polarization.**
contact a. Angle formed by a surface and a tangent to a sessile drop of fluid (usually water) at the point where the drop meets the surface. This angle indicates the degree of **wettability** of that surface. The more wettable (or hydrophilic) the material, the smaller the angle, being equal to 0° for a completely hydrophilic material when water spreads evenly over that surface. Hydrophobic surfaces can have contact angles greater than 90°, e.g. silicone rubber in which the angle is about 120° (Fig. A10). *Syn.* wetting angle.
See **test, sessile drop.**
a. of convergence Angle between the lines of sight of the two eyes which are in a state of convergence. The angle is positive when the lines of sight intersect in front of the eyes, and negative when they intersect behind the eyes. *Note*: Some authors regard the angle of convergence as the

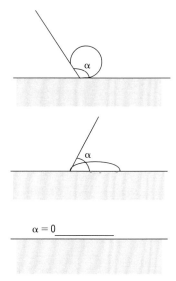

Fig. A10 Different contact angles α between a drop of fluid and a contact lens material.

rotation of one eye only toward the fixation point and refer to the angle of convergence of both eyes, previously defined, as the **total angle of convergence** or the **total convergence**. The total angle of convergence required for binocular fixation of a target is equal to

$$\text{total convergence (in } \Delta) = \frac{\text{PD (in cm)}}{d \text{ (in m)}}$$

or

$$\text{total convergence (in } \Delta) = \text{convergence (in ma)} \\ \times \text{PD (in cm)}$$

where d is the distance between the target and the midpoint of the base line and PD the interpupillary distance. Convergence is given in either prism dioptres (Δ) or metre angles (ma), which is equal to $1/d$ (Table A9). *Syn.* angle of triangulation.
See **angle, metre; dioptre, prism; line of sight.**
critical a. Angle of incidence in which the refracted ray travels along the surface between the two media (angle of refraction equal to 90°). Thus, if the angle of incidence is greater than the critical angle, the ray is totally reflected. If, however, the angle of incidence is smaller than the critical angle, the ray is refracted (with some light reflected). The critical angle i_c is given by the following formula

$$\sin i_c = n/n'$$

where n and n' are the indices of the media on each side of the surface, with the light

Table A8 Critical angle (in degrees) beyond which all the light is reflected at the surface separating various transparent substances from air or water

Substance	Refractive index n	Critical angle i_c	
		In contact with air $n' = 1$	In contact with water $n' = 1.333$
Water	1.333	48.6	–
Spectacle crown glass	1.523	41.0	61.1
Flint glass (dense)	1.62	38.1	55.4
Flint glass (extra dense)	1.706	35.9	51.4
PMMA	1.49	42.2	63.5
Cr-39	1.498	41.9	62.9
Polycarbonate	1.586	39.1	57.2
Diamond	2.42	24.4	33.4

Table A9 Relationship between viewing distance and total convergence in metre angles and prism dioptres for four interpupillary distances (PD in cm)

Object distance from cornea (cm)	Metre angle (ma)	Convergence (in prism dioptres)			
		PD: 6.0	6.4	6.8	7.0
200	0.5	3.0	3.2	3.4	3.5
100	1.0	6.0	6.4	6.8	7.0
67	1.5	9.0	9.6	10.2	10.5
50	2.0	12.0	12.8	13.6	14.0
40	2.5	15.0	16.0	17.0	17.5
33	3.0	18.0	19.2	20.4	21.0
25	4.0	24.0	25.6	27.2	28.0
20	5.0	30.0	32.0	34.0	35.0
16	6.25	37.5	40.0	42.5	43.7
14	7.14	42.8	45.7	48.5	50.0

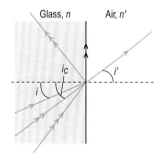

Fig. A11 Critical angle i_c and total internal reflection (i, angle of incidence; i', angle of refraction).

travelling from the high index medium n to the low index medium n' (Fig. A11 and Table A8). *Syn.* limiting angle.
See optics, fibre; prism, reflecting; reflection, total; refractometer.

a. of deviation 1. Angle through which a ray of light is deviated on reflection by a mirror, or on refraction by a lens or prism. 2. Angle between the visual axis, or line of sight, of the deviated eye in strabismus and the straight-ahead position while the other eye fixates straight ahead. It can be assessed **subjectively** by having the patient report simultaneous perception (e.g. the lion in the cage seen in the amblyoscope) or **objectively** as measured by the practitioner either with the amblyoscope or using prisms and cover test, or by the Hirschberg test. *Syn.* angle of squint; angle of strabismus.
See **angle of anomaly; incomitance; method, Hirschberg's; method, Javal's; method, Krimsky's; prism, minimum deviation of a.**
a. of divergence Angle between the lines of sight of the two eyes which are in a state of divergence.
drainage a. See angle of the anterior chamber.
a. of elevation *See* angle of altitude.
a. eta *See* acuity, stereoscopic visual.
external a. *See* canthus.
a. of filtration *See* angle of the anterior chamber.
a. gamma The angle between the optical axis and the fixation axis.
a. of incidence Angle between the incident ray and the normal to the surface at the point of incidence in either reflection or refraction at a surface separating two media.
iridocorneal a. *See* angle of the anterior chamber.
a. kappa Angle between the pupillary axis and the visual axis, measured at the nodal point. *Symbol:* κ.
See angle lambda; line of sight.
a. lambda Angle between the pupillary axis and the line of sight formed at the centre of the entrance pupil. It is this angle which is measured clinically as it is almost equal to angle alpha. *Symbol:* λ.
See axis, pupillary; line of sight.
limiting a. *See* angle, critical.
metre a. (ma) Unit of convergence which is equal to the reciprocal of the distance (in metres)

between the point of fixation assumed to lie on the median line and the base line of the eyes. Thus, if an object is located at 25 cm from the base line, each eye converges through 4 ma; at 1 metre, 1 ma, etc. Metre angles of convergence can be converted into prism dioptres of convergence by multiplying by the subject's interpupillary distance expressed in cm. *Example*: For a PD of 6.0 cm, a convergence of 5 ma is multiplied by 6 = 30 Δ. *See* angle of convergence.

minimum a. of resolution (MAR) The angle subtended at the nodal point of the eye (or the centre of the entrance pupil) by two points or two lines which can just be distinguished as separate.
See acuity, visual; chart, logMAR.

palpebral a. *See* canthus.

pantoscopic a. Angle between the spectacle plane and the frontal plane of the face when the superior edge of the lens is farther away from the face than the inferior edge (Fig. A12). *Syn.* pantoscopic tilt.
See angle, retroscopic.

a. of polarization The angle of incidence at which the reflected light is maximally polarized. At this angle, the reflected and refracted rays are 90° apart (Fig. A13). This angle i is given by the equation

$$\tan i = n_2/n_1$$

and measures 56.7° when the first medium n_1 is air and the second medium n_2 is a glass with an index of refraction equal to 1.523. *Syn.* Brewster's angle.
See law, Brewster's; light, polarized.

prism a. Angle between the two refracting surfaces of a prism. *Syn.* apical angle; refracting angle (this term is deprecated because of the confusion with "angle of refraction").

recession a. A tear between the longitudinal and circular muscles of the ciliary body. It is most often noted following blunt trauma to the anterior segment. It is typically followed by hyphaemia. This form of injury predisposes the individual to elevated intraocular pressure (i.e. increased risk of glaucoma) in the future. With a gonioscope, angle recession appears with an abnormally wide ciliary body band with a prominent scleral spur and some torn iris processes. There are also marked variations in the width and depth of the angle in different quadrants of the eye.
See cyclodialysis; hyphaemia; iridodialysis; muscle, ciliary.

a. of reflection Angle between the reflected ray and the normal to the surface at the point of incidence.

a. of refraction Angle between the refracted ray and the normal to the surface at the point of emergence.

retroscopic a. Angle between the spectacle plane and the frontal plane of the face when the superior edge of the lens is closer to the face than the inferior edge. *Syn.* retroscopic tilt.
See angle, pantoscopic; plane, frontal; plane, spectacle.

a. of squint *See* angle of deviation.

a. of stereopsis The difference between the angles subtended at the centres of the entrance pupils of the two eyes by two points located in space at different distances from the eyes.
See acuity, stereoscopic visual; test, Howard–Dolman; test, three-needle.

a. of strabismus *See* angle of deviation.

total a. of convergence *See* angle of convergence.

a. of triangulation *See* angle of convergence.

viewing a. *See* angle, visual.

visual a. The angle subtended by the extremities of an object at the anterior nodal point of the eye. If the object is far away, the point of reference can be the centre of the entrance pupil or even the anterior pole of the cornea. *Syn.* viewing angle.

wetting a. *See* angle, contact.

refracting a. *See* angle, prism.

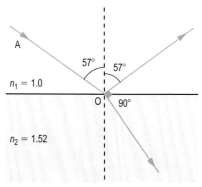

Fig. A13 Ray of non-polarized ordinary light AO is incident to the surface at the polarizing angle. Most of the ordinary light is transmitted across the surface and partially polarized, the rest being reflected and polarized maximally (i.e. vibrating in one plane only).

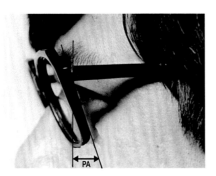

Fig. A12 Pantoscopic angle PA.

angle-closure glaucoma *See* **glaucoma, angle-closure.**

angling Adjusting the angle which the sides of a spectacle frame make with the plane of its front.
See **angle, pantoscopic; angle, retroscopic.**

ångström unit Unit of wavelength of radiant energy. One unit is equal to one ten-thousand-millionth of a metre (10^{-10} m). *Symbol*: A or Å. It is preferable to use the nanometre, which is an SI unit.

aniridia A complete, or almost complete, absence of the iris of the eye. It can be acquired, due to trauma, or inherited as an autosomal dominant trait and caused by mutation in the paired box gene-6 (PAX6) on chromosome 11p13 in which case it is bilateral. The patient is photophobic and in congenital cases there is usually amblyopia and sometimes nystagmus. Glaucoma is a common association caused by anterior synechia resulting from contraction of the remaining iris tissue. Management includes glaucoma therapy, contact lenses incorporating an artificial iris, or tinted spectacle lenses.
See **chromosome; irideremia; lens, cosmetic contact.**

aniseikometer *See* **eikonometer.**

aniseikonia A difference in size and/or shape of the visual images of the two eyes. This may be due either to unequal axial lengths of the two eyes, to an unequal distribution of the retinal elements or an inequality of the cortical representation of the two ocular images (**basic** or **intrinsic aniseikonia**). It is most frequently induced by lenses of different power used in the correction of anisometropia (**refractive aniseikonia**). Symptoms include visual discomfort, visual distortion of space and sometimes difficulty in achieving binocular vision as, for example, in spectacle-corrected unilateral aphakia. Aniseikonia is measured with an eikonometer, although a simple test consists of separating the retinal images of a large target (e.g. a test chart) with prisms and comparing them; placing size lenses in front of one eye until the images appear equal will give an indication of the amount of aniseikonia.
See **lens, aniseikonic; magnification, shape; metamorphopsia; micropsia; test, New Aniseikonia; test, Turville infinity balance.**

aniso-accommodation A condition in which there is unequal accommodative response in the two eyes when fixating an object binocularly. It may result from a disease (e.g. glaucoma, ophthalmoplegia, paralysis of the third nerve, unilateral cataract), uncorrected anisometropia, viewing a near object to the side, toxins affecting one eye more than the other or trauma.

anisoacuity A condition in which there is unequal visual acuity in the two eyes. It occurs in amblyopia and sometimes anisometropia, as well as in an eye with a diseased process (e.g. cataract, keratoconus, uveitis).

anisochromatic Not of uniform colour.

anisochromatopsia Deficiency of colour vision in one eye only or of unequal severity in the two eyes.

anisochromia *See* **heterochromia.**

anisocoria Condition in which the pupils of the eyes are not of equal size. Typically one pupil is abnormal and cannot either dilate or constrict. It may be physiological (e.g. in antimetropia) with a difference in pupil size of about 1 mm or it may be part of a syndrome, the most common being those of Holmes-Adie and Horner's. Physiological anisocoria remains constant irrespective of the level of illumination. Anisocoria can occur as a result of injury (e.g. to the iris sphincter muscle), inflammation (e.g. iridocyclitis), diseases of the iris, paralysis of the third nerve, angle-closure glaucoma, systemic diseases (e.g. diabetes, syphilis) or accidental drug instillation into the eye (if the drug or substance has anticholinergic properties the condition is then referred to as **anticholinergic mydriasis** or **"atropine" mydriasis**). The search for the cause of anisocoria is facilitated by testing the pupil light reflexes and responses to locally instilled drugs (Fig. A14).
See **pupillary defect, efferent; reflex, pupil light; pupillometer.**

anisocycloplegia A condition in which there is unequal reduction of accommodative responses following the binocular instillation of a cycloplegic.

anisohyperopia A condition in which there is unequal amount of hyperopia in the two eyes. *Syn.* compound hyperopic anisometropia.

anisometrope A person who has anisometropia.

anisometropia Condition in which the refractive state of a pair of eyes differs and therefore one eye needs a different lens correction from the other. Correction may induce aniseikonia and, when the eyes deviate from the optical axes of the lenses, anisophoria. Uncorrected anisometropia of low amounts may cause eyestrain or diplopia. Large amounts rarely cause symptoms as one of the retinal images is typically suppressed or there is amblyopia (Table A10). *Syn.* asymmetropia; heterometropia; heteropsia.
See **aniso-accommodation; antimetropia; effect, differential prismatic; isometropia.**

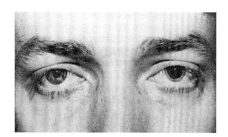

Fig. A14 Anisocoria.

Table A10 Approximate retinal image size differences (in %) for various anisometropias corrected by spectacles (vertex distance = 12 mm)

Anisometropia difference (D)	Axial anisometropia (%)*	Refractive anisometropia† Hyperopic (%)	Myopic (%)
1.0	0.25	1.50	1.25
1.5	0.37	2.25	1.88
2.0	0.50	3.00	2.50
2.5	0.62	3.75	3.12
3.0	0.75	4.50	3.75
3.5	0.87	5.25	4.38
4.0	1.00	6.00	5.00
4.5	1.12	6.75	5.62
5.0	1.25	7.50	6.25
5.5	1.37	8.25	6.88
6.0	1.50	9.00	7.50

*The two eyes are assumed to be of the same refractive power but of different lengths.
†The two eyes are assumed to be of the same length but of different refractive powers.

compound hyperopic a. *See* **anisohyperopia.**

compound myopic a. *See* **antimetropia.**

mixed a. *See* **antimetropia.**

simple a. Anisometropia in which one eye is emmetropic and the other either hyperopic (**simple hyperopic anisometropia**) or myopic (**simple myopic anisometropia**).

anisomyopia A condition in which there is unequal amount of myopia in the two eyes. *Syn.* compound myopic anisometropia.

anisophoria 1. A type of heterophoria in which the amount varies with the direction of gaze. It may be due to: (a) a paresis or spasm of one or more of the extraocular muscles or (b) an anisometropic spectacle correction in which different prismatic effects induce different phorias when the eyes look in different directions of gaze (this type is called **optical anisophoria**). **2.** A latent deviation in which the angular relationship between the visual axes of the two eyes is not equal depending upon which eye is fixating. This is a form of incomitance. *See* **effect, differential, prismatic; incomitance.**

anisopia A condition in which there is unequal vision in the two eyes.

anisotropic State of an optical medium in which the optical properties are not the same in all directions, due to the fact that the refractive index is not the same for all directions. An incident ray will be divided, within a uniaxial anisotropic medium, into two refracted rays: an ordinary ray which obeys Snell's law and an extraordinary ray which follows a different law. Most crystals are anisotropic.
See **birefringence; dichroism; isotropic.**

ankyloblepharon Partial or complete adhesion of the edge of one eyelid to that of the other. It may occasionally result from a cicatrizing lesion of the eyelid margins or following tarsorrhaphy. It may also be congenital in which case the eyelids are joined together by bands of tissue, and this condition is called **ankyblepharon filiforme adnatum.**

ankylosing spondylitis *See* **iridocyclitis; uveitis.**

annealing A process of heating material (glass, metal or polymer) and slowly cooling it to avoid internal strain.
See **glass; strain.**

annular synechia *See* **synechia, annular.**

annulus ciliaris The ring-line structure between the iris and the choroid. *Syn.* ciliary ring.

annulus of Zinn The common tendon from which arise the four recti muscles of the eye. It surrounds the optic foramen and a part of the medial end of the superior orbital fissure. *Syn.* tendon of Zinn.
See **muscle cone.**

anomaloscope An instrument for testing colour vision in which the observer is required to match one-half of a circular field which is illuminated with yellow with a mixture of green and red in the other half. The yellow half can be varied in brightness, while the other may be varied continuously from red to green. A certain combination of the red and green mixture is considered normal, and variations from that mixture indicate anomalous colour vision. With this instrument one can distinguish between a protanope and a protanomal and between a deuteranope and a deuteranomal. *Syn.* Nagel anomaloscope. Some anomaloscopes also test for blue-yellow colour vision deficiencies, e.g. **Pickford–Nicholson anomaloscope.**
See **colour vision, defective; Rayleigh equation.**

anomalous retinal correspondence *See* **retinal correspondence, abnormal.**

anomalous trichromatism *See* **trichromatism, anomalous.**

anoopsia *See* **hypertropia.**

anophthalmos Congenital absence of all tissues of the eyes. It is due to a failure of the outgrowth of the optic vesicle to form the optic cup. However, in many cases some development occurs and there is a rudimentary presence of one or both eyes, such as extreme microphthalmos. *Syn.* anophthalmia; anophthalmus; anopia.
See cup, optic; microphthalmos; monophthalmia; syndrome, Patau's; vesicle, optic.

anophthalmia, unilateral *See* monophthalmia.

anophthalmus *See* anophthalmos.

anopia *See* anophthalmia.

anopsia Defect or loss of vision.
quadrantic a. See quadrantanopia.

anorthopia A perceptual anomaly in which straight lines appear curved.

anorthoscope An apparatus for producing and studying **anorthoscopic perception** which is the veridical perception of an image viewed under very uncommon conditions. It consists of a pair of circular discs mounted one behind the other. A figure is drawn on the rear disc and viewed through a slit in the front disc rotating at a different speed. The shape of the image will be clearly perceived.

anoxia Complete absence of oxygen.
See hypoxia.

antagonism, lateral *See* inhibition, lateral.

antagonist 1. An antagonistic muscle. **2.** A substance (e.g. a drug, hormone or neurotransmitter) that depresses the action of an agonist or binds to a cell receptor without eliciting a physiological response (e.g. excitation or inhibition). *Examples*: atropine and hyoscine, which block the effect of acetylcholine acting on cholinergic receptors, and timolol which blocks adrenergic receptors.
See agonist.

antagonist drug A drug that blocks or reduces the effect of a neurotransmitter.
See beta-blocker; neurotransmitter.

antagonistic muscle *See* muscle, antagonistic.

antazoline phosphate *See* antihistamine.

anterior chamber *See* chamber, anterior.

anterior chamber angle *See* angle of the anterior chamber.

anterior chamber cleavage syndrome *See* Peter's anomaly.

anterior ciliary arteries *See* artery, ciliary.

anterior pole; segment of the eye; synechia; uveitis *See* under the nouns.

antiamoebic agent *See* keratitis, acanthamoeba.

antibacterial *See* antibiotic.

antibiotic 1. Pertaining to the ability to destroy or inhibit other living organisms. **2.** A substance derived from a mould or bacterium, or produced synthetically, that destroys **(bactericidal)** or inhibits the growth **(bacteriostatic)** of other microorganisms and is thus used to treat infections. Some substances have a narrow spectrum of activity whereas others act against a wide range of both gram-positive and gram-negative organisms **(broad-spectrum antibiotics)**. Antibiotics can be classified into several groups according to their mode of action on or within bacteria: (1) Drugs inhibiting bacterial cell wall synthesis, such as bacitracin, vancomycin and the β-lactams-based agents (e.g. penicillin, cephalosporins (e.g. ceftazidime, ceftriaxone, cefuroxime)). (2) Drugs affecting the bacterial cytoplasmic membrane, such as polymyxin B sulfate and gramicidin. (3) Drugs inhibiting bacterial protein synthesis, such as aminoglycosides (e.g. amikacin sulfate, framycetin sulfate, gentamicin, neomycin sulfate and tobramycin), tetracyclines, macrolides (e.g. erythromycin and azithromycin) and chloramphenicol. (4) Drugs inhibiting the intermediate metabolism of bacteria, such as sulfonamides (e.g. sulfacetamide sodium) and trimethoprim. (5) Drugs inhibiting bacterial DNA synthesis, such as nalixidic acid and fluoroquinolones (e.g. ciprofloxacin, levofloxacin, moxifloxacin, norfloxacin and ofloxacin). (6) Other antibiotics such as fusidic acid and the diamidines, such as propamidine isethionate and dibrompropamidine. *Syn.* antibacterial.
See antiinflammatory drug; fusidic acid.

antibody Any of a large variety of proteins normally present in the body or produced in response to an antigen, which is capable of combining with and destroying, thus producing an immune reaction. Antibodies are produced by a type of white blood cell called B cell (B lymphocyte) secreted by lymphatic tissue (e.g. bone marrow, lymph nodes) usually in response to an antigen. Some eye diseases are antibody-dependent (e.g. allergic conjunctivitis, atopic keratoconjunctivitis, vernal conjunctivitis).

anticholinergic *See* acetylcholine; parasympatholytic.

anticholinergic mydriasis *See* anisocoria.

anticholinesterase drugs Parasympathetic drugs that inhibit or inactivate the enzyme acetylcholinesterase, allowing prolonged activity of acetylcholine. They cause miosis and ciliary muscle contraction. There are two groups: reversible which are of short duration (up to 12 hours or so), such as neostigmine, physostigmine and edrophonium chloride, and irreversible which lasts for days or weeks, such as demecarium bromide and diisopropyl fluorophosphate (DFP).
See acetylcholinesterase; miotics.

antifungal agent Any substance which destroys or prevents the growth of fungi. It is one of the antibiotic groups. There are several classes of antifungal drugs: **Polyenes,** which cause an increase in fungal cell wall permeability leading to its death. *Examples*: amphotericin B, natamycin, nystatin. **Azoles,** which act either by inhibiting the synthesis of ergosterol, a component of fungal cell wall or by causing direct wall damage. *Examples*: clotrimazole, econazole, fluconazole, itraconazole, ketoconazole, miconazole. **Pyrimidines,** which interfere with the normal function of fungal cells. *Example*: flucytosine. *Syn.* antimycotic agent.

antigen Any substance that can stimulate an immune response in the body and can react with the products of that response, that is, with specific antibodies or specifically sensitized T lymphocytes, or both. Antigens include bacteria, foreign substance (e.g. dust mite, grass, pollen of trees), toxins and viruses.
See **allergic reactions; hypersensitivity; sensitization.**

antihistamine Any substance that reduces the effect of histamine or blocks histamine receptors, usually the histamine 1 (H1) receptor. It is used in the treatment of allergic conjunctivitis and also in the temporary relief of minor allergic symptoms of the eye. Common agents include antazoline sulfate (this drug is normally combined with a sympathomimetic such as xylometazoline [a vasoconstrictor] in the treatment of allergic conjunctivitis), azelastine hydrochloride, ceti-rizine, chlorphenamine, emedastine, epinastine hydrochloride, ketotifen, levocabastine, loratadine and olopatadine.
See **cell, mast; histamine; hypersensitivity; mast cell stabilizers.**

antiinfective drug A general term indicating either an antibiotic (or antibacterial), an antifungal or an antiviral agent, as well as the sulfonamides.

antiinflammatory drug A drug which inhibits or suppresses most inflammatory responses of an allergic, bacterial, traumatic or anaphylactic origin, as well as being immunosuppressant. They include the corticosteroids (e.g. beta-methasone, dexamethasone, fluorometholone, hydrocortisone acetate, loteprednol etabonate, prednisolone, rimexolone, triamcinolone). They are sometimes combined with an antibiotic drug (e.g. betamethasone combined with neomycin or sulfacetamide, dexamethasone combined with neomycin or polymyxin B). Corticosteroids have side effects, such as enhancing the activity of herpes simplex virus, fungal overgrowth, raising intraocular pressure or cataract formation.
There are other antiinflammatory drugs that are non-steroidal (NSAID) and have little toxicity. They act mainly by blocking prostaglandin synthesis. These include diclofenac sodium, flurbiprofen sodium, indomethacin, ketorolac, nepafenac and oxyphenbutazone.
See **immunosuppressants; steroid.**

antimetropia A condition in which one eye is myopic and the other hyperopic. *Syn.* mixed anisometropia.
See **anisocoria.**

antimongoloid slant A condition in which the nasal corners of the palpebral fissure are higher than the temporal corners, as opposed to the typical mongoloid slant. This occurs when the lateral palpebral ligament is inserted lower than the medial palpebral ligament. It is a feature of the Treacher Collins syndrome.

antimuscarinic drugs *See* acetylcholine; mydri-atic; parasympatholytic.

antimycotic agent *See* antifungal agent.

antioxidant *See* oxidative stress.

anti-reflection coating A thin film of transparent material, usually a metallic fluoride (e.g. mag-nesium fluoride), deposited on the surface of a lens which increases transmission and reduces surface reflection. *Abbreviated*: AR coating. *Syn.* anti-reflection film.
See **coating; Fresnel's formula; image, ghost; lens, coated.**

antisaccade A voluntary eye movement made in the direction opposite to the side where a stimulus is presented. The subject is asked to fixate a small dot for some time. A stimulus is then presented to one side and the subject is asked to inhibit a reflex eye movement towards it but to make a saccade in the opposite direction. Analysis of the errors and/or latencies of the antisaccades indicate dysfunction in the frontal lobe, which controls the saccadic eye movements.
See **movement, saccadic eye.**

antiseptic An agent that kills or prevents the growth of bacteria. This term is generally restricted to agents that are sufficiently non-toxic for superficial application to living tissues. These include the **preservatives** for eye drops and contact lens solutions. Examples of antiseptics are alcohol, benzalkonium chloride, cetrimide, chlorbutanol, chlorhexidine, hydrogen peroxide, iodine and thimerosal (or thiomersalate). Other agents that are too toxic to be applied to living tissues are called **disinfectants** and are used to sterilize instruments and apparatus.
See **disinfection; ethylenediamine tetraacetic acid; neutralization; sterilization.**

anti-VEGF drugs Drugs which bind to vascular endothelial growth factor (VEGF) receptors without causing activation, thus blocking the production of new blood vessels and enhanced vessel permeability by the VEGF. They are used in the treatment of some forms of cancer (administered intravenously) and injected intravitreally in the treatment of choroidal neovascularization, retinal venous occlusion and macular oedema. *Examples*: ranibizumab, bevacizumab, aflibercept, pegaptanib sodium. *Syn.* angiogenesis inhibitors.
See **macular degeneration, age-related; retin-opathy, diabetic; VEGF.**

antiviral agents Substances which block the growth of a virus (e.g. herpes) by inhibiting DNA or RNA synthesis. Common agents include aciclovir (acyclovir), idoxuridine, ganciclovir, trifluoridine (trifluorothymidine) and vidarabine.
See **keratitis, herpetic; virus.**

Anton's syndrome *See* syndrome, Anton's.

A pattern *See* pattern, alphabet.

Apert's syndrome *See* syndrome, Apert's.

aperture An opening, or the area of a lens, through which light can pass.
See **pupil.**

angular a. Half of the maximum plane subtended by a lens at the axial point of an object or image. (Sometimes the full plane angle is taken as the angular aperture, but this is not convenient in optical calculations.)
See **sine condition.**

a. of a lenticular lens That portion of a lenticular lens which has the prescribed power (British Standard).

numerical a. An expression designating the light-gathering power of microscope objectives. It is equal to the product of the index of refraction n of the object space and the sine of the angle u subtended by a radius of the entrance pupil at the axial point on the object, i.e. $n \sin u$.

palpebral a. The gap between the margins of the eyelids when the eye is open. An abnormal increase in the aperture occurs in some conditions, including Graves' disease, buphthalmos, Parinaud's syndrome and retrobulbar tumour. An abnormal decrease in the aperture occurs in some conditions, including ptosis, microphthalmos and ophthalmoplegia (Figs. A15 and A16). *Syn.* interpalpebral fissure (this term is more accurate although used infrequently); palpebral fissure.
See **antimongoloid slant; exophthalmos.**

a. plane *See* **plane, aperture.**

a. ratio *See* **aperture, relative.**

relative a. The reciprocal of the f number. It is therefore equal to the ratio of the diameter of the entrance pupil to the primary focal length of an optical system. *Syn.* aperture ratio. *Note*: The definition of this term is not universally accepted; some authors define it as the reverse of the above definition.
See **f number.**

aperture-stop *See* **diaphragm.**

apex, corneal The most anterior point of the cornea when the eye is in the primary position (Fig. A15). It does not automatically coincide with any common reference point (e.g. line of sight). *Plural*: apices or apexes.
See **bearing, apical; clearance, apical; optical zone of cornea; position, primary.**

apex of a prism The thinnest part of the prism where the two faces intersect.
See **base of a prism.**

aphake Person who is aphakic.

aphakia Ocular condition in which the crystalline lens is absent. It may be congenital but usually it is due to surgical removal of a cataract. As a result the eye has no accommodative power and is usually highly hyperopic.
See **aniseikonia; cataract; eye, pseudophakic; lens, aphakic; phakic; phenomenon, jack-in-the-box; vitreous detachment.**

aphakic eye; lens *See* under the nouns.

aphakic pupillary block *See* **pupillary block.**

apical bearing *See* **bearing, apical.**

apical clearance *See* **clearance, apical.**

aplanatic Pertains to an optical system which is free from spherical aberration and coma.
See **aberration, spherical; focus, aplanatic; lens, aplanatic.**

apochromatic lens *See* **lens, apochromatic.**

apodization A process by which the output intensity profile of an optical system is changed so as to concentrate the illumination of a diffraction pattern in the centre while it becomes almost zero at the edge.

aponeurosis *See* **muscle, levator palpebrae superioris.**

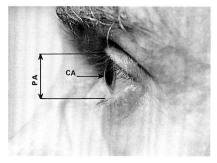

Fig. A15 Palpebral aperture PA and corneal apex CA.

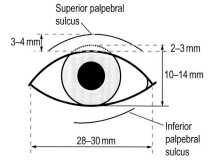

Superior palpebral sulcus
3–4 mm
2–3 mm
10–14 mm
Inferior palpebral sulcus
28–30 mm

Fig. A16 Average dimensions of the normal palpebral aperture of a Caucasian eye.

apoptosis A process of single cell death, which consists of a series of biochemical events including cell shrinkage, condensation of chromatin, formation of cytoplasmic blebs and fragmentation of nuclear DNA into membrane-bound particles that are phagocytosed by other cells. It is an important physiological process that helps keep the number of cells relatively constant by compensating for mitosis. It is necessary to prevent either uncontrolled growth and tumour formation (as may be caused by genetic mutation), or hypotrophy (as in ischaemia) due to excessive apoptosis induced by a stimulus, such as irradiation, toxic drugs, etc. Apoptosis represents a form of programmed cell death. *Example*: Almost all corneal epithelial cells die within 10 days, and are replaced by mitosis.
See **mitosis; nerve growth factor; neuroprotection.**

apostilb The luminance of a perfectly diffusing surface that reflects 1 lumen per square metre. This measure is often used in visual field analysis, where the luminance of the background and targets is measured in apostilb.

apparent frontoparallel plane *See* **plane, apparent frontoparallel.**

apparent pupil *See* **pupil of the eye, entrance.**

apparent size *See* **size, apparent.**

apparent strabismus *See* **strabismus, apparent.**

appendages of the eye The adjacent structures of the eye such as the lacrimal apparatus, the extraocular muscles and the eyelids, eyelashes, eyebrows and the conjunctiva. *Syn.* adnexa oculi; adnexal structures.

apperception The ability to perceive and interpret fully any psychic content or sensory stimuli. *Example*: the apperception aroused by new objects in the visual field that are noticed when entering an unfamiliar room.

applanation tonometer *See* **tonometer, applanation.**

appliance, optical Any optical system which is used in conjunction with the eye. Optical appliances include spectacles, contact lenses to correct sight and/or anomalies of binocular vision and also telescopes or microscopes to magnify an object. *Syn.* optical aid.
See **dispensing, optical; ptosis.**

apraclonidine hydrochloride *See* **sympathomimetic drugs.**

apraxia A disorder of voluntary movement, characterized by the inability, complete or partial (**dyspraxia**) to perform a skilled or purposeful movement, in the absence of motor paralysis, sensory loss or of a general lack of coordination. It is due to a cerebellar disease.
ocular motor a. Congenital inability to perform some voluntary ocular movements. Children with this condition often use head thrusts to move their eyes to the left or to the right.
optical a. Apraxia in which there is an inability to copy or to draw in proper spatial orientation.

It is usually associated with visual agnosia. *Syn.* visual apraxia.
visual a. *See* **apraxia, optical.**

aqueduct of Sylvius A canal in the midbrain that connects the third and fourth ventricles. *Syn.* cerebral aqueduct.

aqueous flare Scattering of light seen when a slit-lamp beam is directed into the anterior chamber, obliquely to the plane of the iris. It occurs as a result of increased protein contents, and usually inflammatory cells, in the aqueous humour. Visual impairment depends on the intensity of the flare. It is a sign of intraocular inflammation.
See **effect, Tyndall; iritis; uveitis.**

aqueous humour Clear, colourless fluid that fills the anterior and posterior chambers of the eye. It is a carrier of nutrients for the lens and to a larger extent the cornea, especially of glucose and essential amino acids. It contributes to the maintenance of the intraocular pressure. It is formed in the ciliary processes, flows into the posterior chamber, then through the pupil into the anterior chamber and leaves the eye through the trabecular meshwork, passing to the canal of Schlemm and then to veins in the intrascleral venous plexus (Fig. A17). A small amount (10% to 15%) also flows out of the eye via the uveoscleral pathway. The aqueous in the anterior chamber is a component of the optical system of the eye. It has an index of refraction of 1.336, slightly lower than that of the cornea, so that the cornea/aqueous surface acts as a diverging lens of low power (less than 6 D). It is a fluid very similar to blood plasma but with a much lower concentration of protein and a higher concentration of ascorbate. The **rate of aqueous humour outflow** varies between 2.0 μl/min and 3.0 μl/min via both the conventional, about 90% (trabecular meshwork and Schlemm's canal), and the unconventional, about 10% (uveoscleral) pathways. This rate is normally equal to the rate of aqueous secretion. If the rate of outflow is lower than the rate of secretion, intraocular pressure increases.
See **ciliary body; ciliary processes; flare, aqueous; pathway, uveoscleral; ultrafiltration.**

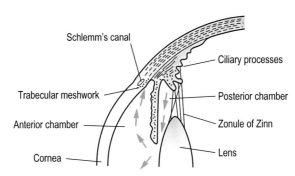

Schlemm's canal

Ciliary processes

Trabecular meshwork

Posterior chamber

Anterior chamber

Zonule of Zinn

Cornea

Lens

Fig. A17 Outflow of aqueous humour.

aqueous outflow *See* aqueous humour; mesh-work, trabecular; pathway, uveoscleral.

AR coating *See* anti-reflection coating.

arachnoid The middle member of the three meninges covering the brain, the spinal cord and the optic nerve. From the optic nerve, it becomes continuous with the sclera.
See **sclera.**

arc eye *See* keratoconjunctivitis, actinic.

arc perimeter *See* perimeter, arc.

arc, pupillary reflex *See* reflex, pupil light.

arc of contact That portion of an extraocular muscle which wraps around the surface of the globe prior to the insertion of its tendon into the sclera. The point where the muscle first comes into contact with the globe is called the **contact point**. The arc of contact continually alters its length as the eye rotates. *Syn.* contact arc.

Archambault's loop *See* loop, Meyer's.

arcs, blue Entoptic phenomenon appearing as two bands of blue light arching from above and below the source toward the blind spot. This phenomenon is induced by a small source of light (preferably red) stimulating the temporal side of the retina near the fovea.
See image, entoptic.

arcuate nerve fibre bundle *See* fibres, arcuate.

arcuate scotoma *See* scotoma, arcuate.

arcus juvenilis *See* corneal arcus.

arcus marginale *See* orbital septum.

arcus, corneal; senilis *See* corneal arcus.

Arden gratings; plates *See* test, Arden grating.

Arden index; ratio *See* electrooculogram.

area 1. Any limited surface or space. **2.** A part of the brain or retina having a particular function.
Brodmann's a's. Areas of the cerebral cortex defined by Brodmann and numbered from 1 to 52. Areas 17, 18 and 19 represent the visual area and visual association areas in each cerebral cortex.
a. centralis See macula lutea.
a. of comfort Zone of comfort.
See criterion, Percival.
extrastriate visual a. See **area, visual association.**
fusion a. See **area, Panum's.**
Panum's a. An area in the retina of one eye, any point of which, when stimulated simultaneously with a single point in the retina of the other eye, will give rise to a single percept. Its diameter in the fovea is about 5 minutes of arc and increases toward the periphery (Fig. A18). *Syn.* fusion area.
See **disparity, retinal; horopter; retinal corresponding points; space, Panum's fusional.**
rod-free a. See foveola.
striate a. See **area, visual.**
visual a. 1. Any region of the brain in which visual information is processed. **2.** This is Brodmann's area 17 in each occipital lobe. The right monocular

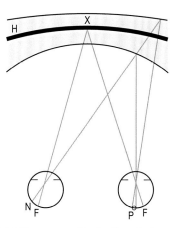

Fig. A18 The eyes are fixating X on the horopter H. Stimulation of point N in the left retina and of any point within Panum's area P of the right retina gives rise to a perception of singleness and stereopsis. Visual lines extrapolated from the limits of Panum's area P indicate the far and near limits of Panum's fusional space (shaded) by their intersection with the visual line of point N in the left eye (F, fovea).

and binocular visual fields are represented in the left area and vice versa. Foveal representation is near the occipital pole while the peripheral retina is mapped farther inward. The area contains six layers of cells numbered 1 to 6 from the top. The upper layers (near the surface) receive input from other cortical regions (V2, V3, V4, etc.). Layer 4 receives most visual input from the lateral geniculate body. It is divided into four sublayers: 4A, 4B, 4Cα and 4Cβ. Layer 4Cα receives most magnocellular input while 4Cβ receives input from the parvocellular pathway. Koniocellular cells from the lateral geniculate body send their axons to layer 3 and 4A. The deeper layers send output to the thalamus and brainstem. The primary visual area is identified by a white striation (**line of Gennari**) on each side of the calcarine fissure. This white line appears in the middle of the fourth layer of the visual cortex and is composed of fibres from the optic radiations. *Syn.* primary visual area; primary visual cortex; striate area; striate cortex; V1; visual cortex. **3.** It also refers to all parts of each occipital lobe related to visual functions. *Syn.* prestriate cortex.
See **column, cortical; cortex, occipital; fissure, calcarine; geniculate body, lateral; magnification, cortical; system, magnocellular; system, parvocellular; visual integration.**
visual association a's. They are the **parastriate area** (**Brodmann's area 18**) and the **peristriate area** (**Brodmann's area 19**) of the occipital cortex surrounding the visual area. Areas 18 and 19 are subdivided into multiple zones (called V2, V3, V4, V5, V6, etc.). They receive projections from the primary visual cortex. They are also connected to other areas of the cortex and via the corpus

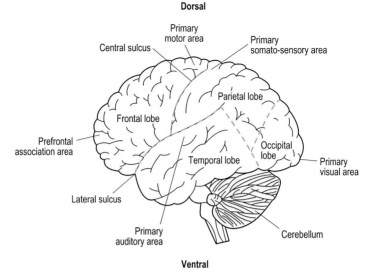

Fig. A19 Lateral surface of the human cortex showing some of the primary areas. Association areas occupy very large portions of the cortex beyond the primary areas. From the primary visual area, information is passed onto the surrounding association areas terminating in the inferior temporal (IT) lobe specialized for object identification (ventral pathway or 'what' system), and the other in the parietal lobe or more precisely near the junction of the temporal, parietal and occipital lobes (referred to as MT) specialized for object localization (dorsal pathway or 'where' system). Integration of information from these pathways is likely further processed ultimately in the frontal lobe. (After Kandel et al 2000, with permission of McGraw-Hill)

callosum with areas 18 and 19 of the opposite hemisphere and receive feedback information. It has been shown that V4 and the inferotemporal cortex or IT (components of the ventral or **temporal** cortex) receive substantial input from the parvocellular pathway. V5 (also called middle temporal cortex or MT, a component of dorsal or **parietal** cortex) receives input from the magnocellular pathway. Processing that occurs in the visual association areas helps to interpret the message that reaches the visual area and to recall memories of previous visual experiences (Fig. A19). *Syn.* extrastriate visual area; extrastriate cortex; prestriate cortex (these terms actually represent all the regions outside the striate cortex where visual processing takes place); secondary visual cortex. *See* **agnosia; magnetic resonance imaging fMRI; prosopagnosia; system, magnocellular visual; system, parvocellular visual.**

argon laser *See* **laser, argon.**

Argyll Robertson pupil *See* **pupil, Argyll Robertson.**

argyrosis The presence of silver in the deep corneal stroma or Descemet's membrane.

Arlt's line *See* **trachoma.**

Arlt's triangle *See* **keratic precipitates.**

arterial circle of the iris, major A vascular circle located in the anterior part of the ciliary body near the root of the iris. It is formed by the anastomosis of the two long posterior ciliary arteries and the seven anterior ciliary arteries. It supplies the iris, the ciliary processes and the anterior choroid.

arterial circle of the iris, minor An incomplete vascular circle located in the region of the collarette of the iris. It is formed by arterial and venous anastomoses. It supplies the pupillary zone of the iris. *See* **collarette.**

arteriosclerosis Thickening and hardening of the walls of arteries which results in an obstruction of the blood flow. It is most frequently the result of hypertension, but in the elderly it can develop in the absence of hypertension. In the retina, the branches of the central retinal artery may become straightened at first, later they become lengthened and tortuous, and the arteriovenous crossings are abnormal. Arteries resemble "**copper wire**" as they become infiltrated with lipid deposits and eventually as "**silver wire**" as the deposits increase and the whole thickness of the artery appears as a bright white reflex. Some retinal oedema may be present and, as the disease progresses, there are retinal haemorrhages and small sharp-edged exudates without surrounding oedema. This retinal condition is called arteriosclerotic retinopathy. *See* **atherosclerosis; neuropathy, arteritic anterior ischaemic optic; ratio, AV; retinopathy, hypertensive; sphygmomanometer.**

arteritis, giant cell An inflammatory disease of the wall of arteries, mainly of the extracranial vessels, which occurs in people who are over 60 years of age. The condition is characterized by headache and pain in muscles and joints, such as those of the jaws; tender or non-pulsating temporal artery; and sometimes fever. A sudden loss of vision in one eye (amaurosis fugax) may occur in the first few weeks after the onset of the disease due to an occlusion of either the central retinal artery or of the short posterior ciliary arteries that supply the optic nerve. Prompt administration of systemic corticosteroids (e.g. hydrocortisone) has been found to be of great value in the management of this condition and to prevent arteritic anterior ischaemic optic neuropathy. *Syn.* temporal arteritis. *See* **amaurosis fugax; neuropathy, arteritic anterior ischaemic optic; pupil, Adie's.**

arteritis, temporal *See* **arteritis, giant cell.**

artery A tubular, elastic vessel which carries blood away from the heart. Its walls are thicker than those of veins to withstand the greater pressure of blood on the arterial side of the circulation.
   anterior ciliary a's. See **artery, ciliary.**
   carotid a. See **amaurosis fugax; artery, internal carotid.**
   central retinal a. Branch of the ophthalmic artery entering the optic nerve some 6–12 mm from the eyeball. It enters the eye through the optic disc and divides into superior and inferior branches. Both these branches subdivide into

nasal and temporal branches which course in the nerve fibre layer, supplying the capillaries feeding the bipolar and the ganglion cell layers of the retina (except for the foveola). The outer third of the retina containing the photoreceptors is supplied by the choriocapillaris.
   See **arteritis, giant cell; retinal artery occlusion; spot, cherry-red; vein, central retinal.**
   ciliary a's. The branches of the ophthalmic artery that supply the whole of the uveal tract, the sclera and the edge of the cornea with its neighbouring conjunctiva. The ophthalmic artery gives rise to one lateral and one medial **posterior ciliary artery**. The latter divides into the short and the long posterior ciliary arteries. The **short posterior ciliary arteries** are some 10–20 branches that pierce the eyeball in an irregular ring around the optic nerve to supply the posterior choroid, the optic disc, the circle of Zinn and the cilioretinal arteries. The **long posterior ciliary arteries** are two branches, which pierce the sclera between 3 and 4 mm from the optic nerve on either side and course in the suprachoroidal space (Fig. A20). They form, with the anterior ciliary arteries, the **major arterial (or iridic) circle of the iris**, which supplies the ciliary body, the anterior choroid and the iris. The **anterior ciliary arteries** are derived from the arteries to the four recti muscles and they anastomose in the ciliary muscle with the long posterior ciliary arteries to

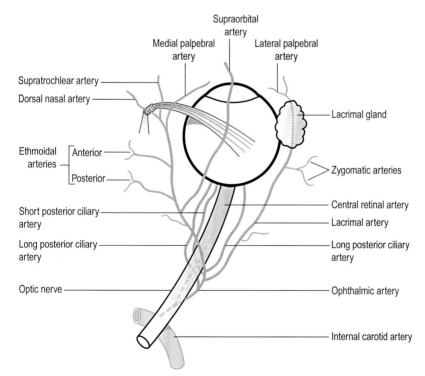

Fig. A20 The ophthalmic artery and its branches. The meningeal and muscular branches are not indicated in the diagram.

form the major arterial circle of the iris. They also give branches that supply the episclera (**episcleral arteries**), sclera, limbus and conjunctiva (**anterior and posterior conjunctival arteries**).
See **anastomosis; arterial circle of the iris, major; plexus, episcleral.**

cilioretinal a. Small artery running from the temporal side of the optic disc to the macular area. It originates from the circle of Zinn and supplies the retina between the macula and the disc. This artery is present in only about a fifth, or less, of human eyes. If a patient possesses this artery, central vision will be spared in case of occlusion of the central retinal artery. In some other eyes, the cilioretinal artery supplies some other region of the retina.
See **circle of Zinn.**

conjunctival a's. *See* **arteries, ciliary.**

copper wire a. *See* **arteriosclerosis.**

episcleral a *See* **artery, ciliary.**

hyaloid a. An artery that is present during the embryological period. It arises from the ophthalmic artery, runs forward from the optic disc to the lens where it spreads over the posterior lenticular surface as a capillary net which in turn anastomoses with a capillary net located on the anterior lens surface. Thus, the lens becomes enveloped by an anastomosing vascular network called the **tunica vasculosa lentis**. The hyaloid artery also gives rise to a large number of branches, the **vasa hyaloidea propria**, which at times almost fills the vitreous cavity. The hyaloid artery degenerates by the eighth month of gestation to become the central retinal artery. *Syn.* persistent hyaloid artery.
See **canal, hyaloid; fissure, optic; hyaloid remnant.**

infraorbital a. Terminal branch of the internal maxillary artery which enters the orbit through the inferior orbital fissure and appears on the face via the infraorbital canal. It supplies the inferior rectus and inferior oblique muscles, the lacrimal sac, the lower eyelid, the upper teeth and lip.

internal carotid a. Branch of the common carotid artery. The internal carotid artery gives rise to many branches and in particular the ophthalmic artery after it passes through the cavernous sinus. It terminates in the anterior and middle cerebral arteries. A partial or total occlusion of the carotid artery can result in stroke or visual loss. The presence of such an insufficiency can be detected with an ophthalmodynamometer (Fig. A20).
See **amaurosis fugax; circle of Willis; ophthalmodynamometer; plaques, Hollenhorst's.**

lacrimal a. It arises from the ophthalmic artery to the outer side of the optic nerve. It supplies the lacrimal gland, the conjunctiva and eyelids, giving origin to the lateral palpebral arteries (Fig. A20).

ophthalmic a. Vessel arising from the internal carotid artery and which enters the orbit through the optic canal. It gives rise to numerous branches: (1) Central retinal artery. (2) Posterior ciliary arteries. (3) Lacrimal artery (and lateral palpebral and zygomatic branches). (4) Muscular branches. (5) Supraorbital artery. (6) Anterior and posterior ethmoidal arteries. (7) Recurrent meningeal artery.

(8) Supratrochlear artery. (9) Medial palpebral arteries. (10) Dorsal nasal artery.
Thus, the ophthalmic artery supplies all the tunics of the eyeball, most of the structures in the orbit, the lacrimal sac, the paranasal sinuses, and the nose (Fig. A20).

persistent hyaloid a. *See* **artery, hyaloid.**

silver wire a. *See* **arteriosclerosis.**

supraorbital a. Branch of the ophthalmic artery which supplies the upper eyelid, the scalp and also sends branches to the levator palpebrae superioris muscle and the periorbita (Fig. A20).

arthritis, juvenile idiopathic An inflammation of a joint or joints beginning in childhood. The entity is commonly divided into several types: **oligoarticular (oligoarthritis)** in which four joints or less are involved. It affects girls much more frequently than boys, especially in early onset, and it is associated with anterior uveitis in about 20% of cases. Complications from the uveitis include posterior synechia, band keratopathy, glaucoma and cataract; **polyarticular (polyarthritis)** in which more than four joints are involved with only a few percent of cases developing uveitis; **polyarticular (rheumatoid factor positive),** which also affects five or more joints with a very low percentage of cases developing uveitis; and the most severe form **systemic (Still's disease)**, which affects boys and girls equally and in which uveitis rarely develops. Treatment of the inflammations is mainly with steroids (and mydriatics may be needed for uveitis). *Syn.* juvenile chronic arthritis; juvenile rheumatoid arthritis. *Note*: Both synonyms were used formerly.

arthritis, rheumatoid An autoimmune systemic inflammatory disease characterized by swelling of the joints causing pain and sometimes deformity. It is often accompanied by ocular inflammations, which include keratoconjunctivitis sicca, episcleritis, scleritis and uveitis, as well as corneal ulceration and scleral thinning (scleromalacia).
See **disease, Reiter's; furrow, marginal; keratoconjunctivitis sicca; keratolysis; keratitis, peripheral ulcerative; scleritis; syndrome, Brown's superior oblique tendon sheath; syndrome, Sjögren's.**

artificial drainage tube A silicone tube implanted into the anterior chamber to facilitate drainage of aqueous humour into the subconjunctival space. It is performed to reduce intraocular pressure.

artificial daylight; eye; pupil; tears *See* under the nouns.

artefact Anything made or introduced artificially which misleads the results of an investigation, image or test. *Example*: in visual evoked cortical potentials, any wave that has its origin elsewhere than in the visual area.

A-scan *See* **ultrasonography.**

aspheric lens *See* **lens, aspheric.**

aspherical Literally "not spherical" but this term is usually restricted to surfaces of revolution having

identical but non-circular (e.g. parabolic) sections in all meridians (British Standard).
See **lens, aspherical.**

asteroid hyalosis Degenerative changes occurring more commonly in males and mainly in one eye. It consists of numerous small stellate or discoid opacities (called **asteroid bodies**) suspended in the vitreous humour. These opacities consisting of fatty calcium globules appear creamy white when viewed by ophthalmoscopy. They rarely affect vision. *Syn.* Benson's disease.
See **synchysis scintillans.**

asthenopia Term used to describe any symptoms associated with the use of the eyes. The causes of asthenopia are numerous: sustained near vision, either when the accommodation amplitude is low or hyperopia is uncorrected (**accommodative asthenopia**), aniseikonia (**aniseikonic a.**), astigmatism (**astigmatic a.**), pain in the eye (**asthenopia dolens**), heterophoria (**heterophoric a.**), ocular inflammation (**asthenopia irritans**), hysteria (**nervous a.**), uncorrected presbyopia (**presbyopic a.**), improper illumination (**photogenous a.**) or retinal disease (**retinal a.**). *Syn.* eyestrain; near point stress (NPS) (although this term is restricted to any symptoms arising from near vision).
See **convergence excess; convergence insufficiency; divergence insufficiency; fatigue, visual; headache, ocular.**

astigmat A person who has astigmatism.

astigmatic Pertaining to astigmatism.

astigmatic dial; fan chart *See* **chart, astigmatic fan.**

astigmatic interval *See* **Sturm, interval of.**

astigmatic lens *See* **lens, astigmatic.**

astigmatism A condition of refraction in which the image of a point object is not a single point but two focal lines at different distances from the optical system. The two focal lines are generally perpendicular to each other. In the eye, it is a refractive error which is generally caused by one or several toroidal shapes of the refracting surfaces, or by the obliquity of the light entering the eye, but it can also develop as a result of subluxation of the lens, diabetes, cataract, keratoconus or trauma (**acquired astigmatism**) (Fig. A21 and Table A11).
See **amblyopia, meridional; chalazion; chart, astigmatic fan; circle of least confusion;** headache, ocular; lens, cross-cylinder; limbal relaxing incision; line, focal; method, fogging; rule, Javal's; stigmatism; Sturm, interval of; test for astigmatism, cross-cylinder; test, fan and block.

accommodative a. Astigmatism induced by accommodation. It is not known whether this is caused by a tilt of the crystalline lens or unequal alterations of the curvatures of the crystalline lens.

against the rule a. Ocular astigmatism in which the refractive power of the horizontal (or near horizontal) meridian is the greatest (Fig. A22). The percentage of people with against the rule astigmatism increases beyond the age of about 45 and becomes more common than with the rule astigmatism in people beyond the age of about 55. Corneal astigmatism is the main cause of this shift. *Syn.* indirect astigmatism; inverse astigmatism.
See **astigmatism, with the rule.**

compound a. Astigmatism in which the two principal meridians of an eye are either both hyperopic (**compound hyperopic astigmatism**) or both myopic (**compound myopic astigmatism**) (Fig. A23).

direct a. *See* **astigmatism, with the rule.**

indirect a. *See* **astigmatism, against the rule.**

induced a. 1. Astigmatism introduced when using contact lenses with toroidal back optic zones. This astigmatism is due to the fact that a toroidal back optic surface separates two media of different refractive indices (the contact lens and tears) and this occurs principally with rigid toric surfaces. Using contact lenses of lower refractive index reduces the amount of induced astigmatism

Table A11 Approximate relationship between uncorrected astigmatism and visual acuity

Astigmatism (D)	Snellen visual acuity	
	(m)	(ft)
4.50	6/60	20/200
3.50	6/36	20/120
2.50	6/24	20/80
1.75	6/18	20/60
1.25	6/12	20/40
0.75	6/9	20/30
0.25	6/6	20/20
0.00	6/5	20/16

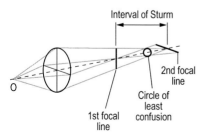

Fig. A21 Astigmatic beam of light (O, object).

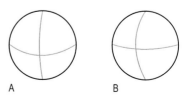

Fig. A22 Types of astigmatism (A, against the rule; B, with the rule).

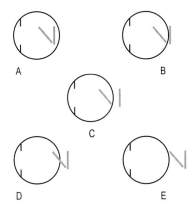

Fig. A23 Clinical types of astigmatism (A, compound myopic; B, simple myopic; C, mixed; D, simple hyperopic; E, compound hyperopic).

(such as gas permeable rather than PMMA). **2.** Astigmatism introduced when a contact lens slips or tilts on the eye. This is due to the fact that the chief ray is deviated and is no longer normal to the front surface of the lens. The amount thus produced is small (about 0.50 D for a slip of 3 mm) but increases if the lens tilts as well as slips. *See* **astigmatism, residual.**

internal a. See **astigmatism, total.**

inverse a. See **astigmatism, against the rule.**

irregular a. Ocular astigmatism in which the two principal meridians are not at right angles to each other. This condition is often the result of injury or disease (e.g. keratoconus), but can also exist in an eye with irregularities in the refractive power in different meridians of the crystalline lens. *See* **lens, combination; lens, piggyback.**

lenticular a. Astigmatism of the crystalline lens. It is usually due to variations in the curvature of one or both surfaces and much less commonly to irregularities in its refractive index. Lenticular astigmatism is typically against the rule.

mixed a. Ocular astigmatism in which one principal meridian is hyperopic and the other myopic (Fig. A23).

oblique a. **1.** Astigmatism in which the two principal meridians are neither approximately horizontal nor approximately vertical. **2.** Aberration of an optical system that occurs when the incident light rays form an angle with the optical axis which exceeds the conditions of gaussian optics. It gives rise to separate **tangential** and **sagittal** line foci instead of a single image point. This relates to optical systems or lenses, which are rotationally symmetrical about the axis. This is not the case in the eye and thus this aberration forms part of the wavefront aberrations of the eye (Table A12). *See* **allometropia; lens, anastigmatic; Petzval surface; ray, paraxial; Sturm, interval of.**

physiological a. Astigmatism not exceeding 0.5–0.75 D in the normal eye.

refractive a. See **astigmatism, total.**

Table A12   Average amount of oblique astigmatism (in dioptres) at different angles to the visual axis (From Millodot M. *Am J Optom Physiol Opt* 1981: 58: 691–695)

Angle (deg)	Nasal retina	Temporal retina
0	0	0
10	0.28	0.29
20	0.55	0.74
30	1.0	1.58
40	1.7	2.45
50	2.7	3.6
60	3.9	4.75

residual a. Astigmatism still present after correction of a refractive error. *See* **astigmatism, induced.**

simple a. Ocular astigmatism in which one principal meridian of the eye is emmetropic and the other myopic (**simple myopic astigmatism**) or hyperopic (**simple hyperopic astigmatism**) (Fig. A23).

total a. Astigmatism of the eye comprising both anterior and posterior corneal surfaces and internal astigmatism (i.e. **lenticular astigmatism**). *Syn.* refractive astigmatism. *See* **rule, Javal's.**

with the rule a. Astigmatism in which the refractive power of the vertical (or near vertical) meridian is the greatest (Fig. A22). *Syn.* direct astigmatism. *See* **astigmatism, against the rule.**

astigmatoscope Instrument for observing and measuring the astigmatism of an eye. *Syn.* astigmometer; astigmoscope.

astringent A chemical substance that causes contraction of soft organic tissues by precipitating proteins from their surfaces. Astringents are incorporated into some artificial tears. *Examples*: acetylcysteine, witch hazel, zinc sulfate. *See* **tears, artificial.**

astrocytes Neuroglial cells with many processes found in the central nervous system, the retina (especially the ganglion cells, the inner plexiform layers and the nerve fibre layer) and the optic nerve. Their function is believed to be nutritional and structural and to be involved in the clearance of neurotransmitters from within the synaptic cleft. *Syn.* Cajal's cells.

astronomical telescope *See* **telescope.**

asymmetropia *See* **anisometropia.**

asymptomatic Having no symptoms of disease or anomaly.

A syndrome *See* **pattern, alphabet.**

ataxia An inability to coordinate muscular activity during voluntary movements.

ataxia, Friedreich's *See* **ataxia, hereditary spinal.**

ataxia, hereditary spinal A hereditary degeneration of the posterior and lateral columns of the spinal cord occurring in childhood. It is characterized by general ataxia, nystagmus and, sometimes, ptosis and external ophthalmoplegia. *Syn.* Friedreich's ataxia.

atheroma Fatty deposits which lead to the formation of plaques in the blood vessels.
See **arteriosclerosis; plaques, Hollenhorst's.**

atherosclerosis A form of arteriosclerosis in which fatty deposits occur in the middle coat of large and medium-sized arteries as, for example, the central retinal artery. The deposits or plaques, which form at the site of arterial damage (due to high blood pressure, smoking, etc.), consist initially of lipid deposits and later of fibrous tissue and insoluble calcium salts. The deposits lead to a reduction and often a blockage of the blood flow resulting in angina, stroke or heart attack. Atherosclerosis occurs usually in elderly people and, in some cases, the condition may lead to retinal artery occlusion.
See **arteriosclerosis; atheroma.**

atopic keratoconjunctivitis *See* **keratoconjunctivitis, atopic.**

atopic reactions *See* **hypersensitivity, keratoconjunctivitis, atopic.**

atopy A genetic predisposition to develop certain hypersensitivity reactions (e.g. hay fever, asthma, allergy, eczema) in response to environmental allergens (e.g. pollen).
See **hypersensitivity; keratoconjunctivitis, atopic.**

atrophy A wasting, shrinking or degeneration of an organ or tissue due to malnutrition, poor blood circulation, loss of nerve supply, disuse, disease or hormonal changes.
choroidal a. See **dystrophy, choroidal.**
gyrate a. An autosomal recessive inherited disorder caused by a deficiency of the mitochondrial matrix enzyme ornithine keto-acid aminotransferase that catalyzes several amino acid pathways. It is caused by mutation in the OAT gene. The signs consist of circular degenerative patches of chorioretinal atrophy beginning near the equator during the teenage years and gradually increasing in number and enlarging to form a whole area with a scalloped border. There is a gradual loss of the visual field, axial myopia, nyctalopia and eventually central vision becomes impaired. Treatment includes pyridoxine (vitamin B6) supplement and arginine-restricted diet.
Kjer-type optic a. An autosomal dominant inherited disorder caused by mutation in the OPA1 gene on chromosome 3q29. It presents with bilateral visual loss and optic atrophy. *Syn.* Kjer's syndrome.
Leber's hereditary optic a. See **neuropathy, Leber's hereditary optic.**
optic a. Degeneration of the optic nerve fibres characterized by a pallor of the optic disc which may appear greyish, yellowish or white. This condition leads to a loss of visual acuity or changes in the visual fields or both. The change in colour of the disc is due to a loss of the normal capillarity of the disc and to a deposition of fibrin or glial tissue which replaces the nerve fibres. **1. Primary** or **simple optic atrophy**. The disc margins are well defined and usually the lamina cribrosa is unobscured. The colour is pale pink to white. Causes include optic neuritis, compression by tumours and Leber's hereditary optic atrophy. **2. Secondary optic atrophy**. The difference with the former is that, in this condition, there is evidence of preceding oedema or inflammation. The margins of the disc appear blurred and glial proliferation is present over the surface of the disc, thus obscuring the lamina cribrosa. The colour is yellowish to grey. Papilloedema gives rise to secondary optic atrophy.
See **neuropathy, Leber's hereditary optic; syndrome, Behr's; syndrome, Foster Kennedy.**
peripapillary a. Atrophy of the area surrounding the optic nerve head in which the sclera and large choroidal vessels become visible, as well as irregular hyperpigmentation and/or hypopigmentation of the retinal pigment epithelium. Although this atrophy is most commonly present in glaucoma, it may be seen in other ocular conditions such as age-related degeneration of the retinal pigment epithelium and Bruch's membrane, long-standing retinitis or choroiditis.

atropine An alkaloid obtained from the belladonna plant. It is an antimuscarinic drug (muscarinic antagonist). In the eye, it acts as a mydriatic and as a cycloplegic. It paralyses the pupillary sphincter and the ciliary muscle by preventing the action of acetylcholine at the parasympathetic nerve endings.
See **acetylcholine; cycloplegia; mydriatic; myopia control.**

atropine-like drug *See* **mydriatic.**

atropine mydriasis *See* **anisocoria.**

attenuation 1. A reduction of intensity of a radiation as it passes through an absorbing or scattering medium. **2.** Narrowing of a blood vessel. **3.** *See* **penalization.**

Aubert's phenomenon *See* **phenomenon, Aubert's.**

Aubert–Förster phenomenon *See* **phenomenon, Aubert–Förster.**

aura, visual Visual sensations that precede an epileptic attack or a migraine. These sensations may appear as light flashes, scintillating scotomata, etc. *See* **migraine.**

auscultation *See* **bruit.**

autofluorescence The ability of certain tissues, such as the optic nerve disc drusen and large lipofuscin deposits, to emit yellow-green light when illuminated with cobalt blue light in the absence of fluorescein.

auto keratometer A keratometer using a microprocessor computer to measure corneal curvature. Such instruments usually provide measurements of the peripheral and central corneal curvatures at different points providing a contour of the cornea in several meridians, as well as of the corneal apex. *See* **corneal topography.**

autokinesis, visual *See* **illusion, autokinetic visual.**

autorefraction 1. A procedure of refraction in which the patient adjusts the controls of the instrument. **2.** Refraction carried out with an electronic optometer which is fully objective, generally using infrared light and which can be operated by a non-specialist. *See* **optometer; refractive error; retinoscopy.**

autorefractor *See* **optometer.**

autorefractometer *See* **optometer.**

AV crossing In cases of arteriosclerosis, the crossing of retinal arteries and veins is abnormal as the arteries compress the underlying veins as a result of the thickening and hardening of its walls. *Syn.* AV nicking. *See* **arteriosclerosis; retinopathy, hypertensive.**

AV nicking *See* **AV crossing.**

avitaminosis A disorder caused by a deficiency of one or more essential vitamins. In the eye, vitamin A and B deficiency may lead to disease. *See* **neuropathy, optic; vitamin A deficiency.**

AV ratio *See* **ratio, AV.**

automated perimeter *See* **perimeter, automated.**

avascular zone *See* **foveola.**

avulsion The forcible separation of two parts or tearing away of a part or of an organ. *Examples*: avulsion of the retina at the ora serrata; avulsion of the eyelid at its insertion.

axanthopsia Yellow blindness. *See* **chromatopsia.**

Axenfeld's intrascleral nerve loop *See* **loop, Axenfeld's nerve.**

Axenfeld's anomaly A rare, inherited developmental abnormality characterized by the adhesion of strands of peripheral iris tissue to a prominent Schwalbe's line (posterior embryotoxon). It forms part of the Axenfeld-Rieger syndrome. *See* **Peter's anomaly; syndrome, Rieger's.**

Axenfeld-Rieger syndrome *See* **syndrome, Axenfeld-Rieger.**

axial length of the eye *See* **length of the eye, axial.**

axial magnification *See* **magnification, axial.**

axial ray *See* **ray, axial.**

axis A real or imaginary straight line about which a body or system can rotate, or about which a body or system is symmetrical.
> **achromatic a.** Line in the eye along which light passes through all the optical elements and emerges without chromatic dispersion. Although it may lie close to the optical axis, it does not necessarily coincide with it. *See* **chromostereopsis; dispersion; parallax, chromatic.**

> **anteroposterior a.** Line passing through the anterior and posterior poles and the centre of rotation of the eye. It is perpendicular to the transverse (or *x*-axis) and the vertical (or *z*-axis). Torsional movements occur around this axis. *Syn.* sagittal axis; *y*-axis. *See* **centre of rotation of the eye; poles of the eyeball; torsion.**

> **cylinder a. 1.** Line of zero curvature on a cylindrical surface. **2.** That principal meridian of a planocylinder in which the power is zero. *See* **lens, astigmatic.**

> **a's. of Fick** Three mutually perpendicular axes that intersect at the centre of rotation of the eye. They are the *x*-, *y*-, and *z*-axes. *Syn.* primary axes of Fick. *See* **axis, anteroposterior; axis, transverse; axis, vertical; plane, sagittal; plane, Listing's; plane, *xy*; plane, *yz*.**

> **fixation a.** Line joining the object of regard to the centre of rotation of the eye. *Syn.* line of fixation.

> **geometrical a.** Line passing through the anterior and posterior poles of the eye. If the refractive surfaces are symmetrical about that axis, it will then coincide with the optical axis.

> **horizontal a.** *See* **axis, transverse.**

> **a. notation** *See* **axis notation, standard.**

> **a. notation, standard** The accepted axis notation for cylinders, the same for each eye, whereby the specified axis direction denotes the angle of the cylinder axis with the horizontal measured anticlockwise from 0° to 180°, the front surface of the lens being viewed (British Standard). (Fig. A24) *Syn.* TABO notation (although the TABO notation specifies the axis direction from 0° to 360°); OCA notation.

> **optical a. 1.** Line joining the optical centres of the refractive surfaces of the eye (a theoretical concept in the eye). A close approximation of this axis is represented by aligning the Purkinje images of a test object. **2.** The line normal to the surfaces of a lens along which light passes undeviated (Fig. P14, p. 265). *See* **images, Purkinje–Sanson.**

> **orbital a.** Line from the middle of the orbital opening to the centre of the optic canal. The orbital axes of a normal adult make an angle of approximately 45° with each other. *See* **orbit.**

> **principal a.** Line passing through the centre of curvature of a surface and through its vertex.

> **pupillary a.** Line passing through the centre of the entrance pupil of the eye and the pole of the cornea. *Syn.* pupillary line.

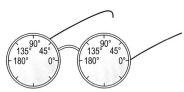

Fig. A24 Illustration of the standard cylinder axis notation.

See **poles of the eyeball.**
sagittal a. See axis, anteroposterior.
transverse a. Horizontal line passing through the centre of rotation of the eye and lying in Listing's plane. *Syn. x*-axis.
See **axis, anteroposterior; plane, Listing's.**
vertical a. Vertical line passing through the centre of rotation of the eye. *Syn. z*-axis.
visual a. The line joining the object of regard to the foveola and passing through the nodal points which are often considered as coincident, as they are very close to each other. Strictly, this axis is not a single straight line as it consists of two parts: one line connecting the object of regard to the first nodal point and the other line parallel and connecting the second nodal point to the foveola. *Syn.* visual line.
See **line of sight.**
x-axis See **axis, transverse.**

y-axis See axis, anteroposterior.
z-axis See axis, vertical.

axometer 1. Instrument used to determine the axis of a cylindrical lens and the optical centre of a lens. **2.** Instrument used in the subjective determination of the principal meridians of an astigmatic eye. *Syn.* axonometer.

axon The threadlike process of a neuron which conducts nerve impulses from the cell body to the neuron's ending (bouton) where it is transmitted via a synapse to another neuron, muscle or gland. *Syn.* nerve fibre (when it is sheathed).
See **neuron; synapse.**

azathioprine See **immunosuppressants.**

azelastine hydrochloride See **antihistamine.**

azithromycin See **antibiotic.**

B

bacillus A large group (genus) of rod-shaped bacteria, which are found in air and soil commonly as spores (a resistant form). Some may cause conjunctivitis, keratitis or endophthalmitis. Some strains produce antibiotics (e.g. bacitracin, gramicidin). *Plural:* bacilli.
See **Gram stain.**

bacitracin An antibiotic drug with similar properties to penicillin and effective principally against gram-positive bacteria, such as Staphylococci and Streptococci. It is mainly used in combination with other agents (e.g. polymyxin B) for treating external eye infections (e.g. blepharoconjunctivitis).

back haptic size See **haptic size, back.**

back of a lens Relating to that surface nearer to the eye (British Standard).

back optic zone diameter See **optic zone diameter.**

back optic zone radius See **optic zone radius, back.**

back vertex focal length See **vertex focal length.**

back vertex power See **power, back vertex.**

backward masking See **metacontrast.**

baclofen An analogue of gamma-aminobutyric acid (GABA) used orally to treat skeletal muscle spasm and in the management of nystagmus, particularly periodic alternating nystagmus.

bacteria Microscopic unicellular organisms that commonly reproduce by cell division (fission) and are contained within a cell wall. Bacteria are either spheres (cocci), rod-shaped (bacilli) or curved. They are further divided into Gram-negative and Gram-positive. They are a natural component of the human body, particularly on the skin, mouth and intestinal tract. Many are beneficial to the environment and living organisms, but some are the cause of many infectious diseases. Infectious bacteria enter the body through torn tissues or by its orifices (e.g. nose, mouth, lungs) and can provoke inflammation. Many bacterial infections may spread from host to host (e.g. contagious conjunctivitis). Infections caused by bacteria are treated with antibiotics. *Singular:* bacterium.
See **antibiotics; Gram stain.**

bacterial conjunctivitis See **conjunctivitis, acute.**

bacteriostatic A term describing substances such as sulfonamides and tetracycline, which inhibit the growth and propagation of bacteria, but do not actually destroy bacteria.
See **antibiotic.**

bactericidal See **antibiotic.**

Badal's optometer See **optometer, Badal's.**

'bag', capsular A sack-like structure remaining within the eye following extracapsular cataract extraction or phacoemulsification. The implanted intraocular lens is placed within this structure to recreate the usual phakic state.
See **cataract extraction; lens, intraocular; phacoemulsification.**

Bagolini's glass; test See **glass, Bagolini's.**

Bailey–Lovie acuity chart See **chart, Bailey–Lovie.**

Bailliart's ophthalmodynanometer See **ophthalmodynanometer.**

Fig. B1 Truncated and prism-ballasted toric contact lens.

balance, binocular Condition characterized by the two eyes being simultaneously in focus or equally out of focus.
See **method, Humphriss; test, balancing; test, Turville infinity.**

balance, muscle The status of the eye muscle function as represented by the phoria measurement.
See **heterophoria.**

balancing lens; test *See* **lens, balancing.**

Baldwin's illusion *See* **illusion, Baldwin's visual.**

Balint's syndrome *See* **syndrome, Balint's.**

ballast Additional weight of material incorporated in a part of a toric contact lens to maintain it in a given orientation (Fig. B1). This is often provided by giving prismatic power to the lens (**prism ballast lens**).

band keratopathy *See* **keratopathy, band.**

band, retinoscopic A strip of light seen in the retinoscopic reflex of an astigmatic eye, especially when neutralizing one of the principal meridians.

band-shaped corneal dystrophy *See* **keratopathy, band.**

bandage lens *See* **lens, therapeutic soft contact.**

Bangerter foils Semitransparent membranes of various degrees of opacification which can be pressed onto a spectacle lens to reduce visual acuity. There are 10 degrees, graded from 1.0 (6/6 or 20/20) to complete occlusion. They are used in the treatment of amblyopia and intractable diplopia. *Syn.* Bangerter graded occluder; Bangerter occluder.
See **occlusion treatment; penalization.**

bar reader *See* **grid, Javal's.**

bar reading *See* **test, bar reading.**

Barany's caloric test *See* **test, caloric.**

Barany's nystagmus *See* **nystagmus.**

Bard's sign *See* **sign, Bard's.**

Bardet–Biedl syndrome *See* **syndrome, Bardet–Biedl.**

baring of the blind spot *See* **spot, baring of the blind.**

barrel-shaped distortion *See* **distortion.**

Barrer A unit of oxygen permeability of a contact lens material. *Symbol*: *Dk*. It is equal to the product of the diffusion coefficient *D* of oxygen through the material (i.e. the speed at which oxygen molecules pass through the material) and the solubility *k* of oxygen in the material (i.e. the number of oxygen molecules that can be absorbed in a given volume of material).
See **oxygen permeability; oxygen transmissibility.**

basal 1. In anatomy, denoting a layer or cells farthest away from the surface. *Example*: the basal cells of the corneal epithelium nearest Bowman's layer. **2.** In optics, denoting the surface opposite to the apex of a prism.

base-apex direction; line *See* **base setting.**

base curve *See* **curve, base.**

base line *See* **line, base.**

base of prism The edge of a prism at which the faces are separated by a maximum distance.
See **base setting.**

base setting The direction of the line from apex to base of a prism in a principal section (a section lying in a plane perpendicular to the refracting edge). The setting position for the base of a prism is normally specified by the direction 'base-up' (or base-down', 'in' or 'out' as the case may be) in which 'up' and 'down' have their ordinary meanings, 'in' means towards the nose and 'out' towards the temple. Base-apex line, base-apex meridian and base-apex direction are deprecated terms (British Standard). Alternatively, the TABO notation is used. Abbreviations for the placement of the base of the prism are **BD** (for base-down), **BI** (for base towards the nose), **BO** (for base towards the temple) and **BU** (for base-up).
See **axis notation, standard; base of prism.**

base of vitreous *See* **vitreous humour.**

Bassen–Kornzweig syndrome *See* **syndrome, Bassen–Kornzweig.**

Batten–Mayou disease *See* **disease, Batten–Mayou.**

beam of light *See* **light, beam of.**

beam splitter An optical system which separates an incident beam of light into two beams of lesser intensity, one reflected and the other transmitted (e.g. a semi-silvered mirror). Some beam splitters are made of birefringent material, which splits the incident light beam into oppositely polarized beams. They are called **polarizing beam splitters**. *Example*: Wollaston prism.

'bear tracks' *See* **retinal pigment epithelium, congenital hypertrophy of the.**

bearing, apical An area of contact between the back surface of a rigid contact lens and the apex of the cornea. It is observed with the fluorescein test.
See **apex, corneal.**

bedewing, endothelial A cluster of inflammatory cells deposited on the posterior surface of the corneal endothelium. They have been noted with anterior eye inflammation and contact lens wear. The symptoms may include slight stinging sensation, some interference with vision and intolerance

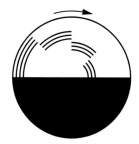

Fig. B2 Benham's top.

to contact lens wear. Reduction of wearing time is usually indicated and, in severe cases, contact lens wear must be ceased.
See blebs, endothelial; corneal endothelium.

Behçet's disease *See* disease, Behçet's.

Behr's pupillary phenomenon; syndrome *See* under the nouns.

belladonna *See* atropine.

Bell's palsy; phenomenon *See* under the nouns.

Benedikt's syndrome *See* syndrome, Benedikt's.

Benham's top A disc, half black and half white, with a number of concentric black bars on the white half which, when rotated, evokes a sensation of colour, called **Fechner's colours** or **Fechner–Benham colours** (Fig. B2). *Syn.* Benham–Fechner top.

benoxinate hydrochloride *See* oxybuprocaine hydrochloride.

Benson's disease *See* asteroid hyalosis.

benzalkonium chloride *See* antiseptic.

Berger's loupe *See* loupe, Berger's.

Berger's postlenticular space *See* space, Berger's postlenticular.

Bergmeister's papilla *See* papilla, Bergmeister's.

Berlin's disease *See* disease, Berlin's.

Bernell clip *See* clipover.

Best's disease *See* disease, Best's.

best vision sphere Adjustment made in the determination of the optimal spherical correction. Low-powered lenses (typically in 0.25 D steps) are placed in front of a patient's eye wearing a corrective lens which has been determined usually objectively, until the best visual acuity is obtained with maximum plus power. This adjustment is generally followed by the plus 1.00 D blur test. *See* method, fogging; test, plus 1.00 blur.

Best's vitelliform macular dystrophy *See* disease, Best's.

best-form lens *See* lens, best-form.

beta-adrenergic blocking agent *See* beta-blocker.

beta-blocker A drug that blocks or reduces the action of neurotransmitters on beta-adrenergic receptors. It reduces secretion of aqueous humour and consequently intraocular pressure and it is used in the treatment of glaucoma. Common beta-blockers include timolol maleate, betaxolol hydrochloride, carteolol hydrochloride, levobunolol hydrochloride and metipranolol. Timolol is often used together with another agent (combination drugs), e.g. timolol and brimonidine, timolol and dorzolamide, timolol and latanoprost. *Syn.* beta-adrenergic antagonist; beta-adrenergic blocking agent.
See adrenergic receptors; miotics; sympatholytic drugs.

betamethasone *See* antiinflammatory drugs.

betaxolol hydrochloride *See* adrenergic receptors; beta-blocker.

bethanechol chloride *See* pilocarpine.

bevacizumab *See* anti-VEGF drugs; macular degeneration, age-related.

Bezold–Brücke phenomenon *See* phenomenon, Bezold–Brücke.

Bianchi's valve *See* lacrimal apparatus; valve of Hasner.

bichrome test *See* test, duochrome.

biconcave lens *See* lens, biconcave.

biconvex lens *See* lens, biconvex.

Bidwell's experiment *See* experiment, Bidwell's.

Bidwell's ghost A special case of a moving positive after-image occurring behind a moving spot of light. This after-image seems like a ghost light trailing behind. *Syn.* Purkinje after-image.
See after-image.

Bielschowsky's head tilt test; phenomenon; phenomenon test *See* under the nouns.

Bietti's band-shaped corneal dystrophy *See* keratopathy, actinic.

bifixation Imaging of an object on the fovea of each eye simultaneously. *Syn.* bifoveal fixation.

bilateral Pertaining to both sides.
See contralateral; ipsilateral; unilateral.

bilateral strip *See* nasotemporal overlap.

billiards spectacles *See* spectacles, billiards.

bimatoprost *See* prostaglandin analogues.

binasal hemianopia *See* hemianopia, binasal.

binocular Pertaining to both eyes.

binocular balance *See* balance, binocular.

binocular disparity *See* acuity, stereoscopic visual; disparity, retinal; perception, depth.

binocular Esterman test *See* test, Esterman.

binocular fusion *See* fusion, sensory.

binocular indirect ophthalmoscope; instability; lock; lustre; parallax *See* under the nouns.

binocular rivalry *See* retinal rivalry.

binocular single vision *See* vision, binocular single.

binocular vision *See* vision, binocular.

binocular visual field *See* **field, binocular visual.**

binoculars A set of two identical telescopes, one for each eye, which gives binocular vision of magnified distant objects. The images are erected using either an eyepiece of negative power, or prisms, or very occasionally, an additional lens system placed between objective and eyepiece. On binoculars, the magnification M and the diameter D of the objective or entrance pupil are shown as $M \times D$ (e.g. 8×30). *Syn.* field glasses; prism binoculars (for those which use prisms as erectors).
See **erector; telescope, galilean; telescope, terrestrial.**

binoculars, prism *See* **binoculars.**

biocompatible Adjective describing a material which is neither harmful nor toxic to living tissue. *Example:* an intraocular lens implant.

biocular Pertaining to the use of the two eyes but without fusion or stereopsis. The term is primarily used in clinical testing and vision therapy in which different prisms are placed in front of each eye.

biofeedback A technique whereby visual (or bodily) processes normally under involuntary control (e.g. accommodation) are displayed to the subject, enabling voluntary control to be learnt. It has been used in myopia control and in acuity improvement but the value of the technique in these conditions is still unproven.
See **response, SILO.**

biological–statistical theory *See* **theory, biological–statistical.**

bioluminescence Emission of light by living organisms, e.g. firefly, certain fungi, etc.
See **luminescence.**

biomarker A substance or a test, sensitive enough to indicate the risk or the early sign of a disease.

biometry of the eye The measurement of the various dimensions of the eye and of its components and their interrelationships. The axial length, anterior chamber depth and the corneal curvature are essential measurements to predict the correct lens power of an intraocular lens. There are several biometers which are used prior to cataract surgery, some based on ultrasound, others on optical systems incorporating the principle of interference.
See **constants of the eye; interferometry, partial coherence; SRK.**

biomicroscope 1. An instrument designed for detailed examination of ocular tissues containing a magnifying system and usually used in conjunction with a slit-lamp. Biomicroscopy can be used to examine both the anterior segment using various illumination techniques and the posterior segment of the eye. **2.** Term commonly used to describe a slit-lamp (although this is not strictly correct).

biomicroscopy, fundus Observation of the fundus of the eye with a biomicroscope. It requires an additional, usually hand-held, lens (+90 D, +78 D, +60 D, etc.) placed between the patient's eye (with the pupil usually dilated) and the slit-lamp, which

is adjusted to be coaxial with the eye. This method provides a real, inverted and reversed stereoscopic view of the fundus.
See **illumination; lens, gonioscopic; lens, Hruby; slit-lamp.**

biomicroscopy, ultrasound *See* **ultrasonography, ophthalmic.**

biomimetic contact lens *See* **lens, biomimetic contact.**

bionic eye *See* **eye, bionic.**

bioptic telescope *See* **telescope, bioptic.**

bipolar cell *See* **cell, bipolar.**

bi-prism, Fresnel's *See* **Fresnel's bi-prism.**

birdshot retinochoroidopathy *See* **retinochoroidopathy, birdshot.**

birefringence Property of anisotropic media such as crystals, whereby an incident light beam is split up into two beams, each plane polarized at right angles to the other. One beam, called **ordinary**, obeys Snell's law, while the other, called **extraordinary**, does not. *Examples:* quartz, tourmaline. *Syn.* birefractive; double refraction.
See **anisotropic; law of refraction; prism, Nicol; prism, Wollaston.**

bitemporal hemianopia *See* **hemianopia, bitemporal.**

Bitot's spot *See* **spot, Bitot's.**

Bjerrum screen *See* **screen, tangent.**

Bjerrum's scotoma; sign *See* **scotoma, Bjerrum's.**

black A visual sensation having no colour and being of extremely low luminosity.

black body; eye *See* under the nouns.

blackout Synonym for amaurosis fugax. It also includes the temporary loss of vision and consciousness occurring in unprotected pilots, due to a reduction of blood supply to the eye and brain at high acceleration.
See **amaurosis fugax.**

blanching, limbal Whitening of the limbal area due to pressure from the edge of a soft lens which fits too tightly.
See **lens, steep; limbus; test, push-up.**

bleaching 1. The process of changing colour from the pink of a dark-adapted retina to a pale yellow colour after it has been exposed to light. This is due to the reaction of the rhodopsin pigment. The process is reversible if the healthy retina is allowed to remain in the dark. **2.** Process to remove a tint from organic lenses.
See **isomerization; pigment, visual; rhodopsin.**

bleary eye *See* **eye, bleary.**

blebs, endothelial Oedema of some cells of the corneal endothelium, which bulge towards the aqueous humour. With specular microscopy or with high magnification biomicroscopy the cells appear as black areas as they do not reflect light towards the observer. Blebs occur within minutes of inserting a contact lens on the eye

and disappear within hours after insertion. They may result from a local acidic pH shift at the endothelium.
See bedewing, endothelial; corneal endothelium; illumination, specular reflection.

blending The process by which the different curvatures of a contact lens or of a bifocal lens are made to merge in a transition zone, with the purpose of eliminating the dividing line.
See optic zone diameter; transition.

blennorrhoea neonatorum *See* ophthalmia neonatorum.

blephara The eyelids. *Singular*: blepharon.

blepharitis A chronic inflammation of the eyelids. The most common of these is marginal blepharitis. Note that the terms anterior and marginal are both used to mean the same, although the word marginal is possibly more specific.
See gland, meibomian; hordeolum, external.
angular b. Inflammation of the canthi, affecting especially the inner canthus.
anterior or marginal b. Chronic inflammation of the eyelid margin accompanied by crusts or scales usually due to a bacterial infection (e.g. **staphylococcal blepharitis** caused by *Staphylococcus aureus,* which is the most common), an allergy, or to excessive secretion of lipid by the meibomian glands and the glands of Zeis (**seborrhoeic blepharitis**). The condition is commonly associated with atopic dermatitis and keratoconjunctivitis sicca. Symptoms and signs include burning, itching, grittiness, mild photophobia and the eyelid is hyperaemic and crusted and usually worse in the morning. Treatment consists mainly of frequent cleaning of the lid margins with a cotton-tipped applicator (or face cloth or cotton ball) dipped in a diluted solution of baby shampoo; warm compresses and an antibiotic ointment (e.g. erythromycin, bacitracin) and occasionally systemic antibiotics such as tetracycline, especially in seborrhoeic blepharitis. In complicated cases, corticosteroids will also be used (Fig. B3).
See acne rosacea; glands, meibomian; glands of Zeis; meibomianitis; trichiasis.

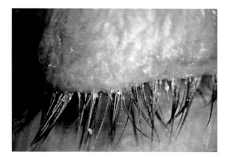

Fig. B3 Hard scales in staphylococcal blepharitis. (From Kanski 2003, with permission of Butterworth-Heinemann)

posterior b. Chronic inflammation resulting from dysfunction and alteration of meibomian glands secretions characterized either by excessive meibomian secretion (**seborrhoeic blepharitis),** or inflammation and obstruction of the meibomian glands (**meibomianitis**). It is characterized by hyperaemia, oily lid margins with scales making the eyelashes stick together and foamy tear film. Posterior blepharitis is associated with acne rosacea.
See meibomianitis.
seborrhoeic b. Inflammation of the eyelids caused by excessive secretion of lipids from the meibomian glands and the glands of Zeis. It is characterized by oily, soft deposits at the lid margins and on the eyelashes. It is typically associated with seborrheic dermatitis, corneal punctate erosions and vascularization. Management includes frequent cleaning of the lid margins with baby shampoo and antibiotic ointment (e.g. erythromycin).
See blepharitis, marginal; meibomianitis.
ulcerative b. Inflammation of the eyelid margin characterized by small ulcers.

blepharochalasis An atrophy of the upper eyelids causing a fold of tissue which often hangs over the eyelid margins. The condition follows recurrent episodes of oedema and inflammation, usually in young people. Treatment is surgical.
See dermatochalasis; epiblepharon.

blepharoconjunctivitis Inflammation of the conjunctiva and eyelids.
See keratitis, herpes simplex.

blepharon *See* blephara.

blepharophimosis A congenital condition characterized by a generalized narrowing of the palpebral fissure. It produces a pseudoptosis, but it commonly forms part of the blepharophimosis syndrome.

blepharoplasty Any operation of the eyelid. It may be done for cosmetic reasons (e.g. to erase the signs of ageing) or for medical reasons (e.g. ptosis, entropion, ectropion).
See blepharochalasis; dermatochalasis.

blepharoplegia Paralysis of an eyelid.

blepharoptosis *See* ptosis.

blepharorrhaphy Suturing of eyelids or of a lacerated lid.
See tarsorrhaphy.

blepharospasm Tonic or chronic spasm of the orbicularis oculi muscle and the upper facial muscles involving involuntary closure of the eyelids. It is more common in women than men and increases with age. It is often provoked by a foreign body in the eye, an abrasion or inflammation of the cornea or conjunctiva, or by excessive exposure to ultraviolet light (e.g. actinic keratoconjunctivitis) or idiopathic (**essential blepharospasm**). Treatment consists chiefly of injection into the muscles around the eyelids of botulinum toxin and treating any underlying ocular disease.

See botulinum toxin; chemodenervation; keratoconjunctivitis, actinic; muscle, orbicularis.

blepharostat *See* eye speculum.

blepharosynechia Adhesion of the eyelids to each other or to the eyeball.

blind Totally or partially unable to see.
  b. spot *See* spot, blind.
  b. test *See* study, single-blind; study, double-blind.

blindness 1. Inability to see. **2.** Absence or severe loss of vision so as to be unable to perform any work for which eyesight is essential. The **World Health Organization (WHO)** defines blindness as the best corrected visual acuity of 3/60 (20/400 or 1.3 logMAR) or less in the better eye. *Syn.* ablepsia; ablepsy; amaurosis.
  blue b. *See* tritanopia.
  colour b. Sometimes this term is incorrectly used to cover all forms of colour vision deficiency, however mild or severe.
  See achromatopsia; colour vision, defective; deuteranopia; monochromat; protanopia; tritanopia.
  congenital stationary night b. Night blindness (nyctalopia) inherited as either autosomal dominant with non-progressive nyctalopia, but normal daylight visual acuity and visual fields and presumed to be due to a defect in neural transmission between the rods and the bipolars in the retina, or autosomal recessive or X-linked with congenital nyctalopia, myopia, nystagmus and reduced visual acuity.
  See disease, Oguchi's; fundus albipunctatus; hemeralopia; retinitis pigmentosa.
  cortical b. Loss of vision due to lesions in the areas of both occipital lobes of the brain associated with visual functions. It may result from trauma or from a vascular disease (e.g. a circulatory occlusion caused by a stroke). A lesion in one occipital lobe may result in homonymous hemianopia, often with macular sparing.
  day b. *See* hemeralopia.
  eclipse b. Partial or complete loss of central vision due to a foveal lesion caused by fixating the sun without adequate eye protection. This condition is caused mainly by the infrared radiations from the sun.
  See actinic.
  flash b. *See* keratoconjunctivitis, actinic.
  green b. *See* deuteranopia.
  hysterical b. Blindness associated with an emotional shock, which occurs without a physical or organic cause. The patient has normal blink and pupillary responses and the fundus appears normal. A placebo therapy and/or psychological counselling may be required.
  legal b. The definition varies from country to country. In the UK, it is equal to either 3/60 (20/400 or 1.3 logMAR) or worse; or 6/60 (20/200 or 1.0 logMAR) or worse, with markedly restricted fields.
  motion b. Very rare condition in which a patient is unable to process information about motion, although other visual functions are unimpaired.

This is believed to be the result of damage to the middle temporal cortex (V5).
  See area, visual association.
  night b. *See* achromatopsia; disease, Oguchi's; fundus albipunctatus; hemeralopia.
  perceptual b. *See* agnosia.
  red b. *See* protanopia.
  river b. *See* onchocerciasis.
  snow b. *See* keratoconjunctivitis, actinic.
  word b. *See* alexia.

blindsight A term used to indicate someone who is totally blind but yet is able, unconsciously, to locate an object on the basis of visual cues. It indicates a lesion which has destroyed the visual cortex but in which the retinotectal pathway to the superior colliculus remains unaffected. This pathway is not involved in conscious vision but receives some information from the retina.
  See pathway, retinotectal.

blink 1. A temporary closure of the eyelids (usually of both eyes). **2.** To close an eye or both, briefly. Blinks are usually involuntary but can be voluntary.

blinking The act of closing the eye, or usually both eyes, temporarily. Blinking plays a protective role against foreign bodies, in moistening the cornea, sweeping it clean and draining tears. The frequency of blinking is conditioned by a number of external and internal factors (e.g. glare, wind, emotion, attention, tiredness, etc.). There are two types of blinking: reflex and spontaneous. Although both are protective and cause lacrimation, it is the principal purpose of spontaneous blinking. Normal spontaneous blink rate is about 10 blinks per minute, although there are wide variations. The duration of a full blink is approximately 0.3–0.4 s. Spontaneous blinking is slower than reflex blinking. Blink rates are often altered with contact lens wear and in some diseased states (e.g. chalazion, Graves' disease). It is important that patients be shown how to blink properly, especially in contact lens wearers to prevent drying of the lens surface, epithelial desiccation, hypoxia and hypercapnia.
  See reflex, blinking; reflex, corneal; wink.

Blivet figure *See* figure, Blivet.

blobs Cluster of cells found in each hypercolumn of the primary visual cortex (V1), which are, in most instances, colour-opponent but insensitive to orientation, shape or movement. They are about 0.2 mm in diameter and separated by an area about 0.5 mm wide called 'interblob'. The reason why these cells are called blobs is because they are easily revealed when stained with the enzyme cytochrome oxidase, as these cells derive energy from the oxidase metabolism, whereas the interblobs stain very lightly.
  See column, cortical; hypercolumn.

Bloch's law *See* law, Bloch's.

Bloch-Sulzberger syndrome *See* incontinentia pigmenti.

blocking The mounting of one or a number of lens blanks on a holder to form a unit (termed a '**block**')

ready for surfacing. The lens blanks are cemented with pitch, wax, etc.
See **surfacing**.

blood–brain barrier A mechanism that prevents some substances in the blood from reaching the brain. It is achieved by brain capillaries, which unlike other capillaries elsewhere in the body, are composed of endothelial cells sealed together in continuous tight junctions and surrounded by astrocytes that contribute to the selective passage of substances. Lipid-soluble substances such as alcohol, caffeine, nicotine and most anaesthetics, as well as glucose, oxygen and water, pass rapidly into brain cells, whereas proteins, most antibiotics and ions do not enter or enter very slowly. The mechanism protects brain cells against harmful substances and pathogens.
See **system, central nervous**.

blood–retina barrier *See* **retina**.

blood pressure *See* **sphygmomanometer**.

bloomed lens *See* **lens, coated**.

blooming *See* **coating**.

blot haemorrhage *See* **haemorrhage, blot**.

'blow-out fracture' *See* **fracture, orbital**.

blue Visual sensation evoked by radiations within the waveband 450–490 nm. It is a primary colour and the complementary of yellow.
See **colour, complementary; colour, primary**.

blue arcs *See* **arcs, blue**.

blue blindness *See* **tritanopia**.

blue field entoptoscope *See* **entoptoscope, blue field**.

blue-yellow blindness *See* **tritanopia**.

blue sclera *See* **sclera, blue**.

blur 1. Degradation of an image formed by an optical system as a result of lack of focusing, aberrations, diffusion of light, etc. **2.** A pattern in which the border is indistinct.
See **lens flare; vision, blurred**.
b. ***back test*** *See* **test, plus 1.00 D blur**.
b. ***circle*** A circular patch of light formed on the retina resulting from a point object whose image is focused either in front of or behind the retina or due to excessive aberrations of the optical system of the eye. The size of the blur circle increases with the distance of the ocular image from the retina and with the diameter of the pupil. Its diameter can be expressed in angular terms (in min arc) as

$$\alpha = 3.48 \times \Delta F \times d$$

where ΔF is the defocus (in dioptres) with respect to the object point, and d is the pupil diameter (in mm) (Figs. B4 and B5). *Example*: An object at infinity is viewed by a 2 D uncorrected myope with a 4.0 mm pupil diameter, i.e. $\alpha = 3.48 \times 2 \times 4 = 28$ min arc. *Syn.* circle of confusion; circle of diffusion.
See **aberration; depth of field**.

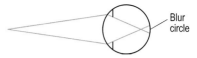

Fig. B4 Blur circle corresponding to an image formed in front of the retina.

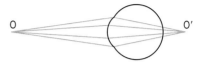

Fig. B5 Effect of pupil size on the blur circle. O′ is the image of object O formed by the optics of the eye. A reduction in pupil size corresponds to a reduction in the size of the blur circle on the retina.

plus 1.00 D b. test *See* **test, plus 1.00 D blur**.
b. ***point*** *See* **point, blur**.
spectacle b. Reduction in visual acuity noticed with spectacles after removal of hard contact lenses (PMMA). This may be due to corneal oedema, alteration of the corneal index of refraction, surface distortion of the cornea, etc. Refitting the patient with gas permeable lenses usually relieves this symptom.

blurred vision *See* **vision, blurred**.

bobbing, ocular Spontaneous, rapid downward movements of both eyes followed by a slow drift to the straight-ahead position. It occurs in patients, usually comatose, who have lesions of the brainstem.

body 1. Any discrete mass. **2.** The main and largest part of a structure. **3.** A substance of any kind.
black b. Thermal radiator which absorbs completely all incident radiation, whatever the wavelength, the direction of incidence or the polarization. This radiator has, for any wavelength, the maximum spectral concentration of radiant flux at a given temperature (CIE). *Syn.* full radiator; planckian radiator.
See **absorption; colour temperature; law, Planck's**.
ciliary b. *See* **ciliary body**.
colloid b's. *See* **drusen**.
cytoid b's. Small swollen white spots found on the retina resembling cells. They are due to degenerated retinal nerve fibres in which cellular components become trapped in the peripheral axons of the optic nerve blocking axonal flow. Collection of cytoid bodies are thought to represent the 'cotton-wool' spots found on or around the optic disc in papilloedema, retinal trauma, diabetic retinopathy, AIDS, systemic lupus erythematosus, etc.
See **exudate**.
lateral geniculate b. *See* **geniculate body, lateral**.
vitreous b. *See* **vitreous humour**.

white b. Sample exhibiting diffuse reflection and having a reflectance of approximately 100%. *Examples*: coating of magnesium oxide; sandblasted opal glass surface; plaster of Paris. *See* **coating; diffusion.**

Bommarito clip *See* **clipover.**

bone spicule A pigmentary configuration in the shape of a bone produced by migration of retinal pigment epithelium cells along blood vessels of the inner retina above areas where there is a loss of photoreceptor function. It is seen in retinitis pigmentosa.

bones of the orbit *See* **orbit.**

book retinoscopy *See* **retinoscopy, dynamic.**

botulinum toxin A poisonous substance which paralyses muscles and leads to inhibition of the release of acetylcholine from presynaptic neuromuscular terminals. The effect can last for weeks after being injected into a muscle. It is used as an alternative or addition to extraocular muscle surgery in the management of strabismus, in particular to assess whether surgery would be helpful. It is also sometimes used in the management of blepharospasm and occasionally nystagmus. *Example*: In lateral rectus paresis, injection into the medial rectus muscle (ipsilateral antagonist) paralyses its action and thus the practitioner can observe the function of the lateral rectus and determine the risk of postoperative diplopia. *See* **chemodenervation.**

bouton *See* **axon; neuron.**

Bowen's disease *See* **disease, Bowen's.**

Bowman's layer *See* **layer, Bowman's.**

boxing centre; system *See* under the nouns.

brachium of the superior colliculus A bundle of nerve fibres that leaves the optic tract below the pulvinar of the thalamus to enter the pretectal nucleus near the superior colliculus. Some fibres also connect the superior colliculus to the lateral geniculate body. Damage to the brachium results in a reduced pupil reflex to light, but does not affect a reflex to near objects. *See* **nucleus, pretectal; reflex, near; reflex, pupil light.**

brachymetropia Term proposed by Donders for myopia.

brachytherapy *See* **radiotherapy, plaque.**

bracketing A procedure used in subjective refraction in which large and equal steps of dioptric changes are made above and below the presumed correct answer, and then reducing the size of the dioptric changes and shifting the centre of the range, until the finest and just detectable blur is induced by equal steps above and below the refractive error. It is commonly used with patients with low vision and also to check the range of clear vision provided by a near addition.

Braille System of printing for blind persons, consisting of points raised above the surface of the paper used as symbols to indicate the letters of the alphabet. Reading is accomplished by touching the points with the fingertips.

brain *See* **meninges.**

brainstem Part of the brain located between the cerebral hemispheres and the spinal cord and comprising the midbrain, the pons and the medulla oblongata. It contains the nuclei of most cranial nerves such as the fourth-trochlear (in the inferior colliculus in the dorsal part of the midbrain), fifth-trigeminal (in the pons), sixth-abducens and seventh-facial (in the lower border of the pons) and the third-oculomotor (in the midbrain). The midbrain integrates information coming from higher brain centres such as the primary visual cortex, the frontal cortex and the superior colliculi and controls many activities (e.g. breathing, heartbeat) as well as eye movements, through a thick bundle of ascending and descending neurons running throughout the brainstem called the **reticular formation.** *See* **fascilus, medial longitudinal; movement, eye; pons.**

break point *See* **point, break.**

break-up time test *See* **test, break-up time.**

Brewster's angle *See* **angle of polarization.**

Brewster's stereoscope *See* **stereoscope, Brewster's.**

bridge The part of a spectacle frame which forms the main connection between the lenses or rims. The bridge assembly is generally taken to include the pads, if any (British Standard). *See* **spectacles.**

flush b. The bridge of a spectacle frame with zero projection.

inset b. A spectacle frame so shaped that the bearing surface of the bridge is behind the plane of the lenses.

keyhole b. Bridge of a spectacle frame with pads, looking like the outline of the upper part of a keyhole.

pad b. Bridge of a spectacle frame with two pads acting as the resting surface on the nose.

saddle b. A bridge so shaped as to rest on the nose over a continuous area, but in which the ends of the bearing surface are extended to lie behind the back plane of the front (British Standard).

brightness Attribute of visual sensation according to which an area appears to emit more or less light. *Syn.* luminosity. *Note 1*: In British recommended practice, the term brightness is now reserved to describe brightness of colour (i.e. the opposite of dullness) as used in the dyeing industry. *Note 2*: This attribute is the psychosensorial correlate, or nearly so, of the photometric quantity luminance (CIE).

Brightness Acuity Tester (BAT) *See* **glare tester.**

b. constancy *See* **constancy, brightness.**

b. enhancement *See* **effect, Brücke–Bartley.**

brimonidine tartrate *See* **alpha-adrenergic agonist.**

brinzolamide *See* carbonic anhydrase inhibitors.

broad H test *See* test, motility.

Broca's pupillometer *See* pupillometer, Broca's.

Broca–Sulzer phenomenon *See* effect, Broca–Sulzer.

Brock's after-image test *See* test, after-image transfer.

Brock's string A white string used to demonstrate physiological diplopia. One end of the string is placed against the bridge of the nose and the other end against a distant object (e.g. a doorknob). The subject should see two strings intersecting wherever the horizontal components of the visual axes meet. Red and green filters, one before each eye, enhance or facilitate the observation of the two strings. Several beads, each of a different colour, are usually threaded on the string so that they can be moved at will. One bead may be used for fixation while the other/s appear double, in crossed diplopia for the one closer to the eyes than the fixation bead and in uncrossed diplopia for the one further away than the fixation bead. Brock's string is commonly used in visual training. The observation of physiological diplopia with Brock's string is often referred to as **Brock's string test**. *Syn.* bead on string.

Brodmann's areas *See* area, Brodmann's.

browlift A cosmetic procedure used to correct sagging eyebrows and remove the wrinkles of the forehead.

Brown's superior oblique tendon sheath syndrome *See* syndrome, Brown's superior oblique tendon sheath.

Bruch's membrane *See* membrane, Bruch's.

Brücke's muscle *See* muscle, ciliary.

Brücke–Bartley effect *See* effect, Brücke–Bartley.

Bruckner's test *See* test, Bruckner's.

bruit A sound heard on auscultation of the heart, lungs, large arteries or veins, or any large cavity (e.g. the orbit). The auscultation is carried out with a stethoscope. *Example*: An occlusive disease of the carotid artery caused by atherosclerosis leads to a reduction in blood flow through the carotid arteries (and a concomitant reduction in blood flow through vessels of the eye and orbit). It gives rise to a swishing sound with the chest piece of the stethoscope on the neck over the carotid artery.
See amaurosis fugax.

brunescent cataract *See* cataract, nuclear.

brushes, Haidinger's *See* Haidinger's brushes.

Brushfield's spots *See* spot, Brushfield's.

B-scan *See* ultrasonography.

buckling, scleral *See* retinal detachment, rhegmatogenous; scleral buckling.

bulbar Pertaining to the eyeball.

bulbar conjunctiva *See* conjunctiva.

bull's eye maculopathy *See* maculopathy, bull's eye.

bulla A fluid-filled blister appearing on the surface of the cornea when it is severely oedematous (increased thickness of more than 25%). It gives rise to a reduction of visual acuity and pain on rupturing. *Example*: bullous keratopathy. *Plural*: bullae.
See keratopathy, bullous.

bullous keratopathy *See* keratopathy, bullous.

bundle of light *See* light, beam of.

Bunsen–Roscoe law *See* law, Bunsen–Roscoe.

buphthalmos A large eye with a megalocornea due to elevated intraocular pressure. The condition affects infants younger than about 3 years, the eye is commonly myopic and there may be lens subluxation. *Syn.* hydrophthalmos.
See glaucoma, congenital; megalophthalmos.

bupivacaine hydrochloride A local anaesthetic of the amide type used in eye surgery. It is used in 0.25–0.75% solution. It is often mixed with lidocaine hydrochloride. Its action starts after about 5 minutes and lasts for about 10 hours.

Burton lamp *See* lamp, Burton.

Busacca's nodules *See* Koeppe's nodules.

button. **1.** The preformed piece of glass which will become the segment of a fused bifocal or multifocal lens. It is ground and polished on one side to the appropriate curvature for fusing to the main lens (British Standard). **2.** The disc of corneal tissue removed from a donor or grafted into a host in keratoplasty.
See keratoplasty; lens, bifocal.

C

CAB Cellulose acetate butyrate is a transparent thermoplastic material that was used in the manufacture of rigid gas permeable contact lenses as it transmits some oxygen. It is a copolymer with varying percentages of cellulose, butyryl and acetyl. It is also used to make spectacle frames. New material containing silicone, fluorine and methyl methacrylate in various proportions have replaced this material for rigid gas permeable lenses.

caecum *See* spot, blind.

'café au lait' spots *See* neurofibromatosis type 1.

calcarine fissure *See* fissure, calcarine.

caliper A device used to measure distances between structures or surfaces. It usually comprises a scale at one end, while at the other end are two legs, which can be adjusted to the appropriate measurement. *Example*: lens thickness caliper.

caloric nystagmus *See* caloric testing.

caloric testing A neuro-ophthalmic technique in which cold and warm water is used to stimulate the vestibular system creating horizontal nystagmus (called **caloric nystagmus** or **Barany's nystagmus**). *See* test, caloric.

camera, fundus A camera attached to an indirect ophthalmoscope aimed at photographing the image of the fundus of the eye. This image is produced by the objective of the ophthalmoscope at the first focal point of the objective of the viewing microscope (and of the camera), which forms an image on the film. A flip mirror within the optical path of the viewing microscope allows the observer to view the image of the fundus and focus it, thus ensuring that the image being photographed is as clear as that being viewed. Fundus cameras usually require a dilated pupil of about 4 mm and their fields of view extend up to 45°. Wide-angle cameras can capture images up to 140°. They provide an objective photographic record of any condition in the fundus. They can also be used to take photographs of the anterior segment of the eye. *See* fundus, ocular; ophthalmoscope, indirect; ophthalmoscope, scanning laser.

camera obscura *See* camera, pinhole.

camera, pinhole A camera in which the lens is replaced by a pinhole (e.g. **the camera obscura**).

campimeter An instrument for the measurement of the visual field, especially the central region (usually within a radius of 30°). *See* chart, Amsler; perimeter; screen, tangent.

campimetry Measurement of the visual field with a campimeter.

Canada balsam A transparent resinous substance produced by the sap of the Canadian balsam fir and used to cement glass (doublet, beam-splitting prisms, the segment of a bifocal lens, etc.). Its index of refraction is equal to about 1.54. It has nowadays been superseded by modern chemical adhesives.

canal A tubular channel which allows the passage of air, food, blood, excretions, secretions or anatomical structures such as nerves or blood vessels.
Cloquet's c. *See* canal, hyaloid.
Hannover's c. A space about the equator of the crystalline lens between the anterior and posterior parts of the zonule of Zinn and containing aqueous humour and zonular fibres (Fig. C1).
hyaloid c. Channel in the vitreous humour, running from the optic disc to the crystalline lens.

In foetal life, this canal contains the hyaloid artery, which nourishes the lens, but it usually disappears prior to birth. *Syn.* central canal; Cloquet's canal; Stilling's canal.
See hyaloid remnant.
infraorbital c. Channel beginning at the infraorbital groove in the floor of the orbit and ending at the infraorbital foramen of the maxillary bone opening onto the face below the inferior orbital margin. It is a channel for the infraorbital artery and the infraorbital nerve.
lacrimal c. *See* canal, nasolacrimal.
nasolacrimal c. Channel that extends from the fossa of the lacrimal sac to the anterior, medial wall of the orbit and ends in the inferior meatus of the nasal cavity. It contains the nasolacrimal duct through which tears drain. *Syn.* lacrimal canal. *See* lacrimal apparatus.
optic c. Canal leading from the middle cranial fossa to the apex of the orbit in the small wing of the sphenoid bone through which pass the optic nerve and the ophthalmic artery. At the entrance of the canal into the orbit is the optic foramen. *See* meninges.
c. of Petit A space between the posterior fibres of the zonule of Zinn and the anterior surface of the vitreous humour (Fig. C1).
Schlemm's c. A circular venous sinus located in the corneoscleral junction, anterior to the scleral spur and receiving aqueous humour from the anterior chamber and discharging into the aqueous and the anterior ciliary veins (Fig. C1). *Syn.* scleral sinus; sinus circularis iridis; sinus venosus sclerae; venous circle of Leber.
See meshwork, trabecular; scleral spur; vein, aqueous.
Stilling's c. *See* canal, hyaloid.

canaliculi *See* lacrimal apparatus.

canaliculitis Inflammation of a lacrimal canaliculus, found most frequently in the lower one. It is caused by an infection usually from a bacterium, the most common being Gram-positive *Actinomyces israelii*, but it may be due to a fungus or a virus. The patient presents with a red, irritated eye with 'pouting' of the punctum and a slight discharge, which can be expressed by compressing the canaliculus. Treatment usually consists of irrigation and topical antibiotics.

candela The candela is the luminous intensity in a given direction of a source emitting monochromatic radiation of frequency 540×10^{12} Hz and the radiant intensity of which in that direction is 1/683 watt per steradian. The candela so defined is the base unit applying to photopic quantities. *Symbol*: cd.

candela per square metre SI unit of luminance. *Syn.* nit. *Symbol*: cd/m^2.
See luminance; SI unit.

candlepower Designates a luminous intensity expressed in candelas.

'can-opener' capsulotomy *See* capsulotomy.

canthal tendon *See* ligament, palpebral.

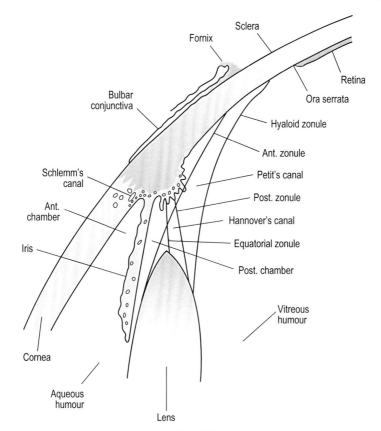

Fig. C1 Section diagram through the anterior portion of the eye.

canthus The angle formed by the upper and lower eyelids at the nasal (**inner canthus** or **medial canthus**) or temporal (**outer canthus** or **external angle**) end. *Plural*: canthi. *Syn*. palpebral angle. *See* **caruncle, lacrimal; conjunctivitis, angular; epicanthus.**

capsular fixation Process of inserting an intraocular lens implant into the capsular bag following cataract extraction.
See **capsulectomy; phacoemulsification.**

capsular opacification This is usually the result of cataract surgery. The most common late complications are posterior capsular opacification and, to a lesser extent, cystoid macular oedema. Soon after the operation, there may be blurring of vision, corneal oedema, as well as Elschnig's pearls and capsular fibrosis.
See **capsulotomy; capsulorhexis; Elschnig's pearls; oedema, cystoid macular.**

capsular tension ring *See* **ring, capsular tension.**

capsule 1. A membrane or sheath enclosing a tissue or organ. **2.** A case, usually made of gelatin, containing a drug for oral administration.
See **'bag' capsular.**

capsule, Bonnet's *See* Tenon's capsule.

capsule, crystalline lens Transparent elastic capsule covering the crystalline lens. It is made of collagen fibrils embedded in a glycosaminogly-can matrix. The thickness of the capsule varies; the anterior portion is thicker than the posterior, and it is also thicker towards the periphery (or equator). This variation in thickness plays a role in moulding the lens substance, contributing to an increase in the curvature of the front surface, in particular, during accommodation. The capsule increases in thickness with age, and its modulus of elasticity decreases with age, which (besides a flattening of the lens and a hardening of the lens substance) contributes to presbyopia (Fig. C2). Under electron microscopy, the capsule appears to have a lamellar structure that disappears with age. The capsule receives the insertion of the zonular fibres. The posterior capsule is liable to rupture following cataract surgery and often results in a loss of vitreous humour.
See **capsular opacification; fibres, lens; modulus of elasticity; shagreen of the crystalline lens; theory, Fincham's; Zinn, zonule of.**

capsule, Tenon's *See* Tenon's capsule.

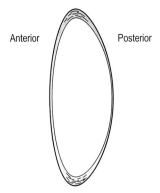

Anterior   Posterior

Fig. C2 Lens capsule of a person about 30 years old. It is thickest near the equator and at the anterior pole. With age, the thickest part of the lens is about halfway between the anterior pole and the equator.

capsulectomy The surgical removal of the capsule of the crystalline lens. In extracapsular cataract extraction, only the anterior portion of the capsule is removed.
See **capsulorhexis; capsulotomy.**

capsulorhexis A form of capsulotomy in which the incision of the anterior capsule is made with a **cystotome** in a smooth circular pattern along the periphery of the lens to enable removal of opaque lens material during phacoemulsification. It is the preferred method of capsulotomy when inserting an intraocular lens because it enables easy removal of the lens capsule due to the smooth circular pattern which is less likely to tear than that made by the jagged 'can-opener' technique.

capsulotomy Incision of the capsule of the crystalline lens. Capsulotomy of the anterior capsule is performed in phacoemulsification and extracapsular cataract extraction (**anterior capsulotomy**) to enable removal of opaque lens matter. The cuts are made with a **cystotome** along the periphery of the lens in a circular configuration or jagged (called **'can-opener' capsulotomy**, which is very rarely performed nowadays). It is also performed on the posterior capsule (**posterior capsulotomy**) when it has become opaque following extraction to regain the loss of visual acuity using a neodymium-yag laser.
See **after-cataract; capsule, crystalline lens; capsulorhexis; cataract extraction, extracapsular.**

carbachol *See* **parasympathomimetic drug.**

carbomer *See* **tears, artificial.**

carbon dioxide *See* **hypercapnia.**

carbonic anhydrase inhibitors Drugs which inhibit the carbonic anhydrase enzyme found in the ciliary epithelium of the ciliary body. This enzyme is essential for the formation of aqueous humour; its reduction results in a decrease in intraocular pressure. Those in use are sulfonamide derivatives. They are administered systemically (e.g. acetazolamide) or topically in the treatment of glaucoma. *Examples*: acetazolamide, brinzolamide, dichlorphenamide, dorzolamide.

carboxymethylcellulose *See* **tears, artificial.**

carcinoma A malignant tumour of the epithelium, the tissue that lines the skin and internal organs of the body. It tends to invade surrounding tissues and to metastasize to distant regions of the body via the lymphatic vessels or the blood vessels. It is a form of cancer. *Plural*: carcinomata. *Example*: carcinoma of the skin.
See **epithelioma; keratosis, seborrhoeic.**
   basal cell c. A slow-growing tumour derived from the basal cells of the epidermis of the skin. It is mainly located on the head and neck and most commonly on the eyelids, especially the lower eyelid. Old people, especially with fair skin, who have had extensive sun exposure are primarily affected. It appears, initially, as a raised nodule with a pearly surface with small dilated blood vessels on its surface, and it may eventually become ulcerated (rodent ulcer) and invade other tissues but rarely metastasizes. Treatment includes surgical excision or cryotherapy.
   lacrimal gland c. Malignant tumour of the lacrimal gland. It presents in middle-aged patients with progressive proptosis, limitation of eye movements and orbital pain. Management consists of exenteration and radiotherapy.
See **gland, pleomorphic adenoma of the lacrimal.**
   sebaceous gland c. Malignant tumour arising from the meibomian glands or occasionally from the glands of Zeis. It frequently affects the upper eyelids of old people. Initially the tumour resembles a chalazion or a chronic blepharitis. However, this tumour is aggressive and may invade the orbit. It may metastasize. Treatment usually consists of thorough surgical excision.
See **blepharitis; chalazion.**
   squamous cell c. Malignant skin cancer that affects the eyelids and conjunctiva. It is aggressive and may metastasize. It occurs most commonly in old people who have had extensive sun exposure. Treatment consists mainly of surgical excision.
See **xeroderma pigmentosum.**

Cardiff acuity test *See* **test, Cardiff acuity.**

cardinal planes; points *See* under the nouns.

cardinal positions of gaze *See* **position, cardinal p's. of gaze.**

cardinal rotation Rotation of the eye from the primary position to a secondary position about either the *x*-axis or the *z*-axis.
See **axis, transverse; axis, vertical; position, primary; position, secondary.**

carmellose *See* **tears, artificial.**

carotene A complex, unsaturated hydrocarbon found as a red or yellow pigment in many fruits and vegetables, including carrots, sweet potatoes, apricots, spinach and dairy products. The two main forms are alpha (α-carotene) and beta (β-carotene), which is the most common form.

They are converted into vitamin A in the liver, where it is bound to a protein and transported through the bloodstream. It produces the molecule retinal of the rod and of the three cone photopigments. *See* **photopigment; vitamin A deficiency.**

carrier 1. *See* **lens, lenticular. 2.** A person who has inherited an allele for a genetic trait but is not affected by the trait associated with the gene. Carriers may pass on the gene to their offspring who display the trait. *Example*: A woman may be a carrier of a red-green colour vision deficiency.

carteolol hydrochloride *See* **sympatholytic drugs.**

caruncle, lacrimal *See* **lacrimal caruncle.**

case study; case-control study *See* under the nouns.

case history *See* **history, case.**

Cassegrain telescope *See* **telescope.**

cast *See* **eye impression.**

cat's eye syndrome *See* **syndrome, cat's eye.**

catadioptric system *See* **system, catadioptric.**

cataphoria *See* **kataphoria.**

cataract Partial or complete loss of transparency of the crystalline lens substance or its capsule, possibly due to alteration in the protein regular arrangement that normally contributes to transparency, and to alteration of protein structure due to oxidation. Cataract may occur as a result of age, trauma, systemic diseases (e.g. diabetes, neurofibromatosis type 2), secondary to ocular diseases (e.g. anterior uveitis), high myopia, long-term steroid therapy, excessive exposure to infrared and ultraviolet light, smoking, heredity, corticosteroid use, maternal infections, Down's syndrome, etc. The incidence of cataract increases with age, amounting to more than 50% in the population over 82 years. It is also more prevalent in Africa, Asia and South America than in Europe and North America. The main symptom is a gradual loss of vision, often described as 'misty'. Some patients may also notice transient monocular diplopia, others notice fixed spots (not floaters) in the visual field and others have better vision in dim illumination. Cataracts can easily be seen with a retinoscope, the ophthalmoscope and especially with the slit-lamp, although, depending on the type, one instrument may be better than the other. At present, the main treatment is surgical. Extraction is performed for one of three reasons: visual improvement, medical or cosmetic. *See* **after-cataract; arthritis, juvenile idiopathic; biometry of the eye; capsule, crystalline lens; disease, Fabry's; disease, Wilson's; dysphotopsia; entoptoscope, blue field; galactosaemia; glare tester; grading scale; hyperacuity; lens, crystalline; lens, intraocular; leukocoria; maxwellian view system, clinical; myopia, lenticular; phacoemulsification; scatter; sight, second; syndrome, Down's; vitreous, persistent hyperplastic primary.**
age-related c. Cataract affecting older persons. It is the most common type of cataract and may

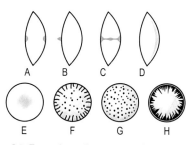

Fig. C3 Examples of cataracts (A, bipolar; B, pyramidal; C, axial; D, subcapsular (cupuliform); E, nuclear; F, coronary; G, snowflake; H, cuneiform).

take several forms: cortical, cuneiform, nuclear, mature or subcapsular. *Syn.* senile cataract.
anterior capsular c. A small central opacity located on the anterior lens capsule, either of congenital origin or due to a perforating ulcer of the cornea. *See* **sign, Vogt's.**
axial c. An opacity situated along the anteroposterior axis of the crystalline lens (Fig. C3).
bipolar c. An opacity involving both the anterior and the posterior poles of the lens (Fig. C3). *See* **cataract, polar.**
blue c. *See* **cataract, blue-dot.**
blue-dot c. A developmental anomaly of the crystalline lens characterized by numerous small opacities located in the outer nucleus and cortex. They appear as translucent bluish dots. The condition is very common and does not usually affect acuity. *Syn.* blue cataract; diffuse cataract; punctate cataract.
brown; brunescent c. *See* **cataract, nuclear.**
capsular c. Opacity confined only to the capsule of the crystalline lens, anteriorly or posteriorly. It is usually congenital, although it may be acquired as a result of trauma or inflammation.
central c. *See* **cataract, nuclear.**
chalky c. A cataract characterized by the presence of lime salt deposits.
Christmas tree c. Rare type of diffuse age-related cataract in which the opacities appear as highly reflective crystals.
complicated c. A cataract caused by or accompanying another intraocular disease, such as glaucoma, cyclitis, anterior uveitis or a hereditary retinal disorder such as retinitis pigmentosa or Leber's disease. *Syn.* secondary cataract. *See* **cataract, cuneiform; Leber's hereditary optic atrophy; retinitis pigmentosa; syndrome, Down's; syndrome, Fuchs'; syndrome, rubella.**
congenital c. Rare type of cataract occurring as a result of faults in the early development of the lens. Some may be hereditary, usually autosomal dominant. The cause of others may be chromosomal abnormalities (e.g. Down's syndrome, Edward's syndrome, Turner's syndrome), sugar metabolic disorders (galactosaemia, galactokinase deficiency), rubella syndrome, or an intrauterine infection (e.g. rubella, varicella, toxoplasmosis). In

many instances, the opacity is located in a discrete zone of the lens and, in half of the cases, it is bilateral. The condition requires urgent treatment to prevent the development of amblyopia.

See **cataract, capsular; cataract, lamellar; cataract, nuclear; cataract, polar; cataract, sutural; galactosaemia; syndrome, Edward's; syndrome, Lowe's; toxoplasmosis.**

coronary c. A cataract characterized by a series of opacities having the shape of a crown or ring near the periphery of the lens (Fig. C3).

cortical c. Cataract affecting the cortex of the lens. The opacities often begin as spokes or isolated dots or clusters forming the cuneiform or subcapsular types of cataract, but eventually the opacity spreads through the entire cortex.

cuneiform c. Age-related cataract characterized by opacities distributed within the periphery of the cortex of the lens in a radial manner, like spokes on a wheel (Fig. C3).

See **cataract, subcapsular.**

cupuliform c. *See* **cataract, subcapsular.**

diabetic c. Cataract associated with diabetes. In old eyes this type is similar to that of a non-diabetic person but in young eyes it is typically of the snowflake type.

diffuse c. *See* **cataract, blue-dot; cataract, Christmas tree.**

electric c. An opacity caused by an electric shock.

c. extraction, extracapsular Surgical procedure for the removal of a cataractous crystalline lens. The anterior capsule is excised after a viscoelastic substance (e.g. sodium hyaluronate) has been injected into the anterior chamber as a protection, especially of the corneal endothelium, the lens nucleus is removed and the residual equatorial cortex is aspirated. The posterior capsule may be polished. An intraocular lens implant may then be inserted.

See **after-cataract; biometry of the eye; capsulectomy; Elschnig's pearls; iodine-povidone; lens, intraocular; phacoemulsification; ring, Soemmering's.**

c. extraction, intracapsular Surgical procedure for the removal of a cataractous crystalline lens. The entire lens, together with its capsule, is removed. This procedure is very rarely performed nowadays.

See **ligament of Wieger.**

fluid c. Hypermature cataract in which the lens substance has degenerated into milky fluid.

glassblower's c. *See* **cataract, heat-ray.**

heat-ray c. Cataract due to excessive exposure to heat and infrared radiation. *Syn.* glassblower's cataract; thermal cataract.

See **exfoliation of the lens; infrared.**

hypermature c. Last stage in the development of age-related cataract. In this case, the lens substance has disintegrated.

See **cataract, incipient; cataract, intumescent cortical; cataract, mature; glaucoma, phacolytic.**

incipient c. First stage in the development of age-related cataract. It is characterized by streaks similar to the spokes of a wheel or with an increased density of the nucleus.

See **cataract, intumescent cortical; cataract, mature; lens, crystalline; sight, second.**

intumescent cortical c. Stage of development of a cataract in which the lens, especially the cortex, absorbs fluid and swells. It may lead to secondary angle-closure glaucoma. The cataract can progress to the hypermature stage in which case the fluid leaks out, resulting in shrinkage of the lens and wrinkling of the anterior capsule, leaving the harder nucleus free within the capsule.

See **cataract, morgagnian.**

lamellar c. Congenital cataract affecting one layer of the crystalline lens only. *Syn.* zonular cataract.

mature c. Middle stage in the development of age-related cataract. It is characterized by a completely opaque lens and considerable loss of vision.

See **cataract, hypermature; cataract, incipient.**

morgagnian c. Hypermature age-related cataract in which the cortex has shrunk and liquefied and the nucleus floats within the lens capsule. Degraded lens proteins may leak into the aqueous humour and cause phacolytic glaucoma. *Syn.* cystic cataract; sedimentary cataract.

See **cataract, intumescent cortical.**

nuclear c. Opacity affecting the lens nucleus. It can be either congenital or age-related in origin. It frequently leads to an increase in myopia (or decrease in hyperopia). In some cases, it reaches such a brown colour that it is called **brunescent cataract** (or **brown cataract**). *Syn.* central cataract (Fig. C3).

polar c. A congenital opacity found at either pole of the crystalline lens. Anterior polar cataract may be flat or project as a conical opacity (**pyramidal cataract**) into the anterior chamber (Fig. C3). Posterior types may be associated with persistent hyaloid remnant (Mittendorf's dot).

See **lentiglobus.**

punctate c. *See* **cataract, blue-dot.**

pyramidal c. *See* **cataract, polar.**

senile c. *See* **cataract, age-related.**

secondary c. 1. *Syn.* for complicated cataract. **2.** *Syn.* for after-cataract.

snowflake c. A cataract characterized by greyish or whitish flake-like opacities. It is usually found in young diabetics or severe cases of diabetes (Fig. C3).

soft c. Cataract in which the lens nucleus is soft.

See **lens, crystalline.**

subcapsular c. An age-related opacity located beneath the anterior or posterior capsule. It may spread from the periphery of the cortex like spokes on a wheel (**cuneiform cataract**). This is the most common type of cortical cataract. The opacities may also be confined to the posterior layers of the cortex with a granular or lace-like appearance (**cupuliform cataract**). Subcapsular cataracts are often the result of radiation exposure, age, toxic damage (e.g. from corticosteroids) or secondary to eye diseases (e.g. uveitis, retinitis pigmentosa). (Fig. C3).

sunflower c. *See* chalcosis lentis.

c. surgery *See* capsulectomy; capsulorhexis; capsulotomy; cataract extraction, extracapsular; cataract extraction, intracapsular; phacoemulsification.

sutural c. Congenital cataract in which the opacities are found along the anterior and/or posterior lens sutures. The opacities may appear Y-shaped or flower-shaped. The condition is often associated with Fabry's disease.

thermal c. *See* cataract, heat-ray.

traumatic c. Cataract following injury to the lens, its capsule or to the eyeball itself. It is commonly unilateral. Penetrating trauma of the lens causes rapid opacification of the cortex or even most of the lens contents. Concussion of the lens may result in capsular, subcapsular or cortical opacities. *See* ring, Vossius'.

zonular c. *See* cataract, lamellar.

catoptric image *See* image, catoptric.

catoptrics The branch of optics which deals with reflection and reflectors.

caudal Term relating to the posterior end of an organism. In the brain, it can also refer to an inferior direction. *See* dorsal; rostral; ventral.

caustic The concentration of light in the caustic surface of a bundle of converging light rays which represents the focal image in an optical system uncorrected for spherical aberration. It appears as a hollow luminous cusp with its apex at the paraxial focus.

cavernous haemangioma; plexus; sinus *See* under the nouns.

cecocentral *See* centrocecal.

ceftazidime *See* antibiotic.

ceftriaxone *See* antibiotic.

cefuroxime *See* antibiotic.

cell 1. In biology, the basic, structural and functional unit from which living organisms and tissues are built. A cell consists of a nucleus surrounded by all the cellular contents (cytoplasm) including various organelles (mitochondria, Golgi apparatus, lysosomes, ribosomes, etc.) and inclusions (glycogen, melanin, triglycerides, etc.) suspended in intracellular fluid (water, proteins, carbohydrates, lipids, inorganic and organic substances) all enclosed in a plasma membrane. There are many types of cells (blood cells, connective tissue cells, epithelial cells, muscle cells, nerve cells, secretory cells, etc.). Living cells are capable of reproduction (for body growth, wound healing, etc.) by mitotic activity. **2.** In optics, a rim in a trial frame or in an optical instrument into which a lens can be placed. *See* protein.

A c. *See* cell, M.

acinar c. A type of cell found within the body of the lacrimal gland. This cell lines the lumens of glands in a lobular pattern and produces a serous secretion.

amacrine c. Retinal cell located in the inner nuclear layer connecting ganglion cells with bipolar cells, as well as with other amacrine cells. Some have an ascending axon synapsing with receptors.

B c. *See* cell, P.

basal c. *See* corneal epithelium.

binocular c. Cell in the visual cortex that responds to stimulation from both eyes. It may, however, show an ocular dominance for either eye. It responds more strongly when corresponding regions of each eye are stimulated by targets of similar size and orientation. *See* column, cortical; hypercolumn.

bipolar c. Retinal cell located in the inner nuclear layer connecting the photoreceptors with amacrine and ganglion cells. There are several types of bipolar cells: **midget bipolar** cells which receive inputs from a single foveal cone and connect with a single ganglion cell, **diffuse bipolar** cells which receive inputs from several cones and connect with many ganglion cells and **rod bipolar** cells which connect several rods to several ganglion cells. *See* potential, receptor.

C c. A retinal ganglion cell with slow axonal conduction which sends information to the superior colliculus and to the centre involved in the control of pupillary diameter, rather than to the lateral geniculate body. There are very few such cells. *Syn.* Pγ cell; W cell (thus called in the cat).

Cajal's c. *See* astrocytes.

clump c. Large pigmented round cells found in the pupillary zone of the iris stroma. They are considered to be macrophages containing mainly melanin granules. The number of these cells increases with age.

colour-opponent c's. Cells which increase their response to light of some wavelengths and decrease their response to others (usually complementary wavelengths). If the light stimulus contains both sets of wavelengths, the two responses tend to cancel each other. Two types of cells have been identified: red-green cells and blue-yellow cells. These cells are found mainly in the lateral geniculate bodies but also among retinal ganglion cells, and they form the blobs in the visual cortex. The responses of these cells support Hering's theory of colour vision. *Syn.* opponent-process cell (although this term also includes a cell that increases its response to white light and decreases its response to dark). *See* blobs; theory, Hering's of colour vision.

complex c. Cell in the visual cortex whose receptive field consists of a large responsive area, approximately rectangular in shape, surrounded by an inhibitory region. The stimulus, which is usually a slit or a straight line, gives an optimum response if appropriately orientated and falling anywhere within the excitatory area. These cells tend to respond optimally to the movement of a specifically orientated slit. Many complex cells also respond better when the optimally orientated slit is moved in one direction rather than in the opposite direction. In general, complex cells show non-linear spatial summation properties.

See area, visual; cell, hypercomplex; cell, simple; field, receptive; summation.

cone c. Photoreceptor of the retina which connects with a bipolar cell and is involved in colour vision and high visual acuity and which functions in photopic vision. The outer segment of the cell is conical in shape, except in the fovea centralis where it is rod-like. The **outer segment** (i.e. the part closest to the pigment epithelium) contains hollow discs (or lamellae), the membranes of which are joined together and are also continuous with the boundary membrane of the cone cell. The visual pigments are contained within these discs. Discs are formed at the base of the outer segment, near the cilium, and older discs are displaced towards the distal end where they are shed within about 2 weeks and phagocytosed by the retinal pigment epithelium. Cone discs form part of the outer segment membrane with which they are continuous. The **inner segments** contain a large amount of mitochondria, as well as Golgi complex and endoplasmic reticulum involved in protein synthesis. There are three types of cones, each containing a different pigment sensitive to a different part of the light spectrum. They are referred to as long-wave-sensitive (or **L-cones**), medium-wave-sensitive (or **M-cones**) and short-wave-sensitive (or **S-cones**). There are about six million cones in the retina, with the greatest concentration in the macular area (Fig. C4).
See **cilium; cone pedicle; effect, Stiles–Crawford; ellipsoid; layer of Henle, fibre; macula; phagocytosis; photopigment; pigment, visual; theory, duplicity; vision, photopic.**

fixed c. See keratocyte.

ganglion c. 1. Retinal cell that connects the bipolars and other cells in the inner plexiform layer with the lateral geniculate body. The axons of the ganglion cells constitute the optic nerve fibres. There are approximately 1.2 million ganglion cells in the human retina. There are many types of retinal ganglion cells. The two major types are the **magno** (**M** or **parasol**) **ganglion cells** which project mainly to the magnocellular layers of the lateral geniculate bodies, and the **parvo** (**P**) **ganglion cells** which project to the parvocellular layers of the lateral geniculate bodies. Two types of P ganglion cells

are noted: P1, which are **midget** cells and have small dendritic fields, and P2, which have large dendritic fields. M and P cells comprise about 10% and 82% of the ganglion cells, respectively (Table C1). **2.** One of a collection of nerve cell bodies found in a ganglion.
See **cell, C; cell, M; cell, P; melanopsin.**

glial c's. Cells found throughout the nervous system. They provide support and nutrition for neurons, as well as being involved in the operation of the brain, especially the fluid surrounding the neurons and their synapses. They are also believed to be involved in the reuptake of neurotransmitters from within the synaptic cleft. There are three types of glial cells: astrocytes, microglia and oligodendroglia. *Syn.* glia; neuroglia.
See **astrocytes; nerve, optic.**

goblet c. Cell of the conjunctival epithelium which secretes mucin.
See **gland, of Henle; mucin; xerophthalmia.**

horizontal c. Retinal cell located in the inner nuclear layer which connects several cones and rods together.

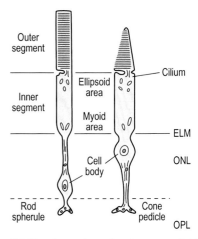

Fig. C4 Structures of a rod and a cone cell of the retina (ELM, external limiting membrane; ONL, outer nuclear layer; OPL, outer plexiform layer).

Table C1	Main distinguishing features of the two principal types of ganglion cells of the retina	
Properties	**P cell (X cell)**	**M cell (Y cell)**
size of cell body	small	large
dendritic spread	small	medium/large
receptive field size	small	medium/large
retinal distribution	90% of these at the macula	5% of these at the macula; about 13% overall
projection	LGN parvocellular layers	LGN magnocellular layers
type of response	sustained	transient
light sensitivity	low	high
wavelength response	selective (except P cells)	non-selective
spatial sensitivity	fine target detail	large target detail
temporal sensitivity	low target velocity	high target velocity

hypercomplex c. Cell in the visual cortex that receives inputs from several simple and complex cells and therefore has an even more elaborate receptive field than a complex cell. It is most effectively stimulated by a stimulus of a specific size and of a specific orientation and which is moved in a specific direction. *See* **cell, complex; cell, simple.**

koniocellular c. *See* **geniculate body, lateral.**

Langerhans' c's. Dendritic cells located mainly in the epidermis, mucous membranes and lymph nodes. They have surface receptors for immunoglobulin (Fc), complement (C3) and surface HLA–DR (Ia) antigen. Langerhans' cells are also found in the conjunctival epithelium and among the basal cells, mainly of the peripheral corneal epithelium. They have antigenic functions, stimulate T-lymphocytes, produce prostaglandin and participate in cutaneous delayed hypersensitivity and corneal graft rejection. Extended wear of contact lenses tends to induce an increase of these cells. They are also found in histiocytic tumours.

M c. Retinal ganglion cell located mainly in the periphery of the retina and which assists in movement perception. M cells tend to give **transient** responses to stimuli and to have non-linear spatial summation properties. This cell transmits information principally to the magno cells of the lateral geniculate bodies. *Syn.* A cell; Pαcell; Y cell (thus called in the cat).

magno c. *See* **cell, ganglion; geniculate body, lateral.**

mast c. Large cell found predominantly in connective tissue, which contains numerous cytoplasmic granules with substances such as heparin, histamine and serotonin that are released during allergic and inflammatory reactions. *See* **antihistamine; histamine; hypersensitivity; mast cell stabilizers.**

midget c. *See* **cell, ganglion.**

Mueller's c. Neuroglial cell in the retina which has its nucleus in the inner nuclear layer and fibres extending from the external to the internal limiting membrane. These cells support the neurons of the retina and possibly assist in their metabolism by storing glycogen thus protecting the retina from fluctuations in systemic glucose levels, uptaking potassium (K⁺) secreted by the photoreceptors and by being involved in phagocytosis following injury. *Syn.* Müller cell.

orientation-specific c. Cell that responds best to specifically orientated lines. This is the case for almost all cells in the visual cortex. *Examples*: complex cell; simple cell. *See* **cell, complex; cell, simple; field, receptive.**

P c. Retinal ganglion cell located mainly in the central region of the retina and which assists in high acuity and colour vision. P cells tend to give **sustained** responses to stimuli and to have linear spatial summation properties. This is the most common type of ganglion cells (about 82%). This cell transmits information principally to the parvo cells of the lateral geniculate bodies. *Syn.* B cell; Pβ cell; X cell (thus called in the cat).

parasol c. *See* **cell, ganglion.**

parvo c. *See* **cell, ganglion; geniculate body, lateral.**

photosensitive retinal ganglion c. (pRGC) A very rare type of ganglion cell comprising about 0.2% of all retinal ganglion cells. It contains a photosensitive pigment melanopsin. Photosensitive ganglion cells project (1) to the suprachiasmatic nucleus of the hypothalamus, which is responsible for the synchronization of the circadian rhythm; (2) to the pretectal olivary nucleus, which controls the pupillary light reflex (constriction and recovery of the pupil in response to light) and (3) to the lateral geniculate nucleus. This neural circuit appears to be independent of the conventional retinal phototransduction in the rods and cones and is not involved in image formation. *Syn.* intrinsically photosensitive retinal ganglion cell (ipRGC); melanopsin retinal ganglion cell (mRGC). *See* **melanopsin; transduction.**

Purkinje c. A type of efferent neuron that has a wide arborisation of dendrites extending towards the surface of the cerebellum with its cell body located in the cortex of the cerebellum and which is involved in eye movements such as the saccades. *See* **cerebellum; movement, eye.**

rod c. Photoreceptor cell of the retina which connects with a bipolar cell. It contains rhodopsin and is involved in scotopic vision. The molecules of rhodopsin are contained in about 1000 hollow discs (double lamellae or membranes), which are isolated from each other and from the boundary membrane of the rod cell. These discs are found in the **outer segment** (i.e. the part closest to the pigment epithelium) of the cell. Discs are formed at the base of the outer segment, near the cilium, and older discs are displaced towards the distal end where they are shed within about 2 weeks and are phagocytosed by the retinal pigment epithelium. The **inner segments** contain a large amount of mitochondria as well as Golgi complex and endoplasmic reticulum involved in protein synthesis. There are about 100 million rod cells throughout the retina; only a small area, the foveola, is free of rods (Fig. C4). *See* **cilium; eccentricity; ellipsoid; foveola; layer of Henle, fibre; phagocytosis; potential, receptor; rhodopsin; rod spherule; theory, duplicity; vision, scotopic.**

Schwann c. A cell whose membrane spirals around the axon with layers of myelin between each coil, as well as being a source of the myelin sheath. The cell provides insulation to the axon. It covers about 1 millimetre, so that hundreds may be needed to completely cover an axon. It also allows for an increase in the speed of the nervous impulse without an increase in axonal diameter. The gaps between the segments covered by the cells are called **nodes of Ranvier**. *See* **potential, action.**

simple c. A cell in the visual cortex whose receptive field consists of an excitatory and an inhibitory area separated by a straight line or by a long narrow strip of one response flanked on both sides by larger regions of the opposite response. Responses occur only to a straight line or a narrow strip orientated approximately parallel to the boundary/ies between the two areas. In general, simple cells show linear spatial summation properties. They are presumably the first cells where the nervous impulses are processed as they enter the visual cortex.
See **area, visual; cell, complex; field, receptive.**

squamous c. *See* **corneal epithelium.**

stem c. Cell that can undergo unlimited division to form other cells of a particular type. This is made possible because they contain a specialized enzyme that allows the stem cell to divide indefinitely and develop into many different cells that comprise various body tissues (e.g. gland, muscle, nerve, skin), the enzyme being different for each tissue.
See **corneal epithelium; limbus; stem cell deficiency, limbal.**

W c. *See* **cell, C.**

wing c. *See* **corneal epithelium.**

X c. *See* **cell, P.**

Y c. *See* **cell, M.**

cellulose acetate butyrate *See* **CAB.**

cellulitis, preseptal Swelling or infection of the eyelid tissue in front of the orbital septum usually caused by a Gram-positive bacterium *Staphylococcus* or *Streptococcus*. There is redness, swelling and tenderness of the eyelid. The condition is treated with systemic antibiotics.

cellulitis, orbital Infection of the orbital contents caused by *Staphylococcus aureus, Streptococcus pneumoniae* or *Haemophilus influenzae*. It is often caused by the spread of infection from adjacent structures, especially the sinuses. The clinical signs are fever, pain, proptosis, redness, swelling of the lid and orbital tissue and restricted eye movements which may occasionally lead to diplopia and, as the condition worsens, visual acuity decreases. Initial management consists of intravenous antibiotics but surgery may become necessary.
See **lamina papyracea.**

central corneal optical zone *See* **optical zone of cornea.**

central fusion *See* **fusion, sensory.**

central retinal artery; vein *See* under the nouns.

central retinal artery occlusion *See* **retinal artery occlusion.**

central retinal vein occlusion *See* **retinal vein occlusion.**

central serous retinopathy; vision; visual acuity *See* under the nouns.

centration distance; near distance; point *See* under the nouns.

centre, boxing The point midway between the two horizontal and the two vertical sides of the rectangle enclosing the lens, in the boxing system. *Syn.* geometric centre of a cut lens.
See **system, boxing.**

centre, optical That point (real or virtual) on the optical axis of a lens which is, or appears to be, traversed by rays emerging parallel to their original direction. Applied to an ophthalmic lens, it is commonly regarded as coinciding with the vertex of either surface (British Standard).
See **point, nodal; vertex.**

centre of rotation of the eye When the eye rotates in its orbit, there is a point within the eyeball that is more or less fixed relative to the orbit. This is the centre of rotation of the eye. In reality, the centre of rotation is constantly shifting but by a small amount. It is considered, for convenience, that the centre of rotation of an emmetropic eye lies on the line of sight of the eye 13.5 mm behind the anterior pole of the cornea when the eye is in the **straight-ahead position (straightforward position)**, that is when the line of sight is perpendicular to both the base line and the frontal plane.
See **axis, anteroposterior; line of sight.**

centre, standard optical position A reference point specific to each spectacle lens shape. The standard optical position is on the vertical line passing through the boxed centre, and it is at the boxed centre.
See **centre, boxing; system, boxing.**

centre, visual Centre of the brain concerned with vision.
See **area, visual; fissure, calcarine.**

centrocecal An area of the retina which includes the macula, the optic disc and the area in between. *Note*: also spelt centrocaecal. *Syn.* cecocentral.

cephalosporin *See* **antibiotic.**

cerebellum A large structure of the hindbrain lying behind the pons and upper medulla in the posterior cranial fossa and connected to the brainstem by three pairs of cerebellar peduncles. It is a major coordinator of movements including eye movements (e.g. pursuit movements) to which afferent impulses come from the visual and vestibular apparatus and the neck and which project to the supranuclear areas involved in eye movements (gaze centres).
See **cell, Purkinje; movement, eye; palsy, supranuclear.**

cerebrohepatorenal syndrome *See* **syndrome, Zellweger's.**

cerium oxide A pink powder derived from the metallic element cerium. It is used to polish lenses and it is also added to ophthalmic glass to absorb ultraviolet radiations.
See **polishing.**

cetirizine *See* **antihistamine.**

cetrimide *See* **antiseptic.**

chalazion A chronic inflammatory lipogranuloma due to retention of the secretion (such as blocked

chart   55

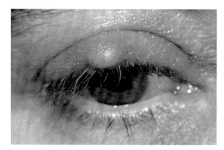

Fig. C5 Upper eyelid chalazion. (From Kanski 2007, with permission of Butterworth-Heinemann)

ducts) of a meibomian gland in the tarsus of an eyelid. It is characterized by a gradual painless swelling of the gland usually without marked inflammatory signs and sometimes astigmatism which is induced by the cyst pressing on the cornea (Fig. C5). Small chalazia may disappear spontaneously but large ones usually have to be incised and **curetted** (i.e. removal of the pus with a scraper) through a tarsal incision. Resolution may also occur after local injection of a corticosteroid drug (e.g. dexamethasone or triamcinolone), an antibiotic if there is a large infection, and hot compresses. *Syn.* meibomian cyst (although it is not a true cyst because its walls are made of granulomatous tissue and not lined with epithelium).
See **hordeolum, internal.**

chalcosis lentis A cataract caused by an excessive amount of copper in the eye. It appears as small yellowish-brown opacities in the subcapsular cortex of the lens and pupillary zone with petal-like spokes that extend towards the equator. It may be due to an intraocular foreign body containing copper, from eyedrops that contain copper sulfate or as part of Wilson's disease. Management consists mainly of removal of the foreign body. *Syn.* sunflower cataract.

chamber In anatomy, a small cavity.
anterior c. Space within the eye filled with aqueous humour and bounded anteriorly by the cornea and posteriorly by the iris and the part of the anterior surface of the lens which appears through the pupil. Its average axial length is 3.2 mm.
See **angle of the anterior chamber; flare, aqueous; gonioscope; method, van Herick, Shaffer and Schwartz; method, Smith's; optics of the eye; test, shadow.**
c's. of the eye The anterior, posterior and vitreous chambers of the eye.
posterior c. Space within the eye filled with aqueous humour and bounded by the posterior surface of the iris, the ciliary processes, the zonule and the anterior surface of the lens.
vitreous c. Space within the eye filled with vitreous humour and bounded by the retina, ciliary body, canal of Petit and the postlenticular space of Berger (see Fig. C1, p. 47).

Chandler's syndrome *See* **syndrome, Chandler's.**

channel A concept relating to the evidence that information about a particular feature of an image is transmitted and processed in the visual pathway approximately independently of information about other domains. The evidence was obtained from various experiments: matching, threshold elevation, after-effect, etc. *Examples*: the three channels of colour vision theory; the spatial frequency channels.
See **after-effect, waterfall.**

chaos, light *See* **light, idioretinal.**

Charles Bonnet syndrome *See* **syndrome, Charles Bonnet.**

chart 1. A tabular presentation of test targets for assessing vision. 2. A recording of clinical data relating to a patient's case.
Amsler c. One of a set of charts used to detect abnormalities in the central visual field which are so slight that they are undetected by the usual methods of perimetry. There are various patterns, each on a different chart, 10 cm square. One commonly used chart consists of a white grid of 5 mm squares on a black background. Each pattern has a dot in the centre, upon which the patient fixates. When fixated at a distance of 30 cm, the entire chart subtends an angle of 20°. If there is any visual impairment (usually as a result of macular disease), it is demonstrated by the absence or irregularities of the lines (Fig. C6). *Syn.* Amsler grid.
See **macular degeneration, age-related; metamorphopsia.**
astigmatic fan c. A test pattern consisting of a semicircle of radiating black lines on a white background for determining the presence and the amount, as well as the axis, of ocular astigmatism. If the chart resembles the 'clock face' type, it is called an **astigmatic dial** or **clock dial chart** (Fig. C7).
Bailey–Lovie c. A visual acuity chart with letter sizes ranging from 6/60 (20/200 or 1.0 logMAR) to 6/3 (20/10 or -0.3 logMAR) in 14 rows of 5 letters. Each row has letters which are approximately 4/5 the size of the next larger letters, and the

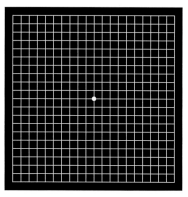

Fig. C6 Amsler chart.

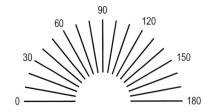

Fig. C7 Astigmatic fan chart.

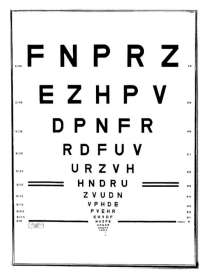

Fig. C8 Bailey–Lovie chart.

letters in each row have approximately the same legibility (within ±10%). It is most useful with low vision patients. This is the most commonly used type of logMAR charts (Fig. C8). There is also a **Bailey–Lovie Word Reading Chart** for near vision. It is composed of words rather than letters. The size progression of each line is logarithmic. The typeface used is the lower case Times Roman customarily used in newspapers and books, and the range of sizes varies between 80-point and 2-point print (or the Snellen equivalent at 40 cm of 6/144 or 20/480 to 6/3.6 or 20/12, respectively). There are 20 such charts, each with a different set of words.
See **acuity, near visual; chart, logMAR.**

clock dial c. *See* **chart, astigmatic fan.**

contrast sensitivity c. A chart designed to test contrast sensitivity. Such a test is useful with patients having low vision and in the early detection of diseases. *Examples*: Pelli–Robson chart; reduced contrast Bailey–Lovie near logMAR letter chart.
See **acuity cards, Teller; chart, Pelli–Robson; sensitivity, contrast; test, Melbourne Edge; test, Arden grating; Vistech.**

E c. Chart for carrying out a subjective visual acuity test on a person who cannot read or on

very young children. It consists of a graduated series of the Snellen letter E orientated in various directions and the subject must report in which direction the 'legs' of the E point. This procedure is sometimes called the **'E' test** or **'E' game**. *Syn.* illiterate E chart; tumbling E chart.
See **acuity cards, Teller; 'E' game; test, Cardiff acuity.**

illiterate E c. *See* **chart, E.**

Landolt broken ring c. A visual acuity chart using a graduated series of Landolt rings in which the target thicknesses and gaps are equal to one-fifth of the outer diameter. The subject must indicate the orientation of the gap, which usually appears in one of four directions: right, left, up or down. This test is less subjective than the Snellen chart. *Syn.* Landolt C chart.

logMAR c. A visual acuity chart in which the rows of optotypes vary in a logarithmic progression. The multiplier of the geometric progression is usually equal to 1.2589 or 0.1 log unit. Each row varies by 0.1 log unit, and each letter read correctly contributes 0.02 log unit. On one side of such a chart, the rows of optotypes are usually labelled with the traditional Snellen notation. On the other side of each row, visual acuity is labelled as the logarithm of the minimum angle of resolution (logMAR), which is the logarithm to the base 10 of the angular subtense of the stroke widths of the optotypes at a standard distance. logMAR charts provide more reliable and discriminative measurements of visual acuity than Snellen charts. It is recommended to report logMAR notation with or without Snellen notation. *Note*: MAR is an abbreviation for Minimum Angle of Resolution (Table C2).
See **chart, Bailey–Lovie; Glasgow acuity cards; test, Lea-Hyvarinen acuity.**

Mars c. *See* **chart, Pelli–Robson.**

Pelli–Robson c. A contrast sensitivity chart consisting of eight lines of letters, all of the same size, subtending 3 degrees at a viewing distance of 1 m. On each line, there are two groups, each containing three different letters; the letters in each group have the same contrast. The contrast of the different letters in each group decreases by a factor of 1/2 and the range of contrast varies between 100% and 0.6% in 16 steps. The subject is asked to read the letters starting with those of high contrast and continuing until two or three letters in one group are incorrectly named. The contrast threshold is represented by the previous group of correctly named letters. The chart gives the results in log contrast sensitivity. This test provides a measurement of contrast sensitivity at low to intermediate spatial frequencies depending upon the viewing distance. A similar chart is the Mars chart. *Syn.* Pelli–Robson contrast sensitivity test.

Raubitschek c. Test target for determining the axis and the amount of astigmatism of the eye. It consists of two parabolic lines (known as wings) in an arrowhead pattern, parallel and closely spaced at one end, and each diverging from each other through a 90° angle at the other end.

Table C2 Relationship between the Snellen fraction and the logMAR notation for distance visual acuity

Snellen fraction		logMAR
(m)	(ft)	
6/150	20/500	1.4
6/120	20/400	1.3
6/95	20/320	1.2
6/75	20/250	1.1
6/60	20/200	1.0
6/48	20/160	0.9
6/38	20/125	0.8
6/30	20/100	0.7
6/24	20/80	0.6
6/19	20/63	0.5
6/15	20/50	0.4
6/12	20/40	0.3
6/9.5	20/32	0.2
6/7.5	20/25	0.1
6/6	20/20	0
6/4.75	20/16	−0.1
6/3.75	20/12.5	−0.2
6/3	20/10	−0.3

Table C3 Relationship between Snellen visual acuity and letter height at two viewing distances (the letter corresponding to an acuity of 6/6 subtends 5' and the gap in the letter 1')

Snellen acuity		Letter height (mm)	
(m)	(ft)	4 m	6 m
6/3	20/10	2.9	4.4
6/4.5	20/15	4.4	6.5
6/6	20/20	5.8	8.7
6/7.5	20/25	7.3	10.9
6/9	20/30	8.7	13.1
6/12	20/40	11.6	17.5
6/15	20/50	14.5	21.8
6/18	20/60	17.5	26.2
6/24	20/80	23.3	34.9
6/30	20/100	29.1	43.6
6/36	20/120	34.9	52.4
6/48	20/160	46.5	69.8
6/60	20/200	58.1	87.3
6/120	20/400	116.4	174.5

There are several methods of using this test. *Syn.* Raubitschek arrows; Raubitschek dial.

reduced contrast Bailey–Lovie near logMAR letter c. A set of 30 Bailey–Lovie charts designed to measure contrast sensitivity. Each chart has a different contrast, half of the charts contains the letters of the distance Bailey–Lovie chart and the other half contains the letters of the near Bailey–Lovie chart. All the charts have the same average reflectance and the contrast of the charts ranges from 0.95% to 0.0013%. The charts are presented to the subject in order of increasing contrast, and the subject reads the letters from the largest to the smallest lines that they are able to. Threshold resolution in log min arc is determined for each of the 30 charts, and a contrast sensitivity curve can thus be determined.

Snellen c. A visual acuity test using a graduated series of **Snellen letters** (or Snellen test types) in which the limbs and the spaces between them subtend an angle of 1 minute of arc at a specified distance. The letters are usually constructed so that they are 5 units high and 4 units wide, although some charts use letters that fit within a square subtending 5 minutes of arc at that distance (Table C3).
See acuity, Snellen; Snellen fraction.

test c. A board externally illuminated, an internally illuminated transparent sheet, a slide for projection or a computer-based system which projects optotypes or other tests used in the subjective determination of refraction. *Syn.* letter chart.
See legibility; optotype.

tumbling E c. See chart E.

Chavasse lens *See* lens, Chavasse.

check ligament *See* ligament, check.

checkerboard pattern *See* pattern, checkerboard.

cheiroscope An instrument used in the management of amblyopia, suppression and hand and eye coordination. It consists of presenting a line drawing to one eye (usually the dominant one), which is traced by a pencil or crayon in the field of view of the other eye. The two fields of view are separated by a septum, and a small mirror is used to reflect the line drawing. Stereoscopes can easily be adapted into cheiroscopes.

chelating agent A compound that renders an ion, usually a metal, biologically inactive by incorporating it into the structure of the molecule. The main chelating agent used in ophthalmic preparations is ethylenediamine tetraacetic acid (EDTA). It is commonly added to preservatives to enhance their efficacy against metal ions.
See ethylenediamine tetraacetic acid; keratopathy, band; wetting agents.

chemical burn An injury caused, usually, by alkali (e.g. ammonia, caustic potash, lime, sodium hydroxide) or acid (e.g. hydrochloric, sulphuric). The type and severity of the injury depends on the properties of the chemical and upon which ocular tissue is involved. However, alkali burns are more severe than acid burns because they penetrate the tissues more rapidly and more deeply. In all cases, immediate copious irrigation is crucial, followed by a topical anaesthetic to relieve pain. Irrigation is continued until repeated measurements of ocular pH reach and retain a normal value. Treatment includes cycloplegics, antibiotics, steroids and ascorbate (only in alkali burns) to restore collagen synthesis. Glaucoma medication may be needed to prevent an increase of intraocular pressure. In some cases, surgery may also be required.

chemodenervation A technique in which a pharmacologic compound (e.g. atropine, botulinum toxin) is used to paralyze a muscle or group of muscles. This technique is most often used in the treatment of certain forms of strabismus as well as blepharospasm.

chemosis Severe oedema of the conjunctiva. *See* **disease, Graves'.**

cherry-red spot *See* **disease, Niemann-Pick; disease, Sandhoff's; disease, Tay-Sachs; spot, cherry-red.**

Cheshire cat effect *See* **effect, Cheshire cat.**

chiasma, optic A structure located above the pituitary gland and formed by the junction and partial decussation (crossing-over) of the optic nerves. The fibres from the nasal half of the retina of the left eye cross over to join the fibres from the temporal half of the right retina to make up the right optic tract and vice versa. About 53% of the axons of the optic nerves cross to the opposite tract (Fig. C9). A lesion of the chiasma produces a typical field defect (heteronymous hemianopia). *Note*: also spelt chiasm.
See **circle of Willis; decussation; pathway, visual; stereo-blindness; tracts, optic.**

chiastopic fusion *See* **fusion, chiastopic.**

Chievitz, transient layer of *See* **layer of Chievitz, transient.**

chlamydial infection *See* **conjunctivitis, adult inclusion; keratitis, epithelial; ophthalmia neonatorum; trachoma.**

chlorambucil *See* **immunosuppressants.**

chloramphenicol A broad-spectrum antibiotic effective against a wide variety of Gram-negative and Gram-positive bacteria (but not *Pseudomonas aeruginosa*). It is commonly used in solution 0.5% or ointment 1% to treat bacterial conjunctivitis or blepharitis.
See **antibiotic.**

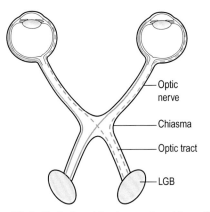

Fig. C9 An illustration of the decussation of the optic nerve fibres occurring in the optic chiasma. Information from one side of the visual field is transmitted to the contralateral, lateral geniculate body (LGB).

chlorbutanol *See* **antiseptic.**

chlorhexidine *See* **antiseptic.**

chlorolabe *See* **pigment, visual.**

chlorphenamine *See* **antihistamine.**

chlorophobia An abnormal aversion to green. *See* **chromatophobia.**

chloropsia *See* **chromatopsia.**

chocolate cyst *See* **lymphangioma.**

choked disc *See* **papilloedema.**

cholinergic Relates to neurons or nerve fibres in which acetylcholine (ACh) is the neurotransmitter, or have actions similar to those caused by ACh. Cholinergic receptors are of two types: **nicotinic** receptors, which are situated in striated muscles (e.g. the extraocular muscles), and **muscarinic** receptors, which are situated in parasympathetically innervated structures (e.g. the iris and ciliary body).
See **acetylcholine; nicotine; parasympathomimetic drug.**

choriocapillaris Layer of the choroid adjacent to Bruch's membrane and consisting of a network of capillaries which supplies nutrients to the retina.

chorioretinitis Inflammation of the retina and the choroid. It originates in the choroid and subsequently spreads to the retina.
See **nystagmus.**

chorioretinopathy *See* **syndrome, white dot.**

chorioretinopathy, central serous Accumulation of serous fluid found in the subretinal space, which leads to retinal detachment. It usually occurs in the central area of the retina and results in a sudden blurring, and/or metamorphopsia and acquired hyperopia. The condition, which is idiopathic, typically affects stressed men between the ages of 20 and 45 years. It subsides by itself within a few months in most cases; otherwise photocoagulation may be necessary.
See **retinal detachment, exudative.**

choristoma A congenital tumour composed of tissue not normally found at the affected site. The main type is dermoid cyst.
See **cyst, dermoid.**

choroid The highly vascular tunic of the eye lying between the retina and sclera. Its main function is to nourish the retina (oxygen and nutrients) and remove waste products. It is a thin membrane extending from the optic nerve to the ora serrata. It contains blood vessels, capillaries, nerves, collagen and melanocytes, as well as fibroblasts, macrophages, mast cells and plasma cells. It consists of five main layers from without inward: the suprachoroid (lamina fusca), the layers of vessels (the large vessels of Haller's layer and the small vessels of Sattler's layer), the choriocapillaris (a capillary bed) and Bruch's membrane (lamina vitrea). The blood supply is provided mostly by the short posterior ciliary arteries and, to a lesser extent, by the long posterior ciliary arteries, as well

as some branches from anterior ciliary arteries. Venous blood drains into the vortex veins. The posterior choroid is thickest in hyperopia and thinnest in myopia. *Note:* Some authors consider the suprachoroid as belonging to the sclera. However, when choroid and sclera are separated, part of the suprachoroid adheres to the choroid and part to the sclera.
See **choroiditis; dystrophy, choroidal; epichoroid; haemangioma, choroidal; melanoma, choroidal; naevus, choroidal; neovascularization, choroidal; space, suprachoroidal.**

choroidal detachment A separation of the choroid from the sclera, usually resulting from intraocular surgery, a severe contusion, hypotony or from a vascular disease. Fluid accumulates in the suprachoroidal space. The ciliary body may be involved. Ophthalmoscopic examination reveals dark, convex, smoothly rounded elevations of both the retina and the choroid. Intraocular pressure may be very low, and some visual field defects may be present. *Syn.* choroidal effusion.
See **hypotony, ocular; syndrome, uveal effusion**.

choroidal flush This is the first evidence of fluorescein dye reaching the eye during the method of fluorescein angiography. It occurs some 10 to 15 seconds after dye injection and approximately 1 second before reaching the retinal circulation because the route from the ophthalmic artery to the choroidal circulation is shorter.

choroidal folds A condition characterized by lines, grooves or striae in the posterior fundus. Clinically, they appear as alternating light and dark lines possibly corresponding to folds in Bruch's membrane and the retinal pigment epithelium. They are most easily seen with fluorescein angiography. They may occur as a result of a retrobulbar tumour, choroidal tumour, posterior scleritis, ocular hypotony, in hyperopic eyes, papilloedema or idiopathic.
See **haemangioma, cavernous**.

choroidal metastasis This is the most common intraocular malignant neoplasm, which usually occurs as a secondary tumour following, for example bronchial or breast cancer. Patient may present with reduced visual acuity, a yellowish, ill-defined lesion in the fundus, which may be associated with exudative retinal detachment. Treatment is with radiotherapy or systemic chemotherapy.

choroidal melanoma; naevus; neovascularization *See* under the nouns.

choroidal rupture A rupture of the choroid, Bruch's membrane and retinal pigment epithelium, which usually occurs in the periphery and results from a blunt trauma to the eye. If it involves the foveal area, permanent visual loss may ensue. Occasionally, choroidal neovascularization develops due to damage to Bruch's membrane.

choroideremia A bilateral, X-linked, inherited progressive degeneration of the choroid and retinal pigment epithelium characterized by night blindness (nyctalopia) which begins in early youth. The condition is caused by mutation in the CHM gene on chromosome Xq21. Males are predominantly affected and usually myopic. The condition is mild and non-progressive in females. Both males and female carriers display a salt-and-pepper appearance of the fundus, but in adult males it advances to tunnel vision, complete retinal pigment and choroidal atrophy and eventually blindness. *Syn.* progressive choroidal atrophy; progressive tapetochoroidal dystrophy.
See **chromosome; field, visual f. expander; inheritance.**

choroiditis Inflammation of the choroid. The ophthalmoscopic appearance is a whitish-yellow area stippled with pigment. However, it is most often associated with an inflammation of the retina (chorioretinitis) and of the other tissues of the uvea. Vision is blurred if the lesion is in the macular area.
See **iritis; uveitis, posterior.**

choroiditis, Tay's *See* **drusen, familial dominant.**

chroma *See* **Munsell colour system.**

chromatic Pertaining to colour.

chromatic aberration; adaptation; dispersion; parallax *See* under the nouns.

chromatic stereopsis *See* **chromostereopsis.**

chromatic vision *See* **vision, colour.**

chromaticity Colour quality of a stimulus defined by its chromaticity coordinates, or by its dominant (or complementary) wavelength and its purity taken together (CIE).
See **saturation; wavelength, dominant.**

chromaticity diagram Plane diagram showing the results of mixtures of colour stimuli, each chromaticity being represented by a single point on the diagram (Fig. C10). Syn. colour triangle.
See **ellipses, MacAdam; illuminants, CIE standard; light, white; purple.**

chromatophobia An abnormal aversion to colours or to certain colours (e.g. **erythrophobia,** an abnormal aversion to red). It may be psychological or physiological, such as an abnormal sensitivity to some short wavelengths following cataract extraction. *Syn.* chromophobia.
See **chlorophobia; cyanophobia.**

chromatopsia Abnormal condition in which objects appear falsely coloured. Depending upon the colour seen, the chromatopsia is called **xanthopsia** (yellow vision), **erythropsia** (red vision), **chloropsia** (green vision) or **cyanopsia** (blue vision). This condition may appear after a cataract operation (blue and red vision) or following exposure to an intense illumination (red vision) or in people suffering from carbon monoxide poisoning and oxygen deprivation. It may cause some damage to the areas of the visual cortex involved in the processing of colour perception, because these areas are supplied with more blood vessels than other areas of the visual cortex. *Syn.* chromopsia.
See **euchromatopsia; xanthopsia.**

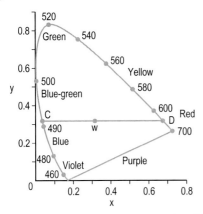

Fig. C10 The CIE chromaticity diagram (1931) (W, white light illuminant C; C and D, complementary wavelengths). Spectral colours are shown on the curved wavelength (or spectral) locus. Non-spectral purples are shown along the straight line joining the spectral limits, 400–700 nm.

chromophobia *See* **chromatophobia.**

chromophore The part of a molecule capable of absorbing light radiations. It is the 11-cis retinal of rhodopsin.
See **rhodopsin.**

chromoretinoscopy An objective method of measuring the longitudinal chromatic aberration of the eye by carrying out retinoscopy through various coloured filters (usually a red and a green filter). However, it is necessary to use a retinoscope source of high luminance (e.g. halogen). The difference in the retinoscopic value obtained with the two coloured filters represents the longitudinal chromatic aberration of the eye between these two dominant wavelengths.

chromosome One of the thread-like structures located within the cell nucleus composed of an extremely long, double-stranded DNA (deoxyribonucleic acid) helix tightly folded around proteins called histones. Each chromosome carries genes that contain the hereditary material that controls the growth and characteristics of the body. There are 46 chromosomes in each human somatic cell organized in 23 pairs, of which 22 pairs are similar in appearance but differ at the molecular level. They are called **autosomal chromosomes or autosomes** and are designated by a number (with chromosome 1 being the longest, followed by chromosome 2, etc.). The other pair, the **sex chromosomes,** determines the sex of the individual. In mammals, the two sex chromosomes of females are alike (homologous) and are referred to as X chromosomes. Males carry one X chromosome along with a much shorter Y chromosome. Each chromosome has a centromere that divides it into two arms, the short arm 'p' and the long arm 'q'. Disorders of chromosome number in which the number of chromosomes is above or below the normal (46) are called **aneuploidy.** Common forms of aneuploidy are **trisomy** in which there is one extra chromosome and **monosomy** in which there is one less than the normal 46. They rarely cause specific eye diseases, but affected individuals present ocular manifestations. *Examples:* Down's syndrome (trisomy of chromosome 21), Edward's syndrome (trisomy 18), Patau's syndrome (trisomy 13), Turner's syndrome (monosomy 45 XO). There are other chromosome abnormalities such as **translocation** (one segment of a chromosome is transferred to another chromosome) as may occur in congenital anterior polar cataract, **deletion** (a loss of a piece of chromosome) as in aniridia, choroideremia, retinoblastoma, etc. Other cases involve damage of a chromosome (e.g. fragile X syndrome).
See **colour vision, defective; DNA; gene; mitosis; mutation.**

chromostereopsis A sensation of apparent depth among coloured objects placed at the same distance from the subject and viewed binocularly, when the pupils are eccentric to the achromatic axes, or the visual axes do not coincide with the achromatic axes. This phenomenon is attributed to the retinal disparity created by the chromatic aberration of the eye. If the objects are red and blue (or green), the red appears closer than the blue (or green) in many people. Other people see the reverse impression and a few others do not see any apparent depth at all. The phenomenon can be enhanced, eliminated or reversed by using prisms or pinhole pupils placed in different regions of the pupil. If the pinhole pupils are decentred symmetrically temporally in front of the natural pupils, the red object will appear closer than the blue (**positive chromostereopsis**), and if they are decentred nasally, the blue object appears closer than the red (**negative chromostereopsis**). Apparent depth is eliminated when the pinholes are centred on the achromatic axes or when using prisms of appropriate power and direction. *Syn.* chromatic stereopsis; colour stereoscopy.
See **aberration, longitudinal chromatic; parallax, chromatic.**

chronic In health care, pertains to a condition of long duration and/or recurs frequently. *Examples:* blepharitis; dry eye.
See **acute.**

chrysiasis A deposition of gold in tissues, especially in the cornea, conjunctiva and the lens, leading to cataract. It occurs as a result of prolonged gold therapy (e.g. gold tablets, which are occasionally used in the treatment of rheumatoid arthritis).

cicatricial ectropion; entropion; pemphigoid *See* under the nouns.

ciclosporin (cyclosporine) An immunosuppressant used in the treatment of the ocular manifestation of autoimmune diseases, uveitis, scleritis, keratoconjunctivitis sicca and ligneous conjunctivitis, and to prevent rejection of corneal grafts, etc. It is believed to exert its immunosuppressive effect by inhibiting the activation of cytotoxic T-lymphocytes. *See* **immunosuppressants**.

CIE standard illuminants *See* **illuminants, CIE standard**.

cilia The eyelashes (*singular*: cilium).

ciliares, striae *See* **stria**.

ciliary arteries *See* **artery, ciliary**.

ciliary block glaucoma *See* **glaucoma, ciliary block**.

ciliary body Part of the uvea, anterior to the ora serrata and extending to the root of the iris where it is attached to the scleral spur. It comprises the ciliary muscle and the ciliary processes and is roughly triangular in sagittal section and extends for about 6 mm. The whole ciliary body forms a ring. The part just beyond the ora serrata is smooth and is thus known as **pars plana** (**orbiculus ciliaris**), about 4 mm. Anterior to this lays a region of ridges, which are the ciliary processes; this region is called the **pars plicata** (**corona ciliaris**), about 2 mm. From the sclera inward the ciliary body consists of: the **supraciliaris** (supraciliary layers) which is made up of strands of collagen containing melanocytes and fibroblasts; the **ciliary stroma** which contains blood vessels, melanocytes and the ciliary muscle; and the **ciliary epithelium** which comprises an inner non-pigmented layer and an outer pigmented layer and is a continuation of the internal limiting membrane of the retina and of the retinal pigment epithelium, respectively. The cells of these layers (particularly those of the non-pigmented layer) appear to be actively engaged in ion and water transport and the production of aqueous humour. *See* **angle, recession; cyclitis; iridodialysis; melanoma, ciliary body; muscle, ciliary; space, supraciliary; stria; ultrafiltration**.

ciliary epithelium *See* **ciliary body**.

ciliary flush *See* **injection, ciliary**.

ciliary ganglion; injection *See* under the nouns.

ciliary margin *See* **iris, plateau**.

ciliary muscle *See* **muscle, ciliary**.

ciliary nerve *See* **nerve, long ciliary**.

ciliary processes About 70 ridges, some 2 mm long and 0.5 mm high, which are arranged meridionally forming the pars plicata of the ciliary body. The ciliary processes consist essentially of blood vessels which are the continuation forward of those of the choroid. The region of the ciliary processes is the most vascular of the whole eye. The ciliary epithelium of the processes, which projects from the ciliary body, is involved in the secretion of aqueous humour. *See* **aqueous humour; diffusion; transport, active; ultrafiltration**.

ciliary ring *See* **annulus ciliaris**.

ciliary spasm *See* **accommodation, spasm of**.

ciliary sulcus *See* **sulcus, ciliary**.

ciliosis Spasmodic twitching of the eyelids.

cilium 1. An eyelash (*plural*: cilia). **2.** A short thin tube that connects the inner to the outer segment of a photoreceptor (Fig. C4, p. 52). *See* **cell, cone; cell, rod**.

ciprofloxacin *See* **antibiotic**.

circadian rhythm *See* **rhythm, circadian**.

circle, blur; of confusion *See* **blur circle**.

circle of Haller *See* **circle of Zinn**.

circle of least confusion The smallest cross-section of a circular bundle of an astigmatic pencil formed by an astigmatic lens and situated between the two focal lines. *See* **astigmatism; Sturm, conoid of**.

circle of Vieth–Müller *See* **horopter, Vieth–Müller**.

circle of Willis Arterial ring surrounding the optic chiasma and hypothalamus. It is formed anteriorly by the anterior cerebral arteries which are linked by the anterior communicating artery; posteriorly, by the division of the basilar artery into the posterior cerebral arteries and, laterally the latter are united by the posterior communicating arteries to the internal carotid arteries. An aneurysm in one part of the circle of Willis may compress the optic chiasma, resulting in a visual field loss. As the terminal branches of the internal carotid arteries are called the middle cerebral arteries, the circle of Willis is sometimes considered to be formed laterally by the latter (Fig. C11). *See* **artery, internal carotid; haemorrhage, preretinal; hemianopia, heteronymous**.

circle of Zinn Anastomosing circle of short ciliary arteries which have pierced the sclera about the optic nerve. Branches pass forward to the choroid, inward to the optic nerve and backward to the pial network. *Syn.* circle of Haller.

citric acid cycle *See* **Krebs cycle**.

City University test *See* **test, City University colour vision**.

CLARE *See* **contact lens acute red eye**.

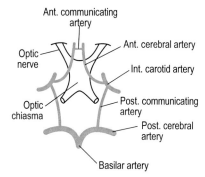

Fig. C11 Diagram showing the circle of Willis and the optic chiasma.

clearance, apical The distance between the posterior surface of a contact lens and the apex of the cornea.
See **bearing, apical.**

cliff, visual A device for testing depth perception. It consists of two identically patterned horizontal surfaces, one well below the other; the upper is extended over the lower by means of a sheet of transparent glass. A subject (usually a newborn of a species) placed in the centre of the upper surface and who is unwilling to move onto the transparent glass that projects over the lower surface is assumed to possess depth perception. Many species have been found to possess depth perception at birth, indicating an innate sense, unaffected by learning experience.

clinical interferometer *See* **maxwellian view system, clinical.**

clinical trial *See* **trial, randomized controlled.**

clinometer Apparatus used to measure ocular torsion.

clip, Halberg Trade name for a plastic device with two cells used for holding trial lenses which are clipped over a lens of a pair of spectacles (Fig. C12).

clip-on *See* **clipover.**

clipover An attachment holding an auxiliary lens or lenses (an add, a prism or a tint) in front of spectacles by spring action. There are many (albeit similar) types of clips that fit over one lens of a pair of spectacles (e.g. Bernell clip, Bommarito clip, Halberg clip, Jannelli clip). They are used extensively in the refraction of low vision patients. *Syn.* clip-on; fit-over; trial lens clip.

clip, trial lens *See* **clipover.**

clobetasone *See* **antiinflammatory drug.**

clock dial chart *See* **chart, astigmatic fan.**

Cloquet's canal *See* **canal, hyaloid.**

closed-angle glaucoma *See* **glaucoma, angle-closure.**

clotrimazole *See* **antifungal agent.**

clouding, central corneal *See* **corneal clouding, central.**

coated lens *See* **lens, coated.**

coating Process of depositing a thin film of transparent material on the surface of an optical element (e.g. lens, mirror, prism) for the purpose of decreasing or increasing its reflection. Reflection from specific wavelengths can be reduced or eliminated by varying the thickness of the film and by **multilayer coating.** *Syn.* blooming.
See **anti-reflection coating; body, white; filter, bandpass; Fresnel's formula.**

Coats' disease; white ring *See* under the nouns.

cobalt blue glass *See* **filter, cobalt blue; lens, cobalt.**

cobblestones *See* **conjunctivitis, giant papillary; conjunctivitis, vernal.**

cocaine Alkaloid derivative from coca leaves used as a local anaesthetic. It also produces a small dilatation of the pupil but does not act on the ciliary muscle.

Cochet–Bonnet aesthesiometer *See* **aesthesiometer.**

Cogan's lid twitch sign *See* **sign, Cogan's lid twitch.**

Cogan's microcystic epithelial dystrophy *See* **dystrophy, epithelial basement membrane.**

Cogan's syndrome *See* **keratitis, interstitial.**

Cogan–Reese syndrome *See* **syndrome, ICE.**

cognitive retinoscopy *See* **retinoscopy, dynamic.**

coherence Property of electromagnetic waves to remain in phase, the maxima and minima of all waves being coincident.

coherent sources If light beams from two independent sources reach the same point in space, there is no fixed relationship between the phases of the two light beams and they will not combine to form interference effects. Such light waves are called

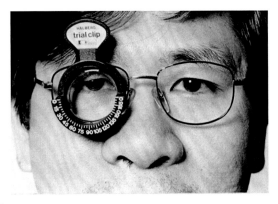

Fig. C12 Halberg clip.

incoherent. If, on the other hand, the two light beams are superimposed after reaching the same point by different paths but are both radiated from one point of a source, **interference** effects will be seen because the phase difference in the two beams is constant. The two virtual sources from which these two beams are apparently coming are called **coherent sources**, and any rays in which there is a constant phase difference are called **coherent rays**. Prior to the advent of the laser, the only way in which one could obtain coherent rays was by dividing the light coming from a point source into two parts.
See **experiment, Young's; holography; maxwellian view system, clinical; tomography, optical coherence.**

collagen The major protein of the white fibres of connective tissue, cartilage, tendons and bones. It is strong, fibrous, insoluble in water, rich in glycine and proline and can be hydrolyzed into gelatin by boiling. In the eye, it forms the primary structural component of the cornea, lens capsule, ciliary body, vitreous base and sclera. Collagen material is also used to make punctal occlusion plugs used to treat keratoconjunctivitis sicca and dissolvable therapeutic contact lenses to deliver high-dose drugs to the cornea. Mutations in collagen genes are a common cause of connective tissue disorders.
See **connective tissue disorders; occlusion, punctal.**

collarette Line separating the pupillary zone from the ciliary zone which can be seen on the anterior surface of the iris. In the normal iris, it is an irregular circular line lying about 1.5 mm from the pupillary margin (Fig. C13).
See **arterial circle of the iris, minor; Fuchs, crypts of.**

colliculi, inferior Two small rounded elevations situated on the dorsal aspect of the midbrain just below the two superior colliculi. They are relay centres for auditory fibres. *Syn.* inferior corpora quadrigemina.

colliculi, superior Two small rounded elevations situated on the dorsal aspects of the midbrain, just below the thalamus. Besides receiving fibres from each other, they receive a small number of axons from the optic tracts and serve as a relay centre for movements of the eyes, head and

neck in response to visual and other stimuli. The deeper layers of the colliculi also receive auditory and somatosensory inputs. Some fibres from the optic tracts pass through the colliculi and end in the pretectal olivary nuclei and are involved in pupil reaction. *Singular*: colliculus. *Syn.* superior corpora quadrigemina.
See **brachium; movement, saccadic eye; pathway, retinotectal; pretectum; reflex, pupil light; syndrome, Parinaud's.**

Collier's sign *See* **sign, Collier's.**

collimation 1. The making of a bundle of light rays parallel. **2.** In radiography, limiting the size of the beam to the required region on the patient, thereby protecting the remainder of the patient from radiation.

collimator An optical apparatus for producing parallel rays of light. It usually consists of a positive achromatic lens with an illuminated object (a slit, a graticule, a scale, etc.) placed at one of its focal points, so that light from any point on the object emerges from the collimator parallel.

colloid bodies *See* **drusen.**

collyrium An eye lotion. It does not, usually, contain any ocular medication. *Example*: physiological saline.

coloboma Congenital, pathological or operative anomaly in which a portion of the structure of the eye is lacking (e.g. coloboma of the choroid, coloboma of the eyelid, coloboma of the iris, coloboma of the lens, coloboma of the retina, etc.). Typical colobomas result from defective closure of the embryonic fissure of the optic cup, a closure which normally occurs within the 5th to the 8th week of gestation. Congenital iris colobomas are usually located inferiorly. They are often associated with Crouzon's syndrome (Fig. C13). Lid colobomas are commonly associated with Treacher–Collins syndrome. **Coloboma of the optic disc** is characterized by a glistening white excavation, decentred inferiorly. There may be reduced visual acuity depending on the severity of the coloboma. It is sometimes confounded with glaucomatous cupping, especially when it is accompanied by a field defect. The condition is often associated with microphthalmia and several syndromes (e.g. Edward's syndrome, Goldenhar's syndrome, Patau's syndrome).

coloboma, Fuchs' *See* **crescent, congenital.**

color *See* **colour.**

colorimeter An instrument for measuring a coloured stimulus by matching it with a known coloured sample.

colorimeter, photoelectric Colorimeter using a photoelectric cell and appropriate filters, instead of the eye.

colorimetric purity The physical property p of a colour stimulus in which the amount of white is evaluated by measuring the luminance of the stimulus wavelength $L\lambda$ and the luminance of the

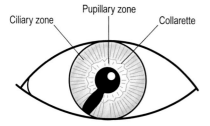

Fig. C13 Coloboma of the iris.

white light Lw which is combined with the stimulus wavelength, as expressed by

$$p = \frac{L\lambda}{L\lambda + Lw}$$

See **saturation.**

colorimetry The measurement of colour in terms of hue, saturation and brightness or other standard (spectral purity, spectral energy, etc.).
See **Munsell colour system.**

colour An aspect of visual perception, characterized by the attributes of hue, brightness and saturation, and resulting from stimulation of the retina by visible photopic light levels (Table C4). *Note*: also spelled color.

achromatic c. Visual sensation resulting from a stimulus having brightness, but devoid of hue or saturation (e.g. white, grey).

c. agnosia See agnosia.

c. blindness See blindness, colour.

complementary c. One of a pair of colours which, when mixed additively, produce white or grey (that is to say an achromatic sensation). *Examples*: Green is the complementary colour of red-purple and yellow is the complementary colour of blue.
See **chromaticity diagram.**

confusion c's. Colours that are confused by a dichromat. The colours confused by a deuteranope, a protanope and a tritanope are not the same. For example, the deuteranope will confuse reds, greens and greys, whereas the protanope will confuse reds, oranges, blue-greens and greys.
See **plates, pseudoisochromatic.**

c. constancy See constancy, colour.

c. contrast See contrast, colour.

c. vision, defective Marked departure of an individual's colour vision aptitude from that of a normal observer. This is indicated by various tests, e.g. anomaloscope, pseudoisochromatic plates, Farnsworth test. The following types of defective colour vision are usually recognized: **anomalous trichromatic vision** or **anomalous trichromatism**; **dichromatic vision** or **dichromatism**; **monochromatic vision** or **monochromatism** (total colour blindness), an anomaly of vision in which there is perception of luminance but not of colour. Both anomalous trichromatism and dichromatism occur in three distinct forms called respectively **protanomalous vision** and **protanopia**, **deuteranomalous vision** and **deuteranopia**, **tritanomalous vision** and **tritanopia** (Table C6). The causes of defective colour vision may be an impairment of a cone pigment or a reduced number of cone cells. The majority of cases of defective colour vision are inherited and thus bilateral. Acquired defects are rare, mostly tritanopic and appear in one eye or are asymmetric, and affect males and females equally. Hence it is essential to test colour vision under monocular conditions. The inherited type occurs as a sex-linked disorder in which the defective gene is on the X chromosome. Because men have only one X chromosome while women have two, sex-linked disorders (most being X-linked recessive) affect mainly males who inherit the genetic defect from their mother (the carrier). Inherited tritanopia and tritanomaly are usually autosomal dominant. For women to show the defect, both of their X chromosomes have to carry the defective gene, a rare occurrence. Defective colour vision occurs in about 8% of the male population and 0.5% of the female population. *Syn.* daltonism.
See **achromatopsia; anomaloscope; acquired colour vision deficiency; deuteranomaly; deuteranopia; inheritance; lens, ChromaGen; lens, X-Chrom; monochromat; pigment, visual; protanomaly; protanopia; rule, Kollner's; sensitivity, spectral; test; test, colour vision; tritanomaly; tritanopia; wavelength discrimination.**

c. fringes Coloured edges around images formed by a lens or an optical system which is not corrected for chromatic aberration.

fundamental c's. See colours, primary.

c. induction See induction, colour.

c. matching Action of making a colour appear the same as a given colour.

metameric c. Spectrally different radiations that produce the same colour under the same viewing conditions. *Note*: The corresponding property is called **metamerism**. *Syn.* metamers (CIE).

c. mixture The production of a colour by mixing two or more lights of different colours (**additive colour mixture**) or two or more pigments (**subtractive colour mixture**).
See **colour, complementary; colour, primary.**

Munsell c. See Munsell colour system.

non-spectral c. Any colour that does not exist as a single wavelength. *Example*: purple, which is a mixture of blue and red radiations (Fig. C10, p. 60).
See **purple.**

primary c's. Any sets of three colours such as, for example, red, green and blue, which, by additive colour mixture of the stimuli in varying proportions, can produce any colour sensation. *Syn.* fundamental colours.

spectral c's. The colours produced by the various radiations of the visible spectrum.
See **light.**

c. space See space, colour.

Table C4	Principal colours of the visible spectrum (approximate range)	
Colour	**Wavelength (nm)**	**Frequency ν (× 10¹⁴ Hz)**
violet	380–450	7.9–6.7
blue	451–490	6.65–6.12
green	491–560	6.1–5.35
yellow	561–590	5.34–5.08
orange	591–630	5.07–4.76
red	631–780	4.75–3.84

c. stereoscopy See **chromostereopsis**.

surface c. Colour perceived as belonging to a surface of an object which is not self-luminous.

c. temperature The temperature of the surface of an ideal black body which emits radiations of the same chromaticity as that from the source being specified. As the temperature increases, the amount of radiations increases and the source changes colour from red through to white to blue-white (Table C5). *Unit*: Kelvin (*symbol*: K). See **body, black; illuminants, CIE**.

c. triangle See **chromaticity diagram**.

c. vision See **vision, colour**.

c. vision, aetiology of See **colour vision, defective**.

colour-opponent cells See **cells, colour-opponent**.

column, cortical In the visual cortex, neurons with similar properties are arranged in columns (about 2 mm high) perpendicular to the surface of the cortex. The columns traverse the six cortical layers until they reach the white matter. Neurons through-out a column respond either to stimuli oriented at the same angle (**orientation column**) or to the inputs from the same eye (**ocular dominance column, ocular dominance slab**). A neighbouring column will then have neurons responding to a slightly different orientation from the one next to it and perhaps the same eye or the other eye. Neurons in layer 4 represent an exception, as they may respond to any orientation or to one eye only. Strabismus in early childhood disrupts the development of ocular dominance columns, thus preventing the development of depth perception. See **area, visual; blobs; hypercolumn**.

coma Monochromatic aberration of an optical system (e.g. a correcting lens) produced when the incident light beam makes an angle with the optical axis. The image appears like a comet with the tail pointing towards the axis. This relates to an optical system or lens, which are rotationally symmetrical about the axis. This is not the case in the eye and thus this aberration forms part of the higher-order wavefront aberrations of the eye. See **aberration; lens, aplanatic; sine condition**.

combination drugs See **antiinflammatory drug**.

combination lens See **lens, combination**.

combination system See **lens, piggy-back**.

comitance See **concomitance**.

commissure Band of nerve fibres connecting cor-responding structures in the brain or spinal cord. See **corpus callosum**.

commotio retinae A blunt trauma to the eye which damages the retina. It is commonly seen in the posterior pole as a dark grey area in the fundus, but may occur in the periphery as well. If confined to the posterior pole it is also called **Berlin's disease**. It is characterized by oedema and, if severe, haemorrhages. If the fovea is involved, a cherry-red spot may appear and visual acuity may be reduced. Generally, the condition subsides within 6 weeks unless very severe and in that case macular pigmentary degeneration may develop. See **disease, Berlin's**.

Table C5 Approximate colour temperature (in K) of some light sources

clear blue sky	12000–26000
overcast sky	6600
sun	5000–6000
electronic flash	about 5600
moonlight	4000
tungsten-halogen lamp	3000
tungsten filament lamp	2600
candle flame	2000

Table C6 Prevalence (%) and classification of colour vision defects

	Anomalous trichromats		
	Deuteranomal	**Protanomal**	**Tritanomal**
male	4.6%	1%	0.0001%
female	0.35%	0.03%	unknown
colour response	slight green deficiency	red deficiency	blue deficiency
	Dichromats		
	Deuteranope	**Protanope**	**Tritanope**
male	1%	1.1%	0.005%
female	0.01%	0.01%	0.003%
colour response	green deficiency	insensitive to red	blue deficiency
neutral point	498 nm	493 nm	570 nm
	Monochromats		
	cone monochromat	rod monochromat	
	unknown	0.003%	

compensated heterophoria *See* heterophoria, compensated.

compensating prism *See* prism, relieving.

compensatory eye movements *See* reflex, static eye.

complementary after-image; colour *See* under the nouns.

complex cell *See* cell, complex.

compliance The willingness to strictly follow the instructions given by a clinician. *Example*: following the cleaning instructions and wearing schedule given after contact lens fitting.

compound astigmatism; eye; optical system *See* under the nouns.

computer vision syndrome *See* syndrome, computer vision.

computerized perimeter; tomography *See* under the nouns.

concave Pertains to a surface shaped like the inside of a sphere.
See lens, diverging; mirror, concave.

concomitance The condition in which the two eyes move as a unit, that is, maintaining a constant angle between them for all directions of gaze when fixating at a fixed distance. *Syn.* comitance. *See* incomitance; strabismus, concomitant.

concretions, conjunctival *See* conjunctival concretions.

condenser An optical system with a large aperture and small focal length used in microscopes and projectors to concentrate as much light as possible onto an object. *Syn.* condensing lens.

condenser, Abbé's A microscope substage condenser consisting of a doublet with a high numerical aperture.
See aperture, numerical; doublet; triplet.

condensing lens *See* condenser.

cone cell *See* cell, cone.

cone degeneration; dystrophy *See* dystrophy, cone.

cone monochromat *See* monochromat.

cone pedicle The wide synaptic terminal of a cone photoreceptor located in the outer molecular (outer plexiform) layer of the retina. There are deep pits (invaginations) in the base of the terminal that contain the dendrites of bipolar and horizontal cells, often two of the former and one of the latter, in each invagination. The neurotransmitter is glutamate, which is stored in vesicles contained in the terminals, and when the photoreceptors are stimulated by light, the release of glutamate is decreased.
See cell, cone; hyperpolarization; neurotransmitter.

cone-rod dystrophy *See* dystrophy, cone-rod.

confocal Having the same focus. *Example*: In a slit-lamp, the microscope and the illumination system have the same focus, i.e. they are confocal. *See* microscope, confocal; ophthalmoscope, confocal scanning laser.

conformer A plastic shell placed in the eye over the orbital implant after enucleation or evisceration. It is used to prevent contraction of the surrounding healing tissues and to avoid rubbing of the palpebral conjunctiva against the sutures made along the conjunctival tissue which encloses the orbital implant. It is worn for some 6 to 8 weeks after surgery prior to fitting an artificial eye. *See* enucleation; orbital implant.

confrontation test *See* test, confrontation.

confusion, circle of *See* blur circle.

confusion colours *See* colour, confusion.

congenital Pertaining to a condition that dates from the time of birth. It may be inherited or caused by an environmental factor.
See acquired; familial; hereditary.

congruous hemianopia; scotomas *See* under the nouns.

conical cornea *See* keratoconus.

conjugate Adjective meaning joined or having formed a pair.
See distance, conjugate; reflex, vestibulo-ocular; version.

conjugate distances *See* distance, conjugate.

conjugate movements *See* version.

conjugate points *See* distance, conjugate.

conjunctiva A thin transparent mucous membrane lining the posterior surface of the eyelids from the eyelid margin and reflected forward onto the anterior part of the eyeball where it merges with the corneal epithelium at the limbus. It thus forms a sac, the **conjunctival sac**, which is open at the palpebral fissure and closed when the eyes are shut. The depths of the unextended sac are 14 to 16 mm superiorly and 9 to 11 mm inferiorly. The conjunctiva consists histologically of three layers: the epithelium, which contains the goblet cells; the stroma, which contains the glands of Krause and Wolfring and the basement membrane, which contains lymphoid tissue and is essential in the regulation of ocular surface immune responses. The conjunctiva is divided into three sections: (1) The portion that lines the posterior surface of the eyelids is called the **palpebral conjunctiva**. It is itself composed of the **marginal conjunctiva**, which extends from the eyelid margin to the **tarsal conjunctiva**; the tarsal conjunctiva, which extends from the marginal conjunctiva to the **orbital conjunctiva** and the orbital conjunctiva, which extends from the tarsal conjunctiva to the fornix. (2) That lining the eyeball is the **bulbar conjunctiva**. It is itself composed of the **limbal conjunctiva**, which is fused with the episclera at the limbus and the **scleral conjunctiva**, which extends from the limbal conjunctiva to the fornix. (3) The intermediate part forming the bottom of the **conjunctival sac**, unattached to the eyelids or the eyeball and joining the bulbar and the palpebral portion is called the **fornix** (or **conjunctival fold, cul-de-sac** or **forniceal conjunctiva**). *See* **conjunctivochalasis; dyskeratosis; eversion, lid; gland, conjunctival; Krause's end bulbs; sulcus, subtarsal.**

conjunctiva, corneal The stratified squamous epithelium of the cornea.

conjunctival concretions Minute, hard, whitish spots of calcium which present in the palpebral conjunctiva due to cellular degeneration. This condition occurs most commonly in the elderly or in people with prolonged conjunctivitis. They are asymptomatic but may be removed with a needle. *Syn.* conjunctival lithiasis.

conjunctival injection *See* **injection, conjunctival.**

conjunctival lithiasis *See* **conjunctival concretions.**

conjunctival naevus *See* **naevus, conjunctival.**

conjunctival sac *See* **conjunctiva.**

conjunctivitis Inflammation of the conjunctiva. It may be acute, subacute or chronic. It may be due to an allergy, an infection (e.g. *Staphylococcus, Streptococcus, Haemophilus*, etc.), a virus inflammation, an irritant (dust, wind, chemical fumes, ultraviolet radiation or contact lenses) or as a complication of gonorrhoea, syphilis, influenzae, hay fever, measles, etc. Conjunctivitis is characterized by various signs and symptoms, which may include conjunctival injection, oedema, small follicles or papillae, secretions (purulent, mucopurulent, membranous, pseudomembranous or catarrhal), pain, itching, grittiness and blepharospasm. The most common type of conjunctivitis is that due to a bacterium. Irrigation of the lid and the use of topical antiinfective agents are the usual treatment. *See* **conjunctival concretions; herpes zoster ophthalmicus; injection, conjunctival; mycophthalmia; ophthalmia neonatorum; syndrome, Stevens–Johnson; trachoma.**

actinic c. *See* **keratoconjunctivitis, actinic.**

acute c. Conjunctivitis characterized by an onset of hyperaemia (most intense near the fornices), purulent or mucopurulent discharge and symptoms of irritation, grittiness and sticking together of the eyelids on waking. In severe cases, there will be chemosis, eyelid oedema, subconjunctival haemorrhages and photophobia. The bacterial type is caused by *Staphylococcus aureus, Haemophilus influenzae* (*H. aegyptius*, Koch–Weeks bacillus) or *Streptococcus pneumoniae* (pneumococcus). A rare form of acute conjunctivitis is caused by the *Neisseria gonorrhoeae* species (gonococcus) or *Neisseria meningiditis* (meningococcus, e.g. **gonococcal conjunctivitis**), which produce a more severe form of the disease referred to as **hyperacute bacterial conjunctivitis** or **acute purulent conjunctivitis**. These require immediate treatment with systemic and topical antibiotics. Acute conjunctivitis is also caused by viruses (**viral conjunctivitis**), such as herpes simplex or adenoviruses. All forms of acute conjunctivitis occasionally spread to the cornea. **Bacterial**

conjunctivitis may in some cases resolve without treatment within 2 weeks. Management consists of topical antibiotic therapy (e.g. chloramphenicol, erythromycin) and cold compresses to relieve symptoms. **Acute allergic conjunctivitis** most typically resolves spontaneously, otherwise treatment includes sodium cromoglicate. **Acute viral conjunctivitis** caused by herpes simplex is treated with antiviral agents (e.g. acyclovir), although viral conjunctivitis caused by other viruses does not respond well to any drug therapy. Supportive treatment such as cold compresses relieves symptoms.

acute haemorrhagic c. Highly contagious viral infection of the anterior segment resulting in haemorrhage of the bulbar conjunctiva. The infection is caused by a picornavirus, often associated with pre-auricular adenopathy and a follicular conjunctivitis. The infection is self-limited and lasts 7 to 10 days. No specific treatment is presently available.

adult inclusion c. An acute conjunctivitis caused by the serotypes D to K of *Chlamydia trachomatis* and typically occurring in sexually active adults in whom the genitourinary tract is infected. Signs in the eye usually appear 1 week following sexual exposure. It may also occur after using contaminated eye cosmetics or soon after having been in a public swimming pool, or in newborn infants (called **neonatal inclusion conjunctivitis** or **neonatal chlamydial conjunctivitis**), which is transmitted from the mother during delivery and appears some 5 to 14 days after birth. The conjunctivitis is mucopurulent with follicles in the fornices, which often spread to the limbal region. The condition is commonly associated with punctate epithelial keratitis, preauricular lymphadenopathy, marginal infiltrates and, in long-standing infection, micropannus in the superior corneal region may also appear. Differentiation from viral follicular conjunctivitis is made through culture, serological and cytological studies. Treatment consists of using both systemic and topical tetracyclines, although in pregnant or lactating women erythromycin is preferable. *Syn.* adult chlamydial conjunctivitis; trachoma-inclusion conjunctivitis. *See* **follicle, conjunctival; keratitis, punctate epithelial; lymphadenopathy; ophthalmia neonatorum; trachoma.**

allergic c. Conjunctivitis which is due to a type 1 hypersensitivity reaction to allergens resulting in the release of histamine from mast cells in response to antigens binding to IgE antibodies on the surface of the mast cells. Common allergens are pollens associated with hay fever (**hay fever conjunctivitis**) and grass (seasonal **allergic conjunctivitis**), air pollutants, house dust mites and smoke (**perennial allergic conjunctivitis**). It is characterized by hyperaemia, itching, burning, swelling, tearing, discharge and small papillae. Conjunctival scrapings contain a large number of eosinophils, and serum IgE is elevated. The condition is commonly associated with rhinitis (**allergic rhinoconjunctivitis**) in which there is

also sneezing and nasal discharge. Treatment commonly includes decongestants, oral antihistamines, mast cell stabilizers (e.g. lodoxamine, sodium cromoglicate) and, if severe, topical corticosteroid eyedrops.
See antihistamine; atopy; conjunctivitis, vernal; decongestants; hypersensitivity; keratoconjunctivitis, atopic.

angular c. Subacute bilateral inflammation of the conjunctiva due to the diplobacillus of Morax–Axenfeld. It involves the conjunctiva in the region of the canthi.

bacterial c. *See* conjunctivitis, acute.

catarrhal c. Type of conjunctivitis associated with the common cold or catarrhal irritation. It can appear in the acute or chronic form.

cicatricial c. *See* erythema multiforme; pemphigoid, cicatricial; syndrome, Stevens-Johnson.

contact lens papillary c. *See* conjunctivitis, giant papillary.

contagious c. Acute conjunctivitis caused by Koch–Weeks bacillus, adenovirus types 3, 7 or 8 and 19, or a pneumococcus infection. It may be transmitted by respiratory or ocular infections, contaminated towels or equipment (e.g. tonometer heads). It is characterized by acute onset, redness, tearing, discomfort and photophobia. The condition is self-limiting in some cases, but keratitis is a common complication. *Syn.* epidemic conjunctivitis; epidemic keratoconjunctivitis; pink eye (colloquial).

eczematous c. *See* conjunctivitis, phlyctenular.

egyptian c. *See* trachoma.

epidemic c. *See* conjunctivitis, contagious.

flash c. Conjunctivitis due to exposure to an electric arc, as from a welder's torch.

follicular c. Conjunctivitis characterized by follicles (usually in one eye only) caused by adenoviruses or chemical or toxic irritation and frequently associated with lymphadenopathy.
See conjunctivitis, adult inclusion; follicle, conjunctival; lymphadenopathy.

fungal c. *See* mycophthalmia.

giant papillary c. Conjunctivitis, characterized by the appearance of 'cobblestones' (large papillae of 0.5 mm or more) on the tarsal conjunctiva of the upper eyelid (and sometimes the lower eyelid). Symptoms include itching, discomfort, mucous discharge and poor vision due to the presence of mucus. The condition may be induced by contact lens wear, ocular prosthesis or exposed sutures following surgery. This conjunctivitis closely resembles vernal conjunctivitis and is also believed to be an allergic condition. In its early stages as a contact lens-induced condition, it is often referred to as **contact lens papillary conjunctivitis** or **contact lens-associated papillary conjunctivitis**. In these cases, the regular use of surfactant and protein removal tablets as well as frequent lens replacement reduce the incidence of this condition, which is less prevalent with the wear of rigid gas permeable than soft contact lenses. Management may also include mast cell stabilizers (e.g. sodium cromoglicate) or antihistamine (e.g. levocabastine) and cessation of lens wear.

See conjunctivitis, vernal; deposits, contact lens; enzyme; surfactant.

gonococcal c. *See* conjunctivitis, acute.

granular c. *See* trachoma.

hay fever c. *See* conjunctivitis, allergic.

lacrimal c. Chronic conjunctivitis caused by an infection of the lacrimal passages.
See lacrimal apparatus.

ligneous c. A rare chronic conjunctivitis characterized by the formation of a firm whitish membrane or pseudomembrane on the tarsal conjunctiva, usually of the upper eyelid. It is typically bilateral, begins in childhood although it may present in patients up to age 85, is more common in females than in males and may persist for months or years. Its cause is unknown but the predisposing factors include bacterial and viral infections, trauma, hypersensitivity reactions and increased vascular permeability, and it is often associated with inflammations of other mucous membranes. The most effective treatment is surgical excision followed by topical cyclosporine drops, but the condition has a tendency to recur.
See conjunctivitis, pseudomembranous.

membranous c. *See* conjunctivitis, pseudomembranous.

neonatal c. *See* ophthalmia neonatorum.

phlyctenular c. *See* keratoconjunctivitis, phlyctenular.

pseudomembranous c. A non-specific inflammatory reaction characterized by the formation on the conjunctiva of a coagulated fibrinous plaque consisting of inflammatory cells and exudates containing mucus and proteins. This plaque forms either a membrane or a pseudomembrane. The latter adheres loosely to the conjunctival epithelium and can be peeled off without bleeding or damage to the underlying epithelium. A true membrane, on the other hand, usually occurs with intense inflammation (**membranous conjunctivitis**). In this case, the conjunctival epithelium becomes necrotic and adheres firmly to the overlying membrane which when peeled leaves a raw bleeding surface. The cause of either condition may be an infection, of which the common sources are herpes simplex virus, adenovirus, beta-haemolytic *Streptococcus*, *Neisseria gonorrhoeae* or as a result of the Stevens–Johnson syndrome, ligneous conjunctivitis, ocular cicatricial pemphigoid, atopic keratoconjunctivitis, chemical burns (especially alkali burns), radiation injury or postsurgical complications.

sun lamp c. *See* keratoconjunctivitis, actinic.

swimming pool c. *See* conjunctivitis, adult inclusion.

vernal c. Chronic, bilateral conjunctivitis which recurs in the spring and summer and is more often seen in boys than girls. Its origin is probably due to an allergy. It is characterized by hard flattened papillae of a bluish-white colour separated by furrows and having the appearance of 'cobblestones' located in the upper palpebral portion of the conjunctiva with mucus deposition between the papillae. A second type of vernal conjunctivitis

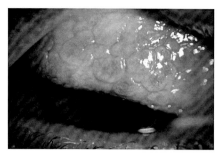

Fig. C14 'Cobblestones' papillae in severe vernal conjunctivitis. (From Kanski 2003, with permission of Butterworth-Heinemann)

exists which affects the limbal region of the bulbar conjunctiva, characterized by the formation of small, gelatinous white dots called **Trantas' dots** or **Horner–Trantas' dots**. The symptoms of the disease are intense itching and watering, and, if keratitis has developed, reduced acuity. Treatment consists mainly of cold compresses and limited (because of side effects) use of topical corticosteroids (e.g. dexamethasone, prednisolone). Sodium cromoglicate or lodoxamide have also been found to be very successful in treating this condition and with fewer side effects than corticosteroids. *Syn.* vernal keratoconjunctivitis (if the condition involves the cornea); spring catarrh; vernal catarrh (Fig. C14).
See **antihistamine; keratoconjunctivitis, atopic; mast cell stabilizers.**
viral c. Conjunctivitis caused by a virus. A variety of viruses can produce the disease, although adenovirus (a double DNA virus) is the most common. It is contagious and can be transmitted by fingers, instruments, in swimming pools or workplaces. It presents with watering, burning, itching, photophobia, eyelid oedema, hyperaemia and follicles and signs of keratitis. Management includes cool compresses and artificial tears, meticulous hand hygiene, and, if condition persists or worsens, topical steroids.
See **conjunctivitis, acute.**

conjunctivochalasis An abnormal fold of the bulbar conjunctiva typically located in the inferior part of the globe. Its cause is unknown, although it is age-related. It can cause symptoms ranging from ocular irritation, epiphora, dryness, to blurred vision. The condition is more common in older eyes. Treatment begins with artificial tears and topical steroids, if inflammation is present, but surgical excision of the redundant conjunctiva may be needed.

connective tissue A tissue of mesodermal origin consisting of fat cells, fibroblasts, mast cells, macrophages and protein fibres (mainly collagen) embedded in a ground surface of mucopolysaccharides. The proportion of the components varies, which accounts for the formation of many different tissues such as bone, cartilage, tendons, ligaments, adipose, aerolar and elastic tissues providing support, protection, binding and structure to the body.

connective tissue disorders Inherited conditions resulting from gene mutations that adversely affect the structure of connective tissues, such as the cornea, sclera, tendons and ligaments. *Examples*: Ehlers–Danlos syndrome, Marfan's syndrome, osteogenesis imperfecta, pseudoxanthoma elasticum, rheumatoid arthritis, scleroderma, Sjögren's syndrome, Stickler's syndrome and Weill-Marchesani syndrome.

conoid of Sturm *See* **Sturm, conoid of.**

consecutive esotropia; exotropia *See* **strabismus, consecutive.**

consensual An adjective descriptive of an involuntary response of one body structure as a result of stimulation of another. *Example*: the reflexive pupillary contraction of both pupils when one eye is stimulated by light.
See **reflex, pupil light.**

consent A voluntary approval from a person to be examined, treated or subjected to any test undertaken upon them. Consent must be obtained prior to any such intervention.

constancy Perceptual phenomenon in which the attributes of certain objects appear to remain relatively constant, despite changes in the stimulus characteristics which induced the perception. All constancies occur only within a limited range.
brightness c. Perceptual phenomenon whereby the brightness of an object appears to remain relatively constant, despite changes in the level of its illumination. *Example*: White paper appears white whether it is seen in sunlight or in the weaker or yellower illumination of a light bulb. *Syn.* lightness constancy.
colour c. Perceptual phenomenon whereby the colour of an object appears to remain relatively constant, despite changes in the spectral composition of the incident light.
shape c. Perceptual phenomenon whereby the shape of an object appears to remain relatively constant, despite changes in the viewing angle. *Example*: A circle held obliquely to the line of sight appears more circular than it should due to shape constancy although its retinal projection is oval.
size c. Perceptual phenomenon whereby the size of an object appears to remain relatively constant, despite changes in the viewing distance (and therefore of its retinal image size), up to a certain distance after which the object appears to change.

constants of the eye Average dimensions of the various parameters of the eye adopted to represent a typical eye. These vary slightly depending upon the authors, such as Donders, Gullstrand, Bennett–Rabbetts, etc (Table C7).
See **eye, reduced; eye, schematic.**

constant, Planck's *See* **photon.**

Table C7   Optical constants of an average adult Caucasian eye

Structure or surface	Refractive index	Radius of curvature (mm)	Distance from ant. surface of cornea (mm)
cornea	1.376	–	–
aqueous humour	1.336	–	–
lens (total)	1.42	–	–
vitreous humour	1.336	–	–
ant. corneal surface	–	7.8	0
post. corneal surface	–	6.5	0.5
ant. lens surface	–	10.6	3.6
accommodated	–	6.1	3.2
post. lens surface	–	–6.2	7.2
accommodated	–	–5.3	7.2
retina	1.363	–	24.1

Table C8   Constringence (V) of some transparent media (index of refraction *n*)

	n	V
Glass		
spectacle crown	1.523	59
dense barium crown	1.620	60
lanthana crown	1.713	54
zinc crown	1.508	61
light flint	1.581	41
dense flint	1.620	36
extra dense flint	1.706	30
titanium oxide	1.701	31
Polymer		
PMMA	1.492	57
CR-39	1.498	59
Polycarbonate	1.586	30
Polystyrene	1.590	31
Water (at 37°C)	1.331	56
Aqueous and vitreous (at 37°C)	1.334	56

constringence   A positive number (*symbol*: V) which specifies any transparent medium. It is equal to

$$V = n_d - 1/n_F - n_C$$

where n_d, n_F and n_C are the refractive indices for the Fraunhofer spectral lines d (587.6 nm), F (486.1 nm) and C (656.3 nm). A material with a high constringence (e.g. V = 50) produces less chromatic aberration than one with a low constringence (e.g. V = 30) (Table C8). The reciprocal of the constringence is called the **dispersive power**. *Syn.* Abbé's number; V-value.
See **dispersion; glass, crown; glass, flint; lines, Fraunhofer's.**

contact arc   *See* **arc of contact.**

contact lens   *See* **lens, contact.**

contact lens acute red eye (CLARE)   An acute corneal inflammation caused by overnight wear of soft contact lenses. It is characterized by pain, usually unilateral, redness, tearing, photophobia, corneal infiltrates and blurred vision that suddenly appears upon waking. The lens is, in most cases, tight or immobile and it is the breakdown of debris accumulated behind the lens that caused the inflammatory reaction. The lens must be removed immediately, and patching of the eye and antiinflammatory therapy may be necessary. *Syn.* immobile lens syndrome; non-ulcerative keratitis; tight lens syndrome.
See **lens, steep; ulcer, corneal.**

contour   The outline of a part of a retinal image where the light intensity changes abruptly corresponding to the boundaries of objects in the visual field. The physiological basis of **contour perception** and **edge detection** is thought to be mediated by the responses of complex and hypercomplex cells in area V1 of the primary visual cortex.
See **area, visual; cell, complex; test, Melbourne Edge.**
illusory c's. (subjective contours)   Contours perceived in the absence of a lightness or colour difference as in the Kanizsa figure (Fig. F5, p. 121). They are thought to be processed in area V2 of the visual cortex.
See **area, visual association; system, parvocellular visual.**
c. interaction   *See* **Glasgow acuity cards; phenomenon, crowding.**

contraindication   The presence of a condition or disease which renders some particular type of treatment undesirable. *Example*: Contact lenses are contraindicated in very dusty, dry and smoky atmospheres.

contralateral   Pertaining to the opposite side.
See **bilateral; geniculate body, lateral; ipsilateral; unilateral.**

contraocular   Pertaining to the opposite eye.

contrast   1. Subjective sense: subjective assessment of the difference in appearance of two parts of a field of view seen simultaneously or successively. Hence, **luminosity contrast, lightness contrast,**

colour contrast, simultaneous contrast, successive contrast. 2. Objective sense: quantities defined by the formulae for **luminance contrast**.

(a) $\dfrac{L_2 - L_1}{L_2}$ (b) $\dfrac{L_2 - L_1}{L_2 + L_1}$ (c) $\dfrac{L_2}{L_1}$

Note: Example (c) is better known as luminance ratio (CIE). L_2 is the maximum luminance and L_1 is the minimum luminance.
See **frequency, spatial; sensitivity, contrast; threshold, difference.**
brightness c. The enhanced apparent darkening of an area when viewed, or following, a lighter stimulus (or lightening, next to it or after a darker stimulus).
colour c. 1. A difference in the appearance of surfaces based on hue or saturation. 2. The enhanced difference in the colour of two surfaces induced by their proximity (**simultaneous colour contrast**) or successive stimulation (**successive colour contrast**). The appearance of the smaller area shifts towards the complementary colour of the surround or background. *Example*: A yellow area appears reddish when surrounded by a green background.
c. sensitivity *See* **sensitivity, contrast.**
c. sensitivity function *See* **function, contrast sensitivity.**
c. sensitivity test *See* **chart, contrast sensitivity; sensitivity, contrast.**
simultaneous c. Difference in the appearance of two adjacent areas occurring at the same time.
successive c. Difference in the appearance of stimuli following each other.
c. threshold *See* **sensitivity, contrast; threshold, difference.**

conus *See* **crescent, myopic.**

convention, sign *See* **sign convention.**

convergence 1. Movement of the eyes turning inward or towards each other (Fig. C15). **2.** Characteristic of a pencil of light rays directed towards a real image point.

See **angle of convergence; vergence.**
c. accommodation *See* **accommodation, convergence.**
accommodative c. That component of convergence which occurs reflexly in response to a change in accommodation. It is easily demonstrated by having one eye fixate from a far point to a near point along its line of sight, while the other eye is occluded. The occluded eye will be seen to make a convergence movement in response to the accommodation. Alternatively, one eye fixates while the other is occluded. If a minus lens is placed in front of the fixating eye, the occluded eye will be seen to converge. *Syn.* accommodative vergence; associative convergence.
See **convergence, fusional; convergence, initial; convergence, proximal; fusion, motor.**
amplitude of c. The angle through which each eye is turned from the far to the near point of convergence. *Syn.* amplitude of triangulation.
See **angle, metre.**
correction induced c. Convergence induced when changing from spectacles to contact lenses in near vision. Spectacles centred for distance vision induce base-in prisms in myopes and base-out prisms in hyperopes, in near vision. Thus, a spectacle-wearing myope converges less and a spectacle-wearing hyperope converges more than an emmetrope fixating at a given distance (Fig. C16). Optically centred contact lenses do not induce any prismatic effect, and the amount of convergence remains the same for all refractive errors. Consequently, myopes require more convergence and hyperopes less convergence when they transfer from spectacles to contact lenses. However, this change in convergence is accompanied by a similar change in accommodation, so that a myope transferring to contact lenses converges and accommodates more than with spectacles, and the reverse applies for a hyperope.
See **accommodation, correction induced; prism, induced.**

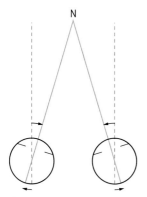

Fig. C15 Convergence from a distant to a near object N.

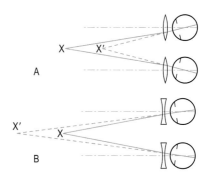

Fig. C16 Prismatic effects induced when an observer fixates a near object X wearing spectacle lenses centred for distance vision (A, plus lenses induce base-out prismatic effects and the hyperope overconverges to X'; B, minus lenses induce base-in prismatic effects and the myope underconverges to X').

c. excess A high esophoria at near, associated with a relatively orthophoric condition at distance. It usually gives rise to complaints of headaches and other symptoms of asthenopia accompanying prolonged close work.
See **accommodative excess.**

far point of c. Farthest point where the lines of sight intersect when the eyes diverge to the maximum.

fusional c. That component of convergence which is induced by fusional stimuli or which is available in excess of that required to overcome the heterophoria. It is usually a **positive fusional convergence**, but in some cases the eyes need to diverge to obtain fusion and this is called **negative fusional convergence**. An example is the movement of the eyes from the passive (one eye covered, the other fixating an object) to the active (both eyes fixating foveally the same object) position. However, as disparate retinal stimuli are a more powerful component of convergence than fusion, the concept of fusional convergence is being substituted by motor fusion (or disparity vergence).
See **convergence, accommodative; convergence, initial; convergence, proximal; convergence, relative; fusion, chiastopic; fusion, motor; fusion, orthopic; vergence facility.**

fusional reserve c. *See* **convergence, relative.**

initial c. Movement of the eyes from the physiological position of rest to the position of single binocular fixation of a distant object in the median plane and on the same level as the eyes. Initial convergence is triggered by the fixation reflex.
See **convergence, accommodative; convergence, fusional; position of rest, physiological.**

instrument c. *See* **convergence, proximal.**

c. insufficiency An inability to converge, or to maintain convergence, usually associated with a high exophoria at near and a relatively orthophoric condition at distance. It results in complaints of fatigue or even diplopia due to the inability to maintain (and sometimes even to obtain) adequate convergence for prolonged close work. Treatment includes orthoptic exercises (e.g. **the pencil-to-nose exercise** or **pencil push-up** in which the tip of a pencil is moved slowly towards the eyes while it is maintained singly for as long as possible; this procedure is repeated until the pencil can be brought within 10 cm before doubling occurs), or a reading addition sometimes with BI prisms.
See **accommodative insufficiency.**

convergence insufficiency symptom survey (CISS) score A method designed to quantify the severity of symptoms associated with convergence insufficiency. It consists of a questionnaire comprising 15 questions to which patients are asked to respond into 4 grades and from which a score is determined. The test has been found to be reliable and valid. A score greater than 16 in individuals less than 18 years of age and greater than 21 in individuals older than 18 years indicates symptoms.

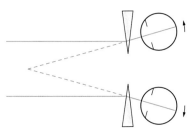

Fig. C17 Base-out prisms cause positive relative convergence movements of the eyes.

near point of c. The nearest point where the lines of sight intersect when the eyes converge to the maximum. This point is normally about 8 to 10 cm from the spectacle plane. If further away, the patient may have convergence insufficiency.

negative c. *See* **divergence.**

proximal c. Component of convergence initiated by the awareness of a near object. For example, when looking into an instrument the image may be at optical infinity yet proximal convergence may be initiated. *Syn.* instrument convergence; psychic convergence; proximal vergence.
See **accommodative, proximal.**

psychic c. *See* **convergence, proximal.**

relative c. That amount of convergence which can be exerted while the accommodation remains unchanged. Clinically, it is measured by using prisms base-out (**positive relative convergence** or **positive fusional convergence**) (Fig. C17) and/or base-in (**negative relative convergence** or **negative fusional convergence**) to the limits of blur but single binocular vision. Beyond that limit, accommodation changes. If the power of the base-out prism is increased, the image, though blurred, will still appear single until the limit of fusional convergence is reached and the image appears double (break point). The prism before the eyes now represents the **positive fusional reserve convergence (positive fusional reserve)**. Similarly, increasing the base-in prism, one reaches the break point, which represents the **negative fusional reserve convergence (negative fusional reserve)**. *Syn.* relative vergence.
See **criterion, Percival; criterion, Sheard; zone of clear, single, binocular vision.**

tonic c. *See* **vergence, tonic.**

total c. *See* **angle of convergence.**

voluntary c. Ability to converge the eyes without the aid of a fixation stimulus. Few people possess this ability, but it can be trained in most people.

convergence-retraction nystagmus *See* **nystagmus, convergence-retraction.**

convex Having a surface curved like the exterior of a sphere.
See **lens, converging; mirror, convex.**

copper deposits *See* **chalcosis lentis; disease, Wilson's.**

copper wire artery *See* **arteriosclerosis.**

coquille An unsurfaced lens, approximately plano, made by allowing sheet material to sag onto a shaped former (British Standard). This lens is often used in goggles.

corectopia A condition in which the pupil is not situated in the centre of the iris. It may occur as a result of iris melanoma, ocular surgery (e.g. trabeculectomy), trauma or from a congenital defect (e.g. coloboma, Rieger's anomaly). *Syn.* ectopia pupillae.
See **luxation of the lens; syndrome, Rieger's.**

coreometer *See* **pupillometer.**

cornea The transparent anterior portion of the fibrous coat of the globe of the eye. It has a curvature somewhat greater than the rest of the globe, so a slight furrow marks its junction with the sclera (the limbus). Looked at from the front, the cornea is about 12 mm horizontally and 11 mm vertically. It is the first and most important refracting surface of the eye, having a power of about 42 D. The anterior surface has a radius of curvature of about 7.8 mm, the posterior surface 6.5 mm and the central thickness is about 0.5 mm and increasing towards the periphery to about 0.68 mm. It consists of five layers, starting from the outside: (1) the stratified squamous epithelium, (2) Bowman's layer, (3) the stroma (substantia propria), (4) Descemet's membrane and (5) the endothelium. The cornea is avascular, receiving its nourishment by permeation through spaces between the lamellae. The sources of nourishment are the aqueous humour, the tears and the limbal capillaries. The cornea is **innervated** by the long ciliary and other nerves of the surrounding conjunctiva, which are all branches of the ophthalmic division of the trigeminal nerve. Innervation is entirely sensory. Within the cornea, there are only unmyelinated nerve endings. The density of nerves in the cornea is very high, making it the most sensitive structure in the body. The major **structural** component of the cornea is collagen, mostly type I, and most of the ground substance between the collagen fibrils in the corneal stroma is proteoglycans whose core proteins bind with keratan sulfate and dermatan sulfate (chondroitin sulfate B). The cornea owes its transparency to the regular arrangement of the collagen fibrils, but any factor that affects this lattice structure (e.g. swelling, pressure) results in a loss of transparency. The cornea contains some 78% water, some 15% collagen and some 5% of other proteins (Fig. C18).
See **bedewing, endothelial; corneal endothelium; corneal epithelium; corneal stroma; corneal topography; dellen; deturgescence; dyskeratosis; field, receptive; glycosaminoglycan; keratitis; keratomycosis; line, Hudson–Stahli; layer, Bowman's; membrane, Descemet's; microcornea; microscope, specular; optical zone of cornea; pachometer; theory, Maurice's; syndrome, Hurler's; tight junction; videokeratoscope.**
conical c. See **keratoconus.**
c. farinata A bilateral corneal degeneration characterized by faint dust-like opacities in the

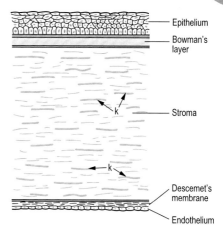

Fig. C18 Diagram showing the various layers of the cornea (k, keratocytes).

deep stroma. They do not impair vision and are usually age-related.
c. guttata Dystrophy of the endothelial cells of the cornea caused by focal accumulation of collagen on the posterior surface of Descemet's membrane. It may result from corneal trauma, cataract surgery, keratic precipitates, tonography, ageing, continuous contact lens wear or as part of the early stages of **Fuchs' endothelial dystrophy** (a disease associated with ageing and with females more than males). It is seen clinically by slit-lamp examination as black spherules in the endothelial pattern. The condition is bilateral, although one eye may be affected more than the other. As the condition progresses, the cornea becomes oedematous with a consequent loss of vision and eventually turns into bullous keratopathy. If the degenerated cells are located at the periphery of the cornea, they are called **Hassall–Henle bodies** and are of no clinical significance except as an indication of ageing. *Syn.* corneal guttae; endothelial corneal dystrophy.
See **illumination, specular reflection; keratic precipitates.**
optical zone of c. See **optical zone of cornea.**
c. plana A rare, congenital, usually bilateral condition in which the corneal curvature is flatter than normal with a significant decrease in refractive power. The eye is usually hyperopic with a shallow anterior chamber often resulting in angle-closure glaucoma. There is some degree of peripheral scleralization and it is closely associated with sclerocornea. Many cases, especially the most severe type, have autosomal recessive inheritance with mutation in the KERA gene on chromosome 12q22. Some mild cases have autosomal dominant inheritance.
See **sclerocornea.**

corneal Pertaining to the cornea.

corneal abrasion An area of the cornea that has been removed by rubbing. The condition ranges

from punctate staining with fluorescein to a total removal of the epithelium. Corneal abrasions may result from overwear of contact lenses, foreign bodies, fingernail scratches, etc. There is pain, photophobia, tearing and blepharospasm. The condition usually heals quickly if not severe and if infection has not occurred. Treatment consists of removal of the foreign bodies, if any, usually by irrigation, tight patching of the eye and antibiotic ointment; if due to contact lenses, discontinue wear until full recovery. Local anaesthetics should not be used in the treatment as they tend to delay the regeneration of the corneal epithelium.
See **Gundersen's conjunctival flap; mitosis; syndrome, overwear; rose bengal.**

corneal acidosis *See* **acidosis.**

corneal apex *See* **apex, corneal; optical zone of cornea.**

corneal arcus A greyish-white ring (or part of a ring) opacity located in the periphery of the cornea in old age. It is due to a lipid infiltration of the corneal stroma. With age, the condition progresses to form a complete ring. That ring is separated from the limbus by a zone of clear cornea. The condition can also appear in early or middle life and is referred to as **arcus juvenilis** (or **anterior embryotoxon**); it is somewhat whiter than corneal arcus. Arcus juvenilis is often associated with heart disease in men (Fig. C19). *Syn.* arcus senilis; gerontoxon.
See **furrow, marginal.**

corneal bullae *See* **bulla; keratopathy, bullous.**

corneal cap *See* **optical zone of cornea.**

corneal clouding, central Diffuse hazy appearance of the cornea due to oedema of the central region of the cornea, usually associated with the wearing of hard contact lenses (mainly PMMA), but it may also occur in keratoconus, Fuchs' endothelial dystrophy, mucolipidosis or disciform keratitis. It is most easily seen with a slit-lamp using retroillumination against the pupil margin or sclerotic scatter illumination. This condition may give rise to Sattler's veil.
See **illumination.**

corneal collagen cross-linking A method used to arrest, or in some cases reverse, the progression of keratoconus by preventing enzymatic degradation of stromal collagen. It consists of anaesthetizing the eye, removing the central 7 to 9 mm of the epithelium, applying a solution of riboflavin (vitamin B2) every 5 minutes for 30 minutes and irradiating the cornea with UVA radiation (370 nm) usually for 30 minutes while continuing to instill riboflavin at 5-minute intervals. After the procedure, antibiotics eyedrops are instilled and a soft contact lens is usually fitted temporarily to mitigate pain. *Note:* Riboflavin is used to prevent damage to the posterior layers of the cornea during the UVA procedure.

corneal corpuscle *See* **keratocyte.**

corneal degeneration *See* **degeneration, pellucid marginal corneal; ectasia, corneal; Vogt's white limbal girdle.**

corneal dellen *See* **dellen.**

corneal dystrophy; ectasia *See* under the nouns.

corneal endothelium The posterior layer of the cornea consisting of a single layer of cells, about 5 μm thick, bound together and predominantly hexagonal in shape. The posterior border is in direct contact with the aqueous humour while the anterior border is in contact with Descemet's membrane. The endothelium acts as a partial barrier to fluid movement maintaining stromal deturgescence while being permeable to nutrients from the aqueous humour. This is accomplished by an active mechanism ('pump') that moves water from the stroma into the aqueous. The endothelium receives most of its energy from the oxidative breakdown of carbohydrates via the Krebs cycle. In the normal adult eye, the cell density varies from between 3000 and 4000 cells/mm^2 in the centre of the cornea to about 2000

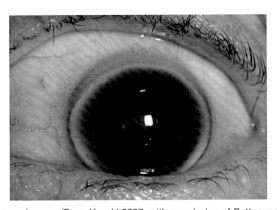

Fig. C19 Advanced corneal arcus. (From Kanski 2007, with permission of Butterworth-Heinemann)

cells/mm^2 in the periphery. With age, cell density progressively diminishes to about half by the age of about 80 years compared to what it was at birth. With disease (e.g. Fuchs' endothelial dystrophy) or trauma, the density of cells decreases further, and when it drops below about 500 cells/mm^2, corneal transparency is compromised as more fluid leaks into the cornea than can be eliminated by the endothelial pump.
See **bedewing, endothelial; blebs, endothelial; cornea guttata; illumination, specular reflection; keratopathy, lamellar; microscope, specular; phacoemulsification; polymegethism, endothelial.**

corneal epithelium The outermost layer of the cornea consisting of stratified epithelium mounted on a basement membrane. It is made up of various types of cells; next to the basement membrane are the **basal cells** (columnar in shape), then two or three rows of **wing cells** and near the surface are two or three layers of thin surface **squamous cells** (or **superficial cells**). The outer surfaces of the squamous cells have projections (called **microvilli** and **microplicae**), which extend into the mucin layer of the precorneal tear film and are presumed to help retain the tear film. The epithelium in humans has a thickness of about 51 µm. Some dendritic cells of mesodermal origin are also normally present. Epithelial **stem cells** are located at the limbus; they give rise to the basal cells and help regulate and regenerate corneal epithelial cells. The corneal epithelium receives its innervation from the conjunctival and the stromal nerves. It also serves as a barrier to the free movement of water from the tears to the stroma due to the presence of tight junctions. The life cycle of epithelial cells is about a week (Fig. C20).
See **cell, Langerhans'; cell, stem; epikeratoplasty; limbus; mitosis; pachometer; palisades of Vogt; tight junction.**

corneal erosion, recurrent Periodic loss of part of the corneal epithelium due to its detachment from the basement membrane, which may be the result of trauma (e.g. fingernail scratch) or of some corneal dystrophy. There is severe pain, redness, lacrimation and photophobia, typically upon awakening. Management usually begins with artificial teardrops and a lubricating ointment, but the acute phase requires antibiotic ointment and pressure patching or a therapeutic soft contact lens or debridement.
See **desmosome; dystrophy, epithelial basement membrane; dystrophy, lattice; dystrophy, Reis–Buckler's.**

corneal exhaustion syndrome *See* **syndrome, corneal exhaustion.**

corneal facet 1. Small flattened depression on the outer surface of the cornea, due to a healed ulcer which has failed to fill with tissue. **2.** The corneal element in the ommatidium of the compound eye.
See **eye, compound; ulcer, corneal.**

corneal fibroblast; fibrocyte *See* **keratocyte.**

corneal fold *See* **oedema.**

corneal fragility The ability of the cornea to withstand damage. It is quantified by measuring the corneal damage threshold (or corneal epithelial fragility threshold) that is the lowest pressure exerted on the cornea (using, e.g., a Cochet–Bonnet aesthesiometer) which produces some ruptured epithelial cells; they can be seen after fluorescein instillation with a slit-lamp and UV filter.

corneal graft *See* **graft, corneal; keratoplasty.**

corneal granular dystrophy *See* **dystrophy, granular corneal.**

corneal hydrops; hyperaesthesia; hypoxia; image *See* under the nouns.

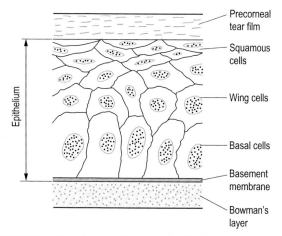

Fig. C20 Diagram showing the various layers of the corneal epithelium.

Precorneal tear film

Squamous cells

Wing cells

Basal cells

Basement membrane

Bowman's layer

Epithelium

corneal infiltrates Small hazy greyish areas (local or diffuse) composed of inflammatory cells, proteins, etc. surrounded by oedema and located in the cornea typically near the limbus. The adjacent conjunctiva is usually hyperaemic. They appear as a result of corneal inflammation (e.g. marginal keratitis, microbial keratitis), reaction to solution preservatives and some contact lens wear (especially extended wear) which causes prolonged hypoxia. Management depends on the cause; for example, if due to contact lenses, cessation of wear is usually indicated, otherwise drug therapy is required.
See **keratitis, acanthamoeba; keratoconjunctivitis, superior limbic.**

corneal keratocyte; limbus *See* under the nouns.

corneal neovascularization *See* pannus.

corneal oedema *See* oedema.

corneal opacity *See* leukoma.

corneal parallelepiped A section of the cornea illuminated by the thin slit of light of a slit-lamp, when viewed obliquely.

corneal reflex *See* reflex, corneal.

corneal sensitivity *See* sensitivity, contrast.

corneal stria *See* oedema; stria.

corneal stroma The thickest layer of the cornea located behind Bowman's layer and in front of Descemet's membrane. It represents approximately 90% of the total corneal thickness and gives the cornea its strength. The stroma consists of about 300 lamellae of parallel collagen fibrils in the centre of the cornea reaching to nearly 500 lamellae at the limbus. In between the fibrils are proteoglycans whose core proteins bind one with keratan sulfate and the other with dermatan sulfate (chondroitin sulfate B). The orientation of the alternate lamellae differs with each other, but they are all parallel with the corneal surface. In the central part of the cornea, the majority of the collagen fibrils are orientated in the inferior-superior and nasal-temporal directions, whereas at the limbus they are orientated circumferentially, providing greater resistance to forces perpendicular to the axes of the fibrils. Between the lamellae are found the elongated flattened keratocytes (corneal corpuscles) from which the collagen fibrils are produced during development. When the cornea becomes oedematous due to trauma, disease or hypoxia, some of the fibrils lose their usual uniform calibre, become displaced and fluid accumulates between the lamellae, the stroma then loses its transparency. *Syn.* substantia propria.
See **keratocyte.**

corneal topography A colour-coded map of the variations in the curvature and power of the anterior surface of the cornea. The typical map shows that the average adult cornea is steeper in the vertical than in the horizontal meridian and has the form of a flattening ellipsoid. It is typically done with a videokeratoscope. Most instruments are based on the analysis of multiple data points from the concentric rings of a Placido disc reflected from the corneal surface, which are compared to the known size of the object. Corneal topography can also be determined with a **scanning-slit topographer** with Scheimpflug imagery, in which a computerized system integrates a series of slit-beam images to produce a map of the curvature and elevation of the anterior and posterior surfaces enabling diagnosis of anterior and posterior keratoconus, and indirectly providing a measurement of corneal thickness. It is also used before and after refractive surgery, monitoring keratoconus progression, orthokeratology, as well as in contact lens management.
See **keratoscope; photokeratoscopy; Scheimpflug photography; videokeratoscope.**

corneal touch threshold The minimum pressure (in force per unit area, such as mg/mm^2) exerted against the cornea which can just be felt.
See **aesthesiometer; hyperaesthesia; sensitivity, corneal.**

corneal transplant *See* keratoplasty.

corneal ulcer *See* ulcer, corneal.

corneal warpage A relative change in the shape of the corneal surface produced by contact lenses, especially rigid lenses with low or no oxygen transmissibility. It affects vision. It is easily observed with corneal topography. The cornea recovers following cessation of contact lens wear.
See **videokeratoscope.**

Cornelia de Lange syndrome *See* syndrome, Cornelia de Lange.

corneoscleral junction *See* limbus, corneal.

corneoscleral meshwork *See* meshwork, trabecular.

corona ciliaris *See* ciliary body.

corpora quadrigemina *See* colliculi, inferior; colliculi, superior.

corpus callosum Transverse white fibres connecting the two cerebral hemispheres allowing the transfer of information from one cerebral hemisphere to the other. It is the largest collection of white matter in the brain and located in its middle.
See **commissure; stereoblindness.**

correction 1. Term used to designate the prescription of spectacle or contact lenses to compensate for ametropia (Figs. C21 and C22). *Syn.* refractive correction. **2.** The process whereby the aberrations of an optical system are minimized.
See **doublet; lens, aplanatic; power, effective; refractive error; triplet.**

correlation In statistics, the degree of association between two variables. The variables are usually shown on a two-dimensional scatter diagram. If there is perfect correlation, r = 1, the relationship is linear. If both variables increase together, the correlation is equal to +1, and if one variable increases as the other decreases, the correlation is equal to −1, both results indicating perfect correlation. Otherwise r takes on various values

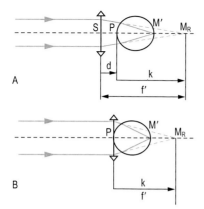

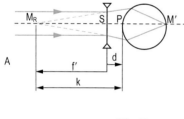

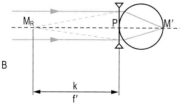

Fig. C21 Optical principle of the correction of a hyperopic eye with A, a spectacle lens, B, a contact lens (M_R, far point of the eye). The principle of distance correction is to arrive at a spectacle or contact lens, the power of which is such that its second principal focus coincides with the far point of the eye (k is the distance from the far point to the reduced eye surface; f′ the focal length of the correcting lens and d the vertex distance).

Fig. C22 Optical principle of the correction of a myopic eye with A, a spectacle lens, B, a contact lens (M_R, far point of the eye). The principle of distance correction is to arrive at a spectacle or contact lens, the power of which is such that its second principal focus coincides with the far point of the eye (k is the distance from the far point to the reduced eye surface; f′ the focal length of the correcting lens and d the vertex distance).

and is equal to 0 when the distribution of the two variables is totally random. The correlation r is also called **Pearson's correlation coefficient** or **product-moment correlation coefficient**. *See* regression; statistics.

correspondence, abnormal retinal *See* retinal correspondence, abnormal.

corresponding points *See* retinal corresponding points.

cortex The outermost layer of tissue of various organs located just below the outer membrane. *Plural*: cortices. *See* area, visual; lens, crystalline.
c. of the crystalline lens See lens, crystalline.
motor c. Area of the frontal lobe of the brain just anterior to the central sulcus which is responsible for voluntary movements of the eyes, as well as other voluntary movements of other parts of the body. The motor cortex in each hemisphere controls mainly muscles on the opposite side of the body. It is laid out according to the parts of the body with the region controlling the feet at the top and the region controlling the legs, the trunk, the arms and the head in descending order.
occipital c. Superficial grey matter on the posterior part of each hemisphere comprising Brodmann's areas 17, 18 and 19. *See* area, visual.
prestriate c. See area, visual association.
striate c.; visual c. See area, visual.

cortical blindness *See* blindness, cortical.

cortical magnification *See* magnification, cortical.

cortical vision screening test *See* test, cortical vision screening.

corticosteroid A class of steroid hormones secreted in the adrenal cortex or produced synthetically. There are two types: **glucocorticoids**, which are essential for the metabolism of carbohydrate, fat and protein and for normal responses to stress, and **mineralocorticoids**, which are necessary for the regulation of salt and water balance. Corticosteroids are used to treat inflammatory and allergic conditions. *See* antiinflammatory drug; gland, adrenal.

cosine law *See* diffusion.

'cotton balls' *See* uveitis, intermediate.

cotton thread test *See* test, phenol red cotton thread.

cotton-wool spot *See* body, cytoid; exudate; retinopathy, background diabetic.

counting fingers A method of recording vision in patients who are unable to identify any optotype on an acuity chart. The patient is asked to count the number of fingers of the examiner placed at a given distance. The number of fingers seen is recorded as, for example, finger counting at 1 metre, three metres, etc.

cover test *See* test, cover.

CR-39 material Allyl diglycol carbonate or Columbia Resin. CR-39 is a light transparent plastic material (refractive index 1.498, V = 59) used in the manufacture of spectacle lenses and much harder than polymethyl methacrylate. It is not quite as hard as glass. *Syn.* hard resin. *See* constringence; lens, plastic.

craniofacial dysostosis *See* syndrome, Crouzon's.

cranium *See* skull; suture.

crescent, congenital A white semilunar patch of sclera seen adjacent to the optic disc due to the fact that the choroid and retinal pigment epithelium do not extend to the optic disc. The condition is present at birth, unlike myopic crescent. *Syn.* Fuchs' coloboma (if located at the lower edge of the disc).
See disc, situs inversus.

crescent, myopic A white semilunar area of sclera located adjacent to the temporal side of the optic disc mainly in pathological myopia, but also sometimes in non-pathological myopia. There is atrophy of the choroid and retinal pigment epithelium in the crescent area, allowing the sclera to be seen. *Syn.* myopic conus; myopic scleral crescent; temporal crescent.

crescent, temporal *See* crescent, myopic.

crest, lacrimal *See* lacrimal crest, anterior; lacrimal crest, posterior.

Crete's prism *See* prism, rotary.

cribbing The process of breaking or chipping of excess glass from an uncut lens blank. It is carried out sometimes prior to edging.

cribriform plate *See* lamina cribrosa.

criterion, Percival Rule proposed by Percival to establish whether a patient is going to experience discomfort in binocular vision. It states that if Donders' line (or demand line) lies within the **zone of comfort**, which is the middle third of the total range of relative convergence (to the blur points), Percival's criterion of comfortable binocular vision is fulfilled. If it is not, appropriate prisms, spherical lenses or visual training can be used to shift the demand point within the zone of comfort. In this criterion, no reference is made to the actual phoria of the subject and for this reason, it has been criticized by several authors. *Syn.* middle third technique.
See convergence, relative; zone of clear, single, binocular vision.

criterion, Rayleigh Observation first made by Rayleigh that the images of two point objects will be resolved when the central maximum in the diffraction pattern of one image coincides with the first minimum of the diffraction pattern of the other image. For a perfect eye, with a 2-mm pupil, this criterion corresponds to a theoretical tolerance in focusing equal to about 0.075 D.
See disc, Airy's; diffraction; resolution, limit of.

criterion, Sheard Rule proposed by Sheard to establish whether a patient is going to experience discomfort in binocular vision. It states that the amount of heterophoria should be less than half the opposing fusional convergence in reserve. If the criterion is not met, appropriate prisms, spherical lenses or visual training can be used. If a patient has 10 Δ of exophoria, the positive fusional vergence should be at least 20 Δ to satisfy this criterion.
See convergence, relative; zone of clear, single, binocular vision.

critical angle *See* angle, critical.

critical fusion frequency *See* frequency, critical fusion.

critical oxygen requirement *See* oxygen requirement, critical.

critical period *See* period, critical.

crocodile shagreen; tears *See* under the nouns.

Crohn's disease *See* disease, Crohn's.

cromolyn sodium *See* mast cell stabilizers.

cross-cylinder lens *See* lens, cross-cylinder.

cross-cylinder test for astigmatism *See* test for astigmatism, cross-cylinder.

cross-fixation A condition often found in infantile large-angle esotropia in which the eyes tend to stay adducted so that the right eye fixates on objects in the left field of gaze and the left eye fixates on objects in the right field of gaze.
See esotropia, infantile.

cross, Maddox *See* Maddox cross.

crossed cylinder, obliquely Two cylindrical lenses combined together with their axes neither parallel nor perpendicular. The combination can be replaced by a single sphero-cylindrical lens in which the two focal lines are perpendicular to each other. The powers and axis of this new lens can be determined graphically or mathematically. An analogous situation is obtained when the cylindrical correction of an eye is corrected by a cylindrical lens placed at an incorrect axis before the eye.

crossed disparity *See* disparity, crossed.

crossed eyes *See* esotropia.

cross-linking, corneal collagen *See* corneal collagen cross-linking.

Cross-Nott retinoscopy *See* retinoscopy, Cross-Nott.

Crouzon's syndrome *See* syndrome, Crouzon's.

crowding phenomenon *See* phenomenon, crowding.

crown glass *See* glass, crown.

crutch, ptosis *See* ptosis.

cryopexy A surgical procedure in which localized freezing is used to reattach the neurosensory retina to the pigment epithelium or to destroy retinal or choroidal tissue. To treat retinal breaks or detachments, an intensely cold metal probe (called a **cryoprobe**) is placed against the sclera causing local protein denaturation and eventually scarring, which results in sealing the retina to the pigment epithelium, while the practitioner is looking into the eye with a binocular indirect ophthalmoscope and pressing the cryoprobe to the areas where the retina needs to be resealed.
See retinal break; retinopexy.

cryosurgery The application of extreme cold (using liquid nitrogen, carbon dioxide or nitrous oxide) as a specialized surgical technique to destroy abnormal tissue (e.g. a tumour or a wart).

cryotherapy A method of treating a disease using intense cold as a destructive medium. It may be used in the treatment of retinal detachment and breaks, conjunctival melanomas, lid tumours, uveitis, distichiasis and trichiasis.

cryptophthalmos A very rare congenital defect in which the eyelids are absent and replaced by a continuous layer of skin over a microphthalmic eyeball, resulting in an absence of palpebral fissure. Eyelashes may or may not be present. The cornea is fused with the overlying skin into one structure. The condition can be either unilateral or bilateral. *Note*: also spelt cryptophthalmia or cryptophthalmus.

crypts of Fuchs *See* Fuchs, crypts of.

crypts of Henle *See* gland, Henle.

crystal, anisotropic A crystal that exhibits birefringence (double refraction).

crystal, dichroic A birefringent crystal which absorbs the ordinary and extraordinary rays unequally. Natural light passing through a plate of a dichroic material becomes partially or totally polarized.
See birefringence; dichroism.

crystal, isotropic A crystal which has the same optical properties in all directions.

crystal, tourmaline *See* polarizer; tourmaline.

crystalline lens *See* lens, crystalline.

crystalline lens, equator of the *See* equator of the crystalline lens.

cues, monocular *See* perception, depth.

cul-de-sac *See* conjunctiva.

cup-disc ratio The ratio of the horizontal diameter of the physiological cup to that of the horizontal diameter of the optic disc. It should be less than 0.6. If it exceeds that value, if there is a difference in ratio between the two eyes or if there is a progressive enlargement of the cup, glaucoma may be suspected (Fig. C23).
See cup, glaucomatous.

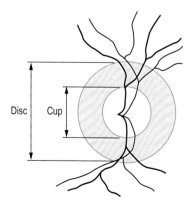

Fig. C23 Diagram of the physiological cup with a cup-disc ratio of 0.5.

cup, glaucomatous A large and deep excavation within the optic disc caused by a raised intraocular pressure. It is characterized by overhanging walls over which the blood vessels bend sharply and reappear at the bottom of the depression.
See cup-disc ratio; disc, cupped.

cup, ocular; ophthalmic *See* cup, optic.

cup, optic 1. A double-layered cup-shaped structure attached to the forebrain of the embryo by means of a hollow stalk. It develops into the retina and inner layers of the ciliary body and iris. It is formed by the invagination of the outer wall of the optic vesicle. Subsequently, nerve cells develop in its invaginated layer and some of these send their axons back along the hollow stalk (**optic stalk** or **lens stalk**) to form the optic nerve. *Syn.* ocular cup; ophthalmic cup; secondary optic vesicle. 2. Synonym for physiological cup.
See anophthalmia; ectoderm; fissure, optic; vesicle, optic.

cup, physiological A funnel-shaped depression at or near the centre of the optic disc, through which pass the central retinal vessels. *Syn.* optic cup (although it would be preferable not to use this synonym since this term has another meaning); physiological excavation.
See disc, cupped; neuroretinal rim.

cupped disc *See* disc, cupped.

curettage *See* chalazion.

curl side *See* side; side, curl.

curvature ametropia *See* ametropia, refractive.

curvature of field Aberration of an optical system due to the obliquity of the incident rays of light relative to the optical axis. The image corresponding to a plane object lies on a curved surface. This aberration does not usually affect the eye, as the retina is itself curved.
See Petzval surface.

curvature of a surface A measure of the shape of a curved surface. It is expressed in a unit called **reciprocal metre**, usually written as m^{-1}, which is equal to the reciprocal of the radius of curvature of a surface in metres. *Example*: If a surface has a radius of curvature r of +0.5 m, its curvature R will be $R = 1/r = 1/+0.5 = 2 \ m^{-1}$.

curve, base 1. The shallower principal meridian of the toroidal surface of a toric lens. The other meridian of the toroidal surface which has the maximum power is called the **cross curve**. 2. In a meniscus lens, the shallower of the two surfaces. 3. Of a range of lenses of different powers, a surface power common to all the lenses in that range.
See lens, periscopic; optic zone radius, back.

cut-off frequency *See* function, contrast sensitivity.

cyanolabe *See* pigment, visual.

cyanophobia An abnormal aversion to blue.
See chromatophobia.

cyanopsia *See* chromatopsia.

cycle, citric acid *See* Krebs cycle.

cycle per degree Unit of spatial frequency. It is equal to the number of cycles of a grating (one dark and one light band) that subtends an angle of one degree at the eye. *Abbreviated*: c/deg; cpd. This unit was developed because there is no finite width in a bar of a sine grating (Fig. C24 and Table C9).

cycle, Krebs *See* Krebs cycle.

cycle, tricarboxylic acid *See* Krebs cycle.

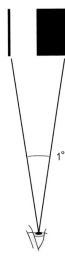

1°

Fig. C24 One cycle per degree.

Table C9 Relationship between the minimum angle of resolution, the Snellen fraction and the equivalent spatial frequency of a sine wave

Resolution (min of arc)	Snellen fraction (m)	(ft)	Spatial frequency (cpd)
0.5	6/3	20/10	60
0.6	6/3.6	20/12	50
0.75	6/4.5	20/15	40
1.0	6/6	20/20	30
1.25	6/7.5	20/25	24
1.5	6/9	20/30	20
2.0	6/12	20/40	15
2.5	6/15	20/50	12
4.0	6/24	20/80	7.5
5.0	6/30	20/100	6
8.0	6/48	20/160	3.8
10.0	6/60	20/200	3
20.0	6/120	20/400	1.5

cyclic heterotropia; strabismus *See* strabismus, cyclic.

cyclitis Chronic or acute inflammation of the ciliary body frequently associated with iritis and choroiditis.
See cataract, complicated; syndrome, Fuchs'; uveitis, intermediate.

cyclodialysis Disinsertion of the ciliary body from the scleral spur which may produce a cyclodialysis cleft resulting in hypotony. It is rarely performed nowadays in the treatment of glaucoma to reduce the intraocular pressure. It formed a communication between the anterior chamber and the suprachoroidal space. It may also occur as a result of trauma or intraocular surgery (e.g. trabeculectomy).
See angle, recession; pathway, uveoscleral.

cyclodiode laser therapy A surgical procedure aimed at lowering intraocular pressure by decreasing aqueous secretion by means of small burns of the ciliary body with pulses of laser energy passed through the eye.

cycloduction Rotation of an eye. *Syn.* cyclorotation; cyclotorsion.

cyclofusion Rotation of the eyes about their anteroposterior axes in an attempt to align the two views of the visual field so as to stimulate corresponding retinal areas, in response to an appropriate stimulus.

cycloparesis A weakness of the ciliary muscle.

cyclopean eye *See* eye, cyclopean.

cyclopentolate hydrochloride An antimuscarinic (or parasympatholytic) drug used as a short duration mydriatic and cycloplegic. Common concentrations are 0.5% and 1.0% as cycloplegic and 0.1% as mydriatic.
See acetylcholine; cycloplegia; mydriasis.

cyclophoria When binocular vision is dissociated (i.e. when stimuli to fusion are eliminated), one eye or both rotate about its/their respective anteroposterior axes to take up the passive position. If the upper portion of the eye rotates inward, it is called **incyclophoria,** and if it rotates outward, it is called **excyclophoria.** It is usually caused by an anomaly of the oblique muscles, most commonly the superior oblique. Cyclophoria is commonly associated with hyperphoria. There are various methods which can be used to detect cyclophoria: the Maddox rod test, the double prism test, the synoptophore with appropriate slides, the fixation disparity unit and Fresnel's bi-prism. *Syn.* periphoria.
See cyclotropia; test, double prism; test, Maddox rod.

cyclophosphamide *See* immunosuppressants.

cycloplegia Paralysis of the ciliary muscle resulting in a loss of accommodation. It is usually accompanied by dilatation of the pupil. It is usually induced by a drug.
See acetylcholine; anisocycloplegia; hyperopia, latent; mydriatic.

cycloplegic 1. Pertaining to cycloplegia. 2. A drug which produces cycloplegia. Cycloplegic drugs, which act by inhibiting the action of acetylcholine at muscarinic receptors in the ciliary muscle, include atropine, cyclopentolate hydrochloride, homatropine hydrobromide, hyoscine hydrobromide (scopolamine hydrobromide) and tropicamide. *Syn.* anticholinergic; antimuscarinic; cholinergic antagonist; cholinergic blocking agent; parasympatholytic.
See **mydriatic.**

cycloplegic refraction *See* refraction, cycloplegic.

cyclorotation *See* cyclotorsion; torsion.

cyclosporine *See* ciclosporin.

cyclotonic A state of constant accommodation. *See* tonus.

cyclotorsion Rotation of an eye about an anteroposterior axis. If, for example, it is inward, it is called **incyclotorsion** and outward, **excyclotorsion**. *Syn.* cycloduction; cyclorotation; torsion (it is often regarded as synonym).
See **test, Maddox rod; torsion.**

cyclotropia Type of strabismus in which one eye is rotated about its anteroposterior axis relative to the other. If the upper pole of the eye is rotated inward, it is called **incyclotropia** and outward, **excyclotropia**.
See **cyclophoria.**

cyclovertical muscles *See* muscles, cyclovertical.

cycloversion Rotation of both eyes in the same direction around their respective anteroposterior axes. *See* **dextrocycloversion; laevocycloversion.**

cylinder axis *See* axis, cylinder.

cylinder lens, cross *See* lens, cross-cylinder.

cylindrical error *See* prescription.

cylindrical lens *See* lens, astigmatic.

cyst An abnormal closed sac containing fluid or soft material. It can happen anywhere on the skin. *dermoid c.* A tumour containing keratin, sebum, collagenous tissue, hair or fat globules which may be found in the cornea, interior of the eye or in the subcutaneous tissue of the superotemporal orbital rim. It presents as a round mass, about 1 to 2 cm in diameter, pink to yellow in colour. **Limbal dermoids** may be associated with Goldenhar's syndrome. There may be induced astigmatism. If vision is impaired or it is cosmetically disfiguring, treatment is by excision.
See **choristoma.**
macular c. See macular cyst.
meibomian c. See chalazion.

c. of Moll A fluid-filled, round, translucent lesion arising from the blockage of the apocrine duct of the gland of Moll and situated on the anterior lid margin.
sebaceous c. A benign yellowish tumour located on the eyelid, usually near the inner canthus. It is most often seen in the elderly. It is caused by blockage of the sebaceous glands of the skin. It may be excised for cosmetic reasons.
c. of Zeis An oily filled lesion arising from blockage of the gland of Zeis and situated on the anterior lid margin.

cystinosis A rare autosomal recessive hereditary metabolic disorder caused by mutation in the gene encoding cystinosin, located on chromosome 17p13 and resulting in an abnormal accumulation of the amino acid cysteine throughout the body. As cystine (formed by union of two cysteine molecules) is poorly soluble, it forms crystals. The child presents with renal failure, hypothyroidism and hypogonadism. Ocular manifestations are corneal cystine crystal deposits and mottling of the retinal pigment epithelium. There is photophobia, pain and eventually reduced vision. Management includes medication with oral and topical cysteamine.

cystoid macular oedema *See* oedema, cystoid macular.

cystotome *See* capsulorhexis; capsulotomy.

cytoid bodies *See* body, cytoid.

cytology A study of cells to detect diseases. The usual procedure is to obtain a sample, to fix it on a glass slide, treat it with various dyes and inspect it under a microscope. Differential staining allows identification of the cells and their state of health.

cytology, impression A simple, non-invasive means of studying cells on the conjunctiva. It is carried out by pressing a small piece of special filter paper against the anaesthetized bulbar conjunctiva for a few seconds, after which it is removed. The operation is usually repeated two or three times over the same area. The filter paper is then fixed to a glass slide, stained and examined under a microscope. Mucin, goblet cells and many epithelial cells which stain in different colours, depending on the dyes used, can be assessed and facilitate the diagnosis of many external eye diseases, such as keratoconjunctivitis sicca and xerophthalmia.

cytomegalovirus retinitis *See* retinitis, cytomegalovirus; syndrome, acquired immunodeficiency.

D

D-15 test *See* test, Farnsworth-Munsell 100 Hue.

dacryoadenitis Inflammation of the lacrimal gland. The acute type is characterized by localized pain, swelling of upper eyelid resulting in an S-shaped ptosis, reduced tear secretion and redness over the upper temporal area of the eye. The chronic type is painless and develops slowly. A frequent cause is an associated systemic infection such as mumps, Epstein-Barr virus, influenza, thyroid eye disease, sarcoidosis or Sjögren's syndrome or it can be idiopathic. Treatment consists mainly of warm compresses and occasionally antibiotics.

dacryocele, congenital A congenital condition in which the infant is born with a swollen lacrimal sac filled with mucoid material. Physical examination reveals a bluish mass located in the nasal canthal region, probably due to an obstruction of the lower end of the nasolacrimal duct, with associated blockage of the canaliculi and puncta. Treatment includes antibiotics as well as nasolacrimal probing and irrigation in many cases. *Syn.* dacryocystocele.

dacryocystectomy Surgical removal of the lacrimal sac.

dacryocystitis Inflammation of the lacrimal sac, most commonly from the staphylococcal or streptococcal infection. It is a rare condition, which may occur when there is a blockage of the nasolacrimal drainage system. The acute type gives rise to redness, tenderness and swelling below the lid margin with intermittent epiphora, while in the chronic type, there is chronic epiphora and, with pressure on the lacrimal sac, pus will come out of the punctum. Treatment includes antibiotics and warm compresses, but surgery may be needed in the chronic type. *See* **dacryocystorhinostomy; epiphora; fistula, lacrimal; lacrimal apparatus.**

dacryocystorhinostomy A surgical operation aimed at unblocking the nasolacrimal duct. A communication channel is performed between the lacrimal sac and the nasal cavity by making an opening through the bone. *See* **dacryocystitis.**

dacryoliths Concretions found in the lacrimal apparatus, in the puncta or canaliculi which it may occlude. The concretions are usually composed of epithelial cells, lipid, non-specific debris as well as calcium.

dacryoma 1. A tumour or swelling anywhere within the lacrimal apparatus. 2. A blockage of a lacrimal punctum.

dacryops 1. A chronic watery eye. 2. A cyst in a tear duct of the lacrimal gland. *See* **epiphora.**

dacryorrhoea An abnormally large flow of tears. *Note*: also spelt dacryorrhea.

Dalen–Fuchs nodules *See* nodule, Dalen–Fuchs.

Dalrymple's sign *See* sign, Dalrymple's.

daltonism Term used formerly to designate colour blindness, usually deutan, so named because John Dalton (1766–1844) was the first to describe his own anomaly. *See* **colour vision, defective.**

dapiprazole *See* alpha-adrenergic antagonist.

dark adaptation *See* adaptation, dark.

dark current *See* electrooculogram.

dark filter test *See* test, neutral density filter.

dark focus *See* accommodation, resting state of.

dark phase *See* electrooculogram.

dark room test *See* test, provocative.

dark vergence *See* vergence, tonic.

dark wedge test *See* test, Bielchowsky's phenomenon.

day blindness *See* hemeralopia.

daylight, artificial Illumination produced by a source of artificial light having a spectral distribution similar to that of daylight. CIE Illuminant C is considered to almost fulfill this criterion. *See* **illuminants, CIE standard.**

daylight, natural Illumination dependent on the sun and the extent of clear sky.

daylight vision *See* vision, photopic.

deaf-blind A person who has a severe hearing impairment in addition to a visual defect. It is usually congenital, but it may result from ageing, some systemic disease or as part of a syndrome (e.g. Usher's syndrome which accounts for about half of all cases of deaf-blind people; rubella syndrome).

debility The state of being feeble or without strength.

debridement Removal of dead or infected tissue or foreign material until surrounding healthy tissue is exposed. This is done to facilitate healing. Corneal debridement is usually performed with a moistened cotton-tipped applicator, a sponge or a spatula. *Example*: debridement of some of the corneal epithelium in dendritic keratitis or in corneal erosion.

decentration (dec) A displacement, horizontal and/or vertical, of the centration point of a spectacle lens from the standard optical centre position (British Standard). *See* **centre, standard optical position; point, centration.**

decibel (dB) 1. Unit used for the measurement of the intensity of a sound. **2.** Light intensities are often presented on a logarithmic (rather than linear) scale. This is done, in particular, to reduce large numbers. Moreover, it has become common, especially in perimetry, to use decibels rather than log units. A decibel scale is a logarithmic scale where 10 decibels are equal to 1 log unit; 20 decibels, to 2 log units, etc. In perimetry, decibels are used to indicate the attenuation of brightness of the stimulus. Thus, a 20 dB stimulus is equal to one-tenth the brightness of a 10 dB stimulus.

decompensation Failure of an organ to fulfill its function adequately. *Examples*: corneal decompensation following years of extended contact lens wear; a failure of the eye movement system to overcome a heterophoria.

decussation Crossing of nerve fibres passing through the mid-sagittal plane of the central nervous system and connecting with structures on the opposite side. Partial decussation occurs at the optic chiasma.

defocus To put or go out of focus.

  hyperopic d. State of the eye in which the retinal image is focused behind the retina. It may occur when placing a negative lens in front of an emmetropic presbyopic eye, in an uncorrected presbyopic hyperope, in a high hyperope unable to overcome the ametropia by accommodating or as an accommodative lag in an uncorrected or corrected myope, as well as in an emmetrope viewing a near object.
  See accommodation, lag of; overcorrection.

  myopic d. State of the eye in which the retinal image is focused in front of the retina. It may occur when placing a positive lens in front of an emmetropic eye, in an uncorrected or undercorrected myopic eye or if there is a lead of accommodation, as is the case in some individuals viewing a distant object.
  See accommodation, lead of; undercorrection.

degeneration Deterioration of tissue or organ resulting in reduced efficiency. *Examples*: degeneration of the cornea, degeneration of the retina.
  See dystrophy, corneal.

  age-related macular d. See macular degeneration, age-related.
  cobblestone d. See degeneration, paving-stone.
  cone d. See dystrophy, cone.
  Doyne's honeycombed d. See drusen, familial dominant.
  hepatolenticular d. See disease, Wilson's.
  lattice d. of the retina See retina, lattice degeneration of the.
  lipid droplet d. See keratopathy, lipid.
  paving-stone d. Discrete yellowish round areas of retinal thinning and depigmentation located near the ora serrata. The underlying choroid may be seen. It is a benign degeneration occurring with advancing age. *Syn.* cobblestone degeneration; peripheral chorioretinal degeneration.
  pellucid marginal d. A rare condition characterized by bilateral, slowly progressive thinning and protrusion of the inferior peripheral cornea. The involved area is clear (hence the word pellucid), but the condition may be complicated by hydrops and the central cornea typically develops against the rule astigmatism. Treatment usually consists of gas permeable scleral lenses, but keratoplasty may be necessary.
  See ectasia, corneal; hydrops; keratoconus.
  peripheral chorioretinal d. See degeneration, paving-stone.
  peripheral cystoid d. Degenerative process in the peripheral retina that occurs almost universally in the elderly. It consists of numerous discrete cystic spaces in the outer plexiform or inner nuclear layer presenting a frothy appearance. The degeneration starts at the ora serrata and slowly progresses to the peripheral retina. If the cysts should join together, degenerative retinoschisis develops. It is not usually associated with retinal tears. The condition does not require any treatment.
  Salzmann's nodular d. A degenerative condition characterized by bluish-white elevated nodules of hyaline tissue on the surface of the cornea. It may occur in people previously affected by trachoma, phlyctenular keratitis, vernal keratitis or keratoconjunctivitis sicca. Most cases are asymptomatic, but if the nodules impair vision, keratoplasty may be necessary.
  senile macular d. See macular degeneration, age-related.
  snailtrack d. Long areas of retinal thinning with a glistening appearance and with round holes that may lead to lattice degeneration of the retina and retinal detachment.
  See retina.
  tapetoretinal d. A hereditary degeneration of the photoreceptors of the retina or of the pigment epithelium layer. Some authors also include the choroid. The fundus presents a granular or honeycomb appearance between the equator and the ora serrata. The condition needs to be differentiated from choroideremia and retinitis pigmentosa, which are far more severe conditions. *Syn.* tapetoretinopathy.
  See choroideremia; retinitis pigmentosa.
  Terrien's marginal d. A rare condition in which the cornea becomes thinner in the periphery along the limbus causing a trough. There is progressive astigmatism, typically against the rule, with a consequent decrease in visual acuity. It affects adult males more commonly than females. Signs are lipid deposition with superficial vascularization. Therapy includes rigid contact lenses and occasionally keratoplasty. *Syn.* Terrien's disease.
  See ectasia, corneal.
  vitreoretinal d. See disease, Wagner's; syndrome, Stickler's.

dehiscence, wound A rupture or splitting open of tissue along natural lines or as a complication of surgery in which the wound separates and some of the contents leak out. It may occur following keratoplasty or retinal surgery.
  See retinal dialysis.

dellen A transient shallow depression in the cornea near the limbus which is caused by a local dehydration of the corneal stroma, leading to a compression of its lamellae. It can occur as a result of strabismus surgery, cataract surgery, swelling of the limbus (as in episcleritis or pterygium), rigid contact lens wear or old age.

DEM test See test, developmental eye movement.

demagnified image See field, visual f. expander; mirror, concave.

demand line See line, demand.

demecarium bromide See anticholinesterase.

demodicosis Infestation of the eyelashes and meibomian glands by the mite *Demodex*. It causes itching and the sensation of burning of the eyelids and occasionally loss of eyelashes. Total removal of the parasites is very difficult; frequent cleaning of the eyelashes with saline water is imperative.

dendrite See neuron.

dendritic keratitis See keratitis, dendritic.

denervation A loss or interference to the nerve supply caused either by a drug, disease or surgery.

densitometry, retinal A technique used to study visual pigments *in vivo*. It consists of measuring the small fraction of light that is reflected by the pigment epithelium of the retina before and after bleaching with a bright source of light. *See* pigment, visual.

density An indication of the compactness of a substance. It is expressed as the ratio of the mass of the substance to its unit volume. The common units are g/cm³ and kg/m³. This property is usually given by lens manufacturers; the greater the density of a material, the greater its weight, all other factors being equal (Table D1).

density, optical The light-absorbing property of a translucent medium such as an optical filter. It is expressed as

$$D = \log_{10}(1/T) = \log_{10}(I/I')$$

where D is the symbol for optical density (*Syn*. absorbance) and T is the transmittance of a medium ($T = I'/I$, where I' is the transmitted light and I the incident light) for a specified wavelength (Table D2). *Example*: A filter has a transmittance of 0.6, its optical density is $\log_{10}(1 / 0.6) = 0.22$. *See* absorption; spectrophotometer; transmittance.

Denver Developmental Screening Test See test, developmental and perceptual screening.

deorsumduction See depression.

deorsumvergence See infravergence.

deorsumversion See version.

depolarization A change in the value of the resting membrane potential towards zero. In the photoreceptors it occurs in darkness. It is caused by a constant influx of Na⁺ (sodium) through binding

Table D1 Density of optical lens materials		
	n	**Density (g/cm³)**
Glass		
spectacle crown	1.523	2.54
dense barium crown	1.620	3.71
dense flint	1.706	3.20
dense barium flint	1.700	4.10
titanium oxide	1.701	2.99
Plastics		
PMMA	1.490	1.19
CR-39	1.498	1.32
polycarbonate	1.586	1.2
cellulose acetate butyrate	1.48	1.2
cellulose propionate	1.46	1.2

Table D2 Relationship between optical density D and light transmitance T of optical filters		
D	**T**	**T (%)**
0.0	1	100
0.1	0.794	79.4
0.2	0.631	63.1
0.3	0.501	50.1
0.4	0.398	39.8
0.5	0.316	31.6
0.6	0.251	25.1
0.7	0.20	20.0
0.8	0.158	15.8
0.9	0.126	12.6
1.0	0.10	10.0
1.5	0.0316	3.16
2.0	0.010	1.0
2.5	0.0032	0.32
3.0	0.0010	0.1
4.0	0.0001	0.01

of 3', 5'–cyclic guanosine monophosphate and opening the channels in the outer segment membrane. The inside of the cell becomes less negative compared to the outside. Depolarization is **excitatory** because the membrane potential shifts towards the neuron's threshold at which an action potential occurs. *See* hyperpolarization; synapse.

depolished glass See glass, ground.

deposits, contact lens Accumulation of materials on or into the matrix of contact lenses. They are mainly tear components (proteins, lipids, mucin, calcium), but other materials can be found (e.g. mercurial or iron deposits, nicotine, hand cream). Deposits reduce comfort, vision, patient tolerance and discolour and spoil the lenses. They may act as antigens for the development of giant papillary conjunctivitis. Most of these deposits can be removed with a surfactant, an enzymatic system and a calcium-preventing solution.

depression Downward rotation of an eye. It is accomplished by the inferior rectus and superior oblique muscles. It can be induced by using base-up prisms. *Syn.* infraduction; deorsumduction.

depressors Extraocular muscles that move the eye downward, such as the inferior rectus and the superior oblique.

deprivation State of being without.
  d. amblyopia *See* amblyopia, deprivation.
  sensory d. The condition produced by a loss of all or most of the stimulation from the visual, auditory, tactile and other sensory systems. Often, deprivation involves only one modality (e.g. vision). Methods used for deprivation include diffusing goggles, white noise, padded gloves, etc. Its effect has shown the necessity of continuous sensory activity to maintain the normal development and functioning of any sensory system.
  visual d. The condition produced by a loss of form vision. It may occur as a result of an anomaly within the eye (e.g. opacification of the cornea) or it can be artificially induced (e.g. by placing a transparent plastic occluder in front of the eye, as used in myopia research with animals).

depth of field For a given setting of an optical system (or a steady state of accommodation of the eye), it is the distance over which an object may be moved without causing a sharpness reduction beyond a certain tolerable amount. (The criterion could be as much as a line of letters on a Snellen chart.) Depth of field increases when the diaphragm (or pupil) diameter diminishes as, for example, in old eyes (Fig. D1). *Examples*: Viewing at infinity, the depth of field ranges between infinity and about 3.6 m for a pupil of 4 mm in diameter and between infinity and about 2.3 m for a 2-mm pupil. At a viewing distance of 1 m, the depth of field ranges from about 1.4 m to 80 cm with a 4-mm pupil and from about 1.8 m to 70 cm with a 2-mm pupil.
  See distance, hyperfocal.

depth of focus For a given setting of an optical system (or a steady state of accommodation of the eye), it is the distance in front and behind the focal point (or retina) over which the image may be focused without causing a sharpness reduction

beyond a certain tolerable amount. (The criterion could be as much as a line of letters on a Snellen chart.) The depth of focus D is represented by the total distance in front and behind the focal point (or the retina) (Fig. D1). As with depth of field, it is inversely proportional to the diameter of the diaphragm (or pupil). It can be calculated, expressed in dioptres, using the equation

$$D = (2b/p)F_e$$

where F_e is the power of the emmetropic eye, p the pupillary diameter and b the maximum size of the retinal image beyond which it is perceived as blurred. *Example*: Assuming a pupil of 3 mm and a retinal image spread over five cones, each 0.002 mm in diameter and spaces between the cones of 0.0005 mm, that is a total size = 0.012 mm, $D = 2 \times 0.012/3 \times 60 = 0.48$ D. Thus an object appears clear if the vergence at the eye varies in the range ±0.24 D. If the eye is focused at infinity, the equation becomes $D = (b/p)F_e$.

depth perception *See* perception, depth.

depth, vertex *See* vertex depth.

dermatitis *See* eczema.

dermatochalasis A condition in which there is a redundancy of the skin of the upper eyelids. It is often associated with a protrusion of fat through a defective orbital septum. The condition occurs usually in old people. The excess skin may cause pseudoptosis. In severe cases, it may obstruct vision. Treatment is surgical. *Syn.* ptosis adiposa; ptosis atrophica.
  See blepharochalasis.

dermoid cyst *See* cyst, dermoid.

dermoid, limbal *See* cyst, dermoid.

desaturated D–15 test *See* test, Farnsworth.

Descartes' law *See* law of refraction.

Descemet's membrane *See* membrane, Descemet's.

descemetocele A forward bulging of Descemet's membrane due to either trauma or a deep corneal ulcer which has eroded the overlying stroma. *Syn.* keratocele.
  See keratolysis.

desiccation The process of becoming dry.
  See eye, dry.

desmosome A small dense body in which the two halves are separated by an intercellular gap filled with extracellular substance. It forms an adhesion of two adjacent cells as, for example, in the corneal epithelium where the basal cells are attached at irregular intervals to the underlying basement membrane (adjacent to Bowman's layer) by **hemidesmosomes** (one half of a desmosome). Thus, scraping off the epithelium usually leaves fragments of the basal cells attached to the basement membrane.

detachment, choroidal *See* choroidal detachment.

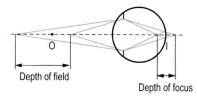

Fig. D1 Schematic representation of the depth of field and the depth of focus of an eye fixating an object at O (I, retinal image size corresponding to the tolerable resolution).

detachment, retinal *See* retinal detachment.

deturgescence State of dehydration existing in the normal cornea as a necessity for transparency. It is maintained by the epithelium, which to a large extent is impermeable to water, and also by a metabolic transport system in the endothelium. *See* turgescence.

deutan A person who has either deuteranomaly or deuteranopia.

deuteranomal Person who has deuteranomaly.

deuteranomaly A type of anomalous trichromatism in which an abnormally high proportion of green is needed when mixing red and green light to match a given yellow. This is the most common type of colour vision deficiency, occurring in about 4.6% of males and 0.35% of the female population. *Syn.* deuteranomalous trichromatism; deuteranomalous vision; green-weakness. *See* anomaloscope; colour vision, defective.

deuteranope Person who has deuteranopia.

deuteranopia Type of dichromatism in which red and green are confused, although their relative spectral luminosities are practically the same as in normals. In the spectrum, the deuteranope only sees two primary colours; the long wavelength portion of the spectrum (yellow, orange or red) appears yellowish, and the short wavelength portion (blue or violet) appears bluish. There is, in between, a neutral point which appears whitish or colourless at about 498 nm. It occurs in slightly over 1% of the male population and only rarely in females. *Syn.* green blindness (although this term is incorrect as green lights appear to a deuteranope as bright as to a normal observer). *See* colour vision, defective; dichromatism; sensitivity, spectral.

developmental and perceptual screening test *See* test, developmental and perceptual screening.

deviating eye *See* eye, deviating.

deviation 1. In strabismus, the departure of the visual axis of one eye from the point of fixation. **2.** A change in direction of a light ray resulting from reflection or refraction at an optical surface.
angle of d. *See* angle of deviation.
conjugate d. Simultaneous and equal rotations of the eyes in any direction. It may be physiological such as versions, or pathological, due to either muscular spasm or paralysis. *See* movements, disjunctive; version.
dissociated vertical d. A form of strabismus in which one eye apparently moves vertically without any compensatory movement from the other eye. Although initially felt to disobey Hering's law, it is now felt that Hering's law is observed if the horizontal, vertical and rotational aspects of the condition are considered together. This form of strabismus often accompanies infantile esotropia and is almost always noted from the period of infancy. The misalignment can be either latent or manifest, and may require operative intervention if of a great degree.

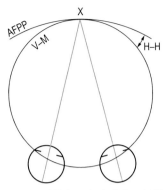

Fig. D2 Hering–Hillebrand deviation H–H (AFPP, apparent frontoparallel plane horopter); V–M (Vieth–Müller circle); X, (fixation point).

See esotropia, infantile; procedure, Faden; test, Bielschowsky's phenomenon.
Hering–Hillebrand d. The deviation of the apparent frontoparallel plane horopter from the Vieth–Müller circle (horopter) (Fig. D2).
minimum d. of a prism *See* prism, minimum deviation of a.
primary d. The deviation found in paralysis of an extraocular muscle when the unaffected eye is fixating.
secondary d. The deviation found in paralysis of an extraocular muscle when the eye with the paralytic muscle is fixating.
skew d. A form of strabismus, typically vertical, that does not follow any standard or typical pattern and is usually difficult to quantify. It may be due to a midbrain disorder, multiple sclerosis or myasthenia gravis.
vertical d. 1. Type of ocular deviation found in strabismus in which the deviating eye is rotated upward with respect to the fixating eye. **2.** Upward ocular deviation of an occluded eye in the cover test, as found in hyperphoria or hypophoria.

Devic's disease *See* disease, Devic's.

dexamethasone *See* antiinflammatory drug.

dextroclination Rotation of the upper pole of the vertical meridian of an eye to the subject's right. *Syn.* dextrocycloduction; dextrotorsion.

dextrocycloversion Rotation of the upper poles of the vertical meridians of both eyes towards the subject's right. *See* laevocycloversion.

dextrodeorsumversion Movement of the eyes down and to the right.

dextroduction Rotation of one eye to the right. *See* duction.

dextrophoria A tendency of the visual axes of both eyes to deviate to the right, in the absence of a stimulus to fusion. *See* heterophoria; laevophoria.

dextrotorsion *See* dextroclination.

dextroversion Movement of both eyes to the right. *See* **version**.

diabetes mellitus A chronic disease that occurs when the pancreas does not produce enough insulin, or alternatively, when the body cannot effectively use the insulin it produces. Insulin is a hormone that regulates blood sugar. Hyperglycaemia, or raised blood sugar, is a common effect of uncontrolled diabetes and, over time, leads to serious damage to many of the body's systems, especially the nerves and blood vessels (definition of the **World Health Organization**). The most common types of diabetes are: **Type 1 diabetes**, which is caused by an autoimmune destruction of the insulin production of beta cells in the pancreas and therefore dependent upon insulin administration, and **Type 2 diabetes**, which is characterized by an ineffective use of insulin. Type 1 diabetes is the most common type in young people whereas Type 2 is the most common diabetes and affects primarily, but not exclusively, adults and is largely the result of obesity and physical inactivity. The main complications in the eye are retinopathy, cataract, rubeosis iridis, ocular motor nerve palsies and xanthelasma. *See* **accommodative insufficiency; anisocoria; cataract; glaucoma, neovascular; glaucoma, open-angle; hypoxia; myopia, lenticular; paralysis of the sixth nerve; paralysis of the third nerve; pupil, Adie's; retinopathy, diabetic; rubeosis iridis; tritanopia; vitrectomy; vitreous detachment.**

diabetic maculopathy; retinopathy *See* under the nouns.

diagnosis 1. Term that indicates the disease (e.g. pulmonary tuberculosis) or the refractive error (e.g. compound myopic astigmatism) that a person has. 2. The art of determining a disease or visual anomaly based on the signs, symptoms and tests.

diagnostic positions of gaze *See* **positions of gaze, diagnostic.**

dialysis, retinal *See* **retinal dialysis.**

diameter, total The linear measurement of the maximum external dimension of a contact lens. It is usually specified in millimetres. It is equal to the back optic zone diameter (BOZD) plus twice the width of each of the back peripheral optic zones (if any) or twice the width of the edge in a spherical lens. Formerly, it was called overall size. *See* **optic zone diameter; v gauge.**

diaphragm 1. In optics, an aperture generally round and of variable diameter placed in a screen and used to limit the field of view of a lens or optical system (**field stop**). It also limits stray light (**light stop**). *Syn.* stop; aperture-stop. 2. In anatomy, a dividing membrane.

diascope An optical apparatus used to project transparencies on a screen. *See* **epidiascope.**

diathermy *See* **retinopexy.**

dibrompropamidine *See* **antibiotic.**

dichlorphenamide *See* **carbonic anhydrase inhibitors.**

dichoptic Viewing a separate and independent field by each eye in binocular vision as, for example, in a haploscope. *See* **masking, dichoptic.**

dichroic Adjective referring to two colours.

dichroism Property exhibited by certain transparent substances of producing two different colours depending upon the thickness of substance traversed, the directions of transmission of light and/or viewing, the concentration of the substance, etc. The most common example is that of crystals (e.g. tourmaline) that absorb unequally the ordinary and extraordinary rays. *See* **anisotropic; crystal, dichroic; pleochrism.**

dichromat Person having dichromatism (i.e. a deuteranope, a protanope or a tritanope).

dichromatism A form of colour vision deficiency in which all colours can be matched by a mixture of only two primary colours. The spectrum appears as consisting of two colours separated by an achromatic area (the neutral point). There are several types of dichromatism: deuteranopia, protanopia and tritanopia. *Syn.* daltonism; dichromatopsia; dichromatic vision. *See* **colour vision, defective; pigment, visual.**

diclofenac *See* **antiinflammatory drug.**

dicoria A condition in which there are two pupils in one iris. It may be congenital or the result of surgery or injury. *Syn.* diplocoria. *See* **polycoria.**

dietary supplements *See* **macular degeneration, age-related; neuropathy, nutritional optic; vitamin A deficiency.**

difference threshold *See* **threshold, difference.**

diffraction Deviation of the direction of propagation of a beam of light, which occurs when the light passes the edge of an obstacle such as a diaphragm, the pupil of the eye or a spectacle frame. There are two consequences of this phenomenon. First, the image of a point source cannot be a point image but a **diffraction pattern**. This pattern depends upon the shape and size of the diaphragm as well as the wavelength of light. Second, a system of close, parallel and equidistant grooves, slits or lines ruled on a polished surface can produce a light spectrum by diffraction. This is called a **diffraction grating**. *See* **disc, Airy's; fringes, diffraction; theory, Maurice's.**

diffractive contact lens *See* **lens, contact.**

diffuser A device used to scatter light. It can be a reflecting surface (e.g. matt paint) or a transmitting medium (e.g. ground glass).

diffusion 1. Scattering of light passing through a heterogeneous medium or being reflected irregularly by a surface such as a sandblasted opal glass surface. Diffusion by a perfectly diffusing surface occurs in accordance with **Lambert's cosine law**.

In this case, the luminance will be the same, regardless of the viewing direction. **2.** The passive movement of ions or molecules through a medium or across a semipermeable membrane (e.g. the ciliary epithelium) in response to a concentration gradient until equilibrium is reached (osmosis). It is one of the three mechanisms that create aqueous humour.
See **light, diffuse; osmosis; reflection, diffuse; ultrafiltration.**

diffusion circle *See* **blur circle.**

diisopropyl fluorophosphate (DFP) *See* **anticholinesterase.**

dilation and irrigation A method of unblocking the lacrimal drainage system, when there is no underlying infection such as canaliculitis or dacryocystitis. It consists of inserting a dilator into one punctum, after topical anaesthesia, to enlarge its opening and then inserting a cannula and passing a small amount of saline water until the patient reports detecting it in the throat.
See **test, dye dilution; test, Jones 1.**

dilator pupillae muscle *See* **muscle, dilator pupillae.**

dioptre 1. A unit proposed by Monoyer to evaluate the refractive power of a lens or of an optical system. It is equal to the reciprocal of the secondary focal length in metres. (*Symbol:* D) Thus a lens with a focal length (in air) of 1 m has a power of 1 D, one with a focal length of 1/2 m, has a power of 2 D, etc (Table D3). **2.** It is also incorrectly used to represent a unit of curvature, being equal to the reciprocal of the radius of curvature expressed in metres.
See **curvature of a surface; myodioptre; paraxial equation, fundamental; refractive error; vergence.**

dioptre, prism 1. A unit specifying the power of an ophthalmic prism based on the amount of light deviation. One prism dioptre (written 1 Δ) represents a deviation of 1 cm on a flat surface 1 m away from the prism. The surface is perpendicular to the direction of the original light ray (Fig. D3). Similarly, a 2 Δ prism deviates light 2 cm at a distance of 1 m, and so on. For small angles, conversion between prism dioptres and degrees is given by the approximate formula (Table D4).

$$7\Delta = 4° \text{ or } 1\Delta = 0.57° \text{ or } 1° = 1.75\Delta$$

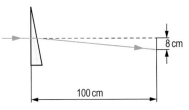

Fig. D3 Effect of an 8 Δ prism.

The exact formula for any angle α less than 90° is

$$\alpha \text{ in } \Delta = 100 \tan \alpha$$

Example: What is the power a prism that deviates an object 20 mm on a wall placed 20 cm away from the prism? α =100 (2/20) = 10Δ.
Note: The current British Standard regarding ophthalmic lenses specifies a deviation (in Δ) of a ray of light of wavelength 587.6 nm incident normally at one surface. **2.** A unit of convergence of the eyes.
See **law, Prentice's; power, prism.**

dioptric power *See* **power, refractive.**

Table D3 Relationship between dioptres and focal length (in air)		
	Focal length	
Dioptre value	**(cm)**	**(in)**
0.25	400	157
0.50	200	79
1.00	100	39
1.50	67	26
2.00	50	20
2.50	40	16
3.00	33.3	13
4.00	25	10
5.00	20	7.9
6.00	16.7	6.6
7.00	14.3	5.6
8.00	12.5	4.9
9.00	11.1	4.4
10.00	10	3.9
12.00	8.3	3.3
14.00	7.1	2.8
16.00	6.2	2.4
20.00	5.0	2.0

Table D4 Relationship between prism dioptres and degrees		
Prism dioptres (Δ)	**Degrees (°)**	**Minutes (')**
1	0.573°	0°34'
2	1.14°	1°8'
3	1.71°	1°43'
4	2.28°	2°17'
5	2.85°	2°51'
6	3.43°	3°26'
7	4.0°	4°0'
8	4.57°	4°34'
9	5.14°	5°8'
10	5.71°	5°43'
15	8.57°	8°34'

dioptrics That branch of optics which deals with the refraction of light (as opposed to reflection). *Example*: the dioptrics of the eye.

dipivefrine hydrochloride *See* sympathomimetic drugs.

diplocoria *See* dicoria.

diplopia The condition in which a single object is seen as two rather than one. This is usually due to images not stimulating corresponding retinal areas. *Syn.* double vision (colloquial). *See* effect, differential prismatic; haplopia; myasthenia gravis; retinal corresponding points; polyopia; sclerosis, multiple; strabismus; test, diplopia; triplopia.

binocular d. Diplopia in which one image is seen by one eye and the other image is seen by the other eye.

crossed d. *See* diplopia, heteronymous.

heteronymous d. Binocular diplopia in which the image received by the right eye appears to the left and that received by the left eye appears to the right. In this condition, the images are formed on the temporal retina. *Syn.* crossed diplopia.

homonymous d. Binocular diplopia in which the image received by the right eye appears to the right and that received by the left eye appears to the left. In this condition, the images are formed on the nasal retina. *Syn.* uncrossed diplopia.

incongruous d. Diplopia present in individuals with abnormal retinal correspondence in which the relative positions of the two images differ from what would be expected on the basis of normal retinal correspondence. *Example*: an exotrope experiencing homonymous diplopia instead of heteronymous diplopia. *Syn.* paradoxical diplopia. *See* retinal correspondence, abnormal.

monocular d. Diplopia seen by one eye only. It is usually caused by irregular refraction in one eye (e.g. in early cataracts, corneal opacity) or by dicoria or polycoria. It may be induced by placing a bi-prism in front of one eye or an incorrect lens centration. *See* image, ghost; luxation of the lens; proptosis.

paradoxical d. *See* diplopia, incongruous.

pathological d. Any diplopia due to an eye disease (e.g. proptosis), an anomaly of binocular vision (e.g. strabismus, uncompensated heterophoria, a variation in the refractive index of the media of the eye (e.g. cataract), a subluxation of the crystalline lens, or to a general disease (e.g. extraocular tumour, multiple sclerosis, myasthenia gravis). *See* exophthalmos; luxation of the lens.

physiological d. Normal phenomenon which occurs in binocular vision for non-fixated objects whose images fall on disparate retinal points. It is easily demonstrated to persons with normal binocular vision: fixate binocularly on a distant object and place a pencil vertically some 25 cm in front of your nose. You should see two rather blurred pencils. The observation of physiological diplopia has been found to be useful in the management

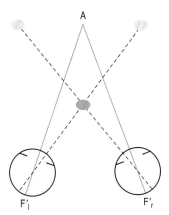

Fig. D4 Physiological diplopia. The subject fixates a distant object A. The near object appears in crossed diplopia (F'_l, F'_r, foveas of the left and right eye, respectively).

of eso or exo deviations, suppression, abnormal retinal correspondence, etc. (Fig. D4). *See* Brock string; disparity, retinal.

d. test *See* test, diplopia.

uncrossed d. *See* diplopia, homonymous.

diploscope Instrument used to evaluate binocular vision and which may be used for the treatment of anomalies of binocular vision.

direct ophthalmoscopy *See* ophthalmoscopy, direct.

direction, oculocentric Direction associated with a particular retinal point. It is always perceived in the same direction if the light is received by the same retinal receptor. The capacity of a receptor to distinguish its excitation from that of its neighbours is referred to as **local sign** (or **Lotze's local sign**). This characteristic means that each retinal receptor has a unique oculocentric direction. *See* line of direction; oculocentre.

disc 1. A flat, circular, coin-shaped structure. 2. In anatomy, the intervertebral disc.

Airy's d. Owing to the wave nature of light, the image of a point source consists of a diffraction pattern. If light passes through a circular aperture, the diffraction pattern will appear as a bright central disc, called Airy's disc, surrounded by concentric light and dark rings. Airy's disc receives about 87% of the luminous flux, the next concentric ring about 8% and the next 3%. The radius of Airy's disc equals

$$1.22\lambda\, f/d$$

where d is the radius of the entrance pupil of the optical system of focal length f and λ the wavelength of the light used. In the eye, with a pupil of 4 mm diameter and $\lambda = 507$ nm, the diameter of Airy's disc is about 5 mm, which

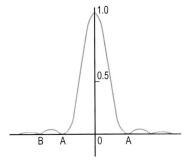

Fig. D5 Point spread function of the intensity of the diffraction pattern from a circular aperture. Airy's disc is represented by the central disc (AA), the radius of which is equal to 1.22 $\lambda f'/d$, the radius of the next concentric light ring (0B) is equal to 2.23 $\lambda f'/d$. The light intensity is maximum in the middle of Airy's disc; it is equal to 1.75% in the middle of the next concentric light ring.

corresponds to a visual angle of about one minute of arc (Fig. D5). *Syn.* diffraction disc.
See **criterion, Rayleigh; function, point-spread; resolution, limit of.**

choked d. *See* **papilloedema.**

cupped d. An enlarged and deepened excavation of the physiological cup. It may be physiological, pathological due to glaucoma (**glaucomatous cup**) in which there is a loss of nerve fibres or following atrophy of the optic nerve (as in papilloedema). *See* **lamina cribrosa.**

diffraction d. *See* **disc, Airy's.**

inversion of the d. *See* **disc, situs inversus of the.**

Maxwell d. A rotating disc onto which differently coloured discs radially slit can be fitted together to overlap and divide the surface into sectors of different colours. It may be used to investigate colour mixture.

morning glory d. A congenital, usually unilateral, anomaly of the optic disc characterized by an excavation. It may be due to a failure of the embryonic fissure such that the optic disc and some peripapillary tissue prolapse posteriorly. The optic disc is abnormally large, and a white-grey tuft of glial tissue covers its centre. The annular zone surrounding the disc has irregular areas of pigmentation and depigmentation. The optic disc thus resembles a morning glory flower. Patients present with reduced visual acuity and strabismus and, in about one-third of patients, retinal detachment.

optic d. Region of the fundus of the eye corresponding to the optic nerve head. It can be seen with the ophthalmoscope as a pinkish-yellow area with usually a whitish depression called the physiological cup. The optic disc has an area of about 2.7 mm², a horizontal width of about 1.75 mm and a vertical height of about 1.9 mm, although there are wide variations in the size of the disc, being smaller in highly hyperopic eyes, pseudopapilloedema and non-arteritic ischaemic optic neuropathy and larger in highly myopic eyes and buphthalmos. The optic disc is the anatomical correlate of the physiological blind spot. It is greatly affected in glaucoma, papillitis and Leber's hereditary optic atrophy. *Syn.* optic nerve head; optic papilla (although this is not strictly correct because the disc is not elevated above the surrounding retina).
See **cup, glaucomatous; drusen, optic disc; haemorrhage, subarachnoid; lamina cribrosa; neuroretinal rim; papilloedema; syndrome, Swann's.**

optic d. pit A rare, unilateral condition characterized by the presence of a depression in the optic nerve head. It appears as a greyish pit, usually larger than in the unaffected eye and situated temporally. Patient is usually asymptomatic unless there are complications (e.g. macular retinoschisis) and peripheral visual field defects are common.

pinhole d. A blank disc with a small aperture (2 mm diameter or less) mounted in a trial lens rim. It is used to reduce the size of the blur circle in an ametropic eye. In this condition, vision will improve giving an indication of the final visual acuity that will be obtained with corrective lenses. If no improvement occurs, the eye is amblyopic. This procedure is called the **pinhole test.**

Scheiner's d. An opaque disc in which there are two pinholes separated by a distance less than the pupil diameter. It is used to measure the dioptric changes during accommodation or to detect the type of ametropia (Fig. D6).
See **experiment, Scheiner's.**

situs inversus of the d. A congenital condition, usually bilateral, in which the retinal blood vessels emerge towards the nasal side of the disc (instead of temporal) and course nasally before turning temporally. It is often associated with congenital crescent, tilted disc and myopic astigmatism.

stenopaeic d. **1.** A pinhole disc. **2.** A blank disc with a slit used in detecting and measuring the astigmatism of the eye (Fig. D7). *Syn.* stenopaeic slit. *Note*: also spelt stenopeic or stenopaic.
See **kinescope; spectacles, stenopaeic.**

tilted d. A congenital bilateral condition in which the optic nerves insert obliquely into the globe. It is often associated with myopia and astigmatism. The signs are a bitemporal visual field defect (often upper temporal), and the disc is usually orientated inferonasally with elevation of the superotemporal margin and situs inversus of the retinal blood vessels.
See **disc, situs inversus of the.**

disciform keratitis *See* **keratitis, disciform.**

disciform scar A subretinal scar, most often located in the macular area. It results from the haemorrhages that sometimes follow choroidal neovascularization (consisting of fibrovascular tissue) in the exudative type of age-related macular degeneration. It causes irreparable damage to vision.
See **macular degeneration, age-related.**

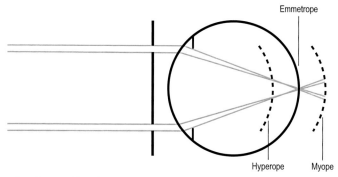

Fig. D6 Images of a distant object formed on the retina of an unaccommodated emmetrope (clear single image), a hyperope and a myope (blurred double images) looking through a Scheiner's disc. To determine the type of ametropia, cover one of the pinholes; if the top hole is covered, a hyperope will report that the lower image disappears (because the retinal image is inverted perceptually), whereas a myope will report that the upper image disappears.

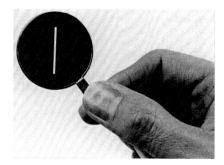

Fig. D7 Stenopaeic slit.

discomfort glare *See* glare, discomfort.

disconjugate movements *See* movement, disjunctive eye.

disease An abnormal process affecting the structure or function of a part, organ or system of the body. It is typically manifested by signs and symptoms, but the aetiology may or may not be known. Disease is a response to a specific infective agent (a microorganism or a poison), to environmental factors (e.g. malnutrition, injury, industrial hazards), or to congenital or hereditary defects, or to a combination of all these factors. *Note*: Illness is sometimes used as a synonym of disease, but it also refers to a person's perception of their health, regardless of whether the person does or does not have a disease.
autoimmune d. A disease produced when the immune response of an individual is directed against its own cells or tissues. It is not yet known exactly what causes the body to react to one's own antigens as if they were foreign. Ocular complications principally involve the cornea but may also include the conjunctiva, sclera, uvea and retina. *Examples*: Crohn's disease; diabetes mellitus type 1; Graves' disease; multiple sclerosis; lupus erythematosus; myasthenia gravis; rheumatoid arthritis; Reiter's disease; Sjögren's syndrome.
Batten–Mayou d. Autosomal recessive metabolic disorder resulting in a juvenile form of amaurotic family idiocy. It is characterized by progressive degeneration of the retina, which eventually leads to blindness. *Syn.* Spielmeyer–Stock disease.
Behçet's d. Idiopathic multisystem disorder consisting of ulceration of the mouth and genital region and vasculitis. Ocular manifestations include acute anterior uveitis typically with hypopyon, vitritis, retinal infiltrates and retinal oedema. The disease tends to recur at regular intervals. It usually affects individuals below the age of 40 and, in a few cases, the eye becomes blind. Treatment is with immunosuppressants and steroids.
See **immunosuppressants**.
Benson's d. *See* asteroid hyalosis.
Berlin's d. A blunt trauma to the globe in which the posterior pole of the retina develops oedema (and, if severe, haemorrhages).
See **commotio retinae**.
Best's d. An autosomal dominant inherited degeneration in which there is an accumulation of lipofuscin within the retinal pigment epithelium, which interferes with its function. It is caused by a mutation in the bestrophin gene (BEST1). The disease is characterized by the appearance on the retina in the first and second decades of life of a bright orange deposit, resembling the yolk of an egg (vitelliform), with practically no effect on vision. It eventually absorbs, leaving scarring, pigmentary changes and impairment of central vision in most cases, although in some cases the retinal lesion may be eccentric with very little effect on vision. The electrooculogram is abnormal throughout the development of the disease from previtelliform, vitelliform to the end-stage when there is scarring or atrophy. *Syn.* Best's macular dystrophy; juvenile vitelliform macular dystrophy; vitelliform macular dystrophy. Mutation in the VMD2 gene can cause **adult vitelliform macular dystrophy**, a condition

characterized by smaller macular lesions and very little impairment of vision.
See **dystrophy, pattern.**
Bourneville's d. *See* **sclerosis, tuberous.**
Bowen's d. A disease characterized by a slow-growing tumour of the epidermis of the skin which may involve the corneal or conjunctival epithelium.
Coats' d. Chronic progressive retinal vascular anomalies, usually unilateral, occurring predominantly in young males. It is characterized by retinal exudates, irregular dilatation (telangiectasia) and tortuosity of retinal vessels and appears as a whitish fundus reflex (leukocoria). Subretinal haemorrhages are frequent and eventually retinal detachment may occur. The main symptom is a decrease in central or peripheral vision, although it may be asymptomatic in some patients. Management may involve photocoagulation or cryotherapy. A less severe form of the disease is called **Leber's miliary aneurysms.** *Syn.* retinal telangiectasia.
See **cryopexy; telangiectasia.**
Crohn's d. Type of inflammatory chronic bowel disease characterized by granulomatous inflammation of the bowel wall causing fever, diarrhoea, abdominal pain and weight loss. The ocular manifestations include acute iridocyclitis, scleritis, conjunctivitis and corneal infiltrates.
Devic's d. A demyelinative disease of the optic nerve, the optic chiasma and the spinal cord characterized by a bilateral acute optic neuritis with a transverse inflammation of the spinal cord. Loss of visual acuity occurs very rapidly and is accompanied by ascending paralysis. There is no treatment for this disease. *Syn.* neuromyelitis optica.
Eales' d. A non-specific peripheral retinal periphlebitis (i.e. an inflammation of the outer coat of a vein) that usually affects mostly young males, often those who have active or healed tuberculosis. It is characterized by recurrent haemorrhages in the retina and vitreous and sudden visual reduction due to vitreous haemorrhage. This disease is a prime example of retinal vasculitis.
Fabry's d. An X-linked recessive disease caused by mutations in the gene encoding alpha-galactosidase A (GLA) and characterized by an abnormal accumulation of glycolipid in the tissues. It appears as small purple skin lesions on the trunk and there may be renal and cardiovascular abnormalities. Ocular signs include whorl-like corneal opacities, spoke-shaped posterior cataract and tortuous conjunctival and retinal blood vessels.
Gaucher's d. An autosomal recessive inherited disorder in which fat metabolism is abnormal due to an enzyme deficiency (e.g. alglucerase). There are three main types. Type 1 is characterized by enlargement of the liver and spleen, anaemia and bone abnormalities. Type 2 and 3 have in addition central nervous system degeneration and ocular signs such as strabismus and yellowish-brown deposits on the bulbar conjunctiva, which may encroach on the cornea. The three types are caused by mutation in the gene encoding acid beta-glucosidase (GBA) on chromosome 1q22.

Goldman-Favre d. An autosomal recessive disorder characterized by a liquefied vitreous with central and peripheral retinoschisis resulting in loss of visual function. A cataract may also develop.
See **retinoschisis.**
Graves' d. An autoimmune disorder in which the thyroid stimulating immunoglobulin (IgG) antibodies bind to thyroid stimulating hormone (TSH) receptors in the thyroid gland and stimulate secretion of too much thyroid hormones (e.g. thyroxine T3 and T4), thus leading to hyperthyroidism (also called **thyrotoxicosis**). The level of TSH in the blood is thus low and this is one test used to diagnose the disease. Between a quarter and a half of people with Graves' disease develop ocular manifestations (called **Graves' ophthalmopathy, thyroid ophthalmopathy**). General symptoms include irritability, fatigue, muscle weakness, sweating, diarrhea, weight loss and swollen neck (goiter). Ocular manifestations include swollen and inflamed extraocular muscles and build-up of fluid and orbital fat, red eyes, lacrimation, exophthalmos, retraction of the eyelids (**Dalrymple's sign**), conjunctival hyperaemia, lid lag in which the upper lid follows after a latent period when the eye looks downward (**von Graefe's sign**), retraction of the upper eyelid on attentive fixation (**Kocher's sign**), defective eye movements (**restrictive myopathy**), convergence weakness (**Moebius sign**) and optic neuropathy. The ocular signs and symptoms vary from mild to moderate in severity. The disease occurs between the ages of 20 and 50 years, more commonly in women than men and in people who smoke heavily. If only the eye signs of the disease are present without clinical evidence of hyperthyroidism, the disease is called **euthyroid** or **ophthalmic Graves' disease**. Treatment begins with control of the hyperthyroidism with radioiodine therapy, antithyroid drugs and beta-blockers. Some cases may recover spontaneously with time. Mild cases of ocular deviations and restrictions may benefit from a prismatic correction. Ocular lubricants provide relief and protection. If there is inflammation and pain, corticosteroids may be used. Surgery is occasionally used when there is diplopia in the primary position of gaze. *Syn.* thyroid-associated orbitopathy; thyroid eye disease.
See **accommodative infacility; exophthalmos.**
Hansen d. *See* **uveitis, bacterial.**
Harada's d. A disease characterized by bilateral uveitis associated with alopecia, vitiligo, meningitis and hearing defects. However, as many aspects of this entity overlap clinically and histopathologically with the Vogt–Koyanagi syndrome it is nowadays combined and called the Vogt–Koyanagi–Harada syndrome.
von Hippel's d. A rare disease, sometimes familial, in which haemangiomata occur in the retina where they appear ophthalmoscopically as one or more round, elevated, reddish nodules. The condition is progressive and takes years before there is a complete loss of vision. *Syn.* angiomatosis retinae.

Huntington's d. A rare disease inherited as an autosomal dominant trait caused by a mutation in the HTT gene which produces a progressive degeneration of nerve cells in the brain and results in involuntary movements and mental deterioration leading to dementia. It affects principally people in midlife. Ocular manifestations include horizontal saccadic palsy and strabismus. *Syn.* Huntington's chorea.

Leber's d. *See* **neuropathy, Leber's hereditary optic.**

Lyme d. *See* **uveitis, bacterial.**

Niemann–Pick d. An autosomal recessive inherited lipid storage disorder characterized by a partial destruction of the retinal ganglion cells and a demyelination of many parts of the nervous system. It is caused by mutation in the NPC1 gene. The condition usually involves children of Jewish parentage. When the retina is involved, there is a reddish central area (cherry-red spot) surrounded by a white oedematous area. The disease usually leads to death by the age of 2. This disease is differentiated from **Tay–Sachs disease** because of its widespread involvement and gross enlargement of the liver and the spleen. *Syn.* sphingomyelin lipidosis.
See **disease, Tay–Sachs.**

Norrie's d. An inherited X-linked recessive disorder characterized by bilateral congenital blindness. It is caused by mutation in the norrin gene (NDP). The initial ocular presentation is leukocoria. It then progresses to cataract, corneal opacification and phthisis bulbi. The condition may be associated with mental retardation and hearing defects. *Syn.* oculoacoustico-cerebral degeneration; Andersen–Warburg syndrome.

Oguchi's d. An autosomal, recessive, inherited night blindness found mainly in Japan. All other visual capabilities are usually unimpaired, but the patient presents an abnormal golden-brown fundus reflex in the light-adapted state, which becomes a normal colour with dark-adaptation (**Mizuo phenomenon**). It is presumed to be due to an abnormality in the neural network of the retina. The disease can be caused by mutation in the arrestin gene (SAG) or the rhodopsin kinase gene (GRK1).

ophthalmic Graves' d. *See* **disease, Graves'.**

Paget's d. A hereditary systemic disorder of the skeletal system accompanied in a few patients with ocular disorders, such as retinal abnormalities including peripapillary atrophy, angioid streaks and choroidal neovascularization.

von Recklinghausen's d. *See* **neurofibromatosis type 1.**

Refsum's d. An autosomal recessive hereditary disorder caused by a defective metabolism of phytanic acid alpha-hydrolase resulting in an accumulation of phytanic acid in the blood and tissues. The principal signs are pigmentary degeneration of the retina, cerebellar ataxia, peripheral neuropathy and deafness. The visual fields are constricted, and there is night blindness. Management with a phytanic acid–free diet (i.e. fat free) may retard the progression of the condition. *Syn.* Refsum's syndrome.
See **syndrome, Zellweger's.**

Reiter's d. *See* **syndrome, Reiter's.**

Sandhoff's d. An autosomal, recessive, inherited disease similar to Tay–Sachs disease with the same signs, but differing in that both the enzymes hexosaminidase A and B are defective. It develops more rapidly and can be found among the general population. It is caused by mutation in the beta subunit of the hexosaminidase (HEXB) gene on chromosome 5q13. The main ocular manifestation is a whitish area in the central retina with a cherry-red spot which eventually fades and the optic disc develops atrophy. *Syn.* Gm2 gangliosidosis type2.

sickle-cell d. A hereditary anaemia encountered among black and dark-skinned people due to a defect in the haemoglobin. It is characterized by retinal neovascularization and haemorrhages, exudates, cataract and subconjunctival haemorrhage. *Syn.* sickle-cell anaemia.

Spielmeyer–Stock d. *See* **disease, Batten–Mayou.**

Stargardt's d. An autosomal recessive inherited disorder of the retina occurring in the first or second decade of life and affecting the central region of the retina. A few cases are inherited as an autosomal dominant trait. Known causes of the disease include a mutation in one of the following genes: ABCA4, CNGB3 and ELOVL4. There is an accumulation of lipofuscin within the retinal pigment epithelium, which interferes with its function. With time, a lesion develops at the macula, which has a 'beaten-bronze' reflex. It is often surrounded by yellow-white flecks. There is a loss of central vision, but peripheral vision is usually unaffected. Myopia is common. Management usually consists of a high plus correction for near to magnify the retinal image and wearing UV-protecting sunglasses. *Syn.* juvenile macular dystrophy; Stargardt's macular dystrophy.
See **dystrophy, macular; fundus flavimaculatus.**

Steinert's d. *See* **dystrophy, myotonic.**

Still's d. *See* **arthritis, juvenile rheumatoid.**

Sturge–Weber d. *See* **syndrome, Sturge–Weber.**

Tay–Sachs d. An autosomal recessive lipid storage disorder caused by a deficiency of the enzyme hexosaminidase A which leads to an accumulation of Gm2 ganglioside (a fatty acid derivative) in the ganglion cells of both the retina and the brain. It is caused by mutation in the alpha subunit of the hexosaminidase A gene (HEXA). It has its onset in the first year of life, vision is affected and the central retina shows a whitish area with a reddish central area (cherry-red spot) which fades and the optic disc develops atrophy. Eventually the eye becomes blind and death occurs, usually at about the age of 30 months. It affects Jewish infants more than others by a factor of about 10 to 1. *Syn.* Gm2 gangliosidosis type 1; infantile amaurotic familial idiocy.
See **disease, Niemann–Pick.**

Terrien's d. *See* **degeneration, Terrien's marginal.**

thyroid eye d. *See* disease, Graves'.

Wagner's d. *See* syndrome, Wagner's.

Wernicke's d. A disease characterized by disturbances in ocular motility, pupillary reactions, nystagmus and ataxia. It is mainly due to thiamin deficiency and is frequently encountered in chronic alcoholics. *Syn.* Wernicke's syndrome.

Wilson's d. A systemic disease resulting from a deficiency of the alpha-2-globulin ceruloplasmin. It begins in the first or second decade of life and is characterized by widespread deposition of copper in the tissues, tremor, muscular rigidity, irregular involuntary movements, emotional instability and hepatic disorders. The ocular features are degenerative changes in the lenticular nucleus and, most noticeably, a Kayser–Fleischer ring. *Syn.* hepatolenticular degeneration; lenticular progressive degeneration; pseudosclerosis of Westphal.

disinfectant *See* antiseptic.

disinfection The process or act of destroying pathogenic microorganisms. However, certain bacterial spores may survive and germinate which could lead to contamination.

See antiseptic; sterilization; surfactant.

chemical d. A method of disinfecting soft contact lenses which uses solutions containing either a preservative or hydrogen peroxide. Preservatives include chlorhexidine, thimerosal (very rarely used nowadays) and more commonly nowadays the preservatives with larger molecules which cannot penetrate into the lens matrix of soft contact lenses, such as the biguanide polyhexanide (polyamino-propyl biguanide or polyhexamethylene biguanide). Hydrogen peroxide has a broad-spectrum efficacy against bacteria, fungi and viruses. It must, however, be neutralized before the lenses can be worn. Rigid gas permeable contact lenses are disinfected with a preservative such as chlorhexidine, benzalkonium chloride, polyhexanide and polixetonium chloride. Failure to disinfect contact lenses may lead to microbial keratitis. Disinfectants for contact lenses have to pass **FDA** and International Organization for Standardization (**ISO**) tests to be approved. They must be effective against three specific bacteria (*Pseudomonas aeruginosa*, *Staphylococcus aureus* and *Serratia marcescens*) and two fungi (*Candida albicans* and *Fusarium solani*).

See neutralization.

heat d. A method of disinfecting soft contact lenses, based on heating the lens to a temperature of at least 80°C for 10 minutes. This is achieved in specially manufactured heating units in which the lenses are kept in physiological saline solution. However, repeated boiling of soft lenses may cause some degradation of the lens material, and tear mucoproteins that have not been previously removed with a surface cleaning agent tend to become coagulated on the lens surface.

disinsertion 1. Rupture of a tendon at the point of insertion into a bone or a tissue. *Example*: rupture of the insertion of the tendon of the levator palpebrae superioris muscle into the upper eyelid. *See* ptosis, involuntional. **2.** *See* myectomy.

disinsertion, retinal *See* retinal dialysis.

disjunctive Adjective meaning disjoined or separated or in opposition.

See movement, disjunctive; reflex, vergence; vergence.

disjunctive movements *See* movements, disjunctive.

disjunctive nystagmus *See* nystagmus.

dislocation of the lens *See* luxation of the lens.

disparate retinal points Non-corresponding retinal points.

disparity The condition of being unequal or totally different. The word is used mainly to refer to non-corresponding points in the retina.

See disparity, retinal; retinal corresponding points.

binocular d. *See* acuity, stereoscopic visual; disparity, retinal; perception, depth.

crossed d. Retinal disparity induced by an object nearer to the eyes than the point of fixation and focused on the temporal retina. Thus, the image received by the right eye appears to the left and that received by the left eye appears to the right. *Syn.* crossed retinal disparity.

fixation d. *See* disparity, retinal.

retinal d. Binocular vision in which the two retinal images of a single object do not fall on corresponding retinal points (i.e. when the object lies off the horopter). If, however, the two retinal images still fall within Panum's area, the object will still be seen single. At the fixation point, this may cause over- or underconvergence of the eyes. This particular case is called **fixation disparity** (or **retinal slip**). The presence of fixation disparity often indicates that binocular vision is under stress and the patient has an uncompensated heterophoria. Optical correction or orthoptic exercises usually eliminate the symptoms. Fixation disparity can be measured either (1) directly (e.g. Disparometer, Wesson Fixation Disparity Card, both consisting of targets with pairs of vernier lines of various angular separation, each line being seen by one eye through polarizing filters) or (2) indirectly by assessing the aligning prism value of a disparity test (e.g. Mallett fixation disparity unit). *Syn.* binocular disparity.

See acuity, stereoscopic visual; anaglyph; esodisparity; exodisparity; fusional movements; Mallett fixation disparity unit; perception, depth; stereogram, random-dot; stereopsis; stereotest.

uncrossed d. Retinal disparity induced by an object farther away from the eyes than the point of fixation and focused on the nasal retina. Thus, the image received by the right eye appears to the right and that received by the left eye appears to the left. *Syn.* uncrossed retinal disparity.

vergence d. *See* fusion, motor.

Disparometer Trade name for a clinical instrument designed to measure fixation disparity at near. The target does not have a binocular fixation point and the fusion lock is parafoveal. The instrument fits on the near point rod of a standard phoropter. The Disparometer has two stimuli: one for vertical

disparity measurement and the other for horizontal disparity measurement. The test consists of successive pairs of vernier lines of increasing angular separation within a structureless field, each line being viewed by one eye through polarizing filters. The edge of the field provides a peripheral fusion stimulus. Fixation disparity is measured when the vernier lines appear to be aligned and the amount is given by the angular separation (in minutes of arc) of the lines indicated on the back of the instrument. A fixation disparity curve can be obtained by determining the fixation disparity for various amounts of prism power placed in front of the eyes.
See **Mallett fixation disparity unit; prism, aligning.**

dispensing, optical The act of issuing an optical appliance which corrects, remedies or relieves defects of vision (definition of the **World Council of Optometry**). *Syn.* dispensing; ophthalmic dispensing.
See **optician, dispensing; optics, ophthalmic.**

dispersion A variation in the velocity of propagation of radiations in a medium, as a function of its frequency, which causes a separation of the monochromatic components of a complex radiation. All optical media cause dispersion by virtue of their variation of refractive index with wavelengths. Dispersion is specified by the difference in the refractive index of the medium for two wavelengths. The difference between the blue F (486.1 nm) and the red C (656.3 nm) spectral lines is called the **mean dispersion**, i.e. $n_F - n_C$. Dispersion is usually represented by its **dispersive power** ω or **relative dispersion** which is equal to the mean dispersion divided by the excess refractive index of the helium d (587.6 nm) spectral line ($n_d - 1$), often called the **refractivity** of the material,

$$\omega = n_F - n_C / n_d - 1$$

The reciprocal of the dispersive power is called the Abbé's number or constringence (Fig. D8).
See **aberration longitudinal chromatic; axis, achromatic; lines, Fraunhoffer's; prism, achromatic.**

dispersion, mean; relative *See* dispersion.

dispersive power *See* dispersion.

disposable contact lens *See* lens, contact.

dissociated nystagmus *See* nystagmus.

dissociated vertical deviation *See* deviation, dissociated vertical.

dissociated vertical divergence *See* hyperopia, alternating.

dissociating test *See* test, dissociating.

dissociation Elimination of the stimulus to fusion. It is usually accomplished by occluding one eye or by inducing gross distortion of the image seen by one eye (e.g. Maddox rod), or by placing a strong prism in front of one eye (e.g. von Graefe's test) with the result that the eyes will move to the passive position (or heterophoria position).
See **heterophoria, dissociated; position, passive; test, diplopia; test, dissociating.**

distal Farthest from a central point.
See **proximal.**

distance The amount of space between two points.
abathic d. *See* plane, apparent frontoparallel.
d. between lenses Horizontal distance between the nasal parts of the spectacle lenses in a frame, measured either along the datum line (datum system) or between the nasal peaks of the bevels of the two spectacle lenses (boxing system).
See **spectacle frame markings; system, boxing.**
d. between rims Horizontal distance between the bearing surfaces of a regular bridge of a spectacle frame, usually measured along the datum line, or at a specified distance below the crest of the bridge.
centration d. The specified horizontal distance between the right and left centration points of a pair of ophthalmic lenses.
See **distance, near centration; point, centration.**
conjugate d's. An optical system will form an image of an object. As the path of light is reversible, the position of object and image are interchangeable. These pairs of object and image points are called **conjugate points** (or **conjugate foci**) and the distances of the object and the image from the optical surface are called the **conjugate distances** (Fig. D9). When an eye is accurately focused for an object, object and retina are conjugate.
See **emmetropia; experiment, Scheiner's.**
d. of distinct vision A conventional distance used in calculating the magnifying power of a loupe or microscope. It is usually taken as 25 cm (or 10 inches) from the eye.
See **magnification, apparent.**
focal d. *See* length, focal.

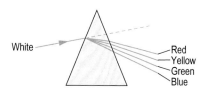

Fig. D8 Dispersion of a white beam of light by a prism.

White → Red / Yellow / Green / Blue

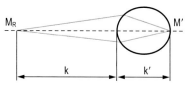

Fig. D9 Conjugate distances k and k′ and conjugate points M_R and M′ in the eye (M_R, far point of the eye; M′, foveola).

hyperfocal d. That distance from a lens or optical system at which the depth of field, on the far side of an object in focus, extends to infinity. On the near side of the object, the depth of field then extends to half that distance. This is a useful distance in photography as it represents the shortest distance on which to focus to obtain a reasonable image definition of an object at infinity and the longest total depth of field. This distance depends on the focal length and the diameter of the entrance pupil of the system as well as the amount of the allowable blur.
See **depth of field.**

image d. Distance along the optical axis of a lens or optical system between the image plane and the secondary principal plane. If the system consists of a single thin lens, the image distance is measured from the optical surface and the reciprocal of this quantity is called the **reduced image vergence** or **image vergence** (in air).
See **plane, principal; power, back vertex.**

interocular d. Distance between the centres of rotation of the eyes, i.e. the length of the base line.

interpupillary d. (PD) The distance between the centres of the pupils of the eyes. It usually refers to the eyes fixating at distance, otherwise reference must be made to the fixation distance (e.g. near interpupillary distance). The average interpupillary distance for men is about 65 mm and for women about 62 mm (in Caucasians). *Syn.* pupillary distance. The interpupillary distance is often measured from the median plane to the centre of the pupil of each eye. This is referred to as the **monocular pupillary distance**; it is a useful measurement, especially in dispensing progressive lenses. The interpupillary distance for near vision can be calculated using the following formula:

near PD = (d/d') distance PD

where d is the distance between the target plane and the spectacle plane and d' the distance between the target plane and the midpoint between the centres of rotation of the eyes (Table D5).
See **pupillometer; rule, PD.**

near centration d. The horizontal distance between the right and left centration points used for near vision.

object d. Distance along the optical axis of a lens or optical system between the object plane and the

primary principal plane. If the system consists of a single thin lens, the object distance is measured from the optical surface and the reciprocal of this quantity is called the **reduced object vergence** or **object vergence** (in air).
See **power, front vertex; vergence.**

reading d. The normal distance at which people read. It is about 33 to 44 cm for men and 29 to 41 cm for women. It is a useful measurement in determining the reading addition, which must be assessed for each patient.

vertex d. *See* **vertex distance.**

d. vision *See* **vision, distance.**

working d. 1. The distance at which a person reads or does close work. **2.** In retinoscopy, the distance between the plane of the sighthole and that of the patient's spectacles. **3.** In microscopy, the distance between an object and the front surface of the objective.

distichiasis Congenital anomaly in which there is a double row of eyelashes in the lid margin, one row being normal and the other row turning inward towards the eye. Distichiasis can also be acquired following scarring or chemical and physical injury. If there are symptoms, treatment consists of removal of the aberrant eyelashes, usually by cryotherapy (removal under extreme cold or freezing conditions) or electrolysis.
See **epilation; polystichia; trichiasis.**

distometer An instrument for measuring the distance between the back surface of a spectacle lens and the apex of the cornea. It is usually carried out by having the patient close the eyes. One end of the instrument or caliper rests against the upper eyelid and the other presses against the back surface of the spectacle lens. The measurements are most commonly given to the nearest 0.5 mm. *Syn.* Lenscorometer (a tradename); vertexometer.

distortion Aberration of an optical system (e.g. a correcting lens) resulting in an image which does not conform to the shape of the object, somewhat resembling the image viewed through a cylindrical lens. This is due to an unequal magnification of the image. Distortion can be barrel-shaped (**barrel-shaped distortion**), in which the corners of the image of a square are closer to the centre than the middle part of the sides, or pincushion (**pincushion distortion**), in which the corners of the image of a square are farther from the centre than the middle

Table D5 Calculated near PD (in mm) as a function of distance PD for three reading distances (target plane to spectacle plane). The distance between the spectacle plane and the midpoint of the base line is assumed to be 27 mm (vertex distance 12 mm).

Distance PD	56	58	60	62	64	66	68	70	72	74
near PD for 45 cm	52.8	54.7	56.6	58.5	60.4	62.3	64.2	66.0	67.9	69.8
difference	3.2	3.3	3.4	3.5	3.6	3.7	3.8	4.0	4.1	4.2
near PD for 40 cm	52.5	54.3	56.2	58.1	59.9	61.8	63.7	65.6	67.4	69.3
difference	3.5	3.7	3.8	3.9	4.1	4.2	4.3	4.4	4.6	4.7
near PD for 35 cm	52.0	53.8	55.7	57.6	59.4	61.3	63.1	65.0	66.8	68.7
difference	4.0	4.2	4.3	4.4	4.6	4.7	4.9	5.0	5.2	5.3

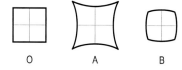

Fig. D10 Distortion (O, object; A, pincushion distortion; B, barrel-shaped distortion).

part of the sides (Fig. D10). *Example of barrel-shaped distortion:* a square object seen through an uncorrected negative spectacle lens. *Example of pincushion distortion:* a square object seen through an uncorrected positive spectacle lens. *See* **aberration; correction; lens, fisheye; sine condition.**

distortion test *See* test, distortion.

diurnal cycle *See* rhythm, circadian.

diurnal variations, in intraocular pressure Normal intraocular pressure varies throughout the day within a range of about 4 mmHg, being higher in the morning than in the evening. In patients with primary open-angle glaucoma this range is greater. This variation must be taken into consideration when measuring intraocular pressure.

diurnal vision *See* vision, diurnal.

divergence 1. Movement of the eyes turning away from each other. **2.** Characteristic of a pencil of light rays, as when emanating from a point source. *Syn.* negative convergence.
See **vergence.**
d. excess A high exophoria at distance associated with a much lower exophoria at near. It may occasionally give rise to diplopia in distance vision.
fusional d. A movement of the eyes away from each other in response to retinal disparity. This is performed to restore single binocular vision. It occurs most commonly when induced by a base-in prism.
d. insufficiency A high esophoria at distance associated with esophoria at near. It often gives rise to symptoms of asthenopia in both distance and near vision.
d. paralysis *See* paralysis, divergence.
vertical d. Relative vertical movement between the two eyes.

diverging lens *See* lens, diverging.

DNA (deoxyribonucleic acid) A type of nucleic acid that constitutes the molecular basis of heredity. It is found principally in the nucleus of all cells where it forms part of the chromosome, or in the cytoplasm of cells lacking a nucleus, such as bacteria. It acts as the carrier of genetic information containing the instructions (code) to make proteins. It consists of two single chains of nucleotides, which are twisted around each other to form a double helix or spiral. The nucleotides contain sugar (deoxyribose), phosphate and the bases (adenine, cytosine, guanine and thymine).

The two strands of DNA are held together by hydrogen bonds located between specific pairs of bases (adenine to thymine and cytosine to guanine). The sequence of bases and consequently gene sequence is sometimes altered, causing mutation. Assessment of DNA has found many applications, including forensic science to help identify a perpetrator (a process called genetic fingerprinting), to establish family relationships or the history of a particular population (phylogenetics) or to differentiate between normal and diseased eyes.
See **chromosome; gene; inheritance; mutation; protein.**

doll's head manoeuvre; phenomenon *See* phenomenon, doll's head.

Dolman's test *See* test, hole in the card.

dominance, ocular The superiority of one eye whose visual function predominates over the other eye. It is that eye (called the **dominant** eye) which is relied upon more than the other in binocular vision. It is not necessarily the eye with the best acuity nor is it fixed as to which eye is dominant as this may depend on the visual task. The lack of ocular dominance is referred to as **ambiocularity** and such a person is **ambiocular.**
See **manoptoscope; occlusion treatment; test, hole in the card.**

dominance, ocular column *See* column, cortical.

dominant eye; inheritance *See* under the nouns.

dominant wavelength (of a colour stimulus, not purple) *See* wavelength, dominant.

Donders' diagram Graphical representation of total convergence as a function of accommodation for any fixation distance. The accommodation in dioptres is represented on the ordinate and the convergence in prism dioptres (or metre angles) on the abscissa. It is used to represent the binocular status of the two eyes, as well as evaluating the patient's visual discomfort at any distance.
See **accommodation, relative amplitude of; convergence, relative; Fig. Z1, p 387; line, demand; zone of clear, single, binocular vision.**

Donders' law *See* law, Donders'.

Donders' line *See* line, demand.

Donders' method *See* method, push-up.

Donders' reduced eye *See* eye, reduced.

donor A person who gives a body part for use in the treatment of another person's disease or injury, or for research. *Example*: a person's cornea donated as a corneal graft to another person.
See **graft, corneal; keratoplasty.**

Doppler's ophthalmodynanometer *See* ophthalmodynanometer.

dorsal Relating to either the back (posterior) or to the top in brain orientation.
See **rostral; system, magnocellular visual; ventral.**

dorsal midbrain syndrome *See* syndrome, Parinaud's.

dorzolamide *See* carbonic anhydrase inhibitors.

dot and blot haemorrhage *See* haemorrhage, dot and blot.

double elevator palsy *See* palsy, double elevator.

double lid eversion *See* eversion, lid.

double Maddox rod test *See* test, Maddox rod.

double refraction *See* birefringence.

double prism test *See* test, double prism.

double vision *See* diplopia.

doublet A combination of two lenses usually cemented to each other used to correct chromatic aberration. It is used in optical instruments. Typically, it consists of a positive crown lens and a negative flint lens.
See lens, achromatizing; triplet.

Dove prism *See* prism, Dove.

Down's syndrome *See* syndrome, Down's.

downbeat nystagmus *See* nystagmus.

Doyne's honeycomb choroiditis *See* drusen, familial dominant.

Draper's law *See* law, Draper's.

drift *See* movement, fixation.

droopy eyelid *See* ptosis.

drusen Small, circular, yellow or white dots located throughout the fundus but more so in the macular region, around the optic disc or the periphery. They consist of deposits of abnormal extracellular material (amyloid P, complement proteins (C3, C5, C5b-9 complex), factors C, apolipoproteins B and E, lipids, vitronectin, zinc, etc.) derived mainly from the retinal pigment epithelium (RPE) and neural retina, and they are located between the basement membrane of the RPE and Bruch's membrane. Drusen interfere with the blood supply to the photoreceptors. Although they may be found in young people, they almost universally occur with ageing but also with retinal and choroidal degeneration (e.g. age-related maculopathy, retinitis pigmentosa, angioid streaks) and primary dystrophy (e.g. fundus flavimaculatus). There are several main types of drusen: (1) **Hard** (or **nodular**) drusen are small, round and discrete. They are deposits of granular material as well as of abnormal collagen. They are the most common type and are usually innocuous. (2) **Soft** (or **diffuse** or **granular**) drusen are often large with indistinct edges and, with time, they may enlarge, coalesce and increase in number. They are due to either a focal thickening of the inner layer of Bruch's membrane or to amorphous material located between that thickened detached part and the rest of Bruch's membrane. Both types (1) and (2) represent an early feature of age-related macular degeneration. (3) **Cuticular** (or **basal laminar**) drusen are small subretinal nodular thickening of the basement membrane of the pigment epithelium. They occur in younger patients more often than hard or soft drusen. (4) With time, the previously described drusen may calcify (**calcific** drusen) and take on a glistening appearance. Drusen rarely produce any symptoms and, if there is a visual loss, it is usually due to an accompanying macular haemorrhage, but if the drusen are very large thus widening the separation between the RPE and Bruch's membrane, there may be a degeneration of the overlying RPE and photoreceptors (Fig. D11). *Syn.* colloid bodies; hyaline bodies.
See macular degeneration, age-related; membrane, Bruch's; naevus, choroidal.

familial dominant d. An autosomal dominant hereditary degeneration of the choroid characterized by light-coloured patches of colloid material located in the area around the macula and often the optic disc. The majority of cases are caused by mutations in the EFEMP1 gene (egf-containing fibulin-like extracellular matrix protein 1). There is no loss of vision unless it is followed by macular degeneration. *Syn.* Doyne's honeycomb choroiditis; Doyne's honeycombed degeneration; Tay's choroiditis (used more commonly for the elderly).

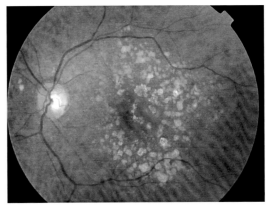

Fig. D11 Calcified drusen. (From Kanski 2007, with permission of Butterworth-Heinemann)

optic disc d. Whitish-yellow spherical excrescences that lie on, within or occasionally around the optic nerve head. They are composed of calcified hyaline-like material possibly resulting from deposition of mucoprotein and calcium that have extruded from degenerating axons. In childhood, they are usually buried within the disc substance and thus not visible on clinical examination but cause elevation of the disc surface resembling papilloedema. With age, they become progressively more superficial. Field defects are common (e.g. generalized constriction, blind spot enlargement) but visual acuity is normal, unless there is some vascular complication. They usually appear bilaterally and affect males and females equally. They are easily diagnosed with fluorescein angiography because exposed drusen are autofluorescent.

dry eye See eye, dry; glands, meibomian; keratoconjunctivitis sicca.

Drysdale's method See method, Drysdale's.

Duane's syndrome See syndrome, Duane's.

duction 1. Movement of one eye alone as in abduction, adduction, depression, elevation, etc. **2.** Disjunctive binocular movements (although it is more correct to call these movements vergences). See **dextroduction; laevoduction; movement, disjunctive eye.**
binocular d. refers to the maximum vergence powers that can be exerted while maintaining single binocular vision through prisms, either in the base-in or base-out direction. Binocular ductions are measured from the passive position (or phoria position) to the break point.

duochrome test See test, duochrome.

duplicity theory See theory, duplicity.

Dutch telescope See telescope, galilean.

Dvorine's pseudoisochromatic plates See plates, pseudoisochromatic.

dye dilution test See test, dye dilution.

dynamic acuity; retinoscopy See under the nouns.

dyschromatopsia General term given to deficiencies of colour vision, especially acquired defects. It may also refer to incomplete achromatopsia. See **colour vision, defective.**

dyscoria Anomaly in the shape of the pupil.

dysgenesis Lack of proper development, as may be the case of the trabecular meshwork in congenital glaucoma. See **Peter's anomaly; syndrome, Axenfeld's; syndrome, Rieger's.**

dysgraphia Difficulty in writing due to a brain lesion. It is not as severe as agraphia.

dyskeratosis Abnormal process which, in the eye, results in hornification of the epithelial layer of the conjunctiva or cornea. It may be hereditary or due to irritation (e.g. radiation) or to prolonged drug administration in the eye. It appears as a dry white plaque (called **leucoplakia** or **leucokeratosis**). It may be benign or malignant, in which case it must be surgically excised. See **pterygium.**

dyslexia A condition characterized by difficulty with reading and spelling. Words may be read but not recognized or understood. It is independent of intelligence, motivation or ocular correction. Its origin may be due to a disorder of the fast processing magnocellular visual system. The condition is commonly associated with the Meares–Irlen syndrome. See **alexia; syndrome, Meares–Irlen; test, developmental and perceptual screening.**

dysmegalopsia A condition in which the perceptual size of objects is abnormal. Objects may appear larger (**macropsia**) or smaller (**micropsia**).

dysmetria, ocular An anomaly of eye movements in which the eyes overshoot (**hypermetria**) or undershoot (**hypometria**) when attempting to fixate an object. It could be a sign of cerebellar disease, ocular motor nerve paresis, myasthenia gravis, internuclear ophthalmoplegia (overshoot of the eye contralateral to the lesion), etc. See **flutter; opsoclonus.**

dysphotopsia Vision of unwanted images seen by some patients who have had an intraocular lens implanted following successful cataract surgery. The unwanted images can be either positive, such as glare, light streaks or halos, or negative, such as shadows or dark objects seen in peripheral vision.

dysplasia A developmental abnormality of cells, tissues or organs, which have become defective, abnormally small, absent or sometimes abnormally large. *Examples*: microphthalmia, anophthalmia, coloboma. See **hyperplasia; hypoplasia.**

dysplasia, septo-optic See syndrome, de Morsier.

dyspraxia See apraxia.

dystrophy A non-inflammatory developmental, nutritional or metabolic disorder.
adult vitelliform foveomacular d. See dystrophy, pattern.
Avellino corneal d. A rare, autosomal dominant disorder in which there are deposits of hyaline amyloid in the stroma. It is caused by a mutation in the gene encoding keratoepithelin TGFB1 on chromosome 5q31. Patients present with reduced visual acuity and occasionally corneal erosions in which case there is pain, lacrimation and photophobia. The disorder presents some features of granular and lattice dystrophy. Syn. granular corneal dystrophy type II.
band-shaped corneal d. See keratopathy, band.
Best's vitelliform macular d. See disease, Best's.
central areolar choroidal d. Autosomal dominant dystrophy of the macula with onset in the third to fifth decades of life. It causes a progressive decrease in visual acuity. It is characterized by

bilateral, atrophic, macular lesions, between one and three disc diameters in size, and through which choroidal vessels can be seen. The prognosis of this condition is poor as it is progressive. *Syn.* central aerolar choroidal sclerosis. *See* **choroideremia.**

central crystalline d. *See* **dystrophy, Schnyder's.**

choroidal d. A group of ocular dystrophies, which are characterized by atrophy of the retinal pigment epithelium and choroid. These lesions have been grouped according to the area involved and the topographical pattern noted. Classical disease states include gyrate atrophy as well as choroideremia. These lesions are often inherited, demonstrating both autosomal recessive and dominant inheritance patterns (Table D6). *See* **atrophy, gyrate; choroideremia.**

Cogan's microcystic epithelial d. *See* **dystrophy, epithelial basement membrane.**

cone d. A degeneration of the cone photoreceptors which, in most cases, is inherited in an autosomal dominant or X-linked recessive fashion, but some cases are sporadic. It appears in the first or second decades of life and is characterized by a progressive loss of visual acuity, colour vision impairment, photophobia and central scotoma. Ophthalmoscopic examination may show a demarcated circular atrophic area in the macular region (**bull's eye maculopathy**). There is no known treatment. *Syn.* cone degeneration. *See* **achromatopsia; monochromat.**

cone-rod d. Bilateral degeneration of the photoreceptors, which affects the cones first and the rods later. It may be inherited in an autosomal dominant fashion caused by mutations in the retinal guanylate cyclase gene GUCY2D or X-linked recessive fashion but many cases are sporadic. It appears in the first to third decades of life. It is characterized by poor visual acuity, colour vision impairment and photoaversion to bright sunlight. The ocular fundus may eventually show an atrophy of the retinal pigment epithelium, which appears as a **bull's eye maculopathy**. Eventually as the rods degenerate, there is progressive night blindness. There is no known treatment.

congenital hereditary endothelial d. A hereditary type of corneal dystrophy occurring in either an autosomal dominant or autosomal recessive form. The autosomal dominant form presents during the first year or two of life causing pain, corneal oedema, tearing and photophobia with slowly progressive corneal opacification. This form does not cause nystagmus because normal corneal function is present during the early period of visual development. The autosomal recessive form presents earlier, usually at birth, and consists of a significantly thickened corneal stroma (oedema) with nystagmus. There is no tearing or photophobia noted. This dystrophy appears to be due to an abnormality in endothelial cell development during the early second trimester of gestation, but does not appear to be related to any other systemic or ocular abnormality.

corneal d. Hereditary disorders affecting both corneas. It is occasionally present at birth, but it develops more frequently during adolescence and progresses slowly throughout life. It varies in appearance and is often described on the basis of which layer is affected (Table D6).

corneal d. of Bowman's layer type 1 *See* **dystrophy, Reis–Buckler.**

Table D6 Classification of ocular dystrophies

Corneal		
Epithelial	**Stromal**	**Endothelial**
epithelial basement membrane d. (Cogan's microcystic epithelial d.)	Avellino d. (granular corneal d. type II)	cornea guttata
Meesmann's d.	granular corneal d. type 1	congenital hereditary endothelial d.
Reis–Buckler d.	lattice d.	Fuchs' endothelial d.
	macular corneal d.	posterior polymorphous d.
	Schnyder's crystalline d.	

Lenticular
myotonic d.*

Choroidal		Retinal
central areolar choroidal d.	cone d.	cone-rod d.
choroideremia (tapetochoroidal d.)	North Carolina macular d.	pattern d. (Best's disease, adult vitelliform foveomacular d., butterfly d., reticular d.)
gyrate atrophy	Sorsby's macular d.	Stargardt's disease. (juvenile macular d.)

*Although this dystrophy is characterized by lenticular opacities, the main signs are muscle wasting, weakness and stiffness.

endothelial corneal d. *See* **cornea guttata.**

epithelial basement membrane d. A bilateral corneal dystrophy located in the corneal epithelium. It occurs most commonly in females. It is characterized by variously shaped greyish-white microcysts and debris, which vary in shape and location over time, coalescing with other microcysts, forming lines and resembling a fingerprint pattern. Symptoms are minimal and vision is unaffected unless the lesions are in the central zone of the cornea. The condition may be associated with **recurrent epithelial erosions**, which cause pain, lacrimation, photophobia and blurred vision. Management normally includes artificial tears, patching, antibiotics and occasionally therapeutic soft contact lenses for frequent or more severe types. *Syn.* Cogan's microcystic epithelial dystrophy; map-dot fingerprint dystrophy. *See* **corneal erosion, recurrent.**

Fuchs' endothelial d. A progressive dystrophy of the corneal endothelium seen more commonly in women than in men, usually in the fifth decade of life. It may be transmitted in an autosomal dominant fashion. It is characterized by wart-like deposits on the endothelial surface. As the condition progresses, there is oedema of the stroma and eventually of the epithelium and bullous keratopathy causing blurring of vision and pain. The stroma may also become vascularized. It is often associated with glaucoma and nuclear lens opacity. Treatment includes hypertonic agents (e.g. sodium chloride 5%), a bandage soft contact lens and, in severe cases, penetrating keratoplasty or posterior lamellar keratoplasty. *See* **cornea guttata; keratopathy, bullous.**

granular corneal d. type 1 An autosomal dominant hereditary condition characterized by the presence of irregularly shaped white granules of hyaline in the stroma of the cornea surrounded by clear areas. It is caused by mutation in the keratoepithelin gene TGFB1 on chromosome 5q31. It usually develops during the first decade of life and progresses slowly throughout life. It rarely results in loss of vision although the granules are located in the centre of the cornea. If severe, keratoplasty is the main treatment. *Syn.* Groenouw's type 1 corneal dystrophy.

granular corneal d. type II *See* **dystrophy, Avellino corneal.**

Groenouw's type 1 corneal d.; type 2 corneal d. *See* **dystrophy, granular corneal type 1; dystrophy, macular corneal.**

juvenile macular d. *See* **disease, Sargardt's.**

juvenile vitelliform macular d. *See* **disease, Best's.**

lattice d. An autosomal dominant, hereditary disorder characterized by the appearance in the corneal stroma of fine branching filaments interlacing and overlapping at different levels, as well as white spots and stellate opacities. These filaments are deposits of amyloid. There are three types of the disease but type 1 is the most common and only affects the eye. It is caused by a mutation in the keratoepithilin gene TGFB1. The onset usually begins in the first decade of life and progresses in the following decades. Recurrent corneal erosions are common. When visual acuity becomes impaired, keratoplasty may be necessary (Fig. D12). *Syn.* Biber–Haab–Dimmer corneal dystrophy; lattice corneal dystrophy type I. *See* **amyloidosis.**

macular d. A group of inherited disorders involving the macular area due to defective metabolism or nutrition in the sensory layer of the retina (e.g. cone dystrophy, cone-rod dystrophy), the retinal pigment epithelium (e.g. Best's disease, Stargardt's

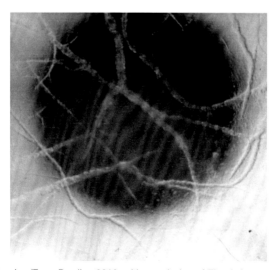

Fig. D12 Lattice dystrophy. (From Bowling 2016, with permission of Elsevier)

disease and pattern dystrophy) or the choroid (e.g. central areolar choroidal dystrophy) (Table D6).

macular corneal d. An autosomal recessive disorder characterized by bilateral, grey-white nodules, which progressively develop into a generalized opacification of the corneal stroma. It is caused by mutations in the gene for a specific sulfotransferase gene CHST6 and depending on the presence or absence of keratan sulfate in the serum and cornea the condition is divided into type 1 and type 2, but they are clinically indistinguishable. By about the fifth decade of life, visual acuity is markedly diminished and penetrating keratoplasty may be necessary. Histological examination shows an accumulation of mucopolysaccharide in the stroma and degeneration of Bowman's layer. *Syn.* Groenouw's type 2 corneal dystrophy.

map-dot fingerprint d. *See* **dystrophy, epithelial basement membrane.**

Meesmann's d. A dominant, hereditary, bilateral disorder characterized by numerous small punctate opacities in the corneal epithelium. It is caused by mutations in the genes encoding the cornea-specific keratins K3 (KRT3) and K12 (KRT12). The condition appears in infancy. It is usually asymptomatic but in some cases there is discomfort and a slight decrease in visual acuity. Ocular lubrication usually suffices but, in very severe cases, keratoplasty may be necessary (Table D6). *Syn.* juvenile epithelial corneal dystrophy; hereditary epithelial dystrophy.

myotonic d. An autosomal dominant hereditary disease characterized by progressive weakness and atrophy of skeletal muscles with delayed muscle relaxation. The main type is caused by mutation in the dystrophia myotonica protein kinase gene, DMPK on chromosome19q13. The main ocular manifestations are cataracts with multicoloured crystals, small dot opacities in the cortex and subcapsular region of the lens, ptosis as well as hyperopia (Table D6). *Syn.* Steinert's disease.

North Carolina macular d. A rare autosomal dominant disorder caused by a mutation in the DHS6S1 gene on chromosome 6q16. It appears soon after birth and varies from normal visual acuity to significant visual impairment with drusen, macular coloboma and choroidal neovascular membrane (Table D6).

pattern d. A group of inherited macular disorders characterized by bilateral yellow or black pigment deposits at the level of the retinal pigment epithelium (RPE) forming a variety of patterns such as butterfly wings (**butterfly dystrophy**), spider-shaped (**reticular dystrophy**) or round slightly elevated (**adult vitelliform foveomacular dystrophy**, which resembles Best's disease but has its onset in the fourth to sixth decades and with only a slight decrease in vision). Pattern dystrophies have been linked to mutations in the peripherin/RDS gene in some patients. The peripherin protein, which is normally present in the photoreceptor outer segments, is disrupted and eventually interferes with RPE metabolism. There may be a slight reduction in visual acuity and mild metamorphopsia, although many patients are asymptomatic. The electrooculogram may show a reduced Arden ratio. *See* **disease, Best's.**

posterior polymorphous d. Autosomal dominant dystrophy of the endothelium and Descemet's membrane, which appears either at birth or in early childhood. It is caused by mutation in the visual system homeobox gene VSX1 or gene OVOL2. The disease is characterized by polymorphous plaques of calcium crystals and vesicular lesions in the endothelium and on its surface. It is usually asymptomatic, but in some cases corneal oedema occurs with a large reduction in visual acuity and this may require penetrating keratoplasty.

retinal d. *See* **dystrophy, macular; retinitis pigmentosa.**

Reis–Buckler d. Autosomal dominant disorder of the cornea, characterized by ring-shaped opacities occurring at the level of Bowman's layer and protruding into the epithelium. It is caused by mutation in keratoepithelin gene TGFB1 on chromosome 5q. The opacities increase in density with time giving rise to a honeycomb appearance. The condition begins in childhood and progresses with frequent recurrent corneal erosions resulting in scarring, decreased visual acuity and reduced corneal sensitivity. In severe cases, keratoplasty may be necessary. Syn. corneal dystrophy of Bowman's layer type 1.

Schnyder's crystalline corneal d. A rare progressive autosomal dominant disorder characterized by abnormal deposition of cholesterol and phospholipids in the stroma, which appear as yellow-white crystals scattered throughout the central cornea. It is caused by mutation in the UBAID1 gene on chromosome 1p36. Visual acuity is reduced and corneal opacification occurs in some cases while others only present a corneal haze. Management include lipid-free diet and may involve keratoplasty (Table D6). Syn. central crystalline dystrophy.

Sorsby's macular d. A rare autosomal dominant disorder caused by a mutation in the gene encoding the tissue inhibitor of metalloproteinase-3, TIMP3 on chromosome 22q12. It presents in the fifth decade of life with reduced visual acuity and exudative maculopathy, subretinal scarring and atrophy and choroidal neovascularization. Prognosis is poor (Table D6).

Stargardt's macular d. *See* **disease, Stargardt's.**

tapetochoroidal d. *See* **choroideremia.**

vitelliform d. *See* **dystrophy, pattern.**

E

Eales' disease See disease, Eales'.

eccentric fixation; viewing See under the nouns.

eccentricity Term referring to the angular distance from the centre of the visual field or from the foveola of the retina. *Example*: The maximum density of rods in the retina is at a retinal eccentricity of about 20°.

ecchymosis See eye, black.

E chart See chart, E.

echo See ultrasonography.

echography See ultrasonography.

echothiophate iodide See acetylcholinesterase.

eclipse blindness See blindness, eclipse.

econazole See antifungal agent.

ectasia A dilatation or distention of a tubular organ or a portion of tissue, which occurs as a result of a pathophysiological process.
   corneal e. A forward bulging and thinning of the cornea. It may result from a disease of the cornea (e.g. keratoconus), trauma, atrophy, raised intraocular pressure or as a complication of photorefractive surgery in which the corneal stroma has been left thinner than about 250 µm. If uveal tissue is included in the protrusion, the condition is called a **staphyloma**. If the ectasia is limited to the peripheral part of the cornea, it is called Terrien's marginal degeneration. *Syn.* keratectasia; keratoectasia; kerectasis.
   See degeneration, pellucid marginal; degeneration, Terrien's marginal; keratoglobus; staphyloma.
   scleral e. A bulging and thinning of the sclera due to disease, trauma, atrophy or raised intraocular pressure. It may be total as in buphthalmos or partial as in staphyloma. *Syn.* sclerectasia.

ectocornea The outermost layer of the cornea, that is, the squamous cell layer of the corneal epithelium.

ectoderm The outermost of the three primary germinal layers of an embryo (the other layers being **mesoderm** and **endoderm**) from which the eye is derived. It differentiates into outer surface ectoderm and inner neuroectoderm, which gives rise to neural crest cells. The **surface ectoderm** gives rise to the crystalline lens, the lacrimal gland, the meibomian glands, the corneal and conjunctival epithelium and the epidermis of the eyelids. The **neuroectoderm (neural ectoderm)** forms the retina, retinal pigment epithelium, the pigmented and non-pigmented layers of the ciliary and iris epithelium, the dilator and sphincter muscles of the iris and the optic nerve fibres. **Neural crest** cells form the corneal stroma and endothelium, sclera, iris and choroidal stroma, ciliary muscle and trabecular meshwork.
   See cup, optic; mesoderm; vesicles, optic.

ectopia lentis An acquired or hereditary abnormality of the crystalline lens characterized by dislocation. It may be complete (called luxation) or partial (called subluxation). Patients present with aphakia, cataract, monocular diplopia, lenticular astigmatism, hyperopia and, if the dislocation is anterior, glaucoma. Treatment is usually optical, although surgery may be necessary if there is glaucoma, cataract or uveitis.
   See luxation of the lens.

ectopia of the macula See macula, ectopia of the.

ectopia pupillae See corectopia.

ectropion Outward turning of the eyelid margin. The most common cause is a loss of tonus of the pretarsal orbicularis muscle combined with laxity of the medial and lateral canthal tendons, which occurs in old people and affects only the lower eyelid (**involutional ectropion**). Tears collect in the lacrimal lake and overflow onto the skin of the face (epiphora). Other causes of ectropion are scarring, burns, trauma (called **cicatricial ectropion**), spasm of the orbicularis muscle, which may affect either the upper or lower eyelid, or paralysis of the orbicularis muscle in which only the lower eyelid is affected or facial nerve palsy (**paralytic ectropion**). Ectropion may lead to exposure keratopathy as the lower part of the cornea remains exposed. Management includes patching the eye during sleep as a temporary measure, but, if severe, the treatment is surgical.
   See keratopathy, exposure.
   cicatricial e.; involutional e. See ectropion.
   congenital e. A rare congenital eversion of the eyelid (most often the lower). It may be due to a deficiency of the anterior eyelid lamina. It is usually associated with other disorders, such as blepharophimosis syndrome or Down's syndrome.
   e. uveae A turning of a portion of the posterior pigment epithelium of the iris growing or being drawn around the pupillary margin onto the anterior iris surface. It may be acquired (e.g. following iris neovascularization, neovascular glaucoma, iris melanoma) or congenital (e.g. neurofibromatosis, Rieger's anomaly).
   paralytic e. See ectropion; syndrome, Rieger's.

eczema An inflammatory disease of the skin characterized by a rash of red spots, rough scaling, dryness and soreness of the skin sometimes leading to the formation of blisters. It often gives rise to itching or to a burning sensation. It may occur on the skin of the face where parts

of spectacles rest. Frames should be cleaned regularly to avoid causing skin irritation. *Syn.* contact dermatitis.
See **atopy; keratoconjunctivitis, atopic,**

edema *See* **oedema.**

edge clearance A small peripheral gap between the edge of a rigid contact lens and the cornea. It is important as it allows tear exchange and eases lens removal. The absence of edge clearance in rigid contact lenses may lead to superficial corneal damage.

edge detection *See* **contour.**

edge lift Deviation of the posterior surface of a contact lens from a sphere at a given diameter. This is produced by either the peripheral curve(s) or the edging process. Edge lift provides **peripheral clearance** of a rigid contact lens, which is assessed by fluorescein pattern. If the edge lift is specified axially (as an extension of the back central optic zone, measured parallel to the axis of symmetry), it is referred to as **axial edge lift**. If specified radially as an extension along the back optic zone radius, it is referred to as **radial edge lift**.
See **optic zone diameter; optic zone radius, back.**

edging Grinding the edge of a lens to the finished shape and size required, at the same time imparting the desired edge form (e.g. flat, bevelled, etc.). This is accomplished with a machine called an **edger**, either by hand with a grinding wheel or automatically operating from a lens pattern or former.
See **cribbing; former; glass cutter; glazing.**

Edinger–Westphal nucleus *See* **nucleus, Edinger–Westphal.**

Edridge–Green lantern An occupational colour vision test that consists of small round and variable-sized coloured lights produced by coloured and neutral density filters.
See **test, lantern.**

edrophonium chloride *See* **anticholinesterase.**

Edward's syndrome *See* **syndrome, Edward's.**

effect The result of an action or condition.
    Aubert's e. *See* **phenomenon, Aubert's.**
    Bezold–Brücke e. *See* **phenomenon, Bezold–Brücke.**
    Broca–Sulzer e. The brightness produced by a flash of a given luminance depends upon its duration. It is maximum for durations around 30 to 40 ms when the flash luminance is photopic and of about 170 lux, but it becomes closer to 70 to 80 ms when the flash is equal to about 120 lux.
    Brücke–Bartley e. An increased brightness produced by an intermittent light source (usually around 8–10 Hz) compared to the same light source viewed in steady illumination. *Syn.* brightness enhancement.
    Cheshire cat e. A form of binocular rivalry in which a moving object seen by one eye can cause the entire image, or parts of the image, of a stationary object seen by the other eye to disappear. The effect can be observed by dividing the field of vision with a mirror placed edge-on in front of the nose at a slight angle. One eye looks straight at a stationary object, such as a sleeping cat, while the other eye sees a reflection through the mirror of a white wall or background. If a hand is waved on the mirror side in the region of the field where the cat is seen, the whole cat or part of it may be seen to disappear.
See **retinal rivalry.**
    Craik–O'Brien–Cornsweet e. A phenomenon in which the brightness of an area on one side of a transition strip appears greater than the brightness of the area on the other side of the strip, although both areas outside the transition strip have exactly the same luminance. The transition strip consists of two opposing luminance gradients that meet along a linear edge (called **Cornsweet edge**); on one side, the luminance gradually increases to the edge and on the other side, the luminance gradually decreases to the edge. The area adjoining the gradient of increasing luminance appears brighter than the area adjoining the gradient of decreasing luminance. One possible explanation is that the edge information predominates and the visual system and brain 'fill-in' the area next to it to construct a higher brightness percept. *Note*: By covering the transition strip, it is easy to confirm that the two areas have the same luminance. *Syn.* Craik–O'Brien–Cornsweet illusion; Cornsweet illusion.
    crowding e. *See* **phenomenon, crowding.**
    differential prismatic e. The difference in prism power induced by a pair of ophthalmic lenses of different power when the eyes look in various directions of gaze (except through the optical centres). Large amounts of differential prismatic effect can hinder fusion and give rise to diplopia. *Example*: A patient's right eye is corrected by +5 D, the left eye by +2 D. When the eye rotates upward so that the visual axes intersect the lenses 1 cm above the optical centres, the induced prism power becomes 5 Δ base down on the right and 2 Δ base down on the left. The differential prismatic effect is 3 Δ base down in front of the right eye, probably too large for fusion to be maintained. *Syn.* prismatic imbalance; relative prismatic effect.
See **anisophoria; law, Prentice's.**
    Gelb e. In a faintly illuminated room a piece of black paper (or a rotating black disc) is illuminated by a high intensity projector. The beam of the projector falls exactly on the area of the black surface. The paper or disc will then appear to be white. A reversal of the perception is accomplished by placing a small piece of white paper near the disc in front of the projected light, at which time the paper or disc reappears in its true colour, i.e. black.
    kinetic depth e. An impression of a three-dimensional structure of a moving two-dimensional shadow cast by a three-dimensional object. It is most easily demonstrated by casting a shadow onto a translucent screen.

Mandelbaum e. A tendency for the accommodative response to be altered when interposing a conflicting visual stimulus to the one being viewed. If the eyes are viewing a distant object through a dirty window or a wire fence, the actual accommodative response will tend to be increased. If the eyes are viewing a near object in front of a dirty window or wire fence, the actual accommodative response will be less than if there were no conflicting stimulus.

McCollough e. A visual after-effect of colour that is seen when viewing, for a minute at least, two differently oriented and differently coloured gratings, such as a vertical grating with blue and black stripes and a horizontal grating with orange and black stripes. After adapting to these, the subject looks at a figure containing a grating of vertical black and white stripes and a grating of black and white horizontal stripes of the same size as the original coloured gratings. The white stripes will then appear to be of the complementary colour, that is, the vertical stripes appear pinkish and the horizontal stripes appear bluish.

moiré e. An illusory shimmering movement produced by moving one pattern superimposed on another pattern very similar to it. The phenomenon occurs because parts of the periodic patterns are in phase in some locations, and out of phase in other locations. *Examples*: passing by a set of railings; if a transilluminated square wave grating is superimposed on an identical grating but cross each other at an angle of less than 45°, moiré fringes will appear at the intersections. *Syn.* moiré pattern.
See **Toposcope.**

oblique e. In central vision, contours with oblique orientations are perceived and discriminated less easily than those close to the horizontal or vertical.
Pulfrich e. *See* **stereophenomenon, Pulfrich.**
Raman e. In certain substances, scattered light may be of a slightly different wavelength from that of the incident light.
Stiles–Crawford e. Variation of the luminosity of a pencil of light stimulating a given receptor depending on the position of entry of the pencil through the pupil. The maximum luminosity occurs for pencils passing through the centre of the pupil and stimulating the receptor along its axis. This phenomenon is attributed to the particular shape of the cone cells of the retina and occurs only in photopic vision.
Tyndall e. Diffusion of light by the particles present in a liquid or gas. It is because of this effect that heterogeneities (e.g. increased proteins) of the media of the eye can be seen, as occurs in iris and/or ciliary body inflammation. *Syn.* Tyndall scatter.
See **aqueous flare.**

effective power *See* **power, effective.**

efferent Carrying nerve impulses away from the central nervous system to the periphery.
See **afferent.**

efficacy, luminous *See* **luminous efficacy.**

efficiency scale, Snell–Sterling *See* visual efficiency scale, Snell–Sterling.

efficiency, spectral luminous (of a monochromatic radiation of wavelength λ) Ratio of the radiant flux at wavelength $λ_m$ to that at wavelength λ such that both radiations produce equally intense luminous sensations under specified photometric conditions and $λ_m$ is chosen so that the maximum value of this ratio is equal to one. *Symbols*: V(λ) for photopic vision. V′(λ) for scotopic vision (Fig. E1 and Table E1). *Note*: Unless otherwise indicated, the values used for the spectral luminous efficiency in **photopic vision** are the values agreed internationally in 1931 by the CIE and adopted in 1933 by the International Committee on Weights and Measures. For **scotopic vision** the CIE in 1951 provisionally adopted new values for young observers (CIE). *Syn.* luminosity curve; spectral sensitivity (commonly used, although there is a slight difference).
See **sensitivity, spectral; vision, photopic; vision, scotopic.**

Efron grading scales *See* **grading scales.**

'E' game A technique used to evaluate visual acuity in young children. The letter 'E' is shown to the child, who is instructed to either state or point his or her fingers in the direction of the open side of the letter. The 'E' is subsequently rotated left, right, up and down randomly as its size is decreased, and acuity is obtained when the smallest letter is just recognizable.
See **chart, illiterate E; Glasgow acuity cards; test, Cardiff acuity; test, Lea-Hyvarinen acuity.**

Egger's line *See* **ligament of Wieger.**

egocentre A point of reference in the self usually located between the eyes. Absolute judgment of distances and visual directions of objects fixated binocularly are referred to the egocentre.
See **localization; oculocentre.**

egocentric localization *See* **localization.**

Ehlers–Danlos syndrome *See* **syndrome, Ehlers–Danlos.**

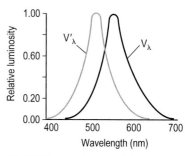

Fig. E1 Relative luminous efficiency curves for photopic $V_λ$ and scotopic $V'_λ$ levels of adaptation for an equi-energy spectrum. These data represent the sensitivity (i.e. 1/threshold energy) compiled from various sources and typically obtained by heterochromatic flicker photometry.

Table E1 Photopic and scotopic relative luminous efficiency factors. The data are based on an average from a large number of individuals agreed by the CIE in 1931 for the photopic factor V_λ and in 1951 for the scotopic factor V'_λ

Wavelength (in nm)	V_λ	V'_λ
380	0.0000	0.000589
400	0.0004	0.009292
420	0.0040	0.09661
440	0.0230	0.3281
460	0.0600	0.5672
480	0.1390	0.7930
500	0.3230	0.9818
507	–	1.0000
520	0.7100	0.9352
540	0.9540	0.6497
555	1.0000	–
580	0.8700	0.1212
600	0.6310	0.03315
620	0.3810	0.007374
640	0.1750	0.001497
660	0.0610	0.0003129
680	0.0170	0.00007155
700	0.0041	0.00001780
720	0.00105	0.00000478
740	0.00025	0.000001379
760	0.00006	0.000000425
780	0.00000	0.000000139

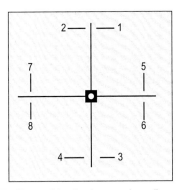

Fig. E2 Target of the direct comparison eikonometer.

eidetic image *See* image, eidetic.

eikonometer Instrument for measuring aniseikonia. The **direct comparison eikonometer (standard eikonometer)** uses as a target a cross with a small white disc at the centre of a black square at its intersection (Fig. E2). Four pairs of opposing arrows are placed four degrees away from the centre of the cross with the even-numbered arrows polarized in one direction and the odd numbered ones in the other direction. The subject wears polarizing lenses so that each set of four arrows

is seen by one eye. If the subject has aniseikonia, one set of arrows will not appear aligned with the other. Aniseikonia in one or more meridians can be measured by means of an adjustable magnifying device before one eye. There is also a **space eikonometer** in which the parts of the target are seen three-dimensionally in space. An office model of this type has been manufactured. The space eikonometer is based on a modification of stereopsis. Aniseikonia will make the target appear tilted. The amount of aniseikonia is indicated by the power of the size lens that swings the target back into a frontoparallel plane. *Syn.* aniseikometer. *See* **lens, aniseikonic; plane, frontoparallel.**

electrodiagnostic procedures Methods such as the electroretinogram, the electrooculogram and the visually evoked cortical potentials which are used to facilitate the diagnosis of some ocular diseases (e.g. retinitis pigmentosa) or the objective measurement of some visual functions (e.g. refractive error, visual acuity).

electroluminescence *See* luminescence.

electromagnetic spectrum *See* spectrum, electromagnetic.

electromyogram Recording of electrical activity of a muscle associated with contraction and relaxation. This is obtained by placing a microelectrode within a muscle. The recording process is called **electromyography**. *See* **law of reciprocal innervation, Sherrington's.**

electrooculogram (EOG) Recording of eye movements and eye position provided by the difference in electrical potential between two electrodes placed on the skin on either side of the eye. The EOG consists of two potentials: the **standing potential (resting potential, dark phase, dark current)**, which is evoked by moving the eyes in the dark and originates from the retinal pigment epithelium, and the **light potential (light rise)**, which is evoked by moving the eyes in a lighted environment and originates from the photoreceptors. Clinically, the ratio between the light and dark potentials (sometimes also called the **Arden index** or **Arden ratio**) is assessed. If that ratio is less than 1.8, it indicates a malfunction of the structures from which the potential originates. The EOG is also used to monitor eye movements (Fig. E3). *See* **disease, Best's; fundus flavimaculatus; potential of the eye, resting.**

electroretinogram (ERG) Recording of mass electrical response of the retina when it is stimulated by light (e.g. a flash). It is recorded by placing an electrode in contact with the cornea or around the eye under the eyelid. A second electrode is placed either on the forehead or the face. The response is complex as many cells of various types contribute to it and varies according to whether the eye is dark or light adapted, the colour and size of the stimulus, the health of the retina, etc. The curve consists of two major components: a negative a-wave and a larger positive b-wave. The a-wave originates in the photoreceptors while the

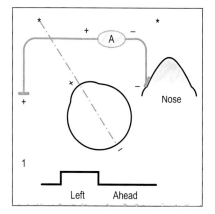

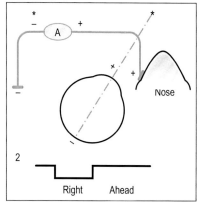

Fig. E3 Principle of electrooculography. The eye acts as a dipole in which the anterior pole is positive and the posterior pole is negative. 1. Left gaze; the cornea approaches the electrode near the outer canthus resulting in a positive-going change in the potential difference recorded from it. 2. Right gaze; the cornea approaches the electrode near the inner canthus resulting in a positive-going change in the potential difference recorded from it (A represents an AC/DC amplifier). Below each diagram is a typical tracing displayed by a pen recorder.

b-wave originates in the bipolar and Mueller cells. Both waves also have a photopic and a scotopic component. A third wave referred to a c-wave may be seen and it reflects activity in the retinal pigment epithelium, as well as the Mueller cells. The ERG is informative in retinitis pigmentosa and optic atrophy. **pERG** indicates that the potential is elicited by a pattern such as an alternating checkerboard of black and white squares, which are temporally modulated and still maintains a constant average luminance across the retina. It measures ganglion cell function as well as macular photoreceptor function. It is useful in evaluating optic nerve disease and macular dysfunction. *See* **alternating checkerboard stimulus; Leber's congenital amaurosis; potential, early receptor; potentials, oscillatory; retinitis pigmentosa.**

electroretinography, multifocal Simultaneous recording of the electroretinogram from small retinal areas (e.g. 103 hexagonal areas in the central 50 degrees of the retina) which are independently light stimulated according to a binary m-sequence (e.g. a random reversal at 75 Hz). This method enables evaluation of specific regions of the retina (e.g. macular degeneration) and mainly of the cone pathway.

elephantiasis oculi 1. Enlargement of the eyelids due to lymphatic obstruction. *Syn.* elephantiasis palpebral. **2.** Extreme exophthalmos.

elephantiasis palpebral *See* **elephantiasis oculi.**

elevation of the eye Upward rotation of an eye. It is accomplished by the superior rectus, inferior oblique, lateral rectus (very slightly) and medial rectus (very slightly) muscles. It can be produced voluntarily or by using base-down prisms. *Syn.* supraduction; sursumduction.

elevator An extraocular muscle involved in rotating the eye upward such as the superior rectus and inferior oblique muscles.

ellipse, Tscherning A graphical representation of the front surface power as a function of total lens power in best-form lenses. There are two possible solutions: (1) Those lenses which are the least curved and represented by the lower portion of the Tscherning ellipse. This portion is called the **Oswalt branch** of the ellipse. (2) Those lenses which are most curved and represented by the upper portion of the ellipse. This latter portion is called the **Wollaston branch** of the ellipse. *See* **lens, best-form.**

ellipses, MacAdam Areas in the CIE chromaticity diagram, each in the form of an ellipse within which the colour appears the same. The size of each ellipse varies in the diagram, being larger for greens than for blues or reds. The ellipses are distorted for colour-deficient individuals.

ellipsoid 1. The refractile outer portion of the inner member of a rod or cone cell. It is located between the myoid and the outer member of the cell, and contains mitochondria. The **myoid** is in contact with the external limiting membrane of the retina while the outer member is next to the pigment epithelium. **2.** Surface of revolution generated by rotating an ellipse about a major or minor axis. *See* **Fig. C4, p. 52.**

Elschnig's membrane; spots *See* under the nouns.

Elschnig's pearls Transparent clusters formed by proliferation of epithelial lens cells found in the remains of the capsule of the crystalline lens following extracapsular cataract extraction or vitritis. They rarely affect vision. *See* **cataract extraction, extracapsular; ring, Soemmering's.**

embolism, retinal *See* **retinal embolism.**

embryotoxon, anterior *See* **arcus, corneal.**

embryotoxon, posterior A condition in which a thickened and anteriorly displaced Schwalbe's line is visible on external examination as a thin greyish ridge adjacent to the limbus. The condition is present in nearly 20% of normal eyes and is a feature of the Axenfeld-Rieger anomaly. *See* **gonioscopy; line of Schwalbe; syndrome, Axenfeld's; syndrome, Alagille; syndrome, Rieger's.**

emedastine *See* **antihistamine.**

Emmert's law *See* **law, Emmert's.**

emmetrope One who has emmetropia.

emmetropia The refractive state of the eye in which, with accommodation relaxed, the conjugate focus of the retina is at infinity. Thus, the retina lies in the plane of the posterior principal focus of the eye and distant objects are sharply focused on the retina. This is the ideal refractive state of the eye. *Note:* The concept of emmetropia is not simple because accommodation is not inactive when fixating at distance (tonic accommodation). In fact, some authors consider hyperopia of up to +1.00 D, in a prepresbyope, as emmetropia. *See* **accommodation, resting state of; ametropia; distances, conjugate.**

emmetropization A process that is presumed to operate to produce a greater frequency of emmetropic eyes than would otherwise occur on the basis of chance. This mechanism would coordinate the development of the various components of the optical system of the eye (e.g. axial length, refracting power of the cornea, depth of the anterior chamber, etc.) to prevent ametropia, especially infant hyperopia, which subsides within the first 3 years of life with the most significant decrease occurring in the first year.

emmetropization theory *See* **theory, emmetropization.**

empirical horopter *See* **horopter, empirical.**

empiricism The belief that knowledge or behaviour stems from experience, learning or data acquired by observation or experimentation. *See* **nativism; theory, empiricist.**

empiricist theory *See* **theory, empiricist.**

Emsley's reduced eye *See* **eye, reduced.**

endophthalmitis Inflammation of the intraocular structures. It can occur after a penetrating wound of the eye (either surgical or accidental), bacterial infection or intraocular foreign bodies. It can occur immediately following cataract surgery or delayed when a microorganism (*Staphylococcus aureus, Staphylococcus epidermis*) remains trapped within the capsular bag causing pain and vision impairment. Management includes intravitreal antibiotics or possibly vitrectomy. Endophthalmitis may also occur as a result of an infection by a fungus (*Candida albicans, Aspergillus*) directly or via intravenous drug abuse, an indwelling catheter, immunosuppression and with *Aspergillus* chronic pulmonary disease. There is usually visual impairment, retinitis and vitritis with yellow-white fluffy 'cotton balls' or 'string of pearls' lesions, which

are more marked with *Aspergillus*. Management includes antibiotic or antifungal agents and vitrectomy. *See* **iodine-povidone; panophthalmitis; vitrectomy.**

endoscope Instrument designed to examine cavities which are not accessible on direct examination with the eye. It usually incorporates fibre optics to increase the flexibility of the instrument. *Examples:* a laryngoscope which is introduced through the mouth to examine the larynx; an ophthalmic endoscope to examine the intraocular structures by inserting a fibre optics system through the sclera, as may be used in ocular surgery.

endothelial bedewing; blebs *See* under the nouns.

endothelial corneal dystrophy *See* **cornea guttata; dystrophy, Fuchs' endothelial; dystrophy, posterior polymorphous.**

endothelial polymegethism; polymorphism *See* under the nouns.

endotheliitis *See* **keratitis, disciform.**

endothelium, corneal *See* **corneal endothelium.**

endpiece That part at either end of a spectacle frame front which contains the pivot for the sides. *Syn.* lug.

enhancement, brightness An increase in brightness resulting either from making a stimulus intermittent or when a surface is surrounded by a dark area, as compared to when it is surrounded by a light area. *See* **contrast; effect, Brücke–Bartley.**

enlargement Term commonly used in low-vision practice to refer to an increase in the size of the retinal image seen by the patient. It can be expressed as the **enlargement ratio**. *See* **magnification, lateral; power, equivalent viewing.**

enophthalmos Recession of the eyeball into the orbit. It is caused by a degeneration and shrinking of the orbital fat, a tumour, an injury to the orbit or to shortening of the extraocular muscles following excessive resections. *See* **entropion; exophthalmometer; exophthalmos.**

entoptic image *See* **image, entoptic.**

entoptoscope, blue field An instrument enabling the visualization, especially in patients with a dense cataract, of the shadows of leucocytes flowing in the retinal capillaries and therefore providing a test of macular function. It consists of a very bright light source, an interference filter with a maximum transmission in the blue end of the spectrum and a diffuser. The instrument is held close to the eye of the patient who is asked to describe his or her observations. The leucocytes appear as flying corpuscles and, if many corpuscles (at least 15) are seen moving in the entire field, the test is considered positive whereas if none or only a few corpuscles are seen, the test is considered negative. Positive responses usually indicate that the patient has good macular function, and negative responses usually indicate that the patient has poor macular function. This test is very useful in predicting central vision before cataract extraction. *See* angioscotoma; maxwellian view system, clinical.

entrance pupil *See* pupil, entrance.

entropion Inward turning of the eyelid. It results in the eyelashes rubbing the cornea (as in trichiasis), which usually causes discomfort. The most common cause of entropion that occurs in old people (called **involutional entropion**) and only affects the lower eyelid is due to a combination of atrophy and weakening of the tarsus, loss of tone of the subcutaneous tissues and loss of elasticity of the skin. Other causes are scarring (e.g. trachoma, Stevens–Johnson syndrome), burns of the palpebral conjunctiva (called **cicatricial entropion**) which may affect either the upper or the lower eyelid, or spasm of the orbicularis muscle often resulting from an ocular inflammation or lid infection (called **acute spastic entropion**) which may subside spontaneously once the original cause has been removed. Temporary relief of entropion may be provided by instilling an ocular lubricant or taping of the lower eyelid to the cheek, but the treatment is usually surgical. *See* ectropion; lens, therapeutic soft contact; spectacles, orthopaedic; procedure, Jones'; procedure, Weis'; pseudotrichiasis; tarsus; trichiasis.

cicatricial e.; involutional e. *See* entropion.
congenital e. A rare congenital inversion of the eyelid usually associated with tarsal hypoplasia or microphthalmia. It may be confused with epiblepharon. If treatment is needed, it is surgical, although many cases resolve spontaneously with time.

enucleation Removal of an eye from its socket. It is usually performed to reduce pain in a blind eye, when there is a serious risk of sympathetic ophthalmia following trauma or when there is a malignant tumour in the eye. Immediately following the operation, a spherical orbital implant is placed into the eye socket with a blank plastic shell in front (a conformer) to hold the eyelids in place and it is replaced several weeks later by an artificial eye. *See* eye, artificial; conformer; evisceration; eye, artificial; orbital implant.

enzyme A protein substance which catalyses (i.e. enhances a chemical reaction in other bodies without undergoing a change in itself) and is formed by living cells but can act independently of their presence. *Example*: enzyme preparations (containing pancreatin, papain or subtilisin A) used to break down tear proteins that become attached to the surface of contact lenses. *See* deposits, contact lens; phagocytosis; surfactant; wetting solution.

ephedrine hydrochloride *See* mydriatic.

epiblepharon A congenital anomaly in which a fold of skin lies across the upper or lower lid margin. In the lower eyelid, it causes a turning inward of the eyelashes without causing entropion. The condition commonly resolves itself with facial growth. *See* blepharochalasis; entropion, congenital.

epibulbar Situated on the eyeball. *Syn.* epiocular.

epicanthus A condition in which a fold of skin that stretches from the upper to the lower eyelid partially covers the inner canthus. It is normal in the fetus, in Down's syndrome and in many infants, especially of oriental origin, where it may give the impression of a convergent strabismus (**pseudoesotropia**). The condition is normally bilateral. As the bridge of the nose develops, the folds eventually disappear. *Plural*: epicanthi. *Syn.* epicanthal fold. *See* strabismus, apparent.

epicanthus inversus A condition in which a fold of skin that stretches from the lower eyelid upward and towards the nose partially covers the inner canthus. It is often associated with ptosis.

epichoroid Synonym for suprachoroid. *See* choroid; sclera.

epidemic An outbreak of a disease, especially infectious but not exclusively, affecting a large number of people in a particular region or in a population. *See* sporadic.

epidemiology A branch of health science that deals with the incidence, prevalence, distribution and control of disease in a population. It is aimed at determining the aetiology of a disease.

epidiascope A projector used to project by reflection pictures (such as the page of a book) onto a screen.

epigenetics The study of traits that are not caused by changes in the DNA code but by environmental stress such as drugs, diet, aging or an extreme life event, which influences gene function and expression.

epikeratophakia *See* epikeratoplasty.

epikeratoplasty A surgical procedure on the cornea aimed at correcting ametropia. The patient's corneal epithelium is removed and a donor's corneal disc (or lenticule) that was previously frozen and reshaped to produce a new anterior curvature is rehydrated and sutured to Bowman's membrane. The lenticule can be removed and exchanged to provide a different power. There are many problems associated with this procedure, in particular the surface re-epithelialization. *Syn.* epikeratophakia; refractive keratoplasty and keratorefractive surgery (both terms also include keratomileusis, keratophakia and radial keratotomy). *See* Intacs; keratomileusis; keratophakia; keratectomy, photorefractive; LASIK; LASEK; lenticule.

epilation The removal of hair by the roots as in the case of ingrowing eyelashes. The eyelashes

are removed with forceps but, unfortunately, they tend to regrow.
See distichiasis; trichiasis.

epinastine hydrochloride *See* antihistamine.

epinephrine *See* adrenaline (epinephrine).

epiocular *See* epibulbar.

epiphora Overflow of tears due to faulty apposition of the lacrimal puncta in the lacrimal lake, scarring of the puncta, paresis of the orbicularis muscle, obstruction of the lacrimal passage, ectropion or increased tear production due to a chronic irritant or disease (e.g. blepharitis, dacryocystitis, thyroid eye disease, viral conjunctivitis). This impairment of the outflow of tears is often unilateral. The main symptoms are discomfort and blurring of vision and sometimes embarrassment. Management depends on the cause. *Syn.* watery eye.
See dacryops; dacryocystitis; hyperlacrimation.

epiretinal membrane *See* membrane, epiretinal.

episclera A loose connective and elastic tissue which covers the sclera and anteriorly connects the conjunctiva to it. The connective tissue consists of collagen fibres and fibroblasts. It is vascularized and gives nutrition to the sclera. Its deeper layers merge with the scleral stroma. It sends connective tissue bundles into Tenon's capsule, which covers the episclera. The episclera becomes progressively thinner towards the back of the eye.
See artery, ciliary; sclera.

episcleritis Inflammation of the episclera. It is a benign, self-limiting, frequently recurring condition that typically affects adults. The disease is characterized by redness (usually in one quadrant of the globe) and varying degrees of discomfort. There are two types of episcleritis: **simple,** which is the most common, and **nodular,** which is localized to one area of the globe forming a nodule. Simple episcleritis usually subsides spontaneously within 1 to 2 weeks while the nodular type usually takes longer. If the discomfort is intense, topical corticosteroids may be used (Fig. E4).
See dellen; scleritis.

epithelial arcuate lesion; plug; splitting *See* staining, fluorescein.

epithelial downgrowth Abnormal growth of corneal or conjunctival epithelium into the interior of the eye as a complication of a penetrating corneal injury and much more rarely following cataract extraction. It may cause secondary glaucoma as a result of cell proliferation through the wound onto the endothelial surface and into the iridocorneal angle.

epithelial keratitis *See* keratitis, punctate epithelial; keratitis, Thygeson's superficial punctate.

epithelial microcysts *See* microcysts, epithelial.

epithelioma A tumour of epithelial cells, ranging from benign to malignant (e.g. carcinoma). *Example:* epithelioma of the conjunctival epithelium that begins near the limbus and spreads to the fornices and cornea. Treatment usually consists of excision, cryotherapy or both, or even enucleation if the tumour invades the eye itself.

epithelium, corneal *See* corneal epithelium.

equalization test *See* test, balancing.

equation, paraxial *See* paraxial equation, fundamental.

equator of the crystalline lens The circle formed by the outer margin of the lens. The equator is not smooth but shows a number of indentations corresponding to the zonular fibres. The indentations tend to disappear during accommodation, when the zonular fibres are loose.
See lens, crystalline; Zinn, zonule of.

equatorial plane of the eye *See* plane, equatorial.

equivalent oxygen pressure *See* oxygen pressure, equivalent.

equivalent points *See* points, nodal.

equivalent power *See* power, equivalent.

equivalent, spherical *See* spherical equivalent.

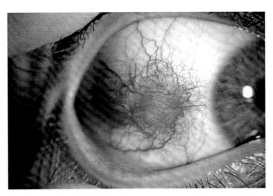

Fig. E4 Simple episcleritis. (From Kanski 2003, with permission of Butterworth-Heinemann)

erector A lens (for example an erecting eyepiece) or prism system (erecting prism such as a **Dove** or a **Porro prism**) placed in an optical system for the purpose of forming an erect image.

error, cylindrical; spherical *See* prescription.

error of refraction of the eye *See* ametropia; refractive error.

erythema multiforme A mucocutaneous disease that occurs as a hypersensitivity to drugs (e.g. sulfonamides) or as a consequence of infection. The condition, which principally affects young people, is characterized by the sudden appearance of various erosions of the mucous membranes and epidermis. A common complication is conjunctivitis, which may become severe with cicatrization, abnormal lid margin function, symblepharon, corneal ulceration and vascularization and keratoconjunctivitis sicca. The patient complains of pain, discharge, photophobia and reduced vision if the cornea is involved. Treatment includes cleansing of the eyelids with antibiotic ointment and, if severe, topical steroids. *Syn.* Stevens–Johnson syndrome (although this term applies to the severe form of the disease).
See syndrome, Stevens–Johnson.

erythrolabe *See* pigment, visual.

erythromycin *See* antibiotic.

erythrophobia *See* chromatophobia.

erythropsia *See* chromatopsia.

erythropsin *See* rhodopsin.

eserine *See* physostigmine.

eso deviation Term referring to either esophoria or esotropia.

esodisparity Fixation disparity characterized by a slight overconvergence of the eyes, while still retaining single binocular vision.
See disparity, retinal.

esophoria (E, ESOP, SOP, eso) Turning of the eye inward from the active position when fusion is suspended. If symptomatic, treatment may be by means of base-out prisms plus spherical lenses or visual training (Fig. E5).
See convergence excess; divergence insufficiency.

esotropia (SOT, ET, esoT) A form of strabismus in which there is a manifest deviation of one eye turned inward. This is the most common type of strabismus in children. The principal categories are accommodative and non-accommodative. *Syn.* convergent strabismus; crossed eyes (colloquial). *See* Fig. S14, p. 328; pattern, alphabet; strabismus; syndrome, Swann's; test, prism adaptation.
accommodative e. Convergent strabismus resulting from abnormal demand on accommodation due to uncorrected hyperopia, accompanied by excessive convergence and insufficient relative fusional divergence. The AC/A ratio (accommodative convergence to accommodation) is normal but the child has high hyperopia

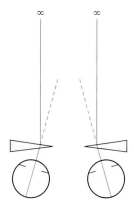

Fig. E5 Prismatic correction of esophoria.

(**refractive accommodative esotropia**). It may also occur in cases in which the AC/A ratio is high and accommodation is accompanied by excessive convergence in a child with a very small amount of hyperopia (**non-refractive accommodative esotropia**). Accommodative esotropia is usually an acquired deviation first presenting in the first decade of life. Children do not usually notice diplopia but instead develop suppression and later amblyopia. Management consists of full hyperopic correction and amblyopia treatment. *Syn.* accommodative strabismus.
See esotropia, non-accommodative; refraction, cycloplegic.
blind spot e. *See* syndrome, Swann's.
consecutive e. *See* strabismus, consecutive.
cyclic e. Very rare and unusual esotropia occurring on a 48-hour rhythm in which a 24-hour period of normal binocular vision is followed by 24 hours of manifest esotropia. The condition, which may have started in early infancy, only becomes apparent during early childhood. With time, cyclic esotropia tends to become constant. *Syn.* alternate day squint.
infantile e. Strabismus which becomes manifest within the first 6 months of life. It is idiopathic and characterized by a large angle of squint, alternate fixation that may become unilateral if amblyopia develops and nystagmus. Management is essentially surgical. A complication following surgery may be dissociated vertical deviation. *Syn.* congenital strabismus; infantile esotropia syndrome.
See cross-fixation; deviation, dissociated vertical.
non-accommodative e. Convergent strabismus not due to abnormal demands on accommodation. There are several types: infantile esotropia, basic esotropia (no significant hyperopia and the deviation is equal for near and distance), microtropia, convergence excess (esotropia for near vision but not for distance), divergence insufficiency (esotropia for distance vision but not for near), consecutive strabismus, sensory strabismus and cyclic esotropia (periodic manifestation of

esotropia as for example on alternate days). Treatment of associated amblyopia and correction of hyperopia are often followed by surgery.
See esotropia, accommodative.

Esterman grid; test *See* test, Esterman.

esthesiometer *See* aesthesiometer.

'E' test *See* 'E' game; chart, illiterate E.

ethmoid bone *See* orbit; sinus, ethmoidal.

ethylenediamine tetraacetic acid (EDTA) A chelating agent used in ophthalmic preparations to remove metals which are essential for the metabolism of bacteria and viruses, and therefore inactivate them. It enhances the bactericidal effect of preservatives and is commonly combined with benzalkonium chloride, chlorhexidine and thiomersalate.
See antiseptic.

etiology *See* aetiology.

euchromatopsia Normal perception of colours.
Syn. euchromatopsy.
See chromatopsia.

euryopia Abnormally wide palpebral aperture.

euthyroid *See* disease, Graves'.

Euthyscope *See* Visuscope.

eversion, lid Turning of the eyelid inside out so as to expose the palpebral conjunctiva. For the upper lid, this is accomplished by grasping the lid by the central eyelashes, pulling it downward and forward and then folding it back over a cotton applicator (or thin plastic rod) placed at the upper margin of the tarsus, while the patient continually maintains downward fixation. Return to the normal lid position is obtained by asking the patient to look up and gently pushing the eyelashes in an outward and downward direction. Foreign bodies and even contact lenses are often lodged under the upper eyelid or in the conjunctival fornix of the upper eyelid. To inspect the superior conjunctival fornix, **double lid eversion** is necessary. Following lid eversion (and usually with local anaesthesia of the conjunctiva), a retractor is placed between the two skin surfaces of the lid with the retractor engaging the tarsus and, after gently pulling outward and upward, the fornix will become visible. Eversion of the lower lid is performed easily by drawing the margin downward while the patient looks upward.
See irrigation; sulcus, subtarsal.

evidence-based healthcare *See* trial, randomized controlled.

evisceration Removal of the inner contents of the eye with the exception of the sclera. It is usually performed when there is intraocular suppuration or pain in a blind eye or sometimes following absolute glaucoma or end-stage diabetes. The intraocular contents are immediately replaced by a spherical orbital implant with a conformer and, several weeks later, the conformer is replaced by an artificial eye.
See eye, artificial; conformer; enucleation; orbital implant.

evoked potential *See* potential, visual evoked.

excavation, physiological *See* cup, physiological.

excimer laser *See* laser, excimer.

excision Surgical removal of a tissue, an organ or a tumour. *Example:* removal of a cyst on the sclera.
See incision.

excyclophoria *See* cyclophoria.

excyclotorsion *See* cyclotorsion; torsion.

excyclotropia *See* cyclotropia.

excyclovergence Rotary movements about their respective anteroposterior axes of one eye relative to the other. If the upper pole of the cornea of one eye moves away from that of the other eye, it is called **excyclovergence**. If, however, the upper pole of the cornea of one eye moves towards that of the other eye, it is called **incyclovergence**.

exenteration Removal of the entire contents of the orbit, including the eyeball, the extraocular muscles, the optic nerve, nerves and blood vessels, the orbital fat and connective tissues. It is performed in cases of invasive malignant tumours.
See enucleation; evisceration.

exfoliation of the lens Shedding of the layers of the lens capsule. It often occurs as a result of exposure to prolonged and intense heat.
See cataract, heat-ray; pseudoexfoliation; syndrome, pseudoexfoliation.

exit pupil *See* pupil, exit.

exo deviation Term referring to either exophoria or exotropia.

exodisparity Fixation disparity characterized by a slight underconvergence of the eyes while still retaining single binocular vision.
See disparity, retinal.

exophoria (X, XOP, exo) Turning of the eye outward from the active position when fusion is suspended. If symptomatic, treatment may be by means of base-in prisms, minus spherical lenses or visual training (Fig. E6).
See convergence, insufficiency; divergence excess.

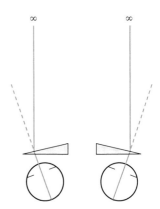

Fig. E6 Prismatic correction of exophoria.

exophoria, physiological The relative exophoria at near when it is compared to the heterophoria in distance vision. It is, on average, of the order of 3 to 4 D at a fixation distance of 40 cm. *Example*: If distance heterophoria is 6 D eso and near heterophoria is 2 D eso, the physiological exophoria is 4 D exo.

exophthalmometer Instrument for measuring the amount of exophthalmos (or enophthalmos). There are several types, the most common being the **Hertel exophthalmometer**; it measures the distance between the corneal apex and the apex of the deepest angle of the lateral orbital margin of both eyes simultaneously, using either mirrors or prisms and a superimposed millimetre scale. The normal range varies between 12 mm and 21 mm, and a difference between the eyes greater than 2 mm is suspicious. The instrument can be used to monitor the progress of Graves' ophthalmopathy.

exophthalmos Abnormal protrusion of the eyeball(s) from the orbit, caused by Graves' ophthalmopathy, endocrine malfunction, paralysis of the extraocular muscles, injury of the orbit, cavernous sinus thrombosis or a tumour behind the eye. The palpebral fissure is usually wider and a rim of sclera may be visible above and below the cornea (Fig. E7). Unilateral displacement is usually referred to as **proptosis**.
See diplopia, pathological; disease, Graves'; elephantiasis oculi; enophthalmos; syndrome, Apert's; syndrome, Crouzon's.

exotropia A form of strabismus in which there is a manifest deviation of one eye turned outward. The principal categories are constant exotropia and intermittent exotropia. **Constant exotropia** may be **congenital,** which is often associated with an underlying neurological anomaly, or **basic,** which appears after 6 months of age with equal exotropia for near and distance vision. Both types are usually treated surgically. **Intermittent exotropia** is the most common form of exotropia. It begins as an exophoria and breaks down to exotropia presenting in children between 2 and 5 years of age. It is characterized by worse exotropia at near (convergence excess) or worse exotropia at distance (divergence excess). As it occurs intermittently, acuities are generally good. Treatment includes spectacle correction, orthoptic exercises or surgery.
See **Fig. S14, p. 328; pattern, alphabet; strabismus.**

exotropia, consecutive *See* strabismus, consecutive.

exotropia, paralytic pontine *See* syndrome, 'one and a half'.

experiment, Bidwell's Experiment aimed at producing the complement of a colour stimulus by viewing it through a rotating disc which presents the sequence: black, colour stimulus and white. *See* colour, complementary.

experiment, Scheiner's A demonstration of the refractive changes occurring in the eye when accommodating. The subject observes a target monocularly (such as a simple point of light) through a **Scheiner's disc** (an opaque disc with two pinholes separated by a distance less than the pupil diameter). It will be seen singly at only one distance where the eye is focused, because target and retina are then conjugate. If the eye accommodates, two points of light are seen. The principle of this experiment is incorporated in several refractometers.
See **Fig. D6, p. 91; optometer, infrared; optometer, Young's.**

experiment, Young's Method of producing interference of light which was shown by Young in 1801. He used two coherent beams of light that were produced by passing light through a very small circular aperture in one screen, then through two small circular apertures very close together in a second screen. On a third screen, behind the second screen, there will be two overlapping sets of waves and, if the original source is emitting monochromatic light, interference fringes will appear on the third screen (Fig. E8).
See **coherent sources; interference fringes.**

exposure keratitis *See* keratitis, exposure.

exposure meter Light measuring instrument for ascertaining the setting (lens aperture, shutter speed, etc.) of a camera for correct light exposure of the photographic material (CIE).

expressivity The extent to which an inherited trait or disease is manifested in the phenotype. It is a qualitative evaluation unlike penetrance. When

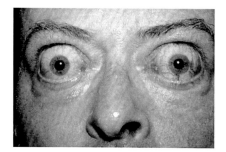

Fig. E7 Severe bilateral exophthalmos and lid retraction in Graves' disease. (From Kanski 2003, with permission of Butterworth-Heinemann)

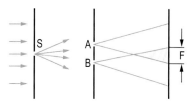

Fig. E8 Young's experiment (S, source of light (illuminated pinhole); A and B, pinholes; F, circular interference fringes).

there is variable expression, only some aspects of the disease appear. *Syn.* expression.

extended object; source; wear lens *See* under the nouns.

external hordeolum; limiting membrane; ophthalmoplegia *See* under the nouns.

extinction phenomenon *See* phenomenon, extinction.

extorsion *See* torsion.

extraocular muscles *See* muscles, extraocular.

extrinsic muscles *See* muscles, extraocular.

exudate A liquid or semisolid which has been discharged through the tissues to the surface or into a cavity. Exudates in the retina are opacities that result from the escape of plasma and white blood cells from defective blood vessels. They usually look greyish-white or yellowish and are circular or ovoid in shape. They are sometimes classified into three groups according to size: (1) **punctate hard** exudates, which often tend to coalesce. They are found in diabetic retinopathy, Coats' disease, etc.; (2) exudates of moderate size, such as 'cotton-wool or soft exudates' as, for example, in branch/central retinal vein occlusion, hypertensive retinopathy, etc. These 'exudates' have ill-defined margins and are actually areas of ischaemia containing cytoid bodies, unlike hard exudates which are generally lipid deposits; (3) larger exudates, as found in the severe forms of retinopathy.
See hypertension; papilloedema.

eye The peripheral organ of vision, in which an optical image of the external world is produced and transformed into nerve impulses. It is a spheroidal body approximately 24 mm in diameter with the segment of a smaller sphere (of about 8 mm radius), the cornea, in front. It consists of an external coat of fibrous tissue, the sclera and transparent cornea; a middle vascular coat, comprising the iris, the ciliary body and the choroid; and an internal coat, the retina, which includes the cones and rods photoreceptors. Within the eye, there are the aqueous humour located between the cornea and the crystalline lens, the crystalline lens held by the zonule of Zinn and the vitreous body located between the crystalline lens and the retina. The movements of the eye are directed by six extraocular muscles (Fig. E9). *Syn.* organ of sight; visual organ.
amaurotic e. *See* amaurosis.
amblyopic e. An eye which has amblyopia. *Syn.* lazy eye (colloquial).
anterior segment of the e. Portion of the eye comprising all the structures situated between the front surface of the cornea and the front surface of the vitreous. The eyelids are sometimes included in this definition.
aphakic e. An eye without the crystalline lens.
artificial e. A prosthesis made nowadays of plastic, usually polymethyl methacrylate, in which the front surface has been painted to resemble an eye and which is placed in the socket in front of the orbital implant to replace the conformer several weeks after enucleation or evisceration. *Syn.* ocular prosthesis.
See conformer; eye impression; ocularist; orbital implant.
axial length of the e. *See* length of the eye, axial.
e. bank An organization that collects, evaluates, stores and distributes eyes from donors. The eyes are used for corneal transplantation and research. *See* keratoplasty.
bionic e. Term referring to the prosthesis implanted in the eye and occipital cortex which, along with a camera to capture light, is intended to restore visual function in a blind patient. There are several systems, most of them experimental.
black e. A colloquial term for a swollen or blue-black spot on the skin of the eyelid caused by effusion of blood as a result of a superficial injury in which the skin is not broken. The correct term is **ecchymosis** of the eyelid. The condition

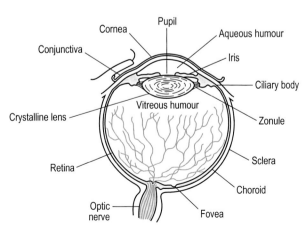

Fig. E9 Cross-section of the eye. (After Millodot 1976, with permission of Aquila Communications Inc)

recovers by itself within 2 to 3 weeks while changing in colour to yellow. Immediately after the injury, application of ice helps minimize the haemorrhage and swelling.
See **haematoma.**

bleary e. A red and watery eye with a lacklustre appearance. Lack of sleep is a common cause. *Syn.* blear eye.

e. blink *See* **blink.**

compound e. The eye of arthropods composed of a variable number of ommatidia.
See **corneal facet; ommatidium.**

crossed e's. *See* **esotropia.**

cyclopean e. Imaginary eye located at a point midway between the two eyes. When the two visual fields overlap and the impressions from the two eyes are combined into a single impression, the apparent direction of a fixated object appears in a direction that emanates from the cyclopean eye.

dark-adapted e. An eye that has been in darkness and is sensitive to low illumination. *Syn.* scotopic eye.

deviating e. The non-fixating eye in strabismus or under heterophoria testing. *Syn.* squinting eye.

dominant e. The eye that is dominant when ocular dominance exists. It is not necessarily the eye with the best visual acuity nor is it fixed, as this may depend on the visual task.
See **dominance, ocular; manoptoscope; test, hole in the card.**

dry e. This term encompasses various tear film disorders or blockage of the puncta resulting in insufficient tear volume and symptoms ranging from a mild form causing discomfort and slight irritation, which is usually relieved with artificial tears, to the most common forms: keratoconjunctivitis sicca, xerophthalmia, xerosis or Sjögren's syndrome. In most instances, the tear film break-up time is shorter than normal.
See **keratoconjunctivitis sicca; tear film; test, break-up time.**

equatorial plane of the e. *See* **plane, equatorial.**

exciting e. *See* **ophthalmia, sympathetic.**

fixating e. The eye that is directed towards the object of regard in strabismus.
See **eye, deviating.**

glass e. An artificial eye made of glass.
See **ocularist; prosthesis, ocular.**

e. impression A negative form or replica of the anterior part of the eye. A substance with rapid gelling properties is held in contact with the eye until gelled. This **impression** (or **mould**) is then used in the preparation of a positive model called a **cast** (or **casting**) of the anterior part of the eye; it is made by filling the impression with a material containing a base which hardens to artificial stone. Using this cast, a **shell** of a scleral contact lens is produced with optimum shape of the back surface. An impression is also made in the preparation of an artificial eye after enucleation to ensure that its back surface fits the orbital implant and covering of the conjunctiva. *Syn.* impression moulding; mould; ocular impression.
See **eye, artificial.**

lazy e. *See* **eye, amblyopic.**

e. lens *See* **eyepiece.**

light-adapted e. An eye that has been exposed to light and is insensitive to low illumination. *Syn.* photopic eye.
See **adaptation, light; theory, duplicity.**

e. movements *See* **movement, eye.**

e. patch A piece of material or plastic that is worn over the eye when it has been injured or over the socket when it is missing.

phakic e. An eye that contains the crystalline lens.
See **phakic.**

photopic e. *See* **eye, light-adapted.**

pink e. *See* **conjunctivitis, contagious.**

e. position Position of the eye in the orbit, maintained by the extraocular muscles.
See **position, primary; position, secondary; position, tertiary.**

posterior segment of the e. Posterior portion of the eye comprising the vitreous humour, the retina, the optic disc, the choroid and most of the sclera.

pseudophakic e. An eye fitted with an intraocular lens implant.
See **lens, intraocular.**

red e. A colloquial term often used for any condition in which the blood vessels of the conjunctiva or ciliary body are congested. Many conditions result in a red eye (e.g. subconjunctival haemorrhage, pterygium, conjunctivitis, episcleritis, corneal abrasion, corneal erosion, ulcerative keratitis, corneal dendritic ulcer, acute iritis, angle-closure glaucoma, orbital cellulitis and possibly contact lens wear).
See **injection, ciliary; injection, conjunctival.**

reduced e. A mathematical model of the optical system of the eye. It consists of a single refracting surface with one nodal point, one principal point and one index of refraction. In the first such model, proposed by **Listing** in 1853, the refracting surface had a power of 68.3 D and was situated 2.34 mm behind the schematic eye's cornea. It had an index of refraction of 1.35, a radius of curvature of 5.124 mm and a length of 20 mm. **Donders'** reduced eye was even more simplified. It has a power of 66.7 D, a radius of curvature of 5 mm, an index of refraction of 4/3 and anterior and posterior focal lengths of −15 and +20 mm, respectively, with a refracting surface situated 2 mm behind the schematic eye's cornea. **Gullstrand's** reduced eye has a radius of curvature of 5.7 mm, an index of refraction of 1.33, a power of 61 D with the refracting surface situated 1.35 mm behind the schematic eye's cornea. **Emsley's** reduced eye has a power of 60 D, an index of refraction of 4/3 and is situated 1.66 mm behind the schematic eye's cornea with anterior and posterior focal lengths of −16.67 and +22.22 mm, respectively.

schematic e. A model consisting of various spherical surfaces representing the optical system of a normal eye based on the average dimensions (called the **constants of the eye**) of the human eye. There are many schematic eyes, although the most commonly used is that of Gullstrand. A great deal of variation among authors stemmed from the difficulty in giving an index of refraction that would represent the heterogeneous character of the crystalline lens. Gullstrand in fact proposed two schematic eyes, one which he called the **exact schematic eye** and the other which he called the **simplified schematic eye** in which the divergent effect of the posterior corneal surface is ignored and the cornea replaced by an equivalent surface; the crystalline lens is homogeneous and the optical system is free from aberrations.

scotopic e. *See* eye, dark-adapted.

e. shield 1. *See* occluder. 2. A protective device to cover the eye against injury, glare or in radiotherapy of the face.

sighting-dominant e. The eye that is preferred in monocular tasks, such as looking through a telescope or aiming a firearm.

e. socket The bony orbit which contains the eyeball, muscles, nerves, vessels, orbital fat and orbital portion of the lacrimal gland.

e. speculum An instrument designed to hold the eyelids apart during surgery. *Syn.* blepharostat.

squinting e. *See* eye, deviating.

e. stone A small, smooth shell or other object that can be inserted beneath the eyelid to facilitate the removal of a foreign body from the eye.

sympathetic e. The uninjured eye in sympathetic ophthalmia that becomes secondarily affected. *Syn.* sympathizing eye.
See ophthalmia, sympathetic.

wall e. A colloquial term referring to (1) a white opaque cornea or (2) a divergent strabismus.

watery e. *See* epiphora.

eyeball The globe of the eye without its appendages. *See* **appendages of the eye.**

eyebrow A transverse elevation covered with hairs and situated at the junction of the forehead and upper lid. *Syn.* supercilium.
See ophryosis.

eyecup A small vessel made of glass, plastic or porcelain, used to bathe the eye.

eyeglass 1. Synonym for monocle. In the plural (**eyeglasses**) it refers to pince-nez or a similar type of eyewear without sides, or to spectacles. 2. The eyepiece of an optical instrument.

eyelashes Rows of stiff hairs (cilia) growing on the margin of the upper and lower eyelids. The upper eyelashes are longer and more numerous and curl upward, while the lower ones turn downward. *Syn.* cilia; lashes.
See distichiasis; epilation; madarosis; polystichia; trichiasis.

eyelid eversion *See* eversion, lid.

eyelid twitch *See* ciliosis; myasthenia gravis; myokymia.

eyelids A pair of movable folds of skin which act as protective coverings of the eye. The upper eyelid extends downward from the eyebrow and is the more moveable of the two. When the eye is open and looking straight ahead, it just covers the upper part of the cornea; when it is closed, it covers the whole cornea. The lower eyelid reaches just below the cornea when the eye is open and rises only slightly when it shuts. Each eyelid consists of the following layers, starting anteriorly: (1) skin, (2) a layer of subcutaneous connective tissue, (3) a layer of striated muscle fibres of the orbicularis muscle, (4) a layer of submuscular connective tissue, (5) a fibrous layer, including the tarsal plates, (6) a layer of smooth muscle, and (7) the palpebral conjunctiva. *Syn.* blephara; lids; palpebrae.
See ablephary; blepharitis; ciliosis; ectropion; entropion; epicanthus; eversion, lid; eyelid lamella; lagophthalmos; lid laceration; ligament, palpebral; myokymia; orbital septum; phthriasis; sign, Cogan's lid twitch; sign, Collier's; sign, Dalrymple's; sulcus, inferior palpebral; sulcus, superior palpebral; tarsorrhaphy; tarsus; xanthelasma.

e. lamella The eyelid is sometimes conceptualized as consisting of an anterior and posterior lamella. The **anterior lamella** consists of the skin, the layer of subcutaneous connective tissue and the layer of striated muscle fibres of the orbicularis muscle. The **posterior lamella** consists of the tarsal plates, a layer of smooth muscle (Müller's palpebral muscle), and the palpebral conjunctiva.

e. retractor muscles The eyelid muscles that open the palpebral aperture. The upper eyelid is elevated by the levator palpebrae superioris muscle and the superior tarsal muscle (of Müller), and the lower eyelid is depressed by the inferior tarsal muscle (of Müller).

eyepiece The lens or combination of lenses in an optical instrument (microscope, telescope, etc.) through which the observer views the image formed by the objective. The most common eyepieces are composed of two single lenses or two doublets; the lens or doublet nearer the eye is called the **eye lens** and the one nearer the objective is called the **field lens**. The role of the eyepiece is to magnify the image and to reduce the aberrations of the image formed by the objective. *Syn.* eye lens; eyeglass; ocular.

Huygens' e. Negative eyepiece used commonly in microscopes. It consists of two planoconvex lenses mounted with their plane surfaces facing the eye. In the most common type, the eye lens has a focal length half that of the field lens and the separation is equal to half the sum of the two focal lengths.

negative e. Eyepiece made up of two lenses, in which the first principal focus of the eyepiece lies between the two lenses, such as in a Huygens' eyepiece.

orthoscopic e. An eyepiece corrected for distortion and which provides a wide field of view and high magnification. It consists of a triplet field lens and a single eye lens. It is used in high-power telescopes and range finders.
See triplet.

positive e. Eyepiece made up of two lenses in which the first principal focus of the eyepiece lies in front of the field lens, such as in a Ramsden eyepiece.

Ramsden e. Positive eyepiece consisting of two planoconvex lenses mounted with their convex side facing each other and having equal focal lengths. The lenses are usually separated by two-thirds the focal length of either.

eyesight Synonym for vision.

eyesize The horizontal dimension of the lens opening of a frame which is bounded by two vertical lines at a tangent to the left and right sides of the opening. *See* spectacle frame markings.

eyestrain *See* asthenopia.

eyewash Any liquid which is used for bathing the eye. *Example*: physiological saline (0.5% sodium chloride).

eyewear *See* spectacles.

eyewire The rim that surrounds the lens of a spectacle frame.

F

facet, corneal *See* corneal facet.

factor, daylight The ratio of daylight illuminance received at a given point inside a room to the simultaneous illuminance on a horizontal plane outside exposed to an unobstructed sky. It is usually expressed as a percentage, 5% or more being considered a well-lit room.

factor, reflection *See* reflectance.

factor, spectral transmission *See* spectrophotometer.

facultative hyperopia *See* hyperopia, facultative.

Faden procedure *See* procedure, Faden.

Falant *See* test, lantern.

fallen eye syndrome *See* syndrome, fallen eye.

false macula *See* macula, false.

false negative A failure to detect a stimulus or a disease when it is actually present. *See* sensitivity; true negative.

false positive An error in which a stimulus or a disease is detected as being present when it is not. *See* specificity; true positive.

familial Pertaining to a condition or trait, either hereditary or acquired, which is found in more members of a family than would be expected by chance. *See* acquired; congenital; hereditary.

familial autonomic dysfunction; dysautonomia *See* syndrome, Riley–Day.

fan and block test *See* test, fan and block.

fan chart *See* chart, astigmatic fan.

far point of accommodation; of convergence; of the eye; sphere *See* under the nouns.

far sight *See* hyperopia.

Farnsworth–Munsell 100 Hue test *See* test, Farnsworth-Munsell 100 Hue.

Farnsworth test *See* test, Farnsworth-Munsell 100 Hue; test, lantern.

fascia A sheet of connective tissue covering, partitioning or binding together muscles and certain other organs, such as the lacrimal sac, the orbital septum and other organs within the orbit, the sclera (e.g. Tenon's capsule), etc.

fascia bulbi *See* Tenon's capsule.

fascia, palpebral *See* orbital septum.

fasciculus A bundle of nerve fibres, all with the same orientation.

fasciculus, medial longitudinal One of a pair of nerve fibres, one on each side of the midline and extending from the upper midbrain to the cervical spinal cord. It is composed largely of ascending fibres from the vestibular nuclei ascending to the motor nuclei (third, fourth and sixth) and innervating the extraocular muscles; and, to a lesser extent, of descending fibres from the medial vestibular nuclei, the reticular formation, the superior colliculi and nucleus of Cajal innervating the musculature of the neck. *Syn.* medial longitudinal bundle; posterior longitudinal bundle. *See* brainstem.

fast eye movements *See* movement, saccadic eye.

fatigue, visual A feeling of weariness resulting from a visual task. It can be of ocular, muscular or psychic origin. However, there does not seem to be objective proof of a reduction in visual aptitude (e.g. visual acuity) accompanying visual fatigue. *See* asthenopia.

feathers A cluster of fine bubbles or particles commonly arising from foreign material or from a fold in the glass in a molten or plastic state (British Standard).

Fechner's colours *See* Benham top.

Fechner's law *See* law, Fechner's.

Fechner's paradox Subjective impression of a decrease in the brightness of a field when viewing it binocularly after one eye that was closed looks through a dark filter (about 5% transmission), the other eye being unobstructed. This is paradoxical because more light is received by the eyes when the field is viewed binocularly, as compared to monocularly.

fenestration *See* lens, fenestrated; lens, scleral contact.

Fermat's law *See* law, Fermat's.

ferning ocular test *See* test, ferning ocular.

Ferry–Porter law *See* law, Ferry–Porter.

fibre A long thread or filament constituting human and animal tissues (e.g. nerve axon, muscle fibre, the filament of connective tissue).

arcuate f's. Axons of the ganglion cells of the retina which are temporal to the optic disc and pass above and below the papillomacular bundle in an arcuate course. *Syn.* arcuate nerve fibres bundle (Fig. F1).
See retinal raphe; scotoma, arcuate.

cilio-equatorial; cilio-posterior capsular f's.
See Zinn, zonule of.

circular f's. See muscle, ciliary.

felderstruktur muscle f's. A type of extraocular muscle fibre whose effect is to produce slow and tonic contractions. They are mainly responsible for maintaining smooth pursuit movements. The fibres are located in the superficial portions of the extraocular muscles and are unique to this type of muscle.

fibrillenstruktur muscle f's. A type of extraocular muscle fibre whose effect is to produce fast and twitch type of contractions. They are mainly responsible for saccadic eye movements. The fibres are located deep within the extraocular muscles and are the type usually found in skeletal muscles.

Henle's f. See layer of Henle, fibre.

lens f's. Long six-sided bands containing few organelles and mostly lacking a nucleus, derived from epithelial cells just within the capsule of the crystalline lens and attached to an anterior and posterior suture. New lens fibres are continuously produced throughout life thus contributing to lens growth with age.

longitudinal f's. See muscle, ciliary.

macular f's. See fibre, papillomacular.

medullated nerve f's. See fibre, myelinated nerve.

meridional f's. See muscle, ciliary.

f's. of Mueller See cell, Mueller's.

myelinated nerve f's. Anomalous congenital extension onto the retina of the myelin sheaths covering the optic nerve fibres. This myelination anterior to the lamina cribrosa normally disappears soon after birth. Ophthalmoscopically, it appears as whitish, striated, feather-shaped patches which may or may not obscure retinal vessels. Vision in these areas may be reduced, although visual acuity is not affected as the patches are most frequently located adjacent to the optic disc and sometimes in the periphery. The most characteristic sign may be an enlargement of the blind spot. *Syn.* medullated nerve fibres; opaque nerve fibres.
See cribriform plate.

f. optics See optics, fibre.

orbiculo-anterior capsular; orbiculo-posterior capsular f's. See Zinn, zonule of.

papillomacular f's. Axons of the ganglion cells of the macular region of the retina which enter the temporal portion of the optic disc and travel in the central region of the optic nerve. In the optic chiasma, the temporal macular fibres remain on the same side, while the nasal ones cross to the other side. These fibres make up the **papillomacular bundle** (Fig. F1).

pupillary f's. Axons of the optic nerve which branch off from the visual portion of the optic tract, before the lateral geniculate body, to run in the superior brachium towards the pretectal region anterior to the superior colliculus. They mediate the pupillary reflexes.
See pretectum; reflex, pupil light.

radial f's. See muscle, ciliary.

visual f's. Axons from the ganglion cells of the retina, making up the optic nerves and optic tracts. There are approximately one million visual fibres in the optic nerve. They synapse in the lateral geniculate body and then project to the region of the calcarine fissure of the cortex conveying the nervous impulses associated with vision.
See pathway, visual.

zonular f's. See Zinn, zonule of.

fibrinoplatelet *See* plaques, Hollenhorst's.

fibrocyte, corneal *See* keratocyte.

fibroplasia, retrolental *See* retinopathy of prematurity.

fibrosis of the extraocular muscles, congenital A rare, congenital disorder characterized by bilateral ptosis, inability to elevate the eyes above the midline and restrictive external ophthalmoplegia with exotropia. It is believed to be due to an abnormal development of the oculomotor nerve.

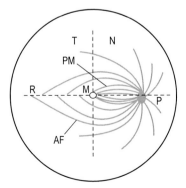

Fig. F1 Diagram of the optic nerve fibres of the right eye seen from the front (M, macula; P, optic disc; R, retinal raphe; PM, papillomacular fibres; AF, arcuate fibres; T, temporal side; N, nasal side).

There are several forms, which are genetically different with variable defects.

fibrosis, preretinal macular *See* **membrane, epiretinal.**

Fick, axes of *See* **axes of Fick.**

Fick's phenomenon *See* **Sattler's veil.**

field A limited area.

binocular visual f. An approximately circular zone of about 120° in diameter centred on the point of fixation (slightly larger in the lower part of the field) in which an object stimulates both retinas simultaneously. Beyond that area on each side, the visual field is monocular. *See* **field, visual.**

f. of excursion *See* **field of fixation.**

f. of fixation The area in space over which an eye can fixate when the head remains stationary. The field of fixation is smaller than the field of vision. It extends to approximately 47° temporally, 45° nasally, 43° upward and 50° downward. *Syn.* field of excursion; motor field. *See* **field of view, apparent; field of view, real; field, visual.**

f. glasses *See* **binoculars.**

keyhole visual f. A term used to describe a visual field defect in which there is a bilateral homonymous hemianopia with macular sparing. An occipital lobe lesion sparing the posterior tips of the occipital lobe usually causes this lesion.

f. lens *See* **eyepiece.**

motor f. *See* **field of fixation.**

receptive f. A sensory area within which a light stimulus (light, mechanical, chemical or thermal) can produce a potential difference in a single cell. Corneal receptive fields are large and overlapping. This accounts for the inability to localize a stimulus accurately. Retinal ganglion receptive fields are circular, often with a response different in the centre than in the periphery (also referred to as on-centre/off-centre or centre/surround organization). Ganglion cell receptive fields are very small in the macular region and large in the periphery of the retina. Receptive fields also exist in the lateral geniculate bodies where they are similar to those of the retina. In the visual cortex, they have various shapes and sizes and may only respond to either a vertical bar or a black dot moving in a given direction and at a given speed, etc. Receptive fields reflect the interaction between excitation and inhibition between neighbouring neurons. The term can also describe the region of space that induces these neural responses (Fig. F2). *See* **cell, complex; cell, hypercomplex; cell, simple; inhibition, lateral; summation.**

f. stop *See* **diaphragm.**

surrounding f. That area of the field of view surrounding any object.

f. of view The extent of an object plane seen through an optical instrument.

f. of view, apparent Angle subtended by the exit port of a sighting instrument or an empty frame aperture at the centre of the entrance pupil of the eye. *Syn.* apparent peripheral field of view. *Note:*

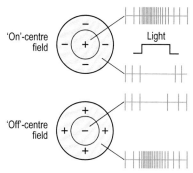

Fig. F2 Typical responses from receptive fields of retinal ganglion cells to a spot of light shone on the area indicated by the bars in each type of receptive field. 'On'-centre cells respond best when stimulated in the central part of the field. 'Off'-centre cells respond best when stimulated in the surround of the field. Note that there are some spontaneous responses even in the absence of illumination.

When referring to the apparent field of fixation, the reference point is the centre of rotation of the eye. *Syn.* apparent macular field of view (Fig. F3). *See* **field of fixation.**

f. of view, real Angle subtended by the effective diameter of a lens at the point conjugate with the centre of the entrance pupil of the eye. *Syn.* real peripheral field of view; true field of view. *Note:* When referring to the real field of fixation, the reference point is the centre of rotation of the eye. *Syn.* real macular field of view (Fig. F3). *See* **phenomenon, jack-in-the-box.**

f. of vision *See* **field, visual.**

visual f. The extent of space in which objects are visible to an eye in a given position. The extent of the visual field tends to diminish with age. The visual field can be measured either monocularly or binocularly. In the horizontal plane meridian, the visual field extends to nearly 190° with both eyes open, the area seen binocularly, that is the region where both eyes can see the stimulus is about 120° and the area seen by one eye only is about 154°. *Syn.* field of vision (Table F1). *See* **field, binocular visual; island of vision; perimetry, kinetic; perimetry, static; test, confrontation.**

visual f. expander An optical system designed to enlarge the field of vision. The most common types are **reverse telescopes** (e.g. looking through the objective of a galilean telescope), which minify objects being viewed but present more information by means of the enlarged visual field. They are usually of low power because of the reduction in visual acuity induced by the minification of the image (**demagnified image**). Another is the **trifield lens** device, which consists of two apex-to-apex prisms (often of different colours) mounted in front of one eye, the apices being fitted to dissect the pupil vertically and a conventional spectacle lens in front of the other eye, However, many patients find

A

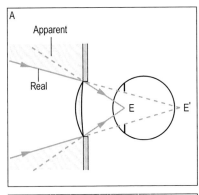

B

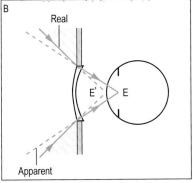

Fig. F3 Apparent and real field of view seen through A, a converging lens and B, a diverging lens, placed in a diaphragm. The apparent field of view is decreased by the converging lens and increased by the diverging lens (E, centre of the entrance pupil; E′, its image formed by the lens). The hatched area is not seen.

Table F1 Average extent of the normal visual field (in degrees) of one eye of a young adult looking in the straight-ahead position, and measured with a white target subtending 1.0° under normal room illumination.	
temporally	94°
down and temporally	88°
down	70°
down and nasally	54°
nasally	60°
up and nasally	56°
up	54°
up and temporally	64°

it difficult to adapt to the visual confusion induced by the prisms as the eyes shift to the side and the patient sees some objects farther away with the eye wearing the prisms than the other eye. These systems are used mainly to improve mobility in patients with glaucoma, retinitis pigmentosa and choroideremia who have constricted visual fields or tunnel vision.

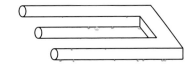

Fig. F4 Blivet figure.

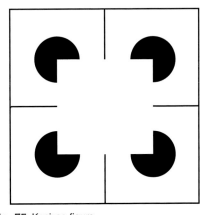

Fig. F5 Kanizsa figure.

fifth cranial nerve *See* nerve, trigeminal.

figure A part or pattern in the visual field which has the perceptual attribute of completeness and is perceived as distinct from the rest of the field which forms the ground. *Example*: a printed word against a background page.
  ambiguous f. An image or drawing arranged in such a way that its perception oscillates or flips involuntarily between, usually, two interpretations even though the retinal image remains constant, thus indicating that higher cortical processing is involved. *Syn.* reversible figure.
  See **figure, Blivet; figure, Kanizsa; illusion; Necker cube; Rubin's vase; Schroeder's staircase.**
  Blivet f. An 'impossible' figure in which three apparently solid tubes are attached at one end of a rectangular base which projects only two bars (Fig. F4).
  See **Necker cube; Schroeder's staircase; Rubin's vase.**
  fortification f. *See* scotoma, scintillating.
  Kanizsa f. An ambiguous figure in which the illusory contour of a square (or triangle) appears in the middle of four (or three) truncated solid squares (or circles). It is an illustration of the perceptual ability to make sense of an incomplete figure by creating a 'whole' image from the separate elements (Gestalt organization). Some people cannot perceive the contour. *Syn.* Kanizsa square (Fig. F5).
  reversible f. *See* figure, ambiguous.

filamentary keratitis *See* keratitis, filamentary.

film, anti-reflection *See* anti-reflection coating.

film, precorneal *See* tear film.

film, tear *See* tear film.

filter Material or device used to absorb or transmit light of all wavelengths equally (**neutral density filter** which is abbreviated **ND filter**) or selectively, such as the **coloured filters** (blue filter transmits only blue light, green filter transmits only green light, etc.). *See* **density, optical; lens, absorptive; test, neutral density filter; wedge, optical.**

bandpass f. A filter that allows the passage of radiations only within a narrow band of wavelengths around a central wavelength. This is done by multilayer coating, which produces destructive interference. *See* **coating; lens, coated.**

cobalt blue f. A filter containing cobalt which only transmits the red and blue ends of the spectrum. It is used in slit-lamps and ophthalmoscopes to produce fluorescence after application of fluorescein to the cornea. *See* **lens, cobalt.**

green f. A filter which transmits only green light. It may be used in ophthalmoscopy to increase the contrast of the blood vessels to the background facilitating the visibility of retinal circulation defects, haemorrhages and microaneurysms and the distinction between retinal and choroidal lesions. However, ophthalmoscopes actually use a filter that transmits a limited amount of red light, as otherwise the observation would be so dark as to make it difficult to see. *Syn.* red-free filter. *See* **ophthalmoscopy, red-free.**

interference f. A coloured filter consisting of five layers, two outside glass, two intermediate evaporated metal films and one central evaporated layer of transparent material. These filters act not by absorption of light but by destructive interference for all except a very narrow band of wavelengths, which are transmitted. *Syn.* coloured filter.

neutral density f. See **filter.**

red f. A filter that transmits only red light. It may be used in ophthalmoscopy to facilitate viewing the yellow macular pigment, but other structures are seen with less contrast. It also produces a larger pupil allowing observation of a larger fundus area. *See* **ophthalmoscopy, red-free.**

red-free f. See **filter, green.**

Wood's f. See **light, Wood's.**

filtration surgery A surgical procedure aimed at lowering the intraocular pressure by producing an outflow of aqueous humour through a drainage passage created in the sclera between the anterior chamber and the subconjunctival space.

See **glaucoma surgery; sclerectomy, deep; trabeculectomy; viscocanalostomy.**

Fincham's theory *See* **theory, Fincham's.**

finger counting *See* **counting fingers.**

fining *See* **smoothing.**

finished lens *See* **lens, finished.**

first-degree fusion *See* **vision, Worth's classification of binocular.**

first-order optics *See* **optics, paraxial.**

Fisher's syndrome *See* **syndrome, Fisher's.**

fisheye lens *See* **lens, fisheye.**

fissure A cleft or a groove found in an organ. In the brain, it usually applies to the deepest cleft. *See* **sulcus.**

calcarine f. Fissure on the medial aspect of the occipital lobe separating the upper and lower halves. Its anterior portion is in front of the parieto-occipital fissure, and the posterior portion extends around the occipital pole and even appears for a short distance on the lateral surface where it ends at the lunate sulcus. *Syn.* calcarine sulcus. *See* **area, visual; line of Gennari.**

embryonic f. See **fissure, optic.**

inferior orbital f. An elongated opening lying between the lateral wall and the floor of the orbit. It is bounded anteriorly by the maxilla and the orbital process of the palate bone and posteriorly by the greater wing of the sphenoid bone. *Syn.* sphenomaxillary fissure. *See* **artery, infraorbital; nerve, zygomatic; Table O4, p. 245.**

interpalpebral f. See **aperture, palpebral.**

optic f. An invagination of the inferior portion of the optic stalk of the embryo. The hyaloid vessels pass through that fissure to supply the developing crystalline lens. In cases in which the invagination (or fissure) fails to fully close, colobomas will be formed. *Syn.* embryonic fissure; choroidal fissure. *See* **artery, hyaloid; cup, optic.**

palpebral f. See **aperture, palpebral.**

sphenoidal f. See **fissure, superior orbital.**

sphenomaxillary f. See **fissure, inferior orbital.**

superior orbital f. An elongated opening lying between the roof and the lateral walls of the orbit, that is, between the two wings of the sphenoid bone. *Syn.* sphenoidal fissure. *See* **nerve, abducens; nerve, oculomotor; nerve, ophthalmic; nerve, trochlear; vein, superior ophthalmic; Table O4, p. 245.**

fistula An unnatural passage from an organ to the body surface or from one organ to another.

carotid-cavernous f. An abnormal interconnection between the internal carotid artery and the cavernous sinus. It may be caused by trauma to the skull or orbit, vascular disease or systemic hypertension. Common signs include pulsating proptosis, eye redness, diplopia, visual loss, dilated epibulbar vessels, anterior segment ischaemia and bruit. The pressure in the orbital veins is elevated as a result of the flow of arterial blood into the cavernous sinus.

lacrimal f. An abnormal opening from the skin onto any part of the lacrimal passage, although most often the lacrimal sac. It may follow a severe acute dacryocystitis.

fit-over *See* **clipover.**

fitted on K Refers to a contact lens in which the back optic zone radius is the same as that of the flattest meridian (or the mean of the two principal meridians) of the cornea. K is a symbol referring to the keratometer reading of the principal meridians of the cornea. *Syn.* alignment fit. *See* **lens, flat; lens, steep.**

fitting Technique and art of selecting and adjusting spectacles or contact lenses following a visual examination.
See dispensing, optical.

fixation The act of directing the eye/s to a given object so that its image is formed on the foveola.
anomalous f. See fixation, eccentric.
f. axis See axis, fixation.
bifoveal f. See bifixation.
binocular f. Fixation on an object with both eyes simultaneously.
f. disparity See disparity, retinal; fusional movements.
f. disparity unit, Mallett See Mallett fixation disparity unit.
eccentric f. Monocular condition in which the image of the point of fixation is not formed on the foveola. In this condition, the patients feel that they are looking straight at the object stimulating the non-foveolar retinal area and the visual acuity of that eye is reduced. The condition occurs most commonly in strabismic amblyopia but can also occur when the fovea has been destroyed by some pathological process. *Syn.* anomalous fixation. *See* Haidinger's brushes; occlusion treatment; penalization; pleoptics; spot, Maxwell's; test, after-image transfer; viewing, eccentric; Visuscope.
foveal f. Normal fixation in which the image of an object falls on the foveola.
line of f. See axis, fixation.
f. movements See movement, fixation.
parafoveal f. Fixation by a retinal area located outside the fovea but within the macula (or fovea centralis), i.e. within 5 degrees of the central visual field. It may occur in amblyopia.
f. pause See reading.
plane of f. See plane of regard.
point of f. Point in space upon which the eye is directed, either monocularly or binocularly. If there is no eccentric fixation, the image of that point is formed on the foveola. *Syn.* object of regard. *See* point of regard.
f. reflex See reflex, fixation.
f. response Eye movement aimed at placing the image of a point of fixation on the foveola.
voluntary f. Conscious fixation of an object as distinguished from the fixation reflex.

flame haemorrhage *See* haemorrhage, preretinal.

flap *See* Gundersen' s conjunctival flap; LASEK; LASIK.

flare, aqueous *See* aqueous flare.

flare, lens *See* lens flare.

flash An intense light of short duration.

flash blindness *See* keratoconjunctivitis, actinic.

flashes Perception of sudden and transient bright spots of light in the absence of light stimuli. Flashes may occur as a result of rhegmatogenous retinal detachment, posterior vitreous detachment, proliferative diabetic retinopathy, papilloedema, retinal break or migraine.
See photopsia.

flat lens *See* lens, flat.

flavimaculatus fundus *See* fundus, flavimaculatus.

Fleischer's ring *See* ring, Fleischer's.

flexure, lens *See* lens flexure.

flicker Perception produced when the retina is stimulated by an intermittent light stimulus which fluctuates between a frequency of a few hertz and the critical fusion frequency.

flicker photometer *See* photometer, flicker.

flight of colours The temporal sequence of after-images of different colours that follow a brief exposure to a bright source of light. It is most easily seen in dark-adapted eyes. The duration of the sequence is much shorter or absent in some patients with retrobulbar optic neuritis or multiple sclerosis.

flint glass *See* glass, flint.

flippers *See* lens flippers.

floaters Heterogeneities in the vitreous humour which may be of embryonic origin or pathological (e.g. in posterior vitreous detachment, retinal detachment, vitritis, asteroid hyalosis). The patient sees spots which float as the eye moves. Floaters are common in normal old eyes. *Syn.* vitreous floaters. *See* iritis; muscae volitantes; myiodesopsia; photopsia; retina, lattice degeneration of the; retinitis, cytomegalovirus; uveitis; vitritis.

floccules of Busacca *See* Koeppe's nodules.

floppy eyelid syndrome *See* syndrome, floppy eyelid.

fluconazole *See* antifungal agent.

flucytosine *See* antifungal agent.

fluid, lacrimal *See* tear film; tears.

fluorescein A fluorescent weak dibasic acid with a molecular weight of 376 whose sodium salt is used in dilute solution as a dye in the fitting of contact lenses, in the detection of corneal abrasions (as it stains epithelial defects), etc. It absorbs blue light and produces a yellowish-red compound, which fluoresces a brilliant yellow-green under ultraviolet or blue illumination. This only occurs when the thickness of the fluorescein dye reaches 15 μm. Tear pooling, eroded areas or discrepancies between the radii of curvature of the cornea and a rigid contact lens appear yellowish-green, whereas if the tear film is very thin, the area appears dark blue or black (Fig. F6). *Syn.* sodium fluorescein. *See* filter, cobalt blue; fluorexon; lamp, Burton; light, Wood's; rose bengal; staining; test, break-up time; test, fluorescein.

fluorescein angiography *See* angiography, fluorescein.

fluorescence Property of a substance that, when illuminated, absorbs light of a given wavelength and re-emits it as radiations of a longer wavelength. *Example*: fluorescein in which the peak excitation is at about 490 nm and the emission at about 530 nm when illuminated with cobalt blue light.

See angiography, fundus fluorescein; law, Draper's; light, Wood's; luminescence.

fluorescent lamp *See* lamp, fluorescent.

fluorexon A staining agent similar to fluorescein but with a much higher molecular weight (710) and which is less readily absorbed by soft contact lens material. It is used in the fitting of soft or hybrid lenses (e.g. a piggyback lens). It stains a pale yellow-brown. However, it is not recommended for use with high water contact lenses (above 65%).

fluorometholone *See* antiinflammatory drug.

fluoroquinolone *See* antibiotic.

flurbiprofen sodium *See* antiinflammatory drug.

flush bridge *See* bridge, flush.

flush, choroidal *See* choroidal flush.

flutter, ocular An involuntary, rapid, horizontal saccadic oscillation of both eyes while attempting to fixate an object. It is a sign of cerebellar disease. *See* myoclonus, ocular; opsoclonus.

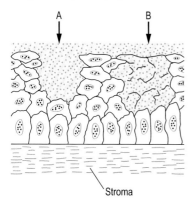

Fig. F6 Fluorescein on the corneal surface staining A, an abraded area and B, some damaged epithelial cells.

flux, luminous *See* luminous flux.

flux, radiant *See* radiant flux.

FM 100 Hue test *See* test, Farnsworth-Munsell 100 Hue.

f number Designation for a photographic lens which gives the ratio of the focal length to the diameter of the effective aperture or entrance pupil. *Example*: f/8 means that the lens has a focal length eight times the diameter of the entrance pupil. *Syn.* f/stop; f-value; focal ratio; lens speed (Table F2). *See* aperture, relative.

focal interval *See* Sturm, interval of.

focal length *See* length, focal.

focal length, equivalent *See* length, equivalent focal.

focal length, vertex *See* vertex focal length.

focal line; plane *See* under the nouns.

focal point *See* focus, principal.

focal power *See* paraxial equation, fundamental; power, refractive.

focal ratio *See* f number.

foci, conjugate *See* distance, conjugate.

focimeter An optical instrument for determining the vertex power, axis direction and optical centre of an ophthalmic lens (Fig. F7). The instrument can be either manual or automated. *Syn.* Lensometer (a tradename); vertexometer; Vertometer (a tradename). *See* lens measure; neutralization; power, back vertex.

focus 1. The point at which rays of light converge after passing through a convex lens to form a real image (**real focus**) or diverge from (**virtual focus**) after passing through a concave lens. **2.** The centre or starting point of a disease process. **3.** To adjust an optical system (e.g. camera or projector) to obtain a sharp image. *Plural*: foci. *Syn.* focusing.

Table F2 Sequence of f numbers used in photography with the corresponding relative image brightness and exposure time to maintain constant film exposure. The relative image brightness is equal to the square of the f number fraction.

f number	Focal length/pupil exact f number	Diameter	Relative image brightness	Relative exposure time
f/0.5	0.5	f/0.500	1/0.25	0.12
f/0.7	0.7	f/0.707	1/0.5	0.25
f/1	1	f/1.000	1/1	0.5
f/1.4	1.4	f/1.414	1/2	1
f/2	2	f/2.000	1/4	2
f/2.8	2.8	f/2.828	1/8	4
f/4	4	f/4.000	1/16	8
f/5.6	5.6	f/5.657	1/32	16
f/8	8	f/8.000	1/64	32
f/11	11	f/11.314	1/128	64
f/16	16	f/16.000	1/256	128
f/22	22	f/22.627	1/512	256
f/32	32	f/32.000	1/1024	512

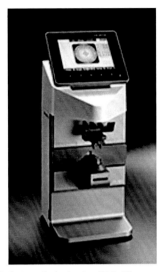

Fig. F7 Automatic focimeter. (Shin Nippon, courtesy of Grafton Optical Co. Ltd.)

See **confocal; focus, principal; line, focal.**
aplanatic foci A pair of conjugate object and image points for which an optical system is free of spherical aberration. *Syn.* aplanatic points.
dark f. *See* **accommodation, resting state of.**
depth of f. *See* **depth of focus.**
principal f. The axial image point produced by an optical system of an infinitely distant object. It is called the **second principal focus** or **posterior principal focus**, or that axial object point for which the image will be formed at infinity (the **first principal focus** or **anterior principal focus**). A converging optical system or lens has two principal foci that are real. A diverging optical system or lens has a second principal focus that is virtual. In curved mirrors, the two principal foci coincide. Depending upon whether the object is at infinity or at the principal focus, this same focal point becomes either the second principal focus or the first principal focus, respectively. *Syn.* focal point. *See* **length, focal; power, equivalent; sign convention.**
real f. *See* **focus.**
sagittal f.; tangential f. *See* **astigmatism, oblique.**
virtual f. *See* **focus.**
focusing *See* **focus.**
fogging method *See* **method, fogging.**
fold, conjunctival *See* **conjunctiva.**
fold, corneal *See* **oedema.**
fold, semilunar *See* **plica semilunaris.**
folds, choroidal *See* **choroidal folds.**
follicle 1. A small gland. 2. A small cavity or deep narrow depression with excretory or secretory function. 3. A small nodule of lymphocytes and other cells occurring as a result of chronic inflammation.

See **papilla.**
conjunctival f. Small localized aggregation of lymphocytes, plasma and other cells appearing as white or grey elevations on the palpebral conjunctiva (tarsal area) as a result of chronic irritation (allergic, viral or mechanical such as contact lenses).
See **conjunctivitis, adult inclusion; conjunctivitis, follicular.**
palpebral f's. *See* **gland, meibomian.**
follicular conjunctivitis *See* **conjunctivitis, follicular.**
footcandle Non-metric unit of illuminance. It is equal to a flux of 1 lumen per ft^2. *Symbol*: fc. 1 fc = 10.764 lux.
footlambert Non-metric unit of luminance. It is equal to the average luminance of a surface emitting or reflecting 1 lumen per ft^2. *Symbol*: fL. 1 fL = 3.426 cd/m^2.
foramen A small aperture usually through a bone or a membranous structure, through which nerves and blood vessels pass.
See **canal, infraorbital; canal, optic; supraorbital notch.**
foramen, ethmoidal; zygomatic *See* Table O4, p. 245
forced duction test *See* **test, forced duction.**
former A pattern, usually made of plastic, used to guide the automatic machines which cut and edge lenses. *Syn.* lens pattern.
See **edging.**
fornix *See* **conjunctiva.**
Forster–Fuchs spot *See* **spot, Fuchs'.**
fortification spectrum *See* **scotoma, scintillating.**
fossa A depression or cavity below the surface level of a part.
hyaloid f. *See* **fossa, patellar.**
f. for the lacrimal gland A depression in the frontal bone in which rests the orbital portion of the lacrimal gland, as well as some orbital fat which itself lies in the posterior part of the fossa called the **accessory fossa of Rochon–Duvigneaud**. The fossa is located behind the zygomatic process of the frontal bone in the anterior and lateral part of the orbital roof.
f. for the lacrimal sac A vertical groove, some 5 mm deep and about 14 mm high, formed by the frontal process of the maxilla and lacrimal bones and which contains the lacrimal sac. The fossa is bounded by the anterior and posterior **lacrimal crests** coming from the maxilla (frontal process) and lacrimal bone respectively with no definite boundary above. It leads downward to the **nasolacrimal canal**, which contains the nasolacrimal duct.
See **lacrimal apparatus.**
patellar f. A cup-shaped depression in the anterior vitreous body that accommodates the posterior part of the crystalline lens. It is actually separated from the lens itself by the postlenticular space of Berger. *Syn.* hyaloid fossa; lenticular fossa.
See **ligament of Wieger.**

trochlear f. A small depression in the frontal bone which contains the pulley (or **trochlea**), a cartilaginous structure surrounded by a thick fibrous sheath 1 mm thick and through which passes the superior oblique muscle. The fossa is located about 4 mm behind the medial upper margin of the orbit. *See* **muscle, superior oblique.**

Foster Kennedy syndrome *See* **syndrome, Foster Kennedy.**

Foucault grating *See* **grating.**

four prism dioptre base out test *See* **test, four prism base out.**

Fourier analysis The mathematical breakdown of waveforms into simple sine wave constituents. Any complex waveform consists of sine waves of different frequencies: the slowest (fundamental) frequency and harmonics thereof (these are frequencies which are odd multiples of the fundamental frequency). It is used in analysis and reconstruction of waveforms as, for example, analysing the spatial frequency components of a visual image. *Syn.* Fourier transform. *See* **sensitivity, contrast.**

fourth cranial nerve *See* **nerve, trochlear.**

fourth nerve paralysis *See* **palsy, fourth nerve.**

fovea *See* **foveola.**

fovea centralis A small area of the retina of approximately 1.5 mm in diameter situated within the macula lutea. At the fovea centralis, the retina is the thinnest as there are no supporting fibres of Mueller, no ganglion cells and no bipolar cells. These cells are shifted to the edge of the depression. The fovea centralis contains mainly cone cells, each one being connected to only one ganglion cell and thus contributing to the highest visual acuity of the retina. The visual field represented by the fovea centralis is equal to about 5° (Fig. F8). *Syn.* foveal pit; macula (term often used by clinicians). *See* **acuity, central visual; foveola; image, retinal; macula lutea.**

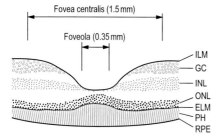

Fig. F8 Cross-section of the retina showing the fovea centralis and foveola (rod-free area). Note that the ganglion cells GC and the cells of the inner nuclear layer INL (bipolar, amacrine and horizontal cells) are shifted to the edge of the depression (ILM, internal limiting membrane; ONL, outer nuclear layer (nuclei of rods and cones); PH, photoreceptors; ELM, external limiting membrane; RPE, retinal pigment epithelium).

foveal avascular zone *See* **foveola.**

foveal fixation *See* **fixation, foveal.**

foveal pit *See* **fovea centralis.**

foveola The base of the fovea centralis with a diameter of about 0.35 mm (or about 1° of the visual field). The image of the point of fixation is formed on the foveola in the normal eye. The foveola contains only cone cells (**rod-free area**). The **foveal avascular zone** is slightly larger (about 0.5 mm in diameter) (Fig. F9). *Syn.* fovea (term often used by clinicians). *See* **eccentricity; fixation; umbo.**

foveation period In congenital nystagmus, it is the amount of time when the image of an object of regard is on or near the fovea and moving so slowly as to enable the patient to acquire useful visual information. The longer the foveation period and the lower the retinal image velocity, the higher the visual acuity.

Foville's syndrome *See* **syndrome, Foville's.**

fracture, orbital *See* **orbital fracture.**

fragile X syndrome *See* **syndrome, fragile X.**

frame A structure in metal, plastic, tortoiseshell, wood, leather, etc. for enclosing or supporting ophthalmic lenses but usually considered without the lenses. *See* **spectacles.**

frame, eyeglass 1. Synonym for spectacles. 2. Synonym for rimless spectacles.

frame heater A device used to warm plastic spectacle frames to soften its material sufficiently to allow insertion of lenses and/or adjustment. Some frame heaters warm air, which is directed to the area of the frame that is to be altered. Others heat salt or glass beads to a given temperature and the part of the frame that is to be altered is placed into the heated material. *Syn.* frame warmer. *See* **spectacle frame, plastic.**

frame markings, spectacle *See* **spectacle frame markings.**

framycetin sulfate *See* **antibiotic.**

Fraunhofer's lines *See* **line, Fraunhofer's.**

free space *See* **space, free.**

frequency, critical fusion Frequency of a flickering light stimulus at which it becomes perceived as a stable and continuous sensation. That frequency depends upon various factors: luminance, colour, contrast, retinal eccentricity, etc. Low-intensity light projected onto the peripheral retina and consequently stimulating mostly rods appear to fuse at approximately 10 Hz. In the central retina, it is about 50 to 60 Hz at high luminance. *Syn.* critical flicker frequency. *See* **effect, Brücke–Bartley; flicker; law, Ferry–Porter; law, Granit–Harper; law, Talbot–Plateau; photometer, flicker.**

frequency, cut-off *See* **function, contrast sensitivity.**

frequency, doubling perimetry *See* **perimetry, frequency doubling.**

frequency of light *See* **hertz; spectrum, electromagnetic; wavelength.**

frequency, Nyquist The maximum spatial frequency of a visual target relative to that of the spacing of the photoreceptors to be able to view it faithfully without distortion or misinterpretation (veridical) resolution). It is equal to a frequency of the photoreceptors spacing twice that of the frequency of the target.
See **aliasing; undersampling.**

frequency, spatial The rate of alternation of the luminance in a visual stimulus (e.g. a grating), usually expressed in cycles per degree.
See **cycle per degree; Fourier analysis; function, contrast sensitivity.**

Fresnel's bi-prism Optical device consisting of two prisms of very small refracting power, set base to base and which forms two images of a single source. It is often used to produce interference fringes. It may also be used to measure cyclophoria. *Syn.* double prism; Fresnel's double prism; Maddox bi-prism; Maddox double prism.
See **interference fringes; prism, Wollaston; test, double prism.**

Fresnel's lens; Press-On prism *See* under the nouns.

Fresnel's formula Formula used to determine the amount of light reflected at the interface between two transparent media. The reflection is

$$\rho = \left(\frac{n_2 - n_1}{n_2 + n_1}\right)^2$$

where n_1 is the index of refraction of the first medium and n_2 that of the second medium. For a lens surface in air, the percentage of light reflected is given by (Table F3)

$$\rho = \left(\frac{n_2 - 1}{n_2 + 1}\right)^2 \times 100\%$$

Table F3 Percentage of light reflected in normal incidence ρ at the surface of several transparent substances of varying refractive indices, in air

Refractive index	ρ (%)
1.333	2.04
1.4	2.78
1.45	3.35
1.5	4.0
1.523	4.3
1.55	4.65
1.60	5.32
1.65	6.02
1.7	6.72
1.75	7.44
1.8	8.16

Example: The reflection from the two surfaces of a glass lens made of crown ($n = 1.523$) is equal to 8.6%.
See **image, ghost; reflectance; reflection, surface.**

Friedreich's ataxia *See* **ataxia, hereditary spinal.**

FRIEND test *See* **test, FRIEND.**

fringes, diffraction A pattern of alternate dark and light bands produced by diffracted light passing the edge of an opening.
See **diffraction.**

fringes, interference *See* **interference fringes.**

Frisby stereotest *See* **stereotest, Frisby.**

front The part of a spectacle frame without the sides.

front silvered mirror *See* **mirror, front surface.**

front vertex focal length *See* **vertex focal length.**

front vertex power *See* **power, front vertex.**

frontal plane *See* **plane, frontal.**

frontalis sling procedure *See* **procedure, frontalis sling.**

frontoparallel plane *See* **plane, frontoparallel.**

frosted lens *See* **lens, frosted.**

Fuchs' adenoma A benign proliferation of small whitish nodules on the pars plicata of the ciliary body which may appear in elderly patients.

Fuchs' coloboma *See* **crescent, congenital.**

Fuchs, crypts of Pit-like depressions or openings found near the collarette and near the periphery of the iris. They allow the passage of aqueous humour from the anterior chamber into the stroma of the iris as the volume of the iris changes with dilatation and contraction.

Fuchs' endothelial dystrophy *See* **dystrophy, Fuchs' endothelial.**

Fuchs' heterochromic iridocyclitis *See* **iridocyclitis, Fuchs' heterochromic.**

Fuchs' spot *See* **spot, Fuchs'.**

Fuchs' spur A few fibres located about midway along the length of the sphincter muscle which join with a few fibres of the dilator muscle of the iris.

Fuchs' syndrome *See* **syndrome, Fuchs'.**

function 1. The particular action of an organ or tissue. 2. Any two variables in which the value of one depends upon the value of the other.
contrast sensitivity f. (CSF) The graphical representation of contrast sensitivity for the detection of a sine wave grating from a uniform field as a function of its spatial frequency. It is done by reducing the contrast of a grating until it can no longer be resolved (this point represents the **contrast threshold**) and repeating the procedure for a number of different spatial frequencies. The contrast sensitivity (1/contrast threshold) is plotted against spatial frequency (Fig. F9). The CSF is greatest at a spatial frequency around 3 cycles/degree, and the point where the curve intercepts the spatial frequency axis (called the **cut-off frequency**) represents the standard visual acuity of the subject at 100% contrast.

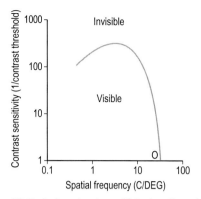

Fig. F9 Typical contrast sensitivity function of an adult human eye (O, cut-off frequency) (both scales are logarithmic).

See **chart, contrast sensitivity; resolution, spurious; sensitivity, contrast.**

line-spread f. A mathematical description of the distribution of light across the image of a very thin bright line object. On the retina, the image of a thin bright slit spreads over a distance subtending about 6 minutes of arc at which point the intensity is less than 2 log units below the maximum.

modulation transfer f. A relationship between the spatial frequency of an image (e.g. in number of cycles per degree or lines per inch) and the modulation amplitude (i.e. the difference between the luminance at the peaks and troughs of a grating). This gives an indication of the ability of a lens to resolve a grating. The greater the quality of a lens, the higher the spatial frequency at which the modulation amplitude falls to zero. At this point the lens can no longer transfer spatial modulation of intensity from the object to the image, and the image appears as a uniform intensity distribution. This technique has been applied to assess the quality of the retinal image by measuring the contrast sensitivity function.

point-spread f. The mathematical description of the light distribution across the image of a point source. The shape and width of the function depends upon the amount of diffraction, aberrations and scatter and, in the eye, the shape of the pupil. The shape of the function, which resembles a normal distribution, is conventionally defined by its 'half-width', being the width of the curve at half the peak luminance. If only diffraction is considered the point-spread function is known as Airy's disc.

See **Fig. D5, p. 90.**

functional Pertaining to a disorder with no detectable lesion to account for the symptoms.
See **amblyopia; organic.**

functional visual loss Reduced vision experienced by an individual but which is not based on objective measurements that could explain the symptom.

See **amblyopia, hysterical; malingering.**

fundoscopy The act of examining the fundus of the eye, as with an ophthalmoscope or with a biomicroscope and slit-lamp.

fundus The bottom or back surface of an organ. The term is used here to refer to the posterior portion of the interior of the eye visible with an instrument (e.g. ophthalmoscope). *Plural:* fundi.

f. albipunctatus A recessively inherited, non-progressive tapetoretinal degeneration caused by mutation in the RDH5 gene and, in few cases, mutation of the RDS gene as a dominant form. It is characterized by a multitude of small, grey or whitish dots scattered throughout the fundus at the level of the pigment epithelium and accompanied by night blindness. The macula is spared, and the retinal blood vessels, optic disc, visual field, colour vision and visual acuity are normal.

f. camera See **camera, fundus.**

f. examination See **biomicroscope; slit-lamp; ophthalmoscope, direct; ophthalmoscope, indirect.**

f. flavimaculatus A retinal degeneration characterized by prominent irregular-shaped whitish or yellow flecks scattered throughout the posterior fundi of both eyes. There is usually little loss of vision unless one of the flecks involves the fovea. It is a variant of Stargardt's disease. The electrooculogram is useful in diagnosing this condition.

leopard f. An ocular fundus marked with dark blotches on its surface as a result of a tapetoretinal degeneration, such as retinitis pigmentosa. *Syn.* leopard retina.

ocular f. The interior of the eye (as may be seen with the aid of an ophthalmoscope) consisting of the retina, the retinal blood vessels and even sometimes the choroidal vessels when there is little pigment in the pigment epithelium (e.g. albinos), the foveal depression and the optic disc. The fundus appears red, owing mainly to the choroidal blood supply. The arteries appear light red and straight while the veins are dark red and tortuous. The size ratio of vein to artery is about 3:2. The colour is lighter in fair people than in darker races and is dependent upon the amount of pigment in the pigment epithelium and in the choroid. In dark races, the fundus is almost dark grey (Fig. F10).

See **biomicroscopy, fundus; camera, fundus; plaques, Hollenhorst's; tapetum lucidum.**

f. reflex See **reflex, fundus.**

salt and pepper f. The appearance of the ocular fundus characterized by a stippling of dark pigmented spots and yellowish-red spots of atrophy, as is found in congenital syphilis, choroideremia, Leber's congenital amaurosis, rubeola, poliomyelitis, etc.

tessellated f. A normal ocular fundus in which the choroidal pattern appears as roughly polygonal dark areas in between choroidal vessels because the retinal pigment epithelium layer is thin and the choroid heavily pigmented. It is usually a sign of

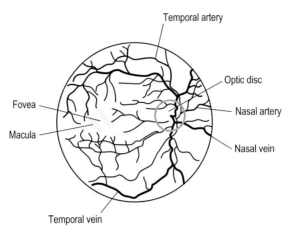

Fig. F10 Diagram of the fundus of the right eye.

pathological myopia. *Syn.* tessellated retina; tigroid fundus; tigroid retina.

tigroid f. *See* fundus, tessellated.

fungal keratitis *See* keratitis, fungal.

furrow, marginal A degenerative process occurring in the peripheral cornea characterized by corneal thinning. It is frequently associated with rheumatoid arthritis in which case there are epithelial defects and progressive ulceration. Furrows may also occur in corneal arcus without epithelial defect or vascularization. *Syn.* limbal furrow.

furrow, palpebral *See* sulcus, inferior palpebral; sulcus, superior palpebral.

fused bifocal *See* lens, bifocal.

fusidic acid A product used as an antibiotic agent in solution 1%. It is synthesized as sodium fusidate from the microorganism *Fusidium coccineum*. It is effective against gram-positive bacteria. It is used in the treatment of bacterial blepharoconjunctivitis, especially staphylococcal infection.

fusion The act or process of mixing or uniting.
   f. area *See* area, Panum's.
   binocular f.; central f. *See* fusion, sensory.
   chiastopic f. Fusion obtained by voluntary convergence on two targets separated in space and such that the right eye fixates the left target and the left eye the right target. This is often facilitated by fixating a small mark above a single aperture placed in front of the two targets and then slowly shifting one's gaze to the targets. The procedure is aimed at improving positive fusional convergence.
   See convergence, fusional; fusion, orthopic.
   critical f. frequency *See* frequency, critical fusion.
   first-degree f.; flat f. *See* vision, Worth's classification of binocular.
   f. field An area around the fovea of each eye within which the fusion reflex is initiated. If the disparate images fall within this area, motor fusion will occur, but if the disparity is too great, there will be no fusional movement. This field is much larger horizontally than vertically.
   flat f. Binocular fusion in which the single percept is two-dimensional and without stereoscopic effect. *Syn.* second-degree fusion.
   See vision, Worth's classification of binocular.
   f. lock *See* lock, binocular; prism, aligning.
   motor f. One of the components of convergence in which the eyes move until the object of regard falls on corresponding retinal areas (e.g. the foveas) in response to disparate retinal stimuli. *Syn.* disparity vergence; fusion reflex.
   See convergence, fusional; fusion, sensory; retinal corresponding points; vergence facility.
   orthopic f. Fusion obtained by voluntary divergence on two targets separated in space and such that the right eye fixates the right target and the left eye the left target. This is often facilitated by looking beyond the targets and then slowly shifting one's gaze to the targets through double apertures placed in front of them. This procedure is aimed at improving negative fusional convergence.
   See convergence, fusional; fusion, chiastopic.
   peripheral f. *See* fusion, sensory.
   f. reflex *See* fusion, motor.
   second-degree f. *See* fusion, flat.
   sensory f. The neural process by which the images in each retina are synthesized or integrated into a single percept. In normal binocular vision, this process occurs when corresponding (or nearly corresponding) regions of the retina are stimulated. This process can occur when the images are either in the central part of the retinae (**central fusion**) or in the peripheral part of the retinae (**peripheral fusion**). *Syn.* binocular fusion.
   See anaglyph; area, Panum's; convergence, fusional; haploscope; response, SILO; retinal corresponding points; stereogram, random-dot; test, bar reading; test, diplopia; test, Worth's four dot.
   third-degree f. *See* vision, Worth's classification of binocular.

fusional convergence *See* convergence, fusional; convergence, relative.

fusional divergence *See* divergence, fusional.

fusional movements Reflex movements of the eyes occurring in response to retinal disparity (even though it may be below the threshold for diplopia to be seen) in order to produce a single image. If the fusional movements are such that, although diplopia is eliminated there is still some disparity, this is called **fixation disparity**.
See disparity, retinal; fusion, motor.

fusional reserve, convergence; vergence *See* convergence, relative; vergence facility.

f-value *See* f number.

G

GABA *See* neurotransmitter.

galactosaemia A rare, autosomal recessive inherited disorder of galactose metabolism caused by the absence of the enzyme galactose-1-phosphate uridyl transferase. The excess galactose is converted by the enzyme aldose reductase to the sugar alcohol galactotol. Systemic signs include lethargy, vomiting and diarrhoea. Cataract in the form of a central 'oil droplet' develops in many cases. Galactose (milk products) should be excluded from the diet to prevent further cataract progression and systemic signs. There can also be cases who suffer from a **galactokinase deficiency** of the enzyme which converts galactose. Systemic signs are absent, but cataract may develop either in infancy or in some older individuals.

galilean telescope *See* telescope, galilean.

galvanic nystagmus *See* nystagmus.

ganciclovir *See* antiviral agents.

ganglion An aggregation of nerve cell bodies found in numerous locations in the peripheral nervous system. *Plural*: ganglia.
  g. cell See cell, ganglion.
  ciliary g. A small reddish-grey body about the size of a pinhead situated at the posterior part of the orbit about 1 cm from the optic foramen between the optic nerve and the lateral rectus muscle. It receives three roots posteriorly: (1) the long nasociliary or sensory root (or ramus communicans), which contains sensory fibres from the cornea, iris and ciliary body and some sympathetic postganglionic axons going to the dilator muscle; (2) the short (or motor or oculomotor) root, which comes from the Edinger–Westphal nucleus through the third nerve (oculomotor) and carries fibres supplying the sphincter pupillae and ciliary muscles; and (3) the sympathetic root, which comes from the cavernous and the internal carotid plexuses and carries fibres mediating constriction of the blood vessels of the eye and possibly mediating dilatation of the pupil. The ciliary ganglion gives rise to 6 to 10 short ciliary nerves. *Syn.* lenticular ganglion; ophthalmic ganglion.
See reflex, pupil light.
  gasserian g. Sensory ganglion of the fifth nerve located in a bony fossa on the front of the apex of the petrous temporal bone. It receives the sensory portion of the fifth nerve (trigeminal) in the posterior part of the ganglion. From its anterior part, the three divisions of the fifth nerve are given off the ophthalmic (which contains the sensory fibres from the cornea and the eye in general), the maxillary and the mandibular nerves. *Syn.* semilunar ganglion; trigeminal ganglion.
See herpes zoster ophthalmicus.
  lenticular g.; ophthalmic g. See ganglion, ciliary.
  semilunar g. See ganglion, gasserian.
  superior cervical g. One of the uppermost and largest ganglion in the two chains of sympathetic ganglia lying alongside the vertebral column. It is located just below the base of the skull between the internal carotid artery and the internal jugular vein. It gives rise to the internal carotid nerve, which forms the internal carotid plexus.
  trigeminal g. See ganglion, gasserian.

gangliosidosis *See* disease, Sandhoff's; disease, Tay–Sachs.

ganzfeld A visual stimulus that consists of completely homogeneous and colourless luminance conditions throughout. It is used especially when recording the standard electroretinogram.

gap junction *See* synapse.

Gardner Reversal-Frequency Test *See* test, developmental and perceptual screening.

Gardner's syndrome *See* syndrome, Gardner's.

gargoylism *See* syndrome, Hurler's.

gasserian ganglion *See* ganglion, gasserian.

Gaucher's disease *See* disease, Gaucher's.

gaussian approximation *See* ray, paraxial.

gaussian optics *See* optics, paraxial.

gaussian points *See* point, cardinal.

gaussian space *See* paraxial region.

gaussian theory *See* theory, gaussian.

gaze To fixate steadily or continuously. *See* position, cardinal p's of gaze.

gaze palsy *See* palsy, gaze.

Gelb effect *See* effect, Gelb.

gene The unit of heredity which determines, or contributes to, one inherited feature of an organism (e.g. eye colour). Physically, a gene is composed of a defined DNA sequence, located at a specific place (**locus**) along the length of a chromosome and transmitted by a parent to its offspring. The DNA sequence of nucleotide bases (adenine, cytosine, guanine and thymine) encodes a specific sequence of amino acids corresponding to a particular protein. If the DNA sequence at one locus is identical on a pair of homologous chromosomes, the organism is referred to as **homozygous (homozygote)**, and if the DNA sequence is not identical, it is referred to as **heterozygous (heterozygote)**. Some genes have several **variants**, each expressing a different phenotype. The total effect of all genes influences the development and functioning of all organs and systems in the body. **Mutations** in some genes may cause diseases. *See* chromosome; genome; inheritance; mutation; pedigree.

gene-environment interaction A term used to indicate that an effect is due to a mixture of environmental factors (nurture) and genetic factors (nature). Most traits show gene-environment interactions, such as myopia, IQ test results, skin colour, etc. Blood type and iris colour are predominantly genetically transmitted, whereas language is predominantly environmental. *See* theory, biological-statistical; theory, nativist.

gene therapy A therapeutic method in which a defective gene is replaced by a normal copy of itself, thus restoring its function. There are several ways in which a new gene is carried into a diseased cell. A common method uses a virus such as a retrovirus, an adenovirus, herpes simplex or an adeno-associated virus as vectors to introduce genes into cells and DNA. This therapy has been used in the treatment of several eye diseases, especially retinoblastoma and retinitis pigmentosa, but so far with limited success.

geniculate body, lateral (LGB) One of two ovoid protuberances lateral to the pulvinar of the thalamus in the diencephalon of the forebrain and into which the fibres of the optic tract synapse on their way to the visual cortex. However, because of the semidecussation of the optic nerve fibres in the optic chiasma, the lateral geniculate body in the right thalamus receives the fibres originating on the temporal retina of the right eye and the nasal fibres of the left. Each body appears, in cross-section, to consist of alternating white and grey areas. The white areas are formed by the medullated nerve fibres of the optic tract, while the grey areas consist largely of the nerve cells in which the fibres of the optic tract terminate (synapses) and from which arises the fibres of the optic radiations. There are six grey areas or layers of cells, with layer 1 being the most ventral and layer 6 the most dorsal (or posterior). Layers 1, 4 and 6 receive the crossed or nasal fibres from the contralateral retina, while layers 2, 3 and 5 receive the uncrossed or temporal fibres from the ipsilateral retina. The neural components of the LGB without the blood vessels and covering layer form the **lateral geniculate nucleus (LGN)**. There are three main types of cells in the LGN. In layers 1 and 2 (those most ventral), the cells are substantially larger than in the other four layers and are called **magno cells (M)** and the layers are called **magnocellular layers**. The main input to these cells are the retinal rods and the magno ganglion cells. In the other four layers (those most dorsal), the cells are smaller and are called **parvo cells (P)** and the layers are called **parvocellular layers**. The main input to these cells are the retinal cones and the parvo ganglion cells. In between each of the main layers is an area with very small and sparsely distributed cells, the **koniocellular cells (K)** and these areas are called koniocellular layers. They receive their input from ganglion cells and process colour. The cells of the parvocellular layers seem to be mainly responsible for transmitting information about visual acuity, form vision, colour perception and low contrast targets. The cells in the magnocellular layers seem to be mainly responsible for transmitting information about motion and flicker perception, stereopsis and high-contrast targets. The M, P and K cells project to different cells in the primary visual cortex (V1), where they retain the same segregation as in the lateral geniculate bodies. The receptive fields of the cells in the LGN are circular with either an 'on' or 'off' centre with the opposite behaviour in the surround, but they are more sensitive to contrast than the retinal ganglion cells. The LGN also receives many other afferents, such as descending afferents from the primary visual cortex, from the brainstem region and from the thalamic reticular nucleus, which may indicate a broader role than a simple relay station (Fig. G1). *See* brachium; cell, M; cell, P; fibre, visual; pathway, visual.

general refraction formula *See* paraxial equation, fundamental.

geniculocalcarine tract *See* radiations, optic.

geniculostriate pathway *See* pathway, geniculostriate.

Gennari, line of *See* line of Gennari.

genome The complete set of genes in an individual. In humans, it is estimated at approximately 30 000

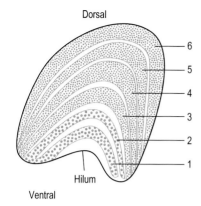

Fig. G1 Section through the lateral geniculate nucleus. The light areas between the main layers are the koniocellular layers.

genes and more than 3 billion base pairs (two nucleotides joined together across a double helix) of DNA.

genotype The complete genetic constitution of an individual at a particular location (locus) in the genome. At many locations (loci) throughout the genome, the chromosomal DNA sequence differs subtly between individuals. Each of the various DNA sequences at one locus is called an **allele**; for instance, if there are three sequence variants present, then there are three alleles. Offspring inherit one homologous chromosome from each parent. Thus, a genotype comprises two alleles: the allele inherited from the father (carried on the paternal chromosome) and the allele inherited from the mother (carried on the maternal chromosome). *See* gene; phenotype.

gentamicin *See* antibiotic.

geometrical axis; optics *See* under the nouns.

gerontopia *See* sight, second.

gerontoxon *See* corneal arcus.

Gerstmann syndrome *See* syndrome, Gerstmann.

ghost image *See* image, ghost.

giant cell arteritis *See* arteritis, giant cell.

giant papillary conjunctivitis *See* conjunctivitis, giant papillary.

giantophthalmos Megalocornea associated with an enlargement of the anterior segment of the eye. *See* keratoglobus.

Giles–Archer lantern *See* test, lantern.

glabella 1. A prominent area of the frontal bone situated above the root of the nose. **2.** The skin between the eyebrows, which is usually hairless. *Syn.* intercilium.

gland An aggregation of cells which secretes or excretes a substance. There are two main groups of glands: (1) The **endocrine** glands which have no duct and whose secretion (a hormone) is absorbed directly into the blood. *Examples*: adrenal gland, pineal gland, pituitary gland, thyroid gland. (2) The **exocrine** glands whose secretion reaches the surface by means of ducts. There are three main types of secretion by exocrine glands: the **serous glands** which secrete a watery substance rich in proteins (e.g. lacrimal gland, sweat glands); the **mucous glands** which secrete mucus, a viscous product (e.g. goblet cells); and the **sebaceous glands** which secrete a lipid substance (e.g. meibomian glands).

accessory lacrimal g's. They are the glands of Krause and Wolfring. These glands are histologically identical to the main lacrimal gland but are located within the eyelids. These glands are responsible for basal (not reflex) tear secretion and appear to be under sympathetic neural control. *See* **tear secretion.**

adrenal g. One of a pair of endocrine glands situated above the kidneys. Each consists of two parts: an inner portion, the **medulla**, which secretes adrenaline and noradrenaline, and an outer portion, the **cortex**, which secretes corticosteroids and sex hormones.

g's. of Ciaccio *See* gland, of Wolfring.

ciliary sebaceous g's. *See* gland, of Zeis.

ciliary sweat g's. *See* gland, of Moll.

conjunctival g. Any gland that secretes a substance into the conjunctiva, such as the lacrimal, meibomian, Krause and Wolfring glands or a goblet cell.

g's. of Henle These are not really glands. They are folds in the mucous membrane of the palpebral conjunctiva, situated between the tarsal plates and the fornices, in which there are goblet cells (Fig. G2). *Syn.* crypts of Henle (strictly speaking, this term refers only to the pit-like depressions).

g's. of Krause Accessory lacrimal glands of the conjunctiva having the same structure as the main lacrimal gland. They are located in the subconjunctival connective tissue of the fornix, especially the superior fornix (Fig. G2).

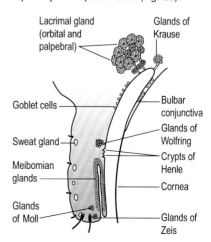

Fig. G2 Section diagram of the upper eyelid showing the various glands.

lacrimal g. A compound gland situated above and to the outer side of the globe of the eye. It consists of two portions: (1) a large orbital or superior portion and (2) a small palpebral or inferior portion. It secretes the middle aqueous layer of the tears through about a dozen fine ducts into the conjunctival sac at the upper fornix although one or two may also open into the outer part of the lower fornix (Fig. G2).
See **carcinoma, lacrimal gland; dacryoadenitis; dacryops; fossa for the lacrimal gland; gland, pleomorphic adenoma of the lacrimal; lactoferrin; nerve, zygomatic; tear duct.**

g's. of Manz Tiny glands located near the limbus. They secrete mucin. The existence of these glands in man is not established.

meibomian g's. Sebaceous glands located in the tarsal plates of the eyelids whose ducts empty into the eyelid margin. They are arranged parallel with each other, perpendicular to the lid margin, about 25 for the upper lid and 20 for the lower. They secrete **sebum**. This sebaceous material provides the outermost oily (or lipid) layer of the precorneal tear film. It prevents the lacrimal fluid from overflowing onto the outer surface of the eyelid. It also makes for an airtight closure of the lids and prevents the tears from macerating the skin. The meibomian glands can be seen showing through the conjunctiva of fair-skinned people as yellow streaks (Fig. G2). **Meibomian gland dysfunction** (MGD) may be induced by blepharitis, chalazion, contact lens wear (particularly soft lenses) and ageing. The most common sign is a cloudy or absent secretion upon expression with symptoms of a mild dry eye. Hot compresses and lid massage will cure more than half of the patients; oral tetracycline will help in many of the others. *Syn.* palpebral follicles; tarsal glands.
See **blepharitis, posterior; chalazion; film, precorneal; hordeolum, internal; keratoconjunctivitis sicca; meibography; meibomianitis; tarsus; Tearscope plus.**

g's. of Moll Sweat glands of the eyelids. They are situated in the region of the eyelashes (Fig. G2). *Syn.* ciliary sweat glands.
See **cyst of Moll.**

pineal g. *See* **pinealoma.**

pleomorphic adenoma of the lacrimal g. A rare tumour of the lacrimal gland. It is derived from proliferation of epithelial cells that form ductal structures with surrounding myoepithelial cells. It is the most common tumour of the gland. It presents in middle age with a visible mass in the suprotemporal corner above the eye, progressing painless proptosis, ophthalmoplegia and choroidal folds. Treatment is by excision of the tumour because of the possibility of malignant transformation. *Syn.* benign mixed tumour.
See **carcinoma, lacrimal gland.**

pituitary g. A pea-sized gland lying at the base of the skull in a depression of the sphenoid bone. It secretes several important hormones including the thyroid-stimulating hormone (TSH), which stimulates the thyroid gland, and the adrenocorticotrophic hormone (ACTH), which stimulates the adrenal glands. A large tumour of the pituitary (pituitary adenoma) compresses the optic chiasma which lies above it and causes a visual field defect, typically bitemporal hemianopia or quadrantanopia.
See **adenoma, pituitary; adrenaline; disease, Graves'; scotoma, centrocecal; syndrome, de Morsier.**

tarsal g's. *See* **gland, meibomian.**

g's. of Wolfring Accessory lacrimal glands of the upper eyelid situated in the region of the upper border of the tarsus (Fig. G2). *Syn.* glands of Ciaccio.

g's. of Zeis Sebaceous glands of the eyelids which are attached directly to the follicles of the eyelashes. Their secretion contributes to the oily layer of the precorneal film (Fig. G2). *Syn.* ciliary sebaceous glands.
See **blepharitis, anterior or marginal; cyst of Zeis; hordeolum.**

glare A visual condition in which the observer feels either discomfort and/or exhibits a lower performance in visual tests (e.g. visual acuity or contrast sensitivity). This is produced by a relatively bright source of light (called the **glare source**) within the visual field. A given bright light may or may not produce glare depending upon the location and intensity of the light source, the background luminance, the state of adaptation of the eye or the clarity of the media of the eye.

direct g. Glare produced by a source of light situated in the same or nearly the same direction as the object of fixation.

disability g. Glare which reduces visual performance without necessarily causing discomfort. Most patients will present little change in visual acuity. However, corneal scars, post-refractive surgery, posterior capsular opacification and cataract may induce a significant decrease in acuity (several lines) and patients may have to be referred. A simple test, called **simple penlight glare test,** consists of using a penlight directed into the patient's eye at an angle of 30° from the fixation axis and remeasuring visual acuity.

discomfort g. Glare which produces discomfort without necessarily interfering with visual performance.

eccentric g. *See* **glare, indirect.**

indirect g. Glare produced by an intense light source situated in a direction other than that of the object of fixation. *Syn.* eccentric glare.

g. source *See* **glare.**

g. tester An instrument for measuring the effect of glare on visual performance. There exist several (e.g. Brightness Acuity Tester (BAT), Miller–Nadler Glare Tester, Optec 1500 Glare Tester). Glare testing is valuable in patients with corneal and lenticular opacities before and after surgery and in elderly patients in whom adaptation to glare is usually more difficult. The **Miller–Nadler Glare Tester** consists of a glare source surrounding a Landolt C. The instrument contains 19 black

Landolt C, all of the same size, 6/120 (or 20/400). Each Landolt C is presented in one of four orientations and from the highest to the lowest contrast at which the subject can no longer judge in which direction the letter appears. The contrast threshold is expressed in percentage disability glare. The **Brightness Acuity Tester (BAT)** is a standardized glare source of light. It is presented in a hemisphere held over one eye. The light source can subtend a visual angle of 8 to 70 degrees at a vertex distance of 12 mm. The patient is asked to read a visual acuity chart through a small aperture in the hemisphere. The chart can be a low-contrast or high-contrast logMAR visual acuity chart or, for example, the Pelli–Robson contrast sensitivity chart.

veiling g. Glare caused by scattered light and producing a loss of contrast.
See **scatter**.

Glasgow acuity cards A visual acuity test composed of a set of cards contained in a flip card format. There are four letters on each card subtending the same visual angle, and of equal legibility. The progression of letter sizes from one card to the next is linear using a logarithmic scale, and the four letters are surrounded by a rectangle providing horizontal and vertical contour interaction. The test is performed at 3 m and is designed for children from 3 years of age and is particularly adapted for the management of amblyopia. *Syn.* logMAR crowded test.
See **test, Cardiff Acuity; test, Lea-Hyvarinen acuity**.

glass 1. Material from which lenses and optical elements may be made. It is hard, brittle and lustrous and usually transparent. It is produced by fusing sand (silica) at about 1400°C with various oxides (potassium, sodium, etc.) and other ingredients such as lead oxide, lime, etc. Glass may be produced in various colours by the addition of different substances (e.g. metal oxides). **2.** A lens.
See **annealing; feathers; lens blank; strain; stria; surfacing**.

absorption g. Glass which transmits only a certain portion of the incident light, the rest being absorbed.

Bagolini's g. A plano lens on which fine parallel striations have been grooved. It produces a slight reduction in acuity, but a punctate light source observed through this lens appears as a streak of light orientated at 90° from the striations. Two such lenses placed in front of the eyes with the striations oriented 90° apart are used to detect sensory and motor anomalies such as retinal abnormal correspondence, suppression, etc. *Syn.* Bagolini's lens; Bagolini's striated glass.
See **test, Bagolini lens**.

cobalt-blue g. See **lens, cobalt**.

crown g. Glass characterized by low dispersion. It has a refractive index of $n = 1.523$ and a constringence or V-value of 59. There are other types of crown glass (e.g. dense barium crown $n = 1.623$, V-value 56; fluor crown $n = 1.485$, V-value

70). When used in ophthalmic lenses, it is called **ophthalmic crown** or **spectacle crown**.
See **doublet; triplet**.

g. cutter A tool with a diamond-tipped edge or hard steel to cut glass.

depolished g. See **glass, ground**.

g. eye See **eye, glass**.

flint g. Glass containing lead or titanium besides the usual ingredients and having a high dispersion (*example*: Total, V-value 31) compared with crown glass and a high refractive index ($n = 1.701$). It is, however, a softer and heavier material than crown. It is used in ophthalmic lenses of high power as it can be made much thinner than a crown glass lens of the same power.
See **doublet; lens, high index; triplet**.

ground g. Glass that has been ground with emery, sandblasted or etched with fluoric acid to give it a matt surface. Such glass is usually translucent but not transparent. *Syn.* depolished glass.
See **lens, frosted**.

magnifying g. See **lens, magnifying**.

opal g. A white or milky translucent glass used to diffuse light.

photochromic g. See **lens, photochromic**.

safety g. **1.** Glass that has been ground and polished and then heated just below its softening point and rapidly cooled. Such treatment renders the glass highly resistant to fracture, and breakage causes it to crumble rather than shatter. Safety glass can also be produced chemically. In this process, the lens is immersed in a molten salt bath (e.g. 99.5% potassium nitrate and 0.5% silicic acid at a temperature of 470°C for some 16 hours). The lens surface thus becomes compressed as larger potassium ions replace the smaller sodium ions which are in the glass. Chemically strengthened lenses have greater impact resistance and can be made thinner than air-tempered glass lenses. However, when broken, the fragments of the chemically strengthened lenses are not as blunt as those of air-tempered glass lenses. *Syn.* toughened glass. **2.** Non-shatterable laminated glass used in automobiles and goggles.
See **lens, safety; polariscope; spectacles, industrial**.

toughened g. See **glass, safety**.

Wood's g. See **light, Wood's**.

glasses *See* **spectacles**.

glasses, field *See* **binoculars**.

glaucoma A progressive neuropathy which leads to retinal ganglion cell death, axon loss and optic neuropathy characterized by optic disc cupping and visual field defects. Risk factors include elevated intraocular pressure (the most important), vascular disease (e.g. progressive ischaemia), connective tissue disorder, positive family history and increased age. It is commonly divided into **open-angle** and **angle-closure** types. If the cause of the glaucoma is a recognized ocular disease or injury (e.g. corneal laceration), it is called **secondary**, whereas if the cause is unknown, it is called **primary**. Glaucoma is present in about 1% of the

Caucasian population over the age of 40 years and about 3% over the age of 70 years, but these figures vary among different populations, tending to be lower in white populations and higher in non-white populations (Table G1).

See cup-disc ratio; cup, glaucomatous; field, visual expander; lamina cribrosa; neuro-protection; syndrome, Marfan's; syndrome, Sturge–Weber; tritanopia.

absolute g. Final stage of the disease which has been either untreated or unsuccessfully treated. The eye is blind and hard, the optic disc is white and the pupil dilated.

acute angle-closure g. (AACG) A form of raised intraocular pressure in which the pressure within the eye increases rapidly due to blockage of the trabecular meshwork obstructing aqueous outflow. Symptoms include intense pain, redness, blurred vision, haloes around lights, as well as nausea. Findings on examination include reduced visual acuity, greatly elevated intraocular pressure (in the range of 40–50 mmHg), corneal epithelial oedema, semidilated and fixed pupil, shallow anterior chamber and mild aqueous cell and flare. Elevated intraocular pressure often causes glaucomatous optic nerve damage, as well as iris atrophy and damage to the anterior epithelial cells of the lens (**glaukomflecken**). Immediate treatment is imperative and includes systemic acetazolamide as well as topical medication. Surgery is often necessary. *Syn.* acute glaucoma; congestive glaucoma.

angle-closure g. (ACG) Glaucoma in which the angle of the anterior chamber is blocked by the root of the iris which is in apposition to the trabecular meshwork and thus the aqueous humour cannot reach the drainage apparatus to leave the eye. This condition occurs usually in anatomically shallow anterior chambers, as is often the case in hyperopes. **Angle-closure** glaucoma can either be **primary angle-closure glaucoma** (PACG) or **secondary** following seclusion pupillae, iridocyclitis, postoperative complications (anterior chamber intraocular lens implant), traumatic cataract, tumours, etc. Moreover, angle-closure glaucoma is divided into **acute** and **chronic**. In **chronic angle-closure glaucoma** (CACG) there may never be an attack but intermittent periods of increased intraocular pressure caused by progressively extensive peripheral anterior synechia. Symptoms may be absent or there may be periodic episodes of mild congestion and blurred vision. Gonioscopy is essential to differentiate this condition from open-angle glaucoma. People most at risk are females, Chinese and South-East Asians, and the average age at presentation is about 60 years. Anatomical predisposing factors are pupillary block and plateau iris. Treatment of angle-closure glaucoma is essentially surgical. However, therapeutic agents may still be needed including miotics hyperosmotic agents, which cause a rapid reduction of the intraocular pressure, beta-blockers and carbonic anhydrase inhibitors. *Syn.* closed-angle glaucoma; narrow-angle glaucoma. A **subacute** form of angle-closure glaucoma may occur as a result of episodes of elevated intraocular pressure caused by anterior synechia, intermittent pupillary block or when in a dark room. Attacks tend to resolve spontaneously, but treatment with prophylactic peripheral laser iridotomy is frequently undertaken.

See anisocoria; cornea plana; iridoschisis; iris bombé; iris, plateau; method, van Herick; Shaffer and Schwartz; method, Smith's; test, provocative; test, shadow.

capsular g. *See* glaucoma, pseudoexfoliation.

chronic g. *See* glaucoma, angle-closure; glaucoma, open-angle.

ciliary block g. *See* glaucoma, malignant.

closed-angle g. *See* glaucoma, angle-closure.

compensated g. *See* glaucoma, open-angle.

congenital g. Glaucoma occurring with developmental anomalies that are manifest at birth and interfere with the drainage of the aqueous humour causing an increase in intraocular pressure. It can also result from a tumour, such as retinoblastoma or persistent fetal vasculature. This in turn causes stretching of the elastic coats of the eye, enlargement of the globe as the sclera and cornea stretch, optic atrophy, marked cupping of the optic disc and loss of vision. Most noticeable is the enlargement of both corneas (buphthalmos). The corneas are oedematous; there are Haab's striae and vascularization as the condition progresses. Immediate treatment is essential, which is typically surgical. *Syn.* hydrophthalmos; infantile glaucoma. Glaucoma occurring after the age of about 3 years is more often referred to as **juvenile glaucoma** as it follows a course similar to adult glaucoma without enlargement of the globe.

See buphthalmos; goniotomy; luxation of the lens; Peter's anomaly; striae, Haab's; syndrome, Rieger's; syndrome, Sturge–Weber; trabeculotomy.

congestive g. *See* glaucoma, angle-closure.

g. detection Tests that are used to diagnose glaucoma. They are ophthalmoscopic viewing of the optic nerve head; tonometry; visual field assessment of typical glaucomatous defects; gonioscopy to assess the width of the anterior chamber; pachometry to measure central corneal thickness and anterior chamber depth as well as providing a correction factor for applanation tonometer results and dimensional analysis of retinal structures including the thickness and topography of the retinal nerve fibre layer (RNFL) and of the optic nerve head. Assessment can be made with **scanning laser polarimetry, confocal scanning laser ophthalmoscopy, optical coherence tomography,** stereoscopic photography of the optic nerve head and red-free photography of the RNFL. Glaucomatous eyes lose retinal nerve fibres with consequent reduction in layer thickness and alteration of the topography of the optic nerve head. These changes frequently precede glaucomatous visual fields losses.

infantile g.; juvenile g. *See* glaucoma, congenital.

Table G1 Glaucoma medications

Class	Drug (common eye drop solution)
Topical Agents	
beta-blockers	betaxolol (0.25% or 0.5%), carteolol (1%), timolol (0.25% or 0.5%, gel 0.1%), levobunolol (0.5%), metipranolol (0.1%)
carbonic anhydrase inhibitors	brinzolamide (1%), dorzolamide (2%)
miotics	carbachol (3%), pilocarpine (0.5,1,2,3,4%)
prostaglandin analogues	latanoprost (0.005%), travoprost (0.004%)
prostamide	bimatoprost (0.03%)
sympathomimetics	apraclonidine (0.5%), brimonidine (0.2%), dipivefrine (0.1%)
combination drugs	timolol (0.5%) with brimonidine (0.2%) timolol (0.5%) with dorzolamide (2%) timolol (0.5%) with latanoprost (0.005%)
Systemic Agents	
carbonic anhydrase inhibitor	acetazolamide (tablet 250 mg)
hyperosmotic agents	glycerol (oral solution) mannitol (intravenous)

inflammatory g. A secondary glaucoma caused by an intraocular inflammation and characterized by elevated intraocular pressure, which may be transient. The most common cause is either active anterior uveitis or following previous episodes of inflammation. Glaucoma may occur as a result of trabecular meshwork blockage due to deposits of inflammatory debris or because of complete posterior synechia (a pupillary block also called **seclusion pupillae**) blocking the flow of aqueous causing iris bombe and angle-closure, or peripheral anterior synechia. The inflammatory process is treated along with a reduction of intraocular pressure.
See **iridocyclitis, Fuchs' heterochromic; syndrome, Posner–Schlossman**.

low tension g. See **glaucoma, normal-tension**.
narrow-angle g. See **glaucoma, angle-closure**.
malignant g. A secondary glaucoma, which occurs when aqueous fluid becomes misdirected into the vitreous cavity. The accumulating fluid then produces a displacement of the lens and iris, causing a narrowing of the anterior chamber angle with resultant raised intraocular pressure. This condition occurs most commonly following intraocular surgery, especially glaucoma surgery, after the cessation of cycloplegic medications or iris melanoma. Treatment consists of medical intervention (cycloplegics, β-adrenergic agents, carbonic anhydrase inhibitors and hyperosmotic agents) or puncture of the vitreous face with the Nd-YAG laser if medical treatment is unsuccessful. In phakic eyes, vitrectomy is sometimes required to open the anterior vitreous face. Syn. ciliary block glaucoma.

neovascular g. A secondary glaucoma due to new vessel formation on the anterior surface of the iris (rubeosis iridis) blocking the exit of the aqueous humour through the angle of filtration. It may occur as a result of central retinal vein occlusion (this type typically develops within 3 months and is sometimes called '**ninety-day glaucoma**') or diabetes. Other causes include central retinal artery occlusion, retinal and choroidal tumours. The condition may initially be open-angle but eventually becomes angle-closure due to anterior synechiae with severe loss of visual acuity, pain, congestion, high intraocular pressure, corneal oedema, aqueous flare, and severe rubeosis iridis. Treatment includes topical steroids to decrease the inflammation, apraclonidine to lower the intraocular pressure and laser treatment of the iris neovascularization and sometimes cyclodestructive procedures (e.g. cyclodiode laser therapy).
See **ectropion uvea; neovascularization, iris**.
ninety-day g. See **glaucoma, neovascular**.
normal-tension g. An ocular condition in which there is a glaucomatous cupping (often accompanied by disc haemorrhages) and visual field defects with an intraocular pressure of 21 mmHg or less. It is commonly regarded as a variant of primary open-angle glaucoma, and it is typically associated with cardiovascular disease or migraine. Treatment with prostaglandin analogues is usually considered the best choice but if there are progressive visual field losses, surgery may be needed. Syn. low-tension glaucoma.
open-angle g. Glaucoma in which the angle of the anterior chamber is open and provides the aqueous humour free access to the drainage apparatus. It can occur in two forms: (1) As a **primary open-angle glaucoma** (POAG) (also called **chronic simple glaucoma, compensated glaucoma, chronic glaucoma**). The increased intraocular pressure (above 21 mmHg) leads to atrophy and excavation of the optic disc and typical defects of the visual field. It is the most common type of glaucoma (opinions of prevalence vary between 0.5% and 3% of the Caucasian population over 40 years and 2%–3% over the age of 70 years). Because of its insidious nature, it is difficult to detect. It tends to occur more

often in people after the age of 40, in people who have a family history of the disease, in African-Caribbeans, in people who have high myopia and in people who have diabetes mellitus. It is characterized by an almost complete absence of symptoms. Haloes around lights and blurring of vision occur in some patients when there has been a sudden increase in intraocular pressure or when the disease is very advanced. The diagnosis of this disease is made by demonstrating that the eye has a characteristic visual field loss (Figs. G3 and G4) and exaggerated diurnal fluctuations in intraocular pressure (0.5 mmHg). POAG has been found to be caused by mutation in genes at several loci, including myocilin gene (MYOC) on chromosome 1q, optineurin gene (OPTN) on chromosome 10p, WD repeat containing protein 36 gene (WDR36) on chromosome 5q22, and others. (2) The other form is **secondary open-angle glaucoma** in which the intraocular pressure is elevated as a result of ocular trauma or iridocyclitis, crystalline lens abnormalities, etc. Management of open-angle glaucoma is usually by medication, unless this proves ineffective and surgery may be necessary. Formerly, pilocarpine (or carbachol) or adrenaline (epinephrine) drops were the most commonly used drugs. Nowadays, β-adrenergic blocking agents such as timolol maleate or betaxolol, which act by reducing aqueous humour formation and do not affect pupil size or accommodation, are employed as the initial treatment. Also used are the carbonic anhydrase inhibitors (e.g. acetazolamide) the α-adrenergic agonist (e.g. brimonidine) and the prostaglandin derivatives (e.g. latanoprost), which enhance the uveoscleral outflow.
See atrophy, optic; cup, glaucomatous; hypertension, ocular; iris, plateau; pseudoexfoliation; spot, baring of the blind; test, provocative; test, shadow; vision, tunnel.

phacolytic g. An open-angle glaucoma secondary to a hypermature or mature cataract. It is due to a leakage of lens proteins into the anterior chamber that blocks the outflow of aqueous humour through the trabecular meshwork. It is characterized by pain, reduced vision because of the cataract and redness with high intraocular pressure.
See trabecular meshwork.

phacomorphic g. A form of secondary angle-closure glaucoma in which the angle of the anterior chamber is closed due to a swollen cataractous lens with pupillary block and iris bombe. The eye presents with a shallow anterior chamber, cataract and elevated IOP.

pigmentary g. A secondary open-angle glaucoma caused by pigment granules released from the posterior surface of the iris and deposited around the anterior segment and impeding the aqueous outflow through the trabecular meshwork. This type of glaucoma develops in about one-third of

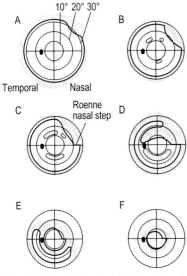

Fig. G3 Typical evolution of field defects in primary open-angle glaucoma of the left eye (A and B, early field defects; C, more field defects with Roenne nasal step; D, Bjerrum scotoma; E and F, advanced field defects).

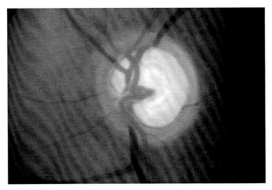

Fig. G4 Advanced glaucomatous cupping in a POAG case. The entire neuroretinal rim has become thinner. Note the large cup-disc ratio. (From Kanski 2007, with permission of Butterworth-Heinemann)

patients with the pigment dispersion syndrome, especially myopic males. The pigments are believed to appear as a result of a posterior bowing of the iris rubbing against the zonule. The intraocular pressure is elevated and sometimes high after a sudden release of pigment following mydriasis or strenuous physical exercise with corneal oedema, redness and haloes. Treatment is usually by medication but if this proves ineffective, surgery may be required. *primary g.* See glaucoma, angle-closure; glaucoma, open-angle.

pseudoexfoliation g. A secondary glaucoma caused by greyish-white, fibrillary amyloid-like material impeding the aqueous outflow through the trabecular meshwork. It usually appears in elderly patients who present with high intraocular pressure, optic disc changes and visual field defects. It is frequently resistant to drug therapy and may require surgery (e.g. laser trabeculoplasty). *Syn.* capsular glaucoma.
See pseudoexfoliation; syndrome, pseudoexfoliation.

secondary g. Glaucoma occurring as a result of intraocular tumour, iritis, iridocyclitis, uveitis, rubeosis iridis, traumatic cataract, tumours, luxation of the lens, etc.
See epithelial downgrowth; hyphaemia; syndrome, Rieger's; syndrome, ICE; syndrome, pseudoexfoliation.

simple g. See glaucoma, open-angle.

g. surgery See artificial drainage tube; cyclodialysis; cyclodiode; filtration surgery; goniotomy; iridectomy; iridotomy; sclerectomy; sclerectomy, deep; trabeculectomy; trabeculoplasty; trabeculotomy; viscocanalostomy.

glaucomatocyclitic crisis See syndrome, Posner–Schlossman.

glaukomfleken See glaucoma, acute angle-closure.

glazing Strictly, the fitting of lenses to a frame or mount, but often to include the cutting and edging processes (British Standard).

glial cell of the retina See cell, glial; cell, Mueller's.

glial veil See papilla, Bergmeister's.

glioma, optic nerve A slow-growing tumour of astrocytes (a type of glial cells) that typically affects children and is associated in about half the cases with neurofibromatosis, type 1. It usually presents with progressive reduction of visual acuity, proptosis, optic nerve head atrophy and may spread to the optic chiasma. Surgical excision may be needed if the tumour has spread beyond the orbit.

glioma, retinal See retinoblastoma.

globe of the eye See eyeball.

gloss Shiny appearance of a surface.
See matt surface.

glossmeter Instrument for measuring the ratio of the amount of light specularly reflected from a surface to that diffusely reflected.
See reflection, diffuse; reflection, regular.

glutamate See cone pedicle; neurotransmitter; rod spherule.

glycerin (glycerol) See hyperosmotic agent.

glycocalyx See mucin.

glycoprotein One of a group of conjugated proteins formed by a protein and a carbohydrate, the most important being the mucins (as found in the lens capsule, vitreous humour) and mucoids (as found in bones, cartilage, tendons).

glycosaminoglycan A complex macromolecule considered to be the 'glue' of the cornea. It is responsible for providing the plasticity and structural support needed for successful corneal function. Along with other molecules, it comprises the solid portion of the cornea (about 22%, the remainder being water). The distribution and arrangement of glycosaminoglycans are responsible for corneal transparency and thickness.

goblet cell See cell, goblet.

goggles Type of large spectacles, with shields and perhaps padding, used as eye protectors from flying particles, dust, wind, chemical fumes or other external hazards.
See glass, safety; shield, eye; spectacles, industrial.

gold deposits See chrysiasis.

Goldenhar's syndrome See syndrome, Goldenhar's.

Goldman-Favre disease See disease, Goldman-Favre.

Goldmann lens See gonioscope.

Goldmann perimeter See perimeter, Goldmann.

Goldmann tonometer See tonometer, applanation.

Goldmann–Weekers adaptometer See adaptometer.

goniolens See lens, gonioscopic.

gonioprism, Allen–Thorpe A prism in which the base is curved so that it can rest on the cornea in gonioscopic examination.

gonioscope Instrument used to observe the angle of the anterior chamber of the eye, usually consisting of a biomicroscope in conjunction with a prismatic contact lens (e.g. Allen–Thorpe gonioprism) or a contact lens and mirror (e.g. Goldmann lens). It facilitates the diagnosis of angle-closure and open-angle glaucoma, as well as the diagnosis of secondary glaucoma (Fig. G5).
See lens, gonioscopic; lens, Koeppe.

gonioscopy Observation of the angle of the anterior chamber of the eye with a gonioscope. When the angle is wide open, all structures are visible (cornea, Schwalbe's line, trabecular meshwork, scleral spur, ciliary body); when the angle is closed, only the cornea is seen. The width of the angle can be described according to either the **van Herick technique**, as to its width or the **Shaffer classification**, which categorizes the angle estimated in degrees, as well as the location of the iris insertion (Table G2).
See method, van Herick, Shaffer and Schwartz.
compression g. See gonioscopy, indentation.

direct g. Observation of the virtual erect image of the angle of the anterior chamber as formed by a gonioscopic lens (e.g. Koeppe lens). The image can be viewed with a hand-held magnification system with the patient in a supine position.

indentation g. Gonioscopy performed when the angle of the anterior chamber is closed to determine whether the closure is appositional or synechial. It is usually done with the four-mirror Zeiss lens by pressing the lens against the cornea forcing the aqueous into the peripheral part of the angle and pushing the iris posteriorly; if the angle is closed by apposition between the iris and cornea (appositional closure), the angle will open. If the angle is closed by adhesion between the iris and cornea (synechial closure), it will remain closed. *Syn.* compression gonioscopy.

indirect g. Observation of the real inverted image of the angle of the anterior chamber as formed by a gonioscopic lens, such as the Goldmann or Zeiss lens. The image is viewed through a biomicroscope. This is the most commonly used gonioscopic method.

goniosynechia Anterior synechia occurring at the angle of the anterior chamber. It is associated with angle-closure glaucoma.

goniotomy A surgical procedure aimed at lowering intraocular pressure by making an incision through the trabecular meshwork to ease the outflow of aqueous humour into Schlemm's canal. This procedure is used principally in congenital glaucoma. *See* glaucoma, congenital.

gonococcal infection *See* conjunctivitis, acute; ophthalmia neonatorum.

Gradenigo's syndrome *See* syndrome, Gradenigo's.

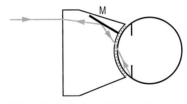

Fig. G5 Optical principle of the Goldmann gonioscopic lens (M, mirror).

grades of binocular vision *See* vision, Worth's classification of binocular.

gradient method; test *See* AC/A ratio.

gradient-index lens *See* lens, gradient-index.

grading scale A method used to present an assessment and recording of the severity of a condition. Grading scales are usually organized in five stages of increasing severity, from grade 0 (normal) to grade 4 (severe). There are several commonly used scales. For example, the **van Herick's** technique and **Shaffer** classification are used for the width of the angle of the anterior chamber and the structure visualized. The **Efron** grading scales for contact lens complications rate a set of 16 anterior ocular complications such as conjunctival redness, corneal neovascularization, corneal oedema, epithelial microcysts, corneal infiltrates, papillary conjunctivitis, etc. The **Lens Opacity Classification System (LOCS)**, which is a method designed to quantify the degree of lens opacification, is performed by viewing the lens through a slit-lamp and comparing the image with a set of photographs. There are separate sets for nuclear, cortical and posterior subcapsular cataracts. Other grading scales are used to evaluate inflammatory cells and flare in the anterior chamber, retinal arteriovenous crossings, cup-disc ratio, etc. *See* method, van Herick Shaffer and Schwartz.

von Graefe's test *See* test, diplopia.

graft, corneal Corneal tissue of a donor used to replace a diseased or opaque cornea. *See* keratoplasty.

Gram stain A procedure for detecting and identifying bacteria and certain other microbes. Microorganisms, such as those found in corneal or conjunctival samples, are stained with crystal violet, rinsed in water, treated with iodine solution, decolorized with ethyl alcohol or acetone and counterstained with a contrasting dye, usually safranin, a pink dye. The preparation is then rinsed with water, dried and examined. Microorganisms that retain the crystal violet stain are said to be **Gram-positive**, while those that retain the counterstain are said to be **Gram-negative**. The stain reveals basic differences in the biochemical and structural properties of living cells. *See* bacteria.

Table G2   Structures of the angle of the anterior chamber as seen by gonioscopy in an individual in whom the angle is open and none of the structures are obscured by the iris

Structure (anterior to posterior)	Anatomy/physiology	Normal appearance
Schwalbe's line	posterior termination of Descemet's membrane	not always discernible off-white ridge; pigment may collect on it
trabecular meshwork	site of aqueous flow; covers internal part of Schlemm's canal	variable degree of pigmentation
scleral spur	strip of scleral tissue	thin white line
ciliary body band	anterior face of ciliary body in the angle recess	pigmented seen more easily if iris is moved backward

Gram-negative A microorganism that takes on the colour of the red counterstain in the Gram stain procedure due to the fact that the cell wall has a thin layer of the protein peptidoglycan. Common Gram-negative bacteria include *Acinetobacter, Chlamydia trachomatis, Enterobacter, Escherichia coli, Haemophilus influenzae, Moraxella lacunata, Neisseria gonorrhoeae, Proteus vulgaris* and *Pseudomonas aeruginosa.*

Gram-positive A microorganism that retains the crystal violet stain in the Gram stain procedure due to the fact that the cell wall has a thick layer of the protein peptidoglycan. Common Gram-positive bacteria include *Actinomyces israelii, Mycobacterium chelonae, Mycobacterium fortuitum, Staphylococcus aureus, Staphylococcus epidermidis, Streptococcus pneumoniae* and *Streptococcus pyogenes.*

gramicidin *See* antibiotic.

Granit–Harper law *See* law, Granit-Harper.

granular dystrophy *See* dystrophy, granular.

granuloma Growth appearing like a nodule, consisting essentially of granulation tissue and occurring as a result of localized inflammation. It can appear on the conjunctiva, the iris, the lacrimal gland or the orbit. *Plural:* granulomata.
See nodule, Busacca's; uveitis, acute anterior.

granulomatosis, Wegener's *See* Wegener's granulomatosis.

Grassman's laws *See* laws, Grassmann's.

graticule Graduated transparent scale engraved or photographed, placed in the front focal plane of the eyepiece of an optical instrument for direct observation of the apparent image size or position in the field of view. *Example*: the focusing screen of a focimeter. *Syn.* reticule.

grating A series of black and white parallel bars of equal width used to measure visual acuity, contrast sensitivity and resolution of optical systems. The grating can be either square-wave (also called **Foucault grating** or **Foucault pattern**), in which the luminance across a bar is constant, or sine-wave, in which the luminance varies sinusoidally. A grating is evaluated by contrast (difference between the luminance of the black bars and that of the white bars), frequency (e.g. number of cycles per degree) and orientation (angle made by the grating relative to a reference plane) (Fig. G6). *See* cycle per degree; frequency, spatial; function, contrast sensitivity.

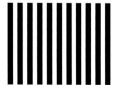

Fig. G6 Square-wave grating.

grating, diffraction *See* diffraction.

Gratiolet, optic radiations of *See* radiations, optic.

Graves' disease *See* disease, Graves'.

green The hue sensation evoked by stimulating the retina with rays of wavelength 490 to 560 nm and situated between blue and yellow. The complementary colour of green is a **non-spectral colour** situated in the red-purple region.

green blindness *See* deuteranopia.

gregorian telescope *See* telescope.

grey A colour said to be achromatic or without hue. It varies in magnitude from white to black. *Note:* also spelt gray.

grid, Amsler *See* chart, Amsler.

grid, Hering–Hermann *See* Hering–Hermann grid.

grid, Javal's A test for simultaneous binocular vision and for detecting central ocular suppression. It consists of five equally spaced opaque parallel bars crossed by two perpendicular bars. It is held between the reader's eyes and a page of print. The bars being perpendicular to the lines of the text occlude some letters (along vertical strips) to one eye, but these letters are seen by the other eye. If binocular vision is present no difficulty is experienced in reading the page. This instrument represents the most common type of **bar reader**. It can be used as an exercise when there is central suppression in heterophoria.
See test, bar reading.

grinding The process of preparing the surface of a lens or of an optical device (a prism, a mirror) by a series of operations which involve roughing, smoothing and polishing.
See blocking; roughing; smoothing; surfacing.

Groenouw's nodular type 1 corneal dystrophy *See* dystrophy, granular.

Grotthus' law *See* law, Draper's.

ground *See* figure.

Gullstrand's reduced eye *See* eye, reduced.

Gullstrand's schematic eye *See* eye, schematic.

Gundersen's conjunctival flap A surgical procedure performed to replace the damaged anterior cornea in cases of painful severe surface disorder (e.g. bullous keratopathy, non-healing corneal ulceration). A thin flap of bulbar conjunctiva is dissected and rotated to cover the corneal surface with its epithelium removed. *Note:* also spelt Gunderson.

Gunn's crossing sign *See* sign, Gunn's crossing.

guttata, cornea *See* cornea guttata.

gyrus One of the prominent rounded elevations between the sulci or grooves on the surface of the hemispheres of the brain. There are numerous gyri. Those associated with the visual association areas are the angular and lingual gyri. *Plural:* gyri.

H

Haab's pupillometer; striae *See* under the nouns.

haemangioma A tumour derived from blood vessels. *Note:* also spelt hemangioma.

capillary h. A tumour of the retinal vasculature, which may be sight-threatening. If there are multiple lesions, it is associated with von Hippel–Lindau syndrome. It presents typically in young adults. The retinal lesion grows from a small red nodule to a larger yellowish mass accompanied by dilatation and tortuosity of the supplying artery and draining vein, and perhaps hard exudates, epiretinal membrane, retinal detachment and vitreous haemorrhage. Treatment, if needed, is with laser photocoagulation, cryotherapy or radiotherapy.

capillary orbital h. A tumour of the orbit, which depending on its size may cause visual impairment and systemic complications. It presents in childhood with bright red lesions (called 'strawberry naevi') or deeper lesions which appear dark blue through the skin and may cause astigmatism and amblyopia and less frequently proptosis. Treatment is for amblyopia but may also include beta-blockers and corticosteroids.

cavernous h. A rare, benign, congenital tumour of the retina and optic nerve head characterized by clusters of intraretinal blood-filled saccules. It is usually asymptomatic, unless there is vitreous haemorrhage. Treatment is not usually necessary.

cavernous orbital h. A benign orbital tumour in adults, mostly females. The tumour is composed of large blood-filled spaces possibly due to dilatation and thickening of the capillary loops. The most common site is the muscle cone behind the globe, causing proptosis, hyperopia and choroidal folds. Visual acuity may be reduced. Treatment is surgical in most cases when the condition is symptomatic.

choroidal h. A congenital benign tumour of the choroid, which usually remains asymptomatic until adulthood when secondary degenerative changes occur in the retinal pigment epithelium and retina, possibly causing visual impairment. It may be localized (**circumscribed**) or **diffuse** in which case it forms part of the Sturge–Weber syndrome. Treatment includes photodynamic therapy, proton beam radiotherapy or plaque radiotherapy.

retinal h. *See* haemangioma, capillary; haemangioma, cavernous; haemangioma, choroidal.

haematoma A swelling containing blood. It may result from injury (e.g. black eye) or from some blood disease, such as leukaemia. *Note:* also spelt hematoma.

haematoma, ocular A swelling due to a large haemorrhage into the tissues of the eye.

haemophthalmia An effusion of blood into the eye.

haemorrhage The escape of blood from any part of the vascular system. *Note:* also spelt hemorrhage.

See hyphaemia.

dot and blot h. A form of intraretinal haemorrhage often noted in background (nonproliferative) diabetic retinopathy, branch retinal vein occlusion, carotid occlusive disease and child abuse (shaken baby). The haemorrhage is located within the inner retina and is limited by the orientation of the inner nuclear and plexiform layers. A small blot haemorrhage is often referred to as a '**dot**' haemorrhage. It is typically a sign of retinal vein occlusion and diabetic retinopathy. *See* retinal vein occlusion; retinopathy, background diabetic; retinopathy, pre-proliferative diabetic.

flame h. *See* haemorrhage, preretinal.

preretinal h. Haemorrhage occurring between the retina and the vitreous body. It is usually large and often shaped like a D with the straight edge at the top. *Syn.* subhyaloid haemorrhage. Others are flame-shaped and occur at the level of the nerve fibre layer and tend to parallel the course of the nerve fibres (**flame haemorrhage**). Retinal haemorrhages occur as a result of retinal vein occlusion, wet form of age-related macular degeneration and diabetic retinopathy. They are usually round and originate in the deep capillaries of the retina. *See* retinopathy, diabetic; retinopathy, proliferative; retinopathy, pre-proliferative diabetic.

subarachnoid h. Haemorrhage within the subarachnoid space due to a rupture of an aneurysm in an intracranial artery, usually in the circle of Willis (most often the anterior communicating artery). It occurs suddenly with severe headache, photophobia, optic disc swelling, altered consciousness and vomiting. It requires immediate medical attention. Subarachnoid haemorrhages form part of Terson's syndrome and are involved in papilloedema. *See* papilloedema; space, subarachnoid; syndrome, Terson's.

subconjunctival h. A red patch of blood on the conjunctiva of the eye, due to the rupture of a small blood vessel beneath it. The condition is nearly always unilateral and the haemorrhage absorbs spontaneously although it frequently alarms the subject. It may be associated with hypertension, especially in people over 50 years of age. *See* disease, sickle-cell.

subhyaloid h. *See* haemorrhage, preretinal.

suprachoroidal h. A rare haemorrhage within the suprachoroidal space due to a rupture of the long or short posterior ciliary artery. It may occur as a complication of intraocular surgery, trauma, advanced age or systemic cardiovascular disease. Signs are pain, increased intraocular pressure, shallowing of the anterior chamber, vitreous prolapse and retinal detachment. Immediate closure of the wound must be performed.

Haidinger's brushes An entoptic phenomenon observed when viewing a large diffusely illuminated blue field through a polarizer. It appears as a pair of yellow brush-like shapes which seem to radiate from the point of fixation. The brushes are believed to be due to double refraction by the radially oriented fibres of Henle around the fovea. This phenomenon is used in detecting and treating eccentric fixation.

Halberg clip *See* clip, Halberg.

half-eyes *See* spectacles, half-eye.

Haller's layer *See* layer, Haller's.

Hallermann–Streiff–Francois syndrome *See* syndrome, Hallermann-Streiff-Francois.

hallucinations, visual Visual perception not evoked by a light stimulus. They may be provoked by some pathological process anywhere along the visual pathway or as a result of an organic brain disease. *See* pseudopsia; syndrome, Charles Bonnet.

halo A coloured ring of light seen around a light source as a result of aberrations, internal reflections, diffraction or scattering. It also appears when the eye is diseased and the cornea is oedematous, as in glaucoma.

hamartoma A malformation resembling a tumour made of a mixture of cells and tissue found at the site of growth.
See retinal pigment epithelium and retina, hamartoma of the.

haplopia Single normal vision, as distinguished from diplopia.

haploscope Instrument used mainly in the laboratory to study various aspects of binocular vision. It presents separate fields of view to the two eyes while allowing changes in convergence or accommodation of one or both eyes, as well as providing for controls of colour, intensity or size of target and field.
See amblyoscope, Worth; dichoptic; masking, dichoptic.

haptic 1. *See* scleral zone. **2.** Pertaining to the sense of touch.
See lens, scleral contact.

Harada's disease *See* disease, Harada's.

Harado-Ito procedure *See* transposition.

hard resin *See* CR-39 material.

harmonious ARC *See* retinal correspondence, abnormal.

Hartman–Shack principle *See* aberration, wavefront.

Hasner's valve *See* valve of Hasner.

Hassall–Henle bodies *See* cornea guttata.

head posture, abnormal A deviation in position of the head, aimed at mitigating the effects of diplopia. It may be due to a field restriction or shyness, but the most frequent reason is an incomitant strabismus. Patients usually adjust their heads to permit fusion. If the deviation is too large to achieve fusion, patients may adjust their heads so as to increase the separation between the diplopic images and thereby making the diplopia less troublesome. If the cause of abnormal head posture remains untreated it may produce torticollis. *Examples*: if the right medial rectus or the left lateral rectus is affected, the face may be turned to the left, and vice versa if the other horizontal muscles are affected; if the left superior oblique is affected, the face may be turned to the right, the chin may be depressed and the head may be tilted to the right.
See palsy, fourth nerve; palsy, sixth nerve; strabismus, paralytic.

head tilt A deviation of the head from its upright position.
See head posture, abnormal; test, Bielschowsky's head tilt.

head tilt test *See* test, Bielschowsky's head tilt.

headache, ocular A headache believed to result from excessive use of the eyes, uncorrected refractive error, especially hyperopia and low grades of astigmatism, binocular vision anomaly or eye diseases (e.g. papilloedema). This headache typically occurs in the brow region but also in the occipital or neck regions.
See accommodative insufficiency; asthenopia.

headlamp 1. Lighting device fitted to a vehicle and used to provide illumination on the road. **2.** A lamp strapped to the forehead of a surgeon or miner, enabling light to be directed where required leaving both hands free.

heliophobia Neurotic fear of exposure to sunlight.

Helmholtz's law of magnification *See* law, Lagrange's.

Helmholtz's theory of accommodation *See* theory, Helmholtz's of accommodation.

Helmholtz's theory of colour vision *See* theory, Young–Helmholtz.

HEMA Transparent hydrophilic plastic used in the manufacture of soft contact lenses. It stands for 2-hydroxyethyl methacrylate.
See index of refraction; lens, contact.

hemangioma *See* haemangioma.

hematoma *See* haematoma.

hemeralopia Term used to mean either **night blindness** in which there is a partial or total inability to see in the dark associated with a loss of rod function or vitamin A deficiency or **day blindness** in which there is reduced vision in daylight while vision is normal in the dark. *Syn.* **nyctalopia** (this term is only synonymous with night blindness); **night sight** (this term is only synonymous with day blindness).
See atrophy, gyrate; blindness, congenital stationary night; choroideremia; disease, Oguchi's; retinitis pigmentosa; vitamin A deficiency.

hemiachromatopsia Colour blindness in one-half of the visual field of one or both eyes.
See achromatopsia.

Fig. H1 Complete bitemporal hemianopia due to a large pituitary tumour compressing the optic chiasma.

hemianopia Loss of vision in one-half of the visual field of one eye (**unilateral hemianopia**) or of both eyes (**bilateral hemianopia**) (Fig. H1). *Syn.* hemianopsia; hemiopia.
See **quadrantanopia; reflex, hemianopic pupillary.**
absolute h. Hemianopia in which the affected part of the retina is totally blind to light, form and colour.
altitudinal h. Hemianopia in either the upper or lower half of the visual field. A common cause is non-arteritic anterior ischaemic optic neuropathy. *See* **neuropathy, non-arteritic anterior ischaemic optic.**
binasal h. Hemianopia in the nasal halves of the visual fields of both eyes.
bitemporal h. Hemianopia in the temporal halves of the visual fields of both eyes. A tumour of the pituitary gland causes this defect.
congruous h. Hemianopia in which the defects in the two visual fields are identical. A common cause is a lesion in the posterior optic radiations.
heteronymous h. A loss of vision in either both nasal halves (**binasal hemianopia**) or both temporal halves of the visual field (**bitemporal hemianopia**). A common cause of the latter is a lesion in the optic chiasma.
homonymous h. A loss of vision in the nasal half of the visual field of one eye and the temporal half of the visual field of the other eye. **Left homonymous hemianopia** is a loss of vision in the temporal half of the visual field of the left eye and the nasal half of the visual field of the right eye. **Right homonymous hemianopia** is a loss of vision in the temporal half of the visual field of the right eye and the nasal half of the visual field of the left eye. Common causes are occlusion of the posterior cerebral artery (stroke), trauma and tumours. Lesions in one optic tract cause incongruous homonymous hemianopia whereas lesions in the optic radiations and visual cortex on one side cause congruous homonymous hemianopia.
See **field, keyhole visual; macular sparing.**
incongruous h. Hemianopia in which the defects in the two affected visual fields differ in one or more ways. A common cause is a lesion in one optic tract.
quadrantic h. See **quadrantanopia.**
relative h. Hemianopia involving a loss of form and colour but not of light.
h. spectacles See **spectacles, hemianopic.**

hemidecussation The rearrangement of the fibres of the optic nerves occurring in the optic chiasma in which about half of them from each optic nerve pass on to the contralateral optic tract. Thus each optic tract contains one-half of the fibres of the ipsilateral optic nerve (representing the ipsilateral half visual field) and one-half from the contralateral optic nerve (representing the contralateral half visual field). *Syn.* semidecussation. *See* **decussation;** Fig. P4, p. 253.

hemidesmosome *See* **desmosome.**

hemifield One-half of the visual field, usually divided vertically through the fovea into the left or the right visual field. It occurs following transection of the optic chiasma. Hemifield neglect sometimes occurs following trauma to the posterior lobe of one hemisphere.
See **visual neglect.**

hemorrhage *See* **haemorrhage.**

Henle, crypts; glands of *See* **gland, of Henle.**

Henle, fibre layer of *See* **layer of Henle, fibre.**

hepatolenticular degeneration *See* **disease, Wilson's.**

Herbert's pits *See* **trachoma.**

hereditary Pertains to a condition that is genetically transmitted from parent to offspring.
See **acquired; congenital; familial; inheritance.**

van Herick, Shaffer and Schwartz method *See* **method, van Herick, Shaffer and Schwartz.**

Hering's after-image; after-image test *See* under the nouns.

Hering's law *See* **law of equal innervation, Hering's.**

Hering's theory of colour vision; visual illusion *See* under the nouns.

Hering–Hermann grid A grid consisting of perpendicularly crossed white stripes on a black background. The observer sees a dark shadow at the intersections of the white stripes. This phenomenon is due to lateral inhibition among peripheral retinal neurons and does not occur for the fixated point (Fig. H2). *Syn.* Hermann's grid; Hermann's visual illusion.
See **inhibition, lateral.**

Hering–Hillebrand deviation *See* **deviation, Hering–Hillebrand.**

herpes simplex of the cornea *See* **herpesvirus; keratitis, herpes simplex; uveitis, viral.**

herpesvirus Any virus belonging to a group of DNA-containing viruses, which have similar structures

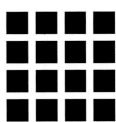

Fig. H2 Hering–Hermann grid.

but few other properties in common. They are: herpes simplex virus 1 (HSV-1) (human herpesvirus 1); herpes simplex virus 2 (HSV-2) (human herpesvirus 2); varicella-zoster virus (VZV) (human herpesvirus 3); Epstein–Barr virus (EBV) (human herpesvirus 4); cytomegalovirus (CMV) (human herpesvirus 5); human herpesvirus 6 (HHV-6); human herpesvirus 7 (HHV-7) and human herpesvirus 8 (HHV-8). Herpesviruses may cause infections including blepharoconjunctivitis, herpes zoster ophthalmicus, iridocyclitis, keratitis, uveitis, retinal necrosis, retinitis and cytomegalovirus retinitis. *See* antiviral agents; herpes zoster ophthalmicus; virus.

herpes zoster A viral infection of the posterior root ganglia of the spinal cord due to a reactivation of the varicella-zoster virus (also called chickenpox virus) which had remained latent. It is characterized by a circumscribed vesicular eruption of the skin and neuralgic pain in the areas supplied by the sensory nerves. This is due to the migration of the virus from the affected ganglia to the sensory nerves. A particular ocular manifestation is herpes zoster ophthalmicus. *Syn.* shingles. *See* uveitis, viral.

herpes zoster ophthalmicus A condition caused by reactivation and infection of the dormant varicella zoster virus (which causes chickenpox) in the sensory ganglion resulting in shingles (herpes zoster) of the innervated sensory fibres of the area of skin (dermatome) supplied by the ophthalmic branch of the trigeminal nerve (fifth cranial nerve). The disease that occurs most commonly in people over 50 years of age begins with a severe, unilateral, disabling neuralgia in the region of distribution of the nerve. It is followed by a vesicular eruption of the epithelium of the forehead, the nose (an involvement strongly correlated with ocular involvement), eyelids and sometimes the cornea. The vesicles rupture leaving haemorrhagic areas that heal in several weeks. Pain usually disappears in about 2 weeks but, in a few cases, neuralgia persists for a long time. **Acute epithelial keratitis** occurs in approximately 50% of all cases of herpes zoster ophthalmicus. Other clinical manifestations include episcleritis, scleritis, conjunctivitis, stromal keratitis, uveitis and more rarely necrotizing retinitis. As the disease progresses, it may give rise to **mucous plaque keratitis**, which occurs usually between the third and the sixth month after the onset of the rash. It is characterized by the plaque lines on the surface of the cornea, which can be easily lifted, and stromal haze. *See* keratitis, acute epithelial; keratitis, disciform; keratitis, interstitial; uveitis, viral.

herpetic keratitis *See* keratitis, herpetic.

Herschel prism *See* prism, rotary.

Hess after-image *See* after-image.

Hertel exophthalmometer *See* exophthalmometer.

hertz A unit of frequency equal to one cycle per second. *Symbol:* Hz.

Hess screen *See* screen, Hess.

Hess–Lancaster test *See* test, Hess–Lancaster.

heterochromatic iridocyclitis *See* iridocyclitis, Fuchs' heterochromic.

heterochromatic stimuli Visual stimuli that give rise to different colour sensations.

heterochromia Difference in colour of the two irides or of different parts of the same iris. It is usually congenital but some cases are associated with eye diseases such as cataract, corneal precipitates, glaucoma, iridocyclitis, iris melanoma or as a result of siderosis. Some cases may form part of a syndrome. *Syn.* anisochromia. *See* iridocyclitis, Fuchs' heterochromic; syndrome, Horner's; syndrome, Marfan's; syndrome, Sturge–Weber; syndrome, Waardenburg's.

heterochromatic flicker photometry *See* photometry, heterochromatic flicker.

heterodeviation A form of ocular alignment that differs from the normal orthophoria. These include the general groups of **heterophoria** (e.g. esophoria, hyperphoria, etc.) and **heterotropia** (e.g. esotropia, exotropia, etc.).

heterometropia *See* anisometropia.

heteronymous diplopia; hemianopia *See* under the nouns.

heterophoria The tendency for the two visual axes of the eyes not to be directed towards the point of fixation, in the absence of an adequate stimulus to fusion. Thus, the active and passive positions do not coincide for that particular fixation distance. This tendency is characterized by a deviation that can take various forms according to its relative direction such as **esophoria, exophoria, excyclophoria, incyclophoria, hyperphoria, hypophoria.** *Syn.* phoria. *See* anisophoria; dextrophoria; dissociation; kataphoria; laevophoria.

associated h. This term has been deprecated and replaced by the term aligning prism. *See* prism, aligning.

compensated h. Any heterophoria that does not give rise to symptoms or to suppression.

decompensated d. See heterophoria, uncompensated.

dissociated h. Any heterophoria which is revealed by methods which produce complete dissociation such as the cover test, the Maddox rod test, the Thorington test, the von Graefe's test, the diplopia test, etc.

uncompensated h. Any heterophoria which gives rise to symptoms or to suppression. The symptoms are associated with visual tasks, especially close work, but also occasionally, inadequate illumination. Resting the eyes will usually lessen the symptoms. Unbalanced spectacle correction, deterioration in the patient's general health, worry and anxiety can also sometimes give rise to an uncompensated heterophoria. This type of heterophoria is presumed to manifest itself as fixation disparity. *Syn.* decompensated heterophoria. *See* Disparometer; Mallett fixation disparity unit; prism, relieving.

heterophthalmia A difference in the appearance of the two eyes as in heterochromia.

heteropsia *See* anisometropia.

heterotopia maculae *See* macula, ectopia of the.

heterotropia *See* strabismus.

hill of vision *See* island of vision.

higher-order aberration *See* aberration, higher-order.

hinge joint of a spectacle frame A joint made up of plates, charniers and a pivot by means of which the sides hinge upon the front of the spectacles.

von Hippel's disease *See* disease, von Hippel's.

von Hippel–Lindau syndrome *See* syndrome, von Hippel–Lindau.

hippus Small rhythmic variations in the size of the pupils. They are present in everybody and increase slightly at high luminances. The frequency of these oscillations is about 1.4 Hz. Hippus may also be associated with systemic disorders such as multiple sclerosis, neurosyphilis and myasthenia gravis.

Hirschberg's test *See* test, Hirschberg's.

histamine A chemical that is present in all body tissues. It is released by mast cells in connective tissues during allergic and inflammatory reactions. *See* antihistamine; cell, mast; hypersensitivity.

histoplasmosis *See* syndrome, presumed ocular histoplasmosis.

history, case A record of a patient's chief complaint, ocular and general health and that of close relatives, and visual requirements. It is a very important part of the examination, which facilitates the diagnosis and treatment of the patient's complaint.

HIV *See* human immunodeficiency virus.

Hodgkin lymphoma *See* lymphoma.

hole in the card test *See* test, hole in the card.

hole in the hand test *See* test, hole in the hand.

Hollenhorst's plaques *See* plaques, Hollenhorst's.

Holmes–Adie syndrome *See* syndrome, Holmes–Adie.

Holmes–Wright lantern *See* test, lantern.

Holmgren's test *See* test, wool.

hologram *See* holography.

holography A technique for obtaining a stereoscopic image of an object without the use of lenses. It consists of recording on a photographic plate the pattern of interference between coherent light reflected from the object and light that comes directly from the same source (or is reflected from a mirror). The coherent light is usually provided by a laser. The photographic recording on the plate (called a **hologram**) when illuminated with coherent light yields an image that is identical in amplitude and phase distribution with the original wave from the object. It thus provides a three-dimensional image of the object in the sense that the observer's eyes must refocus to examine foreground and background and indeed 'look around' objects by simply moving the head laterally.

homatropine hydrobromide Alkaloid derived from atropine. It is an antimuscarinic drug used as a mydriatic and as a weak cycloplegic.

homocentric pencil of rays 1. One in which all rays converge or diverge from a single point. **2.** One in which more than one beam of light share the same pathway. *Example*: In an ophthalmoscope, the illumination and observation paths are shared.

homochromatic after-image *See* after-image, homochromatic.

homocystinuria An autosomal recessive inherited disorder caused by defects of the cobolamin (vitamin B12) dependent pathway that converts homocysteine to methionine and leads to an accumulation of the amino acid methionine and homocysteine. The first signs are ocular; a dislocated lens which may cause diplopia or glaucoma, myopia and occasionally cataract and retinal detachment. Systemic signs are blond hair, intellectual impairment and some of the features of Marfan's syndrome (e.g. tall, thin build). Management includes vitamins B6 (pyridoxine), B9 (folic acid) and B12 supplements.

homonymous diplopia; hemianopia *See* under the nouns.

hordeolum, external An acute suppurative infection (usually caused by staphylococci) of an eyelash follicle or of the sebaceous gland of Zeis or of the sweat gland of Moll (located in the region of an eyelash). The condition occurs most commonly in people who have a lower resistance to staphylococci, as in debility, or who have a blepharitis. It has the appearance of a hyperaemic elevated area, indurated on the eyelid margin where it may rupture and discharge yellowish pus. The symptom is tenderness of the eyelid that may become marked as the suppuration progresses and the eyelid near the margin is red and swollen. Treatment usually consists of hot compresses and application of an antibiotic ointment and perhaps removal of the affected eyelash. Surgical incision is rarely needed. *Plural:* hordeola. *Syn.* stye.

hordeolum, internal An acute purulent infection (usually caused by staphylococci) of the meibomian glands. It usually causes more discomfort than an external hordeolum as it is located on the conjunctival side of the eyelid. Treatment is similar to that of external hordeolum but surgical incision is required more frequently. *Syn.* meibomian stye. *See* chalazion; meibomianitis.

horizontal cell *See* cell, horizontal.

Horner's muscle; syndrome *See* under the nouns.

Horner–Trantas' dots *See* conjunctivitis, vernal.

horopter The locus of object points in space that stimulate corresponding retinal points of the two

eyes when the eyes are fixating binocularly one of these object points. The horopter is a curve that passes through the fixation point and changes shape with fixation distance. Objects closer to the eyes than the horopter are seen double (crossed disparity) and objects further than the horopter are seen double (uncrossed disparity). There are various types of horopters depending upon the method of determination.
See area, Panum's; Fig. D2 p. 86.

apparent frontoparallel plane h. The locus of object points in space which appear to the observer to lie on a plane through the fixation point, parallel to the plane of the face. *Syn.* frontal plane horopter. *See* deviation, Hering–Hillebrand; plane, empirical.

empirical h. A horopter determined experimentally by having an observer judge a series of targets to be neither 'nearer than' nor 'farther than' the fixation point. *Examples*: the frontoparallel plane horopter; the nonius horopter.

longitudinal h. Horopter that is plotted by only considering the longitudinal section where the rods meet the plane of fixation. Thus this horopter is a curve located in that plane and not a surface.

nonius h. Horopter plotted by fixating binocularly a central vertical rod while the other rods located in the periphery have their upper halves seen by one eye only and their lower halves seen by the other eye only. Each rod is moved individually until the two halves are seen aligned. *Syn.* vernier horopter.

rectilinear h. The assemblage of all lines in space that stimulate corresponding retinal lines. It is a pencil of quadratic surfaces with the space horopter as their common curve of intersection.

space h. The horopter consisting of all object points in space which stimulate corresponding retinal points as distinguished from the two-dimensional cases such as the apparent frontoparallel plane, longitudinal or nonius horopters.

theoretical h. A horopter based on theoretical concepts. *Example*: the Vieth–Müller horopter.

vernier h. *See* horopter, nonius.

Vieth–Müller h. A theoretical horopter formed by a circle passing through the point of fixation and the anterior nodal points of the two eyes. Thus any point on this horopter forms an image in the two retinas, which is at equal distances from their respective foveas. *Syn.* Vieth–Müller circle. *See* deviation, Hering–Hillebrand.

horror fusionis Avoidance of fusion resulting from two retinal images which are so different that they are impossible to fuse. This is often the case in strabismus. *Syn.* fusion aversion.

horseshoe tear A type of retinal tear in which a strip of tissue is torn from the retina. The tear commonly follows a vitreous detachment in which the vitreous adheres to the retina and pulls it from the point of adherence during or just after an abrupt eye movement. This type of retinal tear is particularly dangerous since it is often a precursor to a retinal detachment.
See retinal break.

Howard–Dolman test *See* test, Howard–Dolman.

HRR test *See* plates, pseudoisochromatic.

Hruby lens *See* lens, Hruby.

Hudson–Stahli *See* line, Hudson–Stähli.

hue Attribute of colour sensation, such as blue, red, green, etc., which is ordinarily associated with a given wavelength of the light stimulating the retina, as distinguished from the attributes of brightness and saturation.
See phenomenon, Bezold–Brücke; threshold, differential.

human immunodeficiency virus (HIV) An RNA retrovirus of the genus *Lentivirus* that infects and destroys vital cells of the human immune system, such as helper T cells (CD4 cells). It may cause the acquired immunodeficiency syndrome (AIDS) and may lead to complications such as anterior uveitis, viral keratitis, cytomegalovirus retinitis, microvascular abnormalities of the conjunctiva and/or retina, etc.
See syndrome, acquired immunodeficiency (AIDS).

Hummelsheim's procedure *See* transposition.

humour, aqueous *See* aqueous humour.

humour, vitreous *See* vitreous humour.

Humphriss immediate contrast test; method *See* method, Humphriss.

Hurler's syndrome *See* syndrome, Hurler's.

Hutchinson's pupil *See* pupil, Hutchinson's.

Huygens' eyepiece *See* eyepiece, Huygens'.

hyaline bodies *See* drusen.

hyalitis Inflammation of the hyaloid membrane occurring in intermediate uveitis. It sometimes incorrectly refers to inflammation of the vitreous humour.
See vitritis.

hyaloid artery; canal; membrane *See* under the nouns.

hyaloid fossa *See* fossa, patellar.

hyaloid remnant A rare condition in which there remain some parts of the hyaloid artery. Posteriorly there may be a vascular loop or the thread of an obliterated vessel running forward from the optic disc and floating freely in the vitreous. Anteriorly there may be some fibrous remnants attached to the posterior lens capsule and others sometimes floating in the vitreous. The anterior attachment of the hyaloid artery to the lens may also remain throughout life as a black dot, called **Mittendorf's dot**, and can be seen within the pupil by direct ophthalmoscopy (it appears as a white dot with the biomicroscope). There is rarely any visual interference, although patients may sometimes report seeing muscae volitantes. *Syn.* persistent hyaloid artery.
See canal, hyaloid; papilla, Bergmeister's; pseudopapilloedema; vitreous, persistent hyperplastic primary.

hyalosis, asteroid *See* asteroid hyalosis.

hydrocortisone acetate *See* antiinflammatory drug.

hydrogel Type of plastic material which contains water and is commonly mixed with silicone and used in the manufacture of soft contact lenses.

hydrogen peroxide *See* disinfection.

hydrophilic lens *See* lens, contact.

hydrophthalmos *See* buphthalmos; glaucoma, congenital.

hydrops, corneal Excessive accumulation of watery fluid in the stroma of the cornea as a result of rupture of the posterior layers of the cornea (Descemet's membrane and the endothelium). It is often found in advanced keratoconus and may occur as an **acute** form in which case there is pain and visual clouding due to corneal oedema. The oedema usually clears spontaneously, although the scar may interfere with vision. Hyperosmotic agents may be needed to reduce corneal oedema.

hydroxyethylcellulose; hydroxymethylcellulose, hydroxypropylcellulose *See* tears, artificial.

hydroxypropylmethylcellulose *See* hypromellose.

hyoscine hydrobromide An antimuscarinic (or parasympatholytic) drug with actions similar to those of atropine (i.e. mydriasis and cycloplegia) but of shorter duration. It is no longer used. *Syn.* scopolamine hydrobromide.

hyperaccommodation *See* accommodative excess.

hyperacuity The ability of the eye to detect the differences in the spatial locations of two or more stimuli. Hyperacuity thresholds are not based on resolution but on the ability to sense direction. It is extremely sensitive and thresholds are usually below about 15 seconds of arc. Hyperacuity tests include vernier acuity, stereoscopic acuity, orientation discrimination in which differences in the tilts of lines must be detected, the movement displacement threshold, the vertical alignment of a cluster of dots or the ability to bisect two parallel lines. Hyperacuity is less affected by optical defocus or light scattering (as occurs for example in corneal leukoma, cataract, vitreous haemorrhage) than is Snellen acuity and can therefore be helpful in assessing macular function behind a cataract or other media opacity before surgery (Fig. H3).
See maxwellian view system, clinical.

hyperaemia Excessive accumulation of blood in a part of the body. *Note*: also spelt hyperemia. *Syn.* injection.
See injection, ciliary; injection, conjunctival.

hyperaesthesia, corneal Abnormally high corneal sensitivity (threshold less than 15 mg/0.013 mm² near the limbus in the adult eye, if using the Cochet–Bonnet aesthesiometer) as distinguished from **hypoaesthesia** (beyond 70 mg/0.013 mm² near the limbus in the adult eye) which is abnormally low corneal sensitivity.

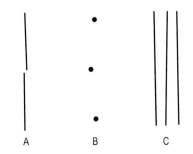

Fig. H3 Examples of hyperacuity tests (A, detection of lack of alignment of two lines; B, of three dots; C, of the tilt of one line).

See aesthesiometer; corneal touch threshold; sensitivity, corneal.

hypercapnia The presence of a raised carbon dioxide content or tension in a milieu (e.g. blood, tears). Contact lens wear tends to give rise to this condition, especially lenses of low gas transmissibility.
See acidosis.

hypercolumn A complete set of orientation columns over a cycle of 180° and of right and left dominance columns in the visual cortex. A hypercolumn may be about 1 mm wide. A hypercolumn of orientation columns is perpendicular to a hypercolumn of ocular dominance columns (Fig. H4).
See blobs; column, cortical.

hypercomplex cell *See* cell, hypercomplex.

hyperfocal distance *See* distance, hyperfocal.

hyperlacrimation Overflow of tears due to excessive secretion by the lacrimal gland. It may be caused by drugs (e.g. pilocarpine), strong emotion, as a reflex from trigeminal stimulation by an inflamed eye, irritation of the cornea or conjunctiva

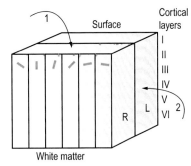

Fig. H4 A hypercolumn consisting of one set of orientation columns and one set of ocular dominance columns in the visual cortex. Electrode 1 penetrating at right angle to the surface encounters neurons responding to the same orientation and the same (right) ocular dominance. Electrode 2 penetrating parallel to the surface encounters neurons responding to the left ocular dominance and to different orientations.

by a chemical irritant in the air, cold wind or a foreign body in the eye. The main symptoms are discomfort and blurring of vision and sometimes embarrassment. Management depends on the cause. *Syn.* hypersecretion.
See epiphora.

hypermetria An abnormally large eye movement. *Example*: a saccade that overshoots its target. *See* dysmetria, ocular; movement, saccadic eye.

hypermetrope A person who has hypermetropia. *See* hyperope.

hypermetropia (H) *See* hyperopia.

hyperope A person who has hyperopia.

hyperopia (H) Refractive condition of the eye in which distant objects are focused behind the retina when the accommodation is relaxed. Thus, vision is blurred. In hyperopia, the point conjugate with the retina, that is the far point of the eye, is located behind the eye (Fig. H5). At birth, the mean refractive error is a hyperopia of about +2.00 D. As the child grows into adolescence, the average refraction tends towards emmetropia. The percentage of people with hyperopia increases beyond the age of 40 (Table H1). *Syn.* far sight; long sight; hypermetropia.
See choroidal folds; chorioretinopathy, central serous; cornea plana; emmetropia; emmetropization; glaucoma, angle-closure; headache, ocular; luxation of the lens; pseudopapilloedema; sclerocornea; test, plus 1.00 D blur.
absolute h. That hyperopia which cannot be compensated for by accommodation (Table H2).
acquired h. Hyperopia resulting from changes in the refractive indices of the media due to age, disease or surgery.
facultative h. That portion of hyperopia which can be compensated for by accommodation.
latent h. That portion of total hyperopia which is compensated for by the tonus of the ciliary muscle. It can be revealed wholly or partially by the use of a cycloplegic.
manifest h. That portion of total hyperopia which can be determined by the strongest convex lens in a subjective routine examination while retaining the best visual acuity.
simple h. Hyperopia uncomplicated by disease, trauma or astigmatism.
total h. The sum of the latent and manifest hyperopia.

hyperopic defocus *See* defocus, hyperopic.

hyperosmotic agent A drug that makes blood plasma hypertonic thus drawing fluid out of the eye and leading to a reduction in intraocular pressure.

It is used in solution in the treatment of angle-closure glaucoma and sometimes before surgery to decrease the intraocular pressure. Common agents include glycerin (glycerol), isosorbide, mannitol and urea.
See solution, hypertonic.

hyperphoria The tendency for the line of sight of one eye to deviate upward relative to that of the other eye in the absence of an adequate stimulus to fusion. If the deviation tends to be downward relative to the other eye or if the other eye in hyperphoria is used as a reference, the condition is called **hypophoria**.
See kataphoria.
left h. (L/R) Hyperphoria in which the line of sight of the left eye deviates upward relative to the other eye.
paretic h. Hyperphoria due to a paresis of one or several of the extraocular muscles.
right h. (R/L) Hyperphoria in which the line of sight of the right eye deviates upward relative to the other eye.

hyperplasia Any condition in which there is an increase in the number of cells in an organ or a tissue. It usually excludes tumour formation. *Example*: choroidal naevus.
See hypoplasia.

hyperpolarization A change in the value of the resting membrane potential towards a more

Table H1 Common ocular and systemic diseases with hyperopia as an associated sign

cornea plana
microphthalmia
sclerocornea
angle-closure glaucoma
branch retinal vein occlusion
fragile X syndrome
growth hormone deficiency
diabetes type 1
hypertension

Table H2 Approximate relationship between uncorrected absolute hyperopia and visual acuity

Hyperopia	Snellen visual acuity	
	(m)	(ft)
+4.5 D	6/120	20/400
+3.5 D	6/90	20/300
+2.5 D	6/60	20/200
+2.0 D	6/36	20/120
+1.5 D	6/24	20/80
+1.0 D	6/18	20/60
+0.75 D	6/12	20/40
+0.50 D	6/9	20/30

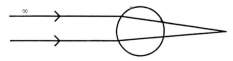

Fig. H5 A hyperopic eye looking at a distant axial point.

negative value. It occurs in the photoreceptors in response to light stimulation. It is caused by a decrease in the level of 3', 5'-cyclic guanosine monophosphate (cGMP), which closes the channels in the outer segment membrane thereby resulting in a closure of the influx of Na^+ (sodium). The inside of the cell becomes more negative than the outside. Hyperpolarization is **inhibitory** because the membrane potential moves away from the neuron's threshold at which an action potential could occur. *See* depolarization; potential, receptor; potential, resting membrane; synapse.

hypersecretion *See* hyperlacrimation.

hypersensitivity An excessive reaction, local or systemic, or inappropriate immune response to an antigen. Four types of immune responses are usually described, but the main reaction involving the eyes is type 1. They are also called **allergic reactions** types 1 through 4.
type 1 hypersensitivity An immediate, abnormal reaction occurring when an antigen reacts with an antibody (e.g. immunoglobulin E (IgE)) attached to a mast cell or basophil. This leads to the release of specific chemical mediators of allergy (e.g. histamine) that react with target organs throughout the body. Systemic signs include itching, lacrimation, skin rash and possibly haemodynamic collapse and shock. Allergic conjunctivitis is an example of this type of hypersensitivity. *Type 2 h. (cytotoxic h.)* is caused by an interaction of antibody and antigens on cell surfaces. *Examples*: cicatricial pemphigoid, Graves' disease, myasthenia gravis. *Type 3 h. (immune-complex mediated h.)* is mediated by a combination of antigen-antibody. *Example*: systemic lupus erythematosus. *Type 4 h. (T cell-mediated h.)* is a delayed reaction (several days to develop) mediated by T lymphocytes. *Example*: rheumatoid arthritis.
See antihistamine; cell, mast; keratoconjunctivitis, atopic; mast cell stabilizers.

hypertelorism, ocular A developmental congenital anomaly in which the distance between the orbits is abnormally large resulting in a large distance between the eyes. This can be associated with mental deficiency, divergent strabismus, exophthalmos or optic atrophy.

See syndrome, Aarskog's; syndrome, Alagille; syndrome, Apert's; syndrome, Crouzon's; syndrome, Waardenbrug's; telecanthus.

hypertension Abnormally high blood pressure beyond 140 to 150 mmHg for systolic blood pressure or beyond 90 to 95 mmHg for diastolic blood pressure. These figures are higher for older people. Elevated blood pressure can give rise to hypertensive retinopathy.
See exudate; palsy, sixth nerve; palsy, third nerve; retinal vein occlusion; retinopathy, hypertensive; sphygmomanometer.

hypertension, ocular A condition in which the intraocular pressure (IOP) is above normal (>21 mmHg) but in which there are neither visual field defects nor optic disc changes. Open-angle glaucoma may or may not develop later; risk factors include thin central corneal thickness, large cup/disc ratio, high IOP and lack of treatment to reduce IOP greater than 30 mmHg.

hypertensive retinopathy *See* retinopathy, hypertensive.

hyperthyroidism *See* disease, Graves'.

hypertonic solution *See* solution, hypertonic.

hypertropia Strabismus in which one eye is directed to the fixation point while the other is directed upward (right or left hypertropia). *Syn.* sursumvergens strabismus; anoopsia (Fig. H6). *See* hypotropia; test, three-step.
alternating h. A condition in which, on dissociation (e.g. by occlusion) of either eye, the eye behind the cover deviates upward but reverts to its fixating position when dissociation ceases. The condition can either occur as an isolated phenomenon or be associated with strabismus or latent strabismus. *Syn.* anaphoria; anatropia; dissociated vertical divergence; double hyperphoria. *See* phenomenon, Bielschowsky's.

hyphaemia Haemorrhage into the anterior chamber of the eye. It usually occurs as a result of trauma to the eye, especially in sports, or as a result of intraocular surgery (e.g. trabeculectomy). It is advisable to have the patient admitted to hospital because of the possibility of recurrent haemorrhage and secondary glaucoma. *Note*: also spelt hyphema.

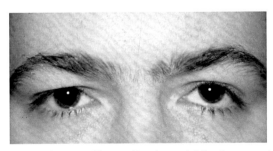

Fig. H6 Left hypertropia in the primary position resulting from a left fourth nerve palsy. (From Bowling 2016, with permission of Elsevier)

hypoaesthesia *See* hyperaesthesia, corneal.

hypoexophoria Combined hypophoria and exophoria.

hypolacrima *See* alacrima.

hypometria *See* dysmetria, ocular.

hypophoria *See* hyperphoria.

hypoplasia Any condition in which there is an underdevelopment or a decrease in the number of cells.
See hyperplasia.

hypoplasia, optic nerve A congenital condition characterized by a reduced number of retinal ganglion cell axons in the optic nerve. Visual acuity varies from normal to severe impairment, and sluggish pupil reactions are also present. The optic disc is smaller than normal with an inner pigmented ring surrounded by a white ring of visible sclera (**double-ring sign**). Many systemic disorders are associated with this condition (e.g. aniridia, blepharophimosis syndrome, de Morsier syndrome, Duane's syndrome, Cornelia de Lange syndrome, Goldenhar's syndrome). Bilateral cases can be caused by mutations in the PAX6 gene.

hypopyon The presence of pus in the anterior chamber of the eye associated with infectious diseases of the cornea (e.g. severe microbial keratitis, corneal ulcer), the iris or the ciliary body (e.g. severe anterior uveitis). The pus usually accumulates at the bottom of the chamber and may be seen through the cornea (Fig. H7).
See keratitis, hypopyon; syndrome, Behçet's.

hypothalamus A group of nuclei at the base of the brain located in the floor of the third ventricle. It consists of the optic chiasma, the paired mammillary bodies, the tuber cinereum, the infundibulum and the pars posterior of the pituitary gland.

hypothesis **1.** A tentative assumption or proposed explanation of a phenomenon made subject to further investigation and proof. **2.** In statistics, it presents as two options; either there is no significant difference between two events or sets of data (e.g. cases vs controls) and the difference is attributed to chance, this is called

the **null hypothesis** (H_0); or there is a significant difference between two sets of data that cannot be explained by chance. This is called the **alternative hypothesis** (H_1).
See significance; statistics.

hypotonic solution *See* solution, hypotonic.

hypotony, ocular Abnormally low intraocular pressure, usually less than 6 mmHg. It may result from trauma in which there is a perforating wound with loss of aqueous, concussion injury or following surgery for glaucoma. **Persistent hypotony** may result in visual impairment due to choroidal folds, choroidal detachment, retinal folds or retinal detachment. *Syn.* ocular hypotonia; ocular hypotonus.
See choroidal folds; cyclodialysis.

hypotropia Strabismus in which one eye fixates while the other is directed downward (right or left hypotropia). *Syn.* deorsumvergens strabismus.
See test, three-step.

hypoxia An inadequate supply of oxygen to tissues. It may occur in some pathological conditions. *Examples*: In long-standing cases of diabetes, there is corneal hypoxia (with consequent high epithelial fragility and some neovascularization) and retinal hypoxia (with consequent neovascularization). Corneal hypoxia (with consequent oedema, loss of sensitivity, etc.) may also occur in contact lens wear.
See anoxia; microcysts, epithelial; mitosis; oedema; oxygen requirement, critical; retinopathy, proliferative; syndrome, corneal exhaustion; syndrome, overwear; tear pumping.

hypoxic stress *See* strain.

hypromellose A highly viscous, water-soluble, nonirritating compound used as a thickening, lubricating and clinging agent. It is used principally as artificial tears (as, for example, in the management of keratoconjunctivitis sicca) and sometimes as a wetting agent. *Syn.* hydroxypropylmethylcellulose.
See alacrima; methylcellulose; staining, 3 and 9 o'clock.

hysteresis, accommodative A term used to indicate an incomplete and temporary relaxation

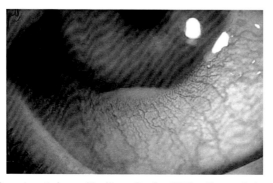

Fig. H7 Hypopyon with acute anterior uveitis. (From Bowling 2016, with permission of Elsevier)

of the accommodation of the eye after a period of fixation. The amount of relaxation varies according to the position of the fixation point relative to the position of the tonic accommodation and to the ametropia of the eye. In general, a sustained near visual task leads to an increase in accommodation, while a sustained distant visual task leads to a decrease in accommodation.
See **accommodation, resting state of.**

hysterical amblyopia *See* **amblyopia, hysterical.**

hysteropia Visual disorder due to hysteria.

iatrogenic Relating to a disorder induced by the treatment itself. *Example*: the development of amblyopia in the good eye following occlusion treatment.

ICE syndrome *See* **syndrome, ICE.**

idiopathic Relating to any primary pathological condition of unknown origin.

idiopathic macular telangiectasia *See* **telangiectasia.**

idoxuridine *See* **antiviral agents.**

illiterate chart *See* **chart, E.**

illuminance Quotient of the luminous flux, F, incident on an element of surface divided by the area, A, of that element of surface. *Symbol*: E. Thus,

$$E = F/A$$

The units are in lux or footcandles. *Syn.* illumination.
See **law of illumination, inverse square; photometer.**

illuminance, retinal *See* **retinal illuminance.**

illuminants, CIE standard The colorimetric illuminants A, B, C and D defined by the CIE in terms of relative spectral energy (power distribution): **standard illuminant A** representing the full radiator with a colour temperature of $T = 2854$ K; **standard illuminant B** representing direct sunlight with a correlated colour temperature of $T = 4874$ K; **standard illuminant C** representing daylight with a correlated colour temperature of $T = 6774$ K; **standard illuminant D** representing daylight with a correlated colour temperature of $T = 6504$ K (CIE). *See* **colour temperature; chromaticity diagram; lamp, Macbeth; light, white.**

illumination 1. The action of brightening an object with light. 2. The science of the application of lighting. 3. Synonym for illuminance.
diffuse i. In slit-lamp examination, it is the illumination obtained with a wide slit and an out-of-focus beam or with a diffuser, thus providing an overall view of the structures of the eye.
direct i. In slit-lamp examination, the slit beam and the microscope are both focused sharply on the structure to be observed. *Syn.* focal illumination.
focal i. *See* **illumination, direct.**
indirect i. In slit-lamp examination, the slit beam is focused on a structure located adjacent to the structure to be observed.
inverse square law of i. *See* **law of illumination, inverse square.**
oscillation i. In slit-lamp examination, it is a technique in which the beam of light is oscillated to provide alternative direct and indirect illumination. It sometimes allows one to see slight changes more easily which otherwise would remain unnoticed under sustained illumination of either kind.
retinal i. *See* **retinal illuminance.**
retro-i. In slit-lamp examination, it is a method of illuminating a structure by using the light that is reflected by the iris or an opaque or senescent lens. This method is closely related to indirect illumination and often in corneal examination part of the cornea will simultaneously be under retro- and indirect illumination. *Syn.* transillumination. As the method is based on light reflected by a posterior surface, it can be used to view a cataract or iris disorder using light reflected from the fundus.
See **corneal clouding, central; oedema.**
sclerotic scatter i. In slit-lamp examination, it is a method in which the slit beam of light is focused on the sclera near the limbus and the cornea remains uniformly dark in the absence of an abnormality as the light is internally reflected and is seen around the limbus on the opposite side of the cornea. However, an abnormality (e.g. a foreign body, oedema or a scar) in the cornea becomes easily visible as it scatters light and will be seen as an area of brightness within the cornea.
See **corneal clouding, central; oedema.**
specular reflection i. In slit-lamp examination, it is a method in which the beam of light and the microscope are placed at equal angles from the normal to the corneal or lens surface to be viewed. This is a method for examining the quality of a surface. This method is particularly useful to observe the corneal endothelium.
See **blebs, endothelial; cornea guttata; shagreen.**

illuminometer *See* photometer.

illusion A false interpretation of an object or figure presented to the eye (visual illusion). Illusions can occur with each of the senses.
See figure, ambiguous.

autokinetic visual i. The apparent motion of a luminous object fixated in the dark or in a large blank field. It is not due to eye movements, and the illusion disappears as soon as the ambient luminance increases so that other objects become visible. *Syn.* visual autokinesis.

Baldwin's i. 1. Illusion in which a line connecting two large squares appears shorter than a line connecting two smaller squares (Fig. I1). **2.** Illusion in which a dot placed halfway between a large disc and a smaller disc appears to be nearer the large one.

café wall i. An illusion induced by a pattern of alternating columns of black and white rectangles (or squares) placed in such a way that the lines that they compose do not appear to be parallel. *Syn.* Munsterberg illusion. A variant of this illusion consists of hollow squares without alternating colour and is called a 'hollow square illusion'.

Cornsweet i. *See* effect, Craik–O'Brien–Cornsweet.

corridor i. Illusion in which images of equal size in a perspective figure of a corridor appear to be of different sizes. The figure that seems further away appears larger than the one in the foreground (Fig. I2).

Craik–Cornsweet i. *See* effect, Craik–O'Brien–Cornsweet.

Delboeuf i. Illusion in which a circle surrounded by a slightly larger concentric circle appears larger than another circle of the same size surrounded by a much larger concentric circle (Fig. I3).

Ebbinghaus i. Illusion in which a circle usually appears larger when surrounded by smaller circles than by larger circles (Fig. I4).

Ehrenstein's brightness i. Illusion in which the erased area at the intersection of radial (or horizontal and vertical) lines appears to be brighter than the background and with an illusory contour (Fig. I5).

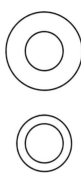

Fig. I3 Delboeuf illusion.

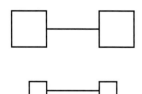

Fig. I1 Baldwin's illusion.

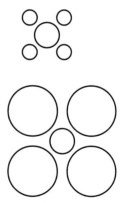

Fig. I4 Ebbinghaus illusion.

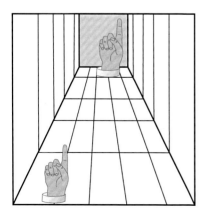

Fig. I2 Corridor illusion.

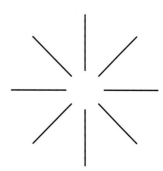

Fig. I5 Ehrenstein's brightness illusion.

floating-finger i. Illusion noted when fixating a point in the distance while the forefingers of each hand are held horizontally about 30 centimetres in front of the eyes with the fingertips nearly touching. A small disembodied finger with two tips appears floating in between and can be shortened or lengthened by varying the distance between the fingertips. It is a peculiar illustration of physiological diplopia (Fig. I6).

frequency doubling i. Illusion in which a grating pattern appears to have twice as many black and white bars than it actually has. This happens when a sinusoidal grating with a low spatial frequency (less than 4 c/deg) flickers in a counterphase fashion (i.e. light bars become dark and vice versa) at a high temporal frequency (more than 15 Hz). This type of stimulation is assumed to stimulate the non-linear mechanism within the magnocellular visual system.
See **perimetry, frequency doubling.**

Helmholtz i. *See* irradiation.

Hering's i. Illusion in which a pair of parallel lines appear bent when placing diagonal lines across them. This illusion is most noticeable when radiating lines are crossing two parallel lines on opposite sides of the point of radiation. In this case, the two parallel lines appear to bend away from each other (Fig. I7).
See **illusion, Wundt's.**

Hermann's i. *See* Hering–Hermann grid.

hole in the hand i. *See* test, hole in the hand.

hollow square i. *See* illusion, café wall.

horizontal-vertical visual i. Illusion in which the vertical line appears longer than the horizontal line when two lines of equal length are placed with the vertical line at the midpoint of the horizontal.
See **illusion, top hat.**

Jastrow i. Illusion in which two identical curved and tapering ring segments placed one above the other appear unequal in size, the band nearer the centres of curvature appearing to be the longest (Fig. I8).

Kundt's i. Illusion occurring when one attempts to bisect a horizontal line with only one eye and the segment on the temporal side of the visual field then appears larger than the other.

moon i. Illusion in which the moon appears much larger at the horizon than when viewed high in the sky. In fact, the actual size of the moon remains constant as does its distance from the earth. One possible explanation is that, at the horizon, there are many other cues in the field of view (e.g. houses, mountains) that make the moon appear to be much closer than when it is high in the sky and thus should be larger.
See **room, Ames.**

Müller–Lyer i. Illusion in which a line with outgoing fins on both ends appears longer than another of equal length but with arrowheads on both ends (Fig. I9).

Munsterberg's i. *See* illusion, café wall.

oculogyral i. Illusion of apparent movement of viewed objects when the body is subjected to rotary acceleration. The initial apparent movement is opposite to that of the direction of rotation of the body and is followed by an apparent movement in the same direction.

Oppel–Kundt i. Illusion in which a divided, interrupted or filled area appears to be larger than an empty area of equal size.

optical i. *See* illusion, visual.

Orbison i. Illusion of a distorted geometric figure such as a square or a circle drawn on a background of radiating lines or concentric lines.

Poggendorff's i. Illusion in which two visible portions of a diagonal line overlaid by a rectangle do not appear to be continuous (Fig. I10).

Ponzo i. Illusion in which two parallel lines of equal length do not appear equal when they are surrounded by two radiating straight lines, one

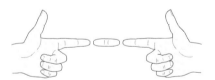

Fig. I6 Floating-finger illusion. (After Colman 2003, with permission of the author)

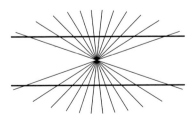

Fig. I7 Hering's illusion.

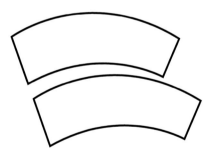

Fig. I8 Jastrow illusion.

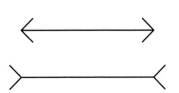

Fig. I9 Müller–Lyer illusion.

on each side. The parallel line nearer the point of radiation appears to be longer (Fig. I11).

Schroeder's staircase visual i. See Schroeder's staircase.

top hat i. Illusion in which a top hat drawn with equal vertical and horizontal dimensions appears to be much greater vertically than horizontally. It is closely related to the horizontal-vertical illusion (Fig. I12).
See **illusion, horizontal-vertical visual.**

visual i. Perception of an object or a figure that does not correspond to the actual physical characteristics of the stimulus. *Syn.* optical illusion; geometrical optical illusion.

waterfall i. See **after-effect, waterfall.**

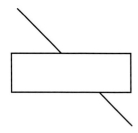

Fig. I10 Poggendorff's illusion.

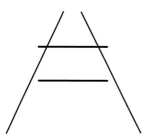

Fig. I11 Ponzo illusion.

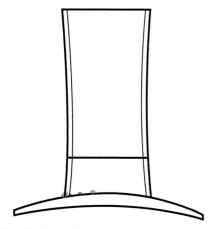

Fig. I12 Top hat illusion.

Wundt's i. Illusion in which a pair of parallel lines appear bent towards each other when crossed by lines radiating from two points, one on each side of the parallel lines.
See **illusion, Hering's.**

Zollner's i. Illusion in which a series of parallel lines appear to converge or diverge from each other when crossed by short diagonal lines.

illusory contours See **contour.**

image A picture of an object formed by a lens, a mirror or other optical system.
See **object; plane, image.**

aerial i. An image found in space and not on a screen, such as the image viewed in indirect ophthalmoscopy.

after-i. See **after-image.**

axial point i. The point of intersection of an image with the optical axis.

catadioptric i. Image formed by both reflecting and refracting surfaces.
See **system, catadioptric.**

catoptric i. Image formed by specular reflection, either from a mirror or by reflection at refracting surfaces such as the optical surfaces of the eye, which form the Purkinje–Sanson images.

corneal i. Catoptric image formed by either the anterior or posterior surface of the cornea. They are also called the first and second Purkinje–Sanson images.

demagnified i. See **field, visual f. expander.**

dioptric i. An image formed by a refracting surface as distinct from a catoptric image.

direct i. A virtual image such as the erect image seen in direct ophthalmoscopy.

double i. A pair of images obtained either optically through a doubling system or due to diplopia.

eidetic i. Visual perception arising from the imagination of the subject or what has previously been seen, and not from immediate retinal stimulation. That image may last from a few seconds to several minutes and appears to be located in front of the eyes.

entoptic i. Visual sensation arising from stimuli within the eye and perceived as in the external world. *Examples*: muscae volitantes; phosphene. *Syn.* entoptic phenomenon.
See **angioscotoma; arcs, blue; entoptoscope, blue field; floaters; Haidinger's brushes; muscae volitantes; phosphene; spot, Maxwell's.**

erect i. Image that is not inverted with respect to the object such as a virtual image produced by a concave lens.
See **images, Purkinje–Sanson.**

extraordinary i. See **birefringence.**

false i. 1. The retinal image in the deviating eye in strabismus. It is less well defined than the true image. 2. See **image, ghost.**
See **image, true.**

ghost i. 1. Unwanted image as may be formed by internal reflection in a lens or an optical system. These images are sometimes annoying to spectacle wearers and even to observers as they detract from the appearance of the spectacle

lens or hide the wearer's eyes behind a veil. The intensity of ghost images is diminished by antireflection coatings. **2.** The faint image seen in monocular diplopia. *Syn.* false image.
See **Fresnel's formula; lens flare; light, stray; mirror, front surface.**
indirect i. A real image, such as the inverted image seen in indirect ophthalmoscopy.
inverted i. Image that is upside down and right for left with respect to its object. *Syn.* reversed image.
See **images, Purkinje–Sanson.**
i. jump See jump.
i. line See line, focal.
ocular i. **1.** The retinal image. **2.** The image formed by the refracting system of the eye, disregarding the presence or the position of the retina.
perceptual i.; psychic i. See image, visual.
Purkinje–Sanson i's. Catoptric images produced by reflection from the optical surfaces of the eye. The **first image** is reflected by the anterior surface of the cornea, the **second image** by the posterior surface of the cornea, the **third image** by the anterior surface of the crystalline lens and the **fourth image** by the posterior surface of the crystalline lens. Only the fourth image is inverted. The third is the largest, but the first is by far the brightest (Fig. I13). During accommodation, the third image becomes smaller while the size of the fourth diminishes only a little. Purkinje–Sanson images are used to measure or calculate various optical dimensions of the eye, to establish angle alpha or lambda and to contribute to some diagnostic tests of strabismus (e.g. Hirschberg's method; Krimsky's method). *Syn.* Purkinje images (Table I2).
See **axis, optical; ophthalmophakometer; phacoscope.**
real i. An image that can be formed on a screen.
See **focus, principal; object, real.**
retinal i. Image formed on the retina by the optical system of the eye. The size of the retinal image h' of a distant object subtending angle u in an emmetropic eye is equal to

$$h' = u/F$$

where h' is in metres, u is in radians and the power of the eye F is in dioptres. The formula is only valid for small angles (Fig. I14 and Table I1). *Example*: A distant object subtends an angle of 5° viewed by an emmetropic eye of power 60 D (π is equal to 3.1416)

$$u = 5 \times \frac{\pi}{180} = 0.0873 \, \text{rad}$$

$$h' = \frac{0.0873}{60} = 0.00145 \, \text{m or } 1.45 \, \text{mm}$$

reversed i. See image, inverted.
i. shell The curved surface containing either all the sagittal or all the tangential foci corresponding to a given object plane.
See **astigmatism, oblique.**
i. space See space, image.
stabilized retinal i. See stabilized retinal image.
true i. The retinal image in the normally fixating eye in strabismus.
See **image, false.**
virtual i. One from which refracted or reflected rays appear to have come. This image can be seen but it is not an actual image and cannot be formed on a screen. *Examples*: the image seen in a plane mirror; the image seen in the cornea.
See **focus, principal; object, virtual.**
visual i. **1.** Perceived image formed by the whole visual system. It includes the physiological and psychological processing. *Syn.* perceptual image; psychic image. **2.** A mental picture based on the recollection of a previous visual experience.
See **aniseikonia; visualization.**

imagery 1. Process of recalling past visual experiences. **2.** Synonym for visualization.
See **image, visual.**

Table I1   Approximate relationship between the retinal image size of an emmetropic eye (in mm) with a power of 60 D and the angular subtense of a distant object

Angle (deg)	Size (mm)
0.017° (or 1′)	0.0048
0.07° (or 4′)	0.0194
0.013° (or 8′)	0.039
0.2° (or 12′)	0.058
0.4° (or 24′)	0.12
0.6° (or 36′)	0.17
0.8° (or 48′)	0.23
1°	0.29
2°	0.58
3°	0.87
4°	1.16
5°	1.45
6°	1.75
8°	2.33
10°	2.91
12°	3.49
15°	4.36

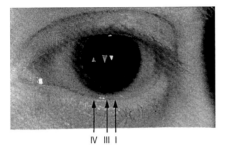

Fig. I13 Purkinje–Sanson images I, III and IV. Image I is authentic; III and IV have been retouched for emphasis.

Table I2 Purkinje–Sanson images (all figures are calculated and rounded off and all distances are referred to the anterior corneal pole)

Source of reflection	Type of image (object is at infinity)	Relative brightness
I anterior corneal surface	– virtual – erect – smaller than object – situated near plane of pupil (about 3.9 mm)	1.0
II posterior corneal surface	– virtual – erect – smaller than I (about × 0.8) – situated near I (about 3.6 mm)	0.01
III anterior lens surface	– virtual – erect – larger than I (about × 2.0) – situated in vitreous (about 10.7 mm)	0.08
IV posterior lens surface	– real – inverted – smaller than I (about × 0.8) – situated in the lens (about 4.6 mm)	0.08

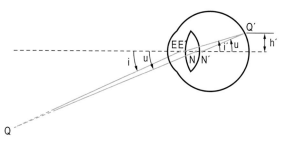

Fig. I14 Retinal image position and size h′ corresponding to an object at infinity. The angles subtended to the axis at the nodal point N and N′ in object and image space are equal (angles u). Also shown are the rays passing through the centre of the entrance and exit pupils, E and E′. Q, off-axis extreme of the distant object. Q′, off-axis extremity of the retinal image.

imbalance, muscular Generic term referring to a defect in the oculomotor system, as in heterophoria or strabismus.
See **test, motility**.

Imbert–Fick law See **law, Imbert–Fick**.

immersion lens See **lens, immersion**.

immune system See **system, immune**.

immunosuppressants Drugs that prevent or reduce the immune response. They are used in the treatment of a variety of severe inflammations such as uveitis, scleritis, keratoconjunctivitis sicca, Behçet's syndrome, Wegener's granulomatosis, sympathetic ophthalmia, and to prevent corneal graft rejection. They include the corticosteroids (e.g. prednisolone), ciclosporin (cyclosporine), tacrolimus and cytotoxic agents (e.g. azathioprine, chlorambucil, cyclophosphamide, methotrexate). It must be noted that immunosuppressants render the patient more susceptible to infection because immunity is reduced.

implant, intraocular lens (IOL) See **lens, intraocular**.

implant, orbital See **orbital implant**.

impression cytology See **cytology, impression**.

impression, eye See **eye impression**.

impression tonometer See **tonometer, impression**.

inadequate stimulus See **stimulus, adequate**.

incandescence Emission of visible radiation by thermal excitation (CIE).
See **lamp, incandescent electric; luminescence**.

incidence 1. The intersection of a ray of light with an optical surface. 2. The number of new cases of a specific disease or condition occurring during a specific period of time (e.g. 1 year) divided by the population at risk during that period. *Example*: The incidence of keratoconus in Olmsted County, Minnesota, was found to be 2 cases per 100 000 population a year.
See **prevalence**.

incidence, angle of See **angle of incidence**.

incidence, plane of See **plane of incidence**.

incident ray See **ray, incident**.

Table I3 Refractive indices of some transparent media at selected wavelengths

Spectral line	G	F	D	C	A
Origin	calcium	hydrogen	sodium	hydrogen	oxygen
Wavelength (nm)	430.8	486.1	589.3	656.3	759.4
Aqueous or vitreous humour	1.3440	1.3404	1.3360	1.3341	1.3317
Crystalline lens	1.4307	1.4259	1.4200	1.4175	1.4144
Spectacle crown	1.5348	1.5293	1.5230	1.5204	1.5163
Dense flint	1.6397	1.6290	1.6170	1.6122	1.6062

incision A surgical cut made into a tissue or organ. *Example*: goniotomy.
See excision.

inclusion conjunctivitis See conjunctivitis, adult inclusion.

incoherent See coherent sources.

incomitance Condition in which the manifest or latent angle of deviation of the lines of sight of the two eyes differs according to which eye is fixating or in which direction the eyes are looking. This condition is usually attributed to a paresis or paralysis of one or more of the extraocular muscles. *Syn.* non-concomitance.
See anisophoria; concomitance; pattern, alphabet; strabismus, incomitant; strabismus, paralytic.

incongruity, retinal See retinal correspondence, abnormal.

incongruous diplopia; hemianopia; scotoma See under the nouns.

incontinenta pigmenti A rare, X-linked, dominant, inherited disorder characterized by pigmented lesions of the skin in bizarre configurations on the trunk and limbs. Ocular manifestations include tractional retinal detachment and occasionally cataract. *Syn.* Bloch-Sulzberger syndrome.

incyclophoria See cyclophoria.

incyclotorsion See cyclotorsion; torsion.

incyclotropia See cyclotropia.

incyclovergence See excyclovergence.

indentation, scleral See scleral indentation.

indentation tonometer See tonometer, impression.

indentor See indentation, scleral.

index case See proband.

index myopia See myopia, lenticular.

index of refraction The ratio of the speed of light in a vacuum or in air, c, to the speed of light in a given medium, v. *Symbol*: n. Hence,

$$n = c/v$$

The speed of light in a given medium depends upon its wavelength. Consequently, the index of refraction varies accordingly, being greater for short wavelengths (blue) than for longer wavelengths (red). The index of refraction forms the basis of

Table I4 Index of refraction n of various media for sodium light ($\lambda = 589.3$)

air	1.00
water (at 20°C)	1.333
spectacle crown glass	1.523
flint glass (dense)	1.62
flint glass (extra dense)	1.65–1.70
titanium oxide glass	1.701
diamond	2.42
Canada balsam	1.53–1.54
CR-39	1.498
Polycarbonate	1.586
silicone rubber	1.44
CAB	1.47
PMMA	1.49
HEMA	1.43
Calcite Crystal	
ordinary ray	1.658
extraordinary ray	1.486
Quartz Crystal	
ordinary ray	1.544
extraordinary ray	1553
Hydrogel Polymer	
20% water content	1.46–1.48
75% water content	1.37–1.38
Eye	
tears	1.336
cornea	1.376
aqueous humour	1.336
crystalline lens (average effect)	1.42
vitreous humour	1.336

Snell's law, which quantitatively determines the deviation of light rays traversing a surface separating two media of different refractive indices (Tables I3 and I4). *Syn.* refractive index. *Plural*: indices.
See dispersion; law of refraction; lens, gradient-index; lens, high index; light, speed of; refractometer.

index of refraction, absolute The ratio of the speed of light in a **vacuum** to the speed of light in a given medium.

index of refraction, relative The ratio of the speed of light in air (or other medium of reference) to the speed of light in a given medium.

indigo The hue evoked by stimulation of the normal eye by light of wavelengths around 430 to 460 nm that is between blue and violet.
See spectrum, electromagnetic.

indirect ophthalmoscope *See* ophthalmoscope, indirect.

indirect vision *See* vision, peripheral.

indocyanine green A dye used in angiography with an excitation peak of about 810 nm and emission at about 830 nm when illuminated in infrared light. It provides better resolution of the choroidal circulation than fluorescein.
See angiography, fluorescein.

indomethacin *See* antiinflammatory drug.

induced astigmatism *See* astigmatism, induced.

induced prism *See* prism, induced.

induction The production of an effect by indirect or asynchronized stimulation.
colour i. The modification or generation of colour perception without direct stimulation of the corresponding cones.
See after-image; Benham's top; Bidwell's ghost.
spatial i. Modification of perception as a result of a simultaneous stimulation in another part of the visual field.
See summation.
temporal i. Modification of perception as a result of a previous stimulus and in some cases a delayed stimulus, as in metacontrast.
See summation.

industrial vision *See* vision, industrial.

infantile esotropia syndrome *See* esotropia, infantile.

infantile glaucoma *See* glaucoma, congenital.

infection An invasion of the body by disease-producing microorganisms (e.g. bacteria, virus, fungus, parasite). Treatment typically includes antiinfective drugs, such as antibiotic, antifungal or antiviral agents.
See inflammation.

inferior oblique muscle; orbital fissure; rectus muscle *See* under the nouns.

inferior tarsal muscle *See* muscle, Muller's palpebral.

infinity, optical In optics, it is the region from which a point on an object sends rays of light which are considered to be parallel onto an optical system. Consequently, it forms a clear image in the focal plane of that system. In clinical optometry, 6 metres is usually regarded as infinity.

inflammation A complex reaction that occurs in response to injury, infection, irritation, toxicity or hypersensitivity. The reaction is characterized by redness, heat, pain and swelling to different degrees. Treatment depends on the cause.
See antiinflammatory drug; cell, mast; infection.

infraduction *See* depression.

infranuclear Situated under a nucleus. In ocular anatomy, it refers to nerve fibres situated below the abducens, oculomotor or trochlear cranial nerve nuclei.

infraorbital canal *See* canal, infraorbital.

Table I5 Divisions of the infrared spectrum	
IR-A (near)	780–1400 nm
IR-B (middle)	1400–3000 nm
IR-C (far)	3000–1 000 000 nm

infrared (IR) Radiant energy of wavelengths between the extreme red wavelengths of the visible spectrum and a wavelength of a few millimetres. The wave band comprising radiations between 780 and 1400 nm is referred to as **IR-A**. Excessive exposure to these radiations can cause visual loss (e.g. eclipse blindness) and cataract. The waveband comprising radiations between 1400 and 3000 nm is referred to as **IR-B**. Excessive exposure to these radiations can cause cataract and corneal opacity. The wave band comprising radiations between 3000 and 1×10^6 nm (or 1 mm) is referred to as **IR-C**. Excessive exposure to these radiations can cause cataract (heat-ray cataract) (Table I5).
See blindness, eclipse; lens, absorptive; optometer, infrared.

infravergence Movement of one eye downward relative to the other. *Syn.* deorsumvergence.
See supravergence; vergence.

infraversion *See* version.

inheritance The acquisition of traits, characteristics and disorders from parents to their children by transmission of genetic information. Genes come in pairs: one originating from the father, the other from the mother. If an individual presents only the hereditary characteristics determined by one gene of the pair on an autosomal chromosome, that gene is called **dominant**. Conditions caused by such genes are said to show **autosomal dominant inheritance**. For instance, for a rare autosomal dominant disease, if one parent is affected, then on average about 50% of their children will also be affected irrespective of the children's sex. *Examples*: Marfan's syndrome, congenital stationary night blindness, neurofibromatosis 1 and 2, von Hippel–Lindau disease. If the individual does not present the hereditary characteristics unless both genes in a pair are of the same type, then the gene is called **recessive**. Conditions caused by such genes are said to **show autosomal recessive inheritance**. For a rare autosomal recessive disease, if a child is affected, then on average about 25% of their siblings will also be affected, irrespective of their sex. *Examples*: Laurence–Moon–Bardet–Biedl syndrome, Tay–Sachs disease, oculocutaneous albinism, galactokinase deficiency. Thirdly, inheritance may be controlled by genes on one of the sex chromosomes, most often the X chromosome. A recessive mutation on the single X chromosome carried by a male will cause a disease, whereas in the female a recessive X chromosome mutation would have to be carried on both of her X chromosomes. Therefore, in **X-linked recessive inheritance (sex-linked recessive inheritance)**, males are affected more

often than females. *Examples*: colour blindness, ocular albinism, choroideremia. A fourth type of inheritance considered in ophthalmic practice is **mitochondrial (maternal) inheritance** in which the inheritance of a trait encoded in the mitochondrial DNA is transmitted through the female line (mother-to-son or mother-to-daughter). *Examples*: Leber's hereditary optic neuropathy; Kearns–Sayre syndrome.
See **acquired; chromosome; colour vision, defective; gene; hereditary.**

inhibition, lateral Action of one neuron (e.g. in the retina) on the neighbouring neuron, the effect of which is to depress or prevent activity in the latter. This mechanism accounts for the increased contrast perception observed at the border of a black and white pattern. In the retina, this is produced by the lateral connections of the amacrine and horizontal cells that interconnect the various retinal cells. *Syn.* lateral antagonism.
See **field, receptive; Hering–Hermann grid; Mach's bands.**

injection 1. A state of visible hyperaemia due to dilatation and engorgement of the small blood vessels. **2.** The act of introducing a drug into the body.
ciliary i. Redness (almost lilac) around the limbus of the eye caused by dilatation of the deeper small blood vessels located around the cornea. It occurs in inflammation of the cornea, iris and ciliary body, and in angle-closure glaucoma. Each of these conditions is associated with loss of vision and usually pain. *Syn.* ciliary flush.
See **decongestant, ocular; eye, red; plexus, pericorneal.**
conjunctival i. Redness (bright red or pink) of the conjunctiva fading towards the limbus due to dilatation of the superficial conjunctival blood vessels occurring in conjunctival inflammations. There is no loss of vision but ocular discomfort and no pain.
See **decongestant, ocular; eye, red; plexus, pericorneal.**
intravitreal i. Injection into the eye posterior to the limbus and directed towards the vitreous. It may be given to administer medication, (e.g. corticosteroids), an antiviral agent (e.g. ganciclovir) in extremely severe ocular inflammations usually of a purulent nature, to inject antibiotics (e.g. amikacin, ceftazidime, vancomycin) immediately after vitrectomy or to inject anti-VEGF drugs in the treatment of wet age-related macular degeneration.
See **anti-VEGF drugs.**
peribulbar i. Injection of a local anaesthetic (e.g. bupivacaine, lidocaine, procaine) around the globe (either single or multiple injections) to produce anaesthesia of the globe and periocular tissues, as well as paralysis of the extraocular muscles (akinesia). Peribulbar injection may also be given to administer medication (e.g. corticosteroids) in posterior segment inflammation. *Syn.* peribulbar block.
retrobulbar i. Injection of a local anaesthetic into the muscle cone behind the eye to produce anaesthesia of the globe and periocular tissues, as well as paralysis of the extraocular muscles (akinesia). It is used less commonly than peribulbar block. *Syn.* retrobulbar block.
subconjunctival i. A method of administering medication (e.g. antibiotics, corticosteroids, mydriatics) postoperatively or in acute anterior segment inflammations. An area of conjunctiva away from the limbus is lifted to form a bleb and an injection is made into it.
sub-Tenon's i. Injection of a local anaesthetic near or beyond the equator using a cannula, which has been inserted under the conjunctiva and Tenon's capsule a few millimetres from the limbus and slid posteriorly to produce anaesthesia of the globe as well as paralysis of the extraocular muscles (akinesia). A sub-Tenon's injection may also be given to administer medication (e.g. corticosteroids) in posterior segment inflammation.

injury *See* **irrigation.**

inner nuclear layer; plexiform layer *See* **retina.**

innervation The supply of nerves to an organ or body part (e.g. the cornea).
See **keratopathy, neurotrophic.**

innervation, reciprocal *See* **law of reciprocal innervation, Sherrington's.**

in phase *See* **phase.**

insertion *See* **muscle, extraocular.**

inside-out test for soft contact lens *See* **test, inside-out.**

instability, binocular A condition in which there is a difficulty in the maintenance of clear single binocular vision. The patient tends to lose the line of text while reading or there is an apparent movement of the text. Clinical features include reduced fusional reserve, unstable heterophoria and unequal visual acuities.
See **convergence, relative.**

Intacs Trade name of an intracorneal implant consisting of two tiny half-ring segments which are inserted into the cornea to reshape its curvature and correct ametropia. The method is presently used to flatten the cornea by a given amount (the thicker the ring segments, the flatter the cornea) to correct low myopia. It is an outpatient procedure carried out under local anaesthesia, takes less than half an hour and is reversible. The ring segments are made of clear biocompatible plastic inserted into the stroma and around the optical zone of the cornea.

integration, visual Term referring to the integration occurring in the brain to give us a final percept, presumably in the prefrontal cortex. Information from the dorsal (parietal or medial temporal) stream dealing with localization or movement is integrated with information from the ventral (inferotemporal) stream dealing with colour or form, so that, for example, we can see a red car moving towards us.

intensity, luminous *See* **luminous intensity.**

intercilium *See* **glabella.**

interface, optical A plane or surface forming a common boundary between two optical media of different refractive indices.

interference Modification of light intensity arising from the joint effects of two or more coherent trains of light waves superimposed at the same point in space and arriving at the same instant. The waves may either reinforce each other, being in phase (**constructive interference**), or cancel each other, being out of phase (**destructive interference**). *See* **coherent sources; experiment, Young's; holography; phase; tomography, optical coherence.**

interference filter *See* **filter, interference.**

interference fringes The alternate light and dark bands produced when two or more coherent rays of light are superimposed on a surface. *See* **Fresnel's bi-prism.**

interferometer **1.** Instrument designed to measure the wavelength of light, the refractive index of a medium, as well as the flatness, thickness, the quality of optical surfaces, etc. The interferometer is based on the phenomenon of interference between two coherent beams of light. The **Michelson interferometer** is a common instrument in which infrared light from a laser source is divided into two beams by partial reflection from a semisilvered mirror (beam splitter) and after reflection from two plane mirrors is recombined to form interference fringes. This principle is used in some commercial instruments. **2.** Name given to several types of clinical maxwellian view systems used to measure visual acuity. *See* **biometry of the eye; maxwellian view system, clinical.**

interferometer, partial coherence A technique used to measure ocular dimensions. It consists of a laser source of infrared light ($\lambda = 780$ nm) directed into the eye via a Michelson-type interferometer, which produces a coaxial dual beam. One of the two components of this dual light beam is delayed with respect to the other by having the plane mirror reflect it at a slightly different distance from the source than the other reflected beam. These components are reflected by several intraocular interfaces. For the axial length, the reflection sites are the cornea and the retinal pigment epithelium. When the delay of the two light beams equals an intraocular distance such as the axial length, an interference signal is detected by the photodetector. The principle is used in some instruments in conjunction with keratometry and Scheimpflug imaging to obtain measurements of anterior chamber depth, lens thickness and corneal curvature including software for the calculation of intraocular lens power. It is not appropriate for eyes with dense cataract or severe corneal oedema. *See* **biometry of the eye; SRK.**

intermittent strabismus *See* **strabismus, intermittent.**

intermuscular membrane *See* **membrane, intermuscular.**

internal hordeolum; ophthalmoplegia *See* under the nouns.

internal limiting membrane *See* **membrane of the retina, internal limiting.**

internal rectus muscle *See* **muscle, medial rectus; muscle, extraocular.**

interneuron *See* **neuron.**

internuclear ophthalmoplegia *See* **ophthalmoplegia, internuclear.**

interocular Situated between the eyes.

interocular distance *See* **distance, interocular.**

interocular transfer Refers to a change in threshold in one eye which had been occluded, similar to, but of lower magnitude, than that in the fixating eye in response to a visual stimulation. *Example*: an elevation of contrast threshold with both eyes following adaptation to high contrast gratings of a given spatial frequency in one eye. The presence of interocular transfer indicates the existence of binocular cortical neurons.

interpalpebral fissure *See* **aperture, palpebral.**

interposition *See* **perception, depth.**

interpupillary distance *See* **distance, interpupillary.**

interpupillometer *See* **pupillometer.**

interstitial keratitis *See* **keratitis, interstitial.**

intertrabecular spaces *See* **meshwork, trabecular.**

interval, astigmatic; focal *See* **Sturm, interval of.**

interval, photochromatic Range of low luminances between the absolute threshold of light perception and the threshold of hue. The length of this interval varies with wavelength, being nearly nil around 650 nm (Fig. I15). *Syn.* achromatic interval. *See* **Purkinje shift; theory, duplicity.**

interval of Sturm *See* **Sturm, interval of.**

intorsion *See* **torsion.**

intracapsular cataract extraction *See* **cataract extraction, intracapsular.**

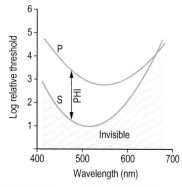

Fig. I15 Photochromatic interval, PHI (P, curve of the threshold of hue; S, curve of the absolute threshold of light).

intraocular Within the eye.

intraocular lens implant *See* lens, intraocular.

intraocular muscles; pressure *See* under the nouns.

intravitreal injection *See* injection, intravitreal.

intrinsic light *See* light, idioretinal.

intrinsic muscles *See* muscle, intraocular.

inverse square law of illumination *See* law of illumination, inverse square.

inverted retina *See* retina, inverted.

involuntary eye movements *See* movement, fixation.

in vitro Term referring to a measurement or a process taking place in a test tube. *Example*: the measurement of the cholesterol content of the crystalline lens done in a test tube.

in vivo Term referring to a measurement or a process taking place in the living body. *Example*: the effect of a contact lens on the cornea.

invisible spectrum *See* spectrum, invisible.

involutional ectropion; entropion *See* under the nouns.

iodine-povidone An antiseptic substance consisting of a combination of iodine with povidone (a water-soluble polymer) used to sterilize the skin and conjunctiva prior to eye surgery to prevent the possible development of endophthalmitis. Application on the skin stains it dark-brown, and an eyedrop instilled into the conjunctival sac gives the eye a reddish-brown tinge. *See* endophthalmitis.

iodopsin A photosensitive pigment found in the retinal cones of the chicken, fishes and many vertebrates. Its maximum absorption is around 562 nm.

ipsilateral Pertaining to the same side of the body. *Example*: The right lateral rectus muscle is the ipsilateral antagonist of the right medial rectus muscle. *See* bilateral; contralateral; geniculate body, lateral; unilateral.

iridaemia Haemorrhage from the iris. *Note*: also spelt iridemia.

iridectomy The surgical removal of part of the iris. The main reasons for iridectomy are to reduce the intraocular pressure, to enlarge an abnormally small pupil, to excise an iris tumour and, in cataract extraction, to prevent possible blockage of the angle of the anterior chamber. Nowadays, **laser iridotomy** is preferred in the treatment of angle-closure glaucoma because the incision obtained by this technique can be carried out as an outpatient procedure with only topical anaesthesia, although the cornea must not be hazy (Fig. I16). *See* **iridotomy.**

irideremia Absence of all or part of the iris. Strictly speaking, a total absence of the iris is called aniridia. *See* **aniridia.**

iridescent Presenting a rainbow-like play of colours as in soap bubbles.

iridiagnosis *See* iridodiagnosis.

iridis rubeosis *See* rubeosis iridis.

iridocorneal angle *See* angle of the anterior chamber.

iridocorneal endothelial syndrome *See* syndrome, ICE.

iridocyclitis Inflammation of both iris and ciliary body. The ciliary body is almost always involved with an inflammation of the iris. The clinical picture of iridocyclitis is practically the same as iritis. The condition is often associated with ankylosing spondylitis or sarcoidosis. *See* **anisocoria; arthritis, rheumatoid; heterochromia; syndrome, Behçet's; uveitis.**

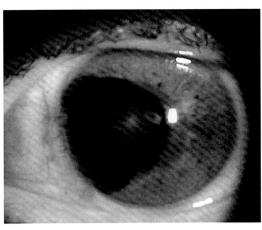

Fig. I16 Large sector iridectomy, which has been performed to excise an iris melanoma. (From Millodot et al 2006, with permission of Blackwell Publishing)

iridocyclitis, Fuchs' heterochromic A chronic, idiopathic, non-granulomatous anterior uveitis characterized by heterochromia, often complicated by cataract which then leads to blurred vision, the main complaint. It is occasionally bilateral; in this case, there is no heterochromia. The condition occurs in about 4% of all cases of uveitis. Keratic precipitates are usually present, being small, round or stellate, grey-white in colour and scattered throughout the posterior surface of the cornea. They do not conglomerate or become pigmented, and filaments may be seen in between them. Iris nodules on the edge of the pupil are common, and glaucoma may develop. Treatment may involve topical steroids as well as cataract or glaucoma therapy. *Syn.* Fuchs' uveitis syndrome; Fuchs' heterochromic cyclitis; heterochromatic iridocyclitis. *See* **keratic precipitates.**

iridodiagnosis Diagnosis of systemic diseases through observation of changes in form and colour of the iris. The validity of this method is questionable. *Syn.* iridiagnosis. *See* **iridology.**

iridodialysis A tearing away (dehiscence) of the iris from its attachment to the ciliary body. It can be seen as a dark area near the limbus and may lead to diplopia. It usually occurs as a result of blunt trauma to the eye.

iridology The study of the iris (colour, shape, etc.), normal and abnormal. *See* **iridodiagnosis.**

iridodonesis A tremulous condition of the iris. It usually occurs in aphakic eyes, when the eye is subluxated or when there has been an injury to the eye. *Syn.* tremulous iris. *See* **luxation of the lens; phacodonesis.**

iridoplasty, laser A procedure performed to widen the angle of the anterior chamber by shrinking the peripheral iris. It is most commonly used in the treatment of iris plateau, but it may also be used in acute angle-closure glaucoma.

iridoplegia Paralysis of the sphincter muscle of the iris resulting in a dilated pupil. The iridoplegia can be partial as in Argyll Robertson pupil or complete in which case the pupil does not react to light or to a near object. It may be due to trauma, drugs (e.g. cocaine instilled in the eye) or a systemic disease (e.g. neurosyphilis).

iridoschisis A condition in which the anterior stroma of the iris atrophies and separates from the posterior layer. It mostly affects the inferior iris in elderly patients. In advanced cases, the ruptured anterior fibres float in the aqueous humour. It commonly accompanies angle-closure glaucoma.

iridotomy Creation of an opening in the iris to allow aqueous humour to flow from the posterior to the anterior chamber. It is commonly performed with a neodymium-YAG or argon laser (**laser iridotomy**) in angle-closure glaucoma, especially that caused by pupillary block. *See* **iridectomy; pupillary block.**

iris The anterior part of the vascular tunic of the eye, which is situated in front of the crystalline lens and behind the cornea. It has the shape of a circular membrane (about 12 mm in diameter) with a perforation in the centre (the **pupil**) and is attached peripherally to the ciliary body. The iris forms a curtain dividing the space between the cornea and the lens into the **anterior** and **posterior chambers** of the eye. The anterior surface of the iris is divided into two portions: the largest peripheral **ciliary zone** and the inner **pupillary zone**. The two zones are separated by a zigzag line, the **collarette**. The iris consists of four layers which are, starting in the front: (1) the layer of fibrocytes and melanocytes; (2) the stroma in which are embedded the following structures: (a) the **sphincter pupillae muscle** which constricts the pupil and is supplied mainly by parasympathetic fibres via the third cranial nerve, (b) the vessels which form the bulk of the iris, and (c) the pigment cells; (3) the posterior membrane consisting of plain muscle fibres which constitute the **dilator muscle** which is supplied mainly by sympathetic motor fibres, via the long ciliary nerves; and (4) the posterior epithelium which is highly pigmented.

Sensory fibres from the iris are contained in the nasociliary branch of the ophthalmic nerve. The blood supply is provided by the ciliary arteries. The colour of the iris is blue in babies belonging to the white races and changes colour after a few months of life as pigment is deposited in the anterior limiting layer and the stroma. Iris colour is caused by variants of the OCA2 gene. Iris patterns are unique for each individual and can be used as a type of identification. The function of the iris and pupil is to regulate the amount of light admitted into the eye, to optimize the depth of focus and to mitigate ocular aberrations. *Plural*: irides. *See* **cell, clump; corectopia; Fig. C13 p. 63; Fuchs, crypts of; heterochromia; inheritance; iridectomy; iridodialysis; iridology; iritis; melanin; melanoma, iris; membrane, pupillary; polycoria; reflex, pupil light; rubeosis iridis.**

iris bombé A condition occurring in posterior annular synechia in which an increase of aqueous humour contained in the posterior chamber causes a forward bulging of the iris. It may provoke an attack of angle-closure glaucoma as the iris may block the drainage angle (Fig. I17).

iris coloboma; melanoma; naevus; nodules *See* under the nouns.

iris naevus syndrome *See* **syndrome, Cogan–Reese.**

iris neovascularization *See* **neovascularization, iris.**

iris, plateau An anatomical anomaly in which the iris lies in a plane rather than bulging anteriorly. This is due to the fact that the **root** (or **ciliary margin**) of the iris is inserted more anteriorly into the ciliary body than is usual. On dilatation of the pupil, the peripheral iris expands against

Table I6   Differential diagnosis* between acute conjunctivitis, acute iritis and angle-closure glaucoma

	Acute conjunctivitis	Acute iritis (anterior uveitis)	Acute angle-closure glaucoma
Signs			
injection	conjunctival	ciliary	conjunctival and ciliary
pupil	normal	contracted	semi-dilated and fixed
intraocular pressure	normal	normal or low, occasionally increased	high
cornea	normal	KP	oedematous
anterior chamber	normal depth	normal depth, aqueous flare	shallow
iris	normal	faded	faded
view of fundus	clear	misty	almost invisible
Symptoms			
pain	irritation	moderate to severe	very severe and radiating
photophobia	slight	marked	slight
lacrimation	watery, purulent or mucopurulent	watery	watery
vision	normal	slightly reduced	much reduced, haloes
onset	gradual	rapid	sudden
systemic complications	none	malaise or fever	nausea and vomiting

*This is a guide, as individual cases vary according to the cause and severity of the disease. KP, keratic precipitates

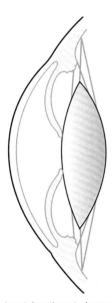

Fig. I17 Iris bombé and posterior synechia.

the trabecular meshwork. It can predispose the eye to angle-closure glaucoma. Iridotomy or laser iridoplasty is commonly performed in iris plateau, but if the angle closure persists, the condition is then referred to as **plateau iris syndrome**. *Syn.* plateau iris.
See **iridotomy; iridoplasty, laser.**

iris processes Fine bands of tissue extending from the anterior surface of the iris, bridging the angle of the anterior chamber from the root of the iris to the scleral spur or more often to the trabecular meshwork into which they usually merge. The processes are found in only about half of the population.

iris, prolapse of the Protrusion of a portion of the iris into a corneal wound. It results from either trauma, a severe corneal ulcer or an operation. In some cases, an anterior synechia may develop as the iris remains fixed in the wound by scar tissue.

iris root *See* **iris, plateau.**

iris sphincter *See* **iris.**

iris, tremulous *See* **iridodonesis.**

iritis Inflammation of the iris. The acute form is usually characterized by pain, photophobia, ciliary injection, exudates in the anterior chamber (aqueous flare), keratic precipitates, oedema, constricted and sluggish pupil, discoloration of the iris, posterior synechia, lacrimation and loss of vision. In some cases, there may be hypopyon and an increase in intraocular pressure due to blocking of the angle of the anterior chamber. Iritis is most often associated with cyclitis (anterior uveitis). The majority of cases are idiopathic or the result of trauma or medication. Treatment includes mydriatics (to prevent synechia) and topical corticosteroid drops. It is essential to differentiate acute iritis from angle-closure glaucoma because of the possible harm of using a mydriatic in the latter (Table I6). *See* **iridocyclitis; photophobia; syndrome, Fuchs';** **uveitis.**

Irlen lens; syndrome *See* **syndrome, Meares–Irlen.**

iron deposits *See* **line, iron; siderosis.**

irradiation 1. Application of electromagnetic radiations to an object. **2.** A phenomenon in which a bright area against a black background appears larger than a darker area of equal size against the same background. *Syn.* Helmholtz illusion.

irregular astigmatism *See* astigmatism, irregular.

irrigation The act of washing or cleansing a cavity or a surface with a stream of water or other solution (e.g. physiological saline) as in chemical or thermal burns or other superficial injuries to the eye, or to dislodge small foreign bodies on the cornea or in the conjunctival sac.
See **corneal abrasion; dilation and irrigation; eversion, lid.**

Irvine–Gass syndrome *See* oedema, cystoid macular.

ischaemia Insufficient blood supply for the need of a part of the body, usually as a result of a disease of the blood vessels supplying that part. It may occasionally affect the anterior segment of the eye, especially in the elderly and present as a dull ache. *Note*: also spelt ischemia.
See **syndrome, ischaemic ocular.**

ischaemia of the retina Lack of blood in the retina due either to arterial narrowing or profuse haemorrhage from any part of the body.
See **arteritis, giant cell.**

ischaemic optic neuropathy; ocular syndrome *See* under the nouns.

iseikonia Condition in which the size and shape of the ocular images of the two eyes are equal, as distinguished from aniseikonia.

iseikonic lens *See* lens, aniseikonic.

Ishihara test *See* plates, pseudoisochromatic.

island of vision A description of the visual field as a three-dimensional hill surrounded by a sea of darkness. Stimuli that fall within the island can be seen, whereas stimuli that fall outside the island cannot be seen. The height of the island represents the sensitivity of the eye with the highest acuity at the top of the hill corresponding to foveal vision and declining progressively towards the periphery (when the eye is light-adapted) (Fig. I18). *Syn.* hill of vision.
See **field, visual.**

isoacuity area 1. An area surrounding the fixation point in which visual acuity is approximately constant. The width of this area varies with the test target, being smallest with resolution of two dots and largest with Landolt rings or gratings. **2.** An area of the visual field in which visual acuity is more or less constant.

isoametropia Condition in which the ametropia is similar in the two eyes. *Syn.* isometropia.

isoametropic amblyopia *See* amblyopia.

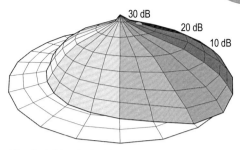

Fig. I18 Island of vision. The sensitivity declines more steeply in the nasal field than in the temporal field. The peak represents foveal vision. (From Rosenfield and Logan 2009, with permission of Butterworth-Heinemann)

isochromatic Possessing the same colour.

isocoria Having two pupils of equal size.
See **anisocoria.**

isoluminant Possessing the same luminance. *Example*: red and green bars of a grating which have the same luminance. If such a grating is moving sideways, many observers will barely perceive its motion or fail to notice it altogether. *Syn.* equiluminant.

isomerization A process occurring in the disc membranes of photoreceptors in which the energy of incident photons raises the energy level in the retinal molecule to such a degree that it changes its shape from the 11-*cis* isomer to the all-*trans* isomer of retinal. This process in which light activates rhodopsin is designated as R → R*. The photopigment is then bleached. This is the initiating step of the visual process.
See **bleaching; rhodopsin; transduction.**

isometropia *See* isoametropia.

isophoria Constancy of the heterophoria in various directions of gaze.
See **heterophoria.**

isopia Identical vision in the two eyes.

isopter In the determination of visual fields, it is the contour line representing the limits of equal retinal sensitivity to a given test target.
See **field, visual; perimeter.**

isotonic solution *See* solution, isotonic.

isotropic Having the same properties of refraction in all directions.
See **anisotropic; birefringence.**

itraconazole *See* antifungal agent.

ivermectin *See* onchocerciasis.

J

J *See* Jaeger test types.

jack-in-the-box phenomenon *See* phenomenon, jack-in-the-box.

Jackson's crossed cylinder test *See* lens, cross-cylinder; test for astigmatism, cross-cylinder.

Jaeger test types Test types for measuring visual acuity at near. They consist of ordinary printers' types of various sizes and are arranged as words and phrases. Depending on the size of test types read, acuity is recorded as J.1, J.2 in ascending size up to J.20. The smallest Jaeger (J.1) subtends an angle of 5' at 450 mm from the eye (Table J1). *See* acuity, near visual.

Jannelli clip *See* clipover.

Javal's grid *See* grid, Javal's.

Javal's method *See* method, Javal's.

Javal's rule *See* rule, Javal's.

Javal–Schiotz keratometer *See* keratometer, Javal–Schiotz.

jaw-winking phenomenon *See* phenomenon, jaw-winking.

Table J1 Approximate relationship between the Jaeger system, the point system (or N notation) and the Snellen equivalent

		Snellen equivalent at 40 cm	
Jaeger	Point	(m)	(ft)
1	3.5	6/7	20/23
2	4.5	6/8	20/27
3	5.5	6/11	20/37
4	6.5	6/13	20/43
5	7.5	6/14	20/47
6	8	6/15	20/50
7	9.5	6/17	20/57
8	11	6/20	20/67
9	12	6/24	20/80
10	13	6/26	20/87
11	14	6/28	20/93
12	16	6/30	20/100
13	18	6/36	20/120
14	22	6/45	20/150

Jensen's procedure *See* transposition.

jerk nystagmus *See* nystagmus.

jnd *See* threshold, differential.

joint *See* hinge.

Jones' procedure *See* procedure, Jones'.

Jones I test *See* test, Jones I.

Jones II test *See* test, Jones II.

Joubert's syndrome *See* syndrome, Joubert's.

Julesz random-dot stereogram *See* stereogram, random-dot.

jump The displacement of the image of an object occurring when viewing across the borderline between two portions of different power in a bifocal or trifocal lens. The jump is eliminated by placing the optical centres on the dividing line; the lens is then called a **no jump** bifocal (e.g. a monocentric bifocal with a straight dividing line) (Fig. J1). *Syn.* image jump; prismatic jump. *See* monocentric.

just noticeable difference *See* threshold, difference.

juvenile epithelial corneal dystrophy *See* dystrophy, Meesmann's.

juvenile glaucoma *See* glaucoma, congenital.

juvenile retinoschisis *See* retinoschisis.

juvenile idiopathic arthritis *See* arthritis, juvenile idiopathic.

juvenile xanthogranuloma *See* xanthogranuloma, juvenile.

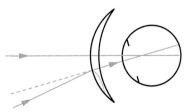

Fig. J1 Image jump upward caused by the segment of a bifocal lens, as the direction of gaze is lowered across the dividing line.

K

Kanizsa figure *See* figure, Kanizsa.

kataphoria 1. A tendency of the visual axes of both eyes to deviate below the horizontal plane in the absence of a stimulus to fusion. **2.** Synonym of alternating deorsumduction. *Note*: also spelt cataphoria.
See depression; hyperphoria.

Kayser–Fleischer ring *See* ring, Kayser–Fleischer.

Kearns–Sayre syndrome *See* ophthalmoplegia, chronic progressive external.

Keith–Wagener–Barker classification *See* retinopathy, hypertensive.

Kennedy's syndrome *See* syndrome, Foster Kennedy.

Kepler telescope *See* telescope.

keratectasia *See* ectasia; staphyloma, anterior.

keratectomy, photorefractive A surgical procedure on the cornea aimed at correcting ametropia. The epithelium is completely removed over a central diameter of about 7 mm, and excimer laser ablation is then carried out on the stroma. A bandage soft contact lens is usually worn afterward for a few days while the epithelium regenerates. Complications are more common than with either LASEK or LASIK. Useful vision recovers more slowly and pain lasts longer than with the latter procedures. *Syn.* keratorefractive surgery; laser refractive keratoplasty (LRK); refractive keratoplasty.
See ectasia, corneal; keratotomy, radial; LASEK; LASIK.

keratic precipitates Cells (e.g. leukocytes) deposited on the endothelium of the cornea which occur as a result of inflammation of the iris or the ciliary body. They often collect in a triangular pattern with the base down (**Arlt's triangle**) on the inferior portion of the endothelial surface. They may also be distributed diffusely over the endothelium, as in Fuchs' heterochromic iridocyclitis or anterior uveitis, or concentrated in one area, as in disciform keratitis or herpes simplex keratitis. In granulomatous uveitis, they are larger than in non-granulomatous uveitis and greasy in appearance (called '**mutton fat**'). Following treatment of the primary cause, they usually disappear.
See cornea guttata; sarcoidosis; uveitis, acute anterior.

keratitis Inflammation of the cornea. It can arise from various sources, the most common being infection by bacteria, fungi or viruses; hypersensitivity to staphylococcal exotoxins; nutritional deficiencies; failure of the eyelids to cover the cornea; deficiencies in the precorneal tear film; contact lens wear (especially extended wear); mechanical, radiation or chemical trauma; or interruption of the ophthalmic branch of the trigeminal nerve. It is usually characterized by a dullness and loss of transparency of the cornea due to infiltrates, neovascularization or oedema and is accompanied by ciliary injection. The discomfort varies from a foreign body sensation to severe pain with lacrimation, photophobia, blepharospasm and an impairment of vision. If the condition is severe, ulcers and pus (hypopyon) will appear, and the iris and ciliary body may become involved. It is important to identify the cause and the organism to treat the condition. Keratitis of bacterial origin is treated with antibiotic drugs. Keratitis of viral origin (e.g. herpes) is treated with antiviral agents and that of fungal origin with antifungal agents.
See **corneal infiltrates; keratomalacia; keratomycosis; keratopathy.**

acanthamoeba k. A rare type of keratitis caused by the microorganism acanthamoeba, which invades the cornea. The symptoms begin with a foreign body sensation, which turns into pain, photophobia, tearing, blepharospasm and blurred vision. The signs are infiltrates that develop into a ring, and the cornea may eventually become opaque. Diagnosis of the disease is made by laboratory analysis of a corneal scraping. Contact lens wear has been found to be associated with this disease in about three-quarters of the cases, especially when the patient has used homemade or unpreserved saline. The other cases were due to contact with stagnant water or following an abraded cornea. The therapy is with repetitive doses of antiamoebic agents (e.g. biguanide) and an antibiotic (e.g. propamidine isethionate) or a combination of propamidine and neomycin. However, strict compliance with contact lens regimens and avoidance of exposure to dirty stagnant water diminish the risks of contracting the disease.
See **corneal infiltrates; disinfection; propamidine isethionate.**

actinic k. *See* **keratoconjunctivitis, actinic.**

acute epithelial k. A condition associated with herpes zoster ophthalmicus. It is characterized by small fine dendritic or stellate lesions in the peripheral cornea in association with a conjunctivitis. This keratitis usually resolves within a week.
See **herpes zoster ophthalmicus.**

acute stromal k. A complication of scleritis in which there are superficial and mid-stromal infiltrates in the limbal region. Lesions can also be noted in the central cornea and may develop vascularization and permanent opacification. In cases of scleritis that are limited (i.e. not diffuse), corneal changes are noted only in the bordering corneal region.

bacterial k. See **keratitis, microbial**.
dendritic k. See **keratitis, herpes simplex**.
disciform k. A deep localized keratitis involving the stroma and the endothelium (**endotheliitis**), usually characterized by central stromal oedema, Descemet's folds, keratic precipitates, a disc-shaped grey area (Wessley's ring) that may spread to the whole thickness of the cornea and occasionally elevated intraocular pressure. Symptoms are blurred vision, sometimes with haloes around lights, discomfort and redness. It may be due to a viral infection (e.g. herpes simplex virus or herpes simplex) or an immune reaction, or it may also occur as a sequel to trauma. It may heal without residue or may cause scarring and vascularization of the cornea. Treatment is with steroid and antiviral agents.
See **corneal clouding, central; herpes zoster ophthalmicus; keratic precipitates; ring, Wessley's**.
epithelial k. See **keratitis, punctate epithelial**.
exposure k. See **keratopathy, exposure**.
filamentary k. Keratitis characterized by the presence of strands (filaments) made up of degenerated epithelial cells and mucus deposited on the corneal surface. It can occur as a result of long-term contact lens wear, thyroid dysfunction, corneal abrasions, keratoconjunctivitis sicca, etc. Management includes lubricants, temporary bandage contact lens, preferably with a topical antibiotic and removal of the filaments.
fungal k. A keratitis caused by a fungus, such as *Fusarium*, *Aspergillus*, or *Candida albicans*. The condition may develop after eye injury (e.g. finger-nail or contact lens scratch, tree branch), especially in agricultural areas. However, it has become more common since the use of corticosteroids. It may also occur in eyes suffering from corneal disease, after keratoplasty, diabetes or extended-wear contact lenses. It is characterized by greyish-white filaments with indistinct and feathery edges infiltrating into the stroma (filamentary keratitis), and the patient complains of pain, photophobia, blurred vision and watery or mucopurulent discharge. There is ciliary and conjunctival injection, and it may be accompanied by ring abscesses and, in severe cases, hypopyon. Differential diagnosis is facilitated by corneal scraping or biopsy of the ulcer. Management consists mainly of antifungal agents. *Syn.* mycotic keratitis.
See **keratomycosis**.
herpetic k. Keratitis caused by either herpes simplex or herpes zoster viruses.
See **herpesvirus; keratitis, herpes simplex**.
herpes simplex k. An inflammation of the cornea, which occurs occasionally as a result of a blepharoconjunctivitis caused by the herpes simplex virus (usually type HSV-1) and may affect the epithelium (**epithelial keratitis**), the stroma (**stromal keratitis**) or the endothelium (**disciform keratitis** or **endotheliitis**). The disease begins with skin vesicles typically spread over the lids, conjunctiva and periorbital area. Symptoms include irritation, photophobia, tearing, reduced corneal

sensation and blurred vision if the central cornea is involved. The characteristic sign of epithelial keratitis is a **dendritic ulcer**, which enlarges progressively resulting in a configuration referred to as a geographical ulcer. Treatment is with an antiviral agent (e.g. aciclovir) or debridement of the epithelium if unresponsive to antiviral agents, usually with topical steroids. *Syn.* dendritic ulcer. See **herpesvirus; keratitis, disciform; keratitis, interstitial; keratitis, punctate epithelial; keratitis, ulcerative**.
herpes zoster k. See **herpes zoster ophthalmicus**.
hypopyon k. Purulent keratitis with ulcer resulting in the presence of pus in the anterior chamber, which gravitates to the bottom. The ulcer is a dirty grey colour and the conjunctiva is also inflamed. The usual cause of the infection is the pneumococcus which gives rise to a corneal ulcer (often called **serpiginous ulcer** because of its tendency to creep forward in the cornea).
See **hypopyon; keratitis, ulcerative; ulcer, corneal**.
interstitial k. Keratitis involving the stroma. It is characterized by deep vascularization and scarring of the cornea and is often associated with iridocyclitis. Formerly, the most common cause was congenital syphilis (**syphilitic keratitis**). However, nowadays it is usually the result of a herpes simplex or herpes zoster infection, or it may be part of a syndrome (Cogan's) or other systemic diseases (e.g. leprosy, tuberculosis). Management involves cycloplegics, topical antiviral agents and, in severe cases, corticosteroids. *Syn.* stromal interstitial keratitis.
See **herpes zoster ophthalmicus; sign, Hutchinson's**.
lagophthalmic k. See **keratopathy, exposure**.
marginal k. A condition characterized by subepithelial peripheral corneal infiltrates which may spread circumferentially and are separated from the limbus by a clear zone, which may eventually become invaded by blood vessels. It is a hypersensitivity response to staphylococcal exotoxins. There is discomfort, pain, redness and photophobia. Treatment is with topical steroids.
microbial k. A keratitis caused by a microorgan-ism such as a bacteria (e.g. *Neisseria gonorrhoeae*, *Pseudomonas aeruginosa*, *Serratia marcescens*, *Staphylococcus aureus*), amoeba (e.g. *Acan-thamoeba*) or, less commonly, a virus or fungus. The most common risk factor is disease of the cornea (e.g. bullous keratopathy) or of the lid (e.g. entropion) and contact lens wear although the incidence of the condition among contact lens wearers is relatively low. It has been estimated to be 2 to 5 individuals with daily wear of soft lenses, and 10 to 20 with extended wear of soft lenses per 10 000 per year. High oxygen permeability leads to less infection. Signs and symptoms include pain, infiltrates, redness, lacrimation, photophobia, corneal oedema, reduced vision, discharge, swollen lids and aqueous flare. The condition may have been precipitated by non-compliance,

poor hygiene, dirty lens case, etc. Immediate management is imperative as the condition could be sight-threatening. It includes cessation of lens wear and drug therapy. *Syn.* bacterial keratitis.

mucous plaque k. *See* herpes zoster ophthalmicus.

mycotic k. *See* keratitis, fungal.

necrotizing stromal k. A rare form of severe stromal keratitis caused by a virus and characterized by stromal necrosis, anterior uveitis with opacification, vascularization and scarring. It is commonly associated with uveitis. Treatment is with steroid and antiviral agents. *See* keratitis, herpes simplex; keratitis.

non-ulcerative k. *See* contact lens acute red eye.

neuroparalytic k. Keratitis caused by a failure of blinking or infrequent or incomplete blinking causing inadequate spread of tears. *See* keratopathy, exposure.

neurotrophic k. *See* keratopathy, neurotrophic.

peripheral ulcerative k. A severe form of keratitis most often associated with a systemic disease, the most common being rheumatoid arthritis, Wegener's granulomatosis, lupus erythematosus and polyarteritis nodosa. It is characterized by pain, usually redness and peripheral ulceration with corneal thinning. Treatment is urgent and directed towards the primary cause (Fig. K1). *See* ulcer, Mooren's.

phlyctenular k. *See* keratoconjunctivitis, phlyctenular.

punctate epithelial k. (PEK) An inflammation of the cornea characterized by either multiple, small, superficial, punctate lesions or minute, flat, epithelial dots resulting from bacterial infection (e.g. chlamydial, staphylococcal), vitamin B_2 deficiency, virus infection (e.g. herpes zoster) and also from exposure to ultraviolet light, injury to the eye with aerosol products or contact lens solutions or wear. The condition is usually associated with conjunctivitis. Treatment depends on the causative agent (e.g. antiviral agents will be used to suppress symptoms in herpes simplex keratitis; cessation of contact lens wear). *Syn.* superficial punctate keratitis, although this term is more often used to describe a PEK of viral origin. *See* conjunctivitis, adult inclusion; keratitis, Thygeson's superficial punctate; staining, 3 and 9 o'clock.

rosacea k. Keratitis associated with acne rosacea of the face. It is characterized by marginal vascularization at the limbus. The vessels extend into the cornea surrounded by a zone of grey infiltration. The infiltrates and vascularization are in the cornea proper and not raised above the surface (unlike phlyctens). There is little tendency to ulcerate. It is usually associated with an inflammation of the conjunctiva (**keratoconjunctivitis**). Treatment involves topical steroid drops as well as systemic antibiotic therapy. *See* acne rosacea; keratoconjunctivitis, phlyctenular.

k. sicca *See* keratoconjunctivitis sicca.

superficial punctate k. *See* keratitis, punctate epithelial.

stromal k. *See* keratitis, disciform; keratitis, herpes simplex; keratitis, interstitial.

stromal necrotizing k. *See* keratitis, necrotizing stromal.

Thygeson's superficial punctate k. A rare type of punctate epithelial keratitis. It is characterized by circular or oval greyish-white epithelial lesions commonly located centrally and slightly elevated with a cluster of granular dots. The lesions show punctate staining with fluorescein. The cause is unknown, although a virus is suspected. It gives rise to mild irritation, photophobia and slight blurring of vision. Treatment includes artificial tears, corticosteroids (but this may induce recurrence) and therapeutic soft contact lenses. Untreated, it may subside within a few years.

ulcerative k. Any keratitis in which there is an ulcer of the cornea. The cause may be bacterial

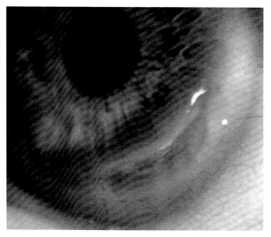

Fig. K1 Early peripheral ulcerative keratitis. (From Bowling 2016, with permission of Elsevier)

or viral infection, trauma or contact lens wear (particularly extended wear). The ulcer is a dirty grey-coloured area on the cornea, the eye is red, the pain can be severe, there is photophobia and lacrimation and vision may be affected. Immediate treatment is necessary: if due to contact lenses, cessation of wear and topical antibiotics will be used.
See **herpes zoster ophthalmicus; keratitis, herpes simplex; ulcer, corneal.**
ultraviolet k. *See* keratoconjunctivitis, actinic.

keratocele Hernia of Descemet's membrane through a hole in the cornea caused by a perforating corneal ulcer or wound.

keratocentesis Puncture of the cornea to remove aqueous humour for analysis and identification of inflammatory cell types, microbes or specific antibodies. It may also be performed to reduce intraocular pressure temporarily.

keratoconjunctivitis Inflammation of the conjunctiva and the cornea.
See **keratitis, punctate epithelial; keratitis, rosacea.**
actinic k. Inflammation of the cornea and conjunctiva caused by exposure to ultraviolet light as, for example, sun lamps, welder's arc or reflection from the snow. Both cornea and conjunctiva are usually involved, although one tissue may be more affected than the other, hence the terms 'actinic conjunctivitis' or 'actinic keratitis'. Some time after exposure (4–8 hours) to the ultraviolet radiations, the patient experiences a marked sandy feeling in the eye, lacrimation, photophobia, blepharospasm with congestion of the conjunctiva and swelling of the eyelids. The condition is usually self-limited and heals within 48 hours. Symptoms are relieved with cold compresses, firm patching and an analgesic. A local anaesthetic may sometimes be used, but this delays the regeneration of the corneal epithelium and is not usually recommended. A topical antibiotic may also be used to prevent secondary infection. Sunglasses or suitable protection may prevent the condition. *Syn.* arc eye; flash blindness; photokeratitis; photokeratoconjunctivitis; photophthalmia; snow blindness (although this is not a strictly correct synonym it is often used as such); sun lamp conjunctivitis; ultraviolet keratitis. *See* **actinic.**
atopic k. A rare but serious inflammation of the conjunctiva and the cornea caused by a reaction of the tissues to an allergen (e.g. pollen, dust mite) in which there is an exaggerated immune response. This hypersensitivity is often associated with a family history of allergic diseases, such as asthma, atopic dermatitis or eczema. Patients are usually young adults. Common signs are redness, lid eczema and small papillae found on the lower and upper tarsal conjunctiva (unlike the large papillae of vernal conjunctivitis which occur only on the upper conjunctiva). Common symptoms are itching, photophobia, a burning sensation and blurred vision if there is keratitis. The condition

may be associated with keratoconus. Treatment includes mast cell stabilizers and antihistamines and, in severe cases, corticosteroids.
See **atopy; conjunctivitis, allergic.**
epidemic k. *See* conjunctivitis, contagious.
phlyctenular k. A condition characterized by the presence of phlyctenules (nodules) on the conjunctiva, limbus or even the cornea. It is a delayed hypersensitivity response to bacterial antigens (e.g. *Staphylococcus aureus, Candida albicans, Chlamydia trachomatis*). Symptoms are soreness, lacrimation and, if the cornea is involved, photophobia. The nodules are pinkish-white on the conjunctiva surrounded by hyperaemia and greyish-white at the limbus and on the cornea. They leave a scar on the cornea (but not on the conjunctiva) when healed. The condition may resolve spontaneously, but therapy is with topical corticosteroids. It is often associated with blepharitis or bacterial conjunctivitis. *Syn.* phlyctenulosis.
k. sicca (KCS) A condition affecting the cornea and conjunctiva due to either a tear deficiency, which is divided into two categories: **Sjögren syndrome hyposecretive KCS** and **non-Sjögren syndrome hyposecretive KCS**, or to an excessive evaporation of tears (**evaporative KCS**). KCS linked to Sjögren's syndrome occurs in two forms: **primary,** in which there is KCS with xerostomia (dry mouth), and **secondary,** in which there is KCS with a systemic autoimmune connective tissue disease such as rheumatoid arthritis, systemic lupus erythematosus and systemic sclerosis. KCS without the association with Sjögren's syndrome is most commonly age-related, but some cases may be due to injury to the lacrimal tissue by tumour, inflammation (e.g. trachoma), systemic disease (e.g. cicatricial pemphigoid, sarcoidosis), systemic medications (e.g. antihistamines, antidepressants), xerophthalmia, photorefractive keratectomy, LASIK or congenital disease (e.g. congenital alacrima, Riley–Day syndrome). **Evaporative KCS** occurs due to an absence of the oily outer surface of the tear film, often as a result of meibomian gland dysfunction or blepharitis, or to abnormal lid-globe congruity, defective blinking, contact lens wear, air-conditioning environment or wind.
Common diagnostic tests are tear film break-up time test, Schirmer's test and rose bengal dye evaluation. Symptoms and signs of the various forms are similar, although they are more severe in patients who have Sjögren's syndrome. Symptoms are burning, foreign body sensation, itching, photophobia and blurred vision (due to corneal involvement). Signs are mucus discharge (plaques and filaments), decreased tear meniscus and conjunctival injection. Management includes artificial tears, corticosteroids, punctal occlusion and, in severe cases, closure of the lacrimal puncta or tarsorrhaphy. *Syn.* dry eye; keratitis sicca.
See **alacrima; cytology; impression; eye, dry; glands, meibomian; immunosuppressants; keratitis, filamentary; keratopathy, exposure; lactoferrin; occlusion, punctual; test, non-invasive break-up time.**

superior limbic k. Chronic inflammation of the superior cornea and conjunctiva. It is characterized by hyperaemia, hazy epithelium and, often, corneal filaments near the upper limbus and the adjacent conjunctiva, and with the sensations of burning, itching, photophobia and hazy vision. The condition is bilateral in 50% of cases. Detection of the disease in its mild form is difficult, as it requires lifting the upper eyelid. The condition typically affects middle-aged women with thyroid dysfunction. The aetiology of the disease is unknown, although contact lens wear may have precipitated the condition in some cases. Management involves several options: application of silver nitrate, topical medication (e.g. sodium cromoglicate), thermal cauterization of the superior bulbar conjunctiva, or occlusion of the lacrimal puncta/um to increase tear volume over the conjunctiva.
See **disease, thyroid eye.**

vernal k. *See* **conjunctivitis, vernal.**

keratoconus (KC) A developmental anomaly in which the central portion of the cornea becomes thinner and bulges forward in a cone-shaped fashion. Two types of cones are commonly described: a round cone and an oval (or sagging) cone. It usually appears around puberty, is bilateral, although one eye may be involved long before the other. Common other corneal signs may be Vogt's striae, Fleischer's ring, scarring and corneal hydrops, as well as myopia and irregular astigmatism. The condition may result from a combination of genetic and environmental factors, especially eye rubbing or atopy. It may be associated with osteogenesis imperfecta, ectopia lentis, aniridia, retinitis pigmentosa, Down's syndrome, Ehlers–Danlos syndrome, and Marfan's syndrome. The main symptom is a loss of visual acuity due to irregular astigmatism and myopia. Correction is usually best achieved with contact lenses, especially rigid gas-permeable, but if these cannot be worn or the condition is very severe, a corneal transplant is carried out (Fig. K2). Corneal collagen cross-linking has been found successful in arresting the progression and is recommended to be performed as soon as the condition is diagnosed (Table K1). *Syn.* conical cornea.
See **corneal clouding, central; corneal collagen cross-linking; corneal topography; degeneration, pellucid marginal; ectasia, corneal; hydrops, acute; keratoconjunctivitis, atopic; keratoscope; lens, combination; lens, piggyback; lenticonus; sclera, blue; sign, Munson's; sign, Rizzuti's; stria; syndrome, Ehlers–Danlos.**

keratoconus fruste Term referring to subtle irregular astigmatism or moderate to high regular astigmatism usually measured by automated corneal topography and simulating keratoconus. However, the condition is usually stationary, corneal thickness is normal and there are none of the biomicroscopic signs of keratoconus (e.g. Vogt's striae, Fleischer's ring). It may develop into manifest keratoconus.

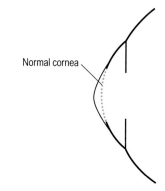

Normal cornea

Fig. K2 Schematic diagram of a keratoconus cornea.

Table K1   Differential diagnosis between keratoconus and related thinning disorders. (Adapted from Krachmer JH, Feder RS, Belin MW. *Surv Ophthalmol* 1984; 28:293–322)

	Keratoconus	Pellucid marginal degeneration	Keratoglobus	Posterior keratoconus
Frequency	most common	less common	rare	least common
Laterality	usually bilateral	bilateral	bilateral	usually unilateral
Age of onset	puberty/early adulthood	age 20 to 40s	usually at birth	birth
Corneal thinning	central or paracentral	inferior crescent-shaped band 1–2 mm wide	generalized and slightly more in periphery	paracentral posterior excavation
Protrusion	apical	above band of thinning	generalized	none
Iron line (Fleischer's ring)	common	rare	none	occasional
Scarring	common	only after hydrops	rare	common
Progression	yes	yes	usually no	no
Induced astigmatism	irregular	high, irregular and varies with location	none	very slight effect

keratoconus, posterior A steep and irregular curvature of the posterior surface of the cornea, usually forming a depression in the central or paracentral area. The anterior surface is normal and vision is rarely affected. The condition is typically congenital, non-progressive and unilateral, but some cases are associated with some ocular abnormalities, such as anterior polar cataract, lenticonus, ectopia lentis, iris atrophy, and it is often the first sign of manifest keratoconus. As the cornea is much thinner, it represents a contraindication to LASIK procedure. The majority of cases do not require treatment.
See **mesenchymal dysgenesis; videokeratoscope.**

keratocyte Main cellular element of the corneal stroma. It is a flattened dendritic cell located between the collagen lamellae with a large flattened nucleus and lengthy processes which may communicate with neighbouring cells. Keratocytes contribute to corneal transparency by regulating the production and maintenance of stromal collagen, as well as having phagocytic functions. They occupy 3% to 5% of the stromal volume. *Syn.* corneal corpuscle; corneal fibrocyte; corneal fibroblast; fixed cell.

keratoectasia *See* **ectasia, corneal.**

keratoglobus A rare, usually bilateral, protrusion of the cornea with general thinning, especially in the periphery. The condition is usually present at birth and generally does not progress. Some cases may be acquired perhaps as the end-stage of keratoconus. The diameter of the cornea is normal or slightly increased, and the intraocular pressure is normal as the condition is not associated with congenital glaucoma. Complications include perforation after minor trauma and corneal hydrops. It is sometimes associated with Leber's congenital amaurosis, Ehlers–Danlos syndrome and blue sclera (Table K1). *Syn.* macrocornea.
See **megalocornea.**

keratolysis A severe corneal disorder in which the corneal stroma melts, which may result in descemetocele or even perforation. It is believed to be due to an altered epithelial barrier, which results in inflammatory mediators entering the stroma. The condition may occur as a complication of necrotizing scleritis or a severe inflammation of the peripheral cornea, especially in patients with a severe dry eye.
See **scleritis, anterior.**

keratomalacia Vitamin A deficiency in which the cornea becomes desiccated at first and then softens and, if the deficiency is long-standing, it presents with infiltration, pannus, necrosis, and opacification and the eye may become blind. There is also a lack of reaction to inflammation leading to a destruction of the eye if infection occurs. It is part of a general systemic condition due to malnutrition. Associated with this condition are conjunctival xerosis, corneal ulceration, night blindness, faulty growth of bone and xerophthalmia.
See **hemeralopia; xerophthalmia.**

keratome A surgical instrument with a sharp edge for incising the cornea.
See **keratomileusis; LASIK.**

keratometer Optical instrument for measuring the radius of curvature of the cornea in any meridian. By measuring along the two principal meridians, corneal astigmatism can be deduced. The principle is based on the reflection by the anterior surface of a luminous pattern of **mires** in the centre of the cornea in an area of about 3.6 mm in diameter. Knowing the size of the pattern h and measuring that of the reflected image h' and the distance d between the two, the radius of curvature r of the cornea can be determined using the approximate formula.

$$r = 2d\,(h'/h)$$

In addition, a doubling system (e.g. a bi-prism) is also integrated into the instrument to mitigate the effect of eye movements, as well as a microscope to magnify the small image reflected by the cornea. The amount of doubling produced by the bi-prism is dependent on its position relative to the objective; if it is near the objective, the amount of doubling is greater than if it is farther away. There are two main types of keratometers: one in which the bi-prism is moved called variable doubling with fixed mires, and the other in which the amount of doubling is fixed but the size of the mires is altered called variable mire with fixed doubling. Moreover, some instruments require rotation to measure the second meridian (two-position) and in others this is unnecessary (one-position). The instrument is used in the fitting of contact lenses and the monitoring of corneal changes occurring as a result of contact lens wear, although corneal topography is most often replacing keratometers (Fig. K3). The range of the instrument can be extended approximately 9 D by placing a +1.25 D lens in front of the objective to measure steeper corneas. The range in the other direction can be extended by approximately 6 D using a −1.00 D lens to measure flatter corneas (Table K2). *Syn.* ophthalmometer.
See **corneal topography; fitted on K; keratoscope; lens, liquid; photokeratoscopy; prism, Wollaston; rule, Javal's; videokeratoscope.**
Javal-Schiotz k. A fixed doubling with variable mire sizes, two-position instrument. Doubling is done with a Wollaston prism. Measurement of each meridian is achieved by rotating the instrument about its optical axis.
Reichert k. A one-position variable doubling with fixed mire size. Doubling is done with two independent adjustable prisms. After focusing the mires, the measurement is made in one meridian and, after refocusing, in the second meridian (Fig. K3).

keratomileusis A surgical procedure on the cornea aimed at correcting ametropia. An anterior layer of the cornea is sliced off with a microkeratome, frozen, ground to a new curvature and sutured back in the same location. There are many complications and technical difficulties associated

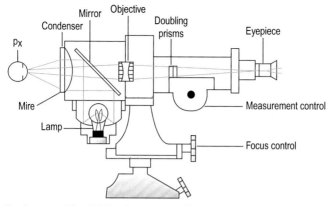

Fig. K3 Schematic diagram of the Reichert keratometer. Px, patient.

Table K2 Extended keratometer range			
with −1.00 D		**with +1.25 D**	
Actual drum reading (D)	Extended value (D)	Actual drum reading (D)	Extended value (D)
36.00	30.87	45.00	52.46
36.50	31.30	45.50	53.05
37.00	31.73	46.00	53.63
37.50	32.16	46.50	54.21
38.00	32.59	47.00	54.80
38.50	33.02	47.50	55.38
39.00	33.45	48.00	55.96
39.50	33.88	48.50	56.55
40.00	34.30	49.00	57.13
40.50	34.73	49.50	57.71
41.00	35.16	50.00	58.30
41.50	35.59	50.50	58.88
		51.00	59.46
		51.50	60.04
		52.00	60.63

with this procedure. *Syn.* refractive keratoplasty and keratorefractive surgery (both terms also include epikeratoplasty, keratophakia and radial keratotomy).
See **epikeratoplasty; Intacs; keratectomy, photorefractive; keratome; keratophakia; LASEK; LASIK.**

keratomycosis A fungus infection of the cornea, which may result in keratitis and ulceration. It is usually introduced by injury and is characterized by an ulcer, which appears as a fluffy white elevated protuberance surrounded by a shallow crater on the edge of which is a sharply demarcated halo. There is ciliary and conjunctival injection. Diagnosis is best provided by laboratory analysis of a specimen of these fungal organisms, which are obtained by scraping the base of the ulcer. *See* **keratitis, fungal; ulcer, corneal.**

keratopathy A non-inflammatory disease of the cornea. *See* **dystrophy, corneal.**

actinic k. See **keratopathy, lipid.**
aphakic bullous k. See **keratopathy, bullous.**
band k. A disorder characterized by the deposition of calcium salts in the anterior layers of the cornea, such as the basement membrane, Bowman's layer and the anterior stromal lamellae. They appear as opacities forming a more or less horizontal band with clear holes within the band giving it a Swiss cheese appearance. The causes may be systemic (e.g. hypercalcaemia, familial, old age, chronic renal failure) or ocular (e.g. chronic anterior uveitis, interstitial keratitis, silicone oil in the anterior chamber, phthisis bulbi). It is commonly associated with juvenile idiopathic arthritis and sarcoidosis. Symptoms include irritation and blurring of vision. Treatment may be necessary for cosmetic or visual reasons. It consists of removal of the calcium salts by scraping the corneal epithelium followed by irrigation with EDTA or laser keratectomy. *Syn.* band-shaped corneal dystrophy.
See **arthritis, juvenile idiopathic; ethylenediamine tetraacetic acid (EDTA).**

bullous k. Degenerative condition of the cornea characterized by the formation of epithelial blebs or bullae, which burst after a few days. This condition may follow cataract surgery (**aphakic bullous keratopathy**) or in which there is an intraocular lens implant (**pseudophakic bullous keratopathy**), corneal trauma, severe corneal oedema, glaucoma, iridocyclitis, etc. Soft contact lenses have often been found useful to relieve pain in this condition by protecting the denuded nerve endings. *See* **cornea guttata; dystrophy, Fuchs' endothelial; lens, therapeutic soft contact.**

climatic droplet k.; Labrador k. *See* **keratopathy, lipid.**

crystalline k. A rare keratopathy characterized by feathery stromal opacities without significant inflammation. It results from a bacterial infection, most frequently after penetrating keratoplasty, but also in ocular surface disease as, for example, ocular pemphigoid or Stevens–Johnson syndrome.

exposure k. A disorder caused by the failure of the eyelids to cover the globe, resulting in improper wetting of the ocular surface by the tears with consequent desiccation of the corneal epithelium. This condition may be caused by facial nerve disorders, in which the orbicularis oculi muscle is paralyzed, or sleep lagophthalmos, thyroid eye disease, proptosis or as a result of hard contact lens wear. The cornea presents punctate epithelial erosions which may develop into ulcers. Treatment is with frequent lubrication and, if severe, lid surgery (e.g. tarsorrhaphy) may be required. *Syn.* lagophthalmic keratitis; neuroparalytic keratopathy. *See* **keratitis, neuroparalytic; staining, 3 and 9 o'clock; disease, Graves'.**

lipid k. A form of corneal degeneration characterized by white or yellowish stromal deposits consisting of cholesterol, fats and phospholipids and, in some cases, corneal vascularization. The condition may be caused by exposure to sunlight (especially ultraviolet radiations) or trauma. The deposits are usually present within the pupillary area, often as elevated nodules distributed in a band-shaped configuration, and can have a dramatic effect on visual function. The damage is similar to that found in pterygium and pinguecula. Treatment consists of resorbing the lipid infiltrates and, in severe cases, keratoplasty. *Syn.* actinic keratopathy; Bietti's band-shaped nodular dystrophy; climatic droplet keratopathy; Labrador keratopathy; lipid droplet degeneration.

neurotrophic k. Condition which results from a loss or damage to the trigeminal innervation to the cornea and leads to a partial or complete anaesthesia of the cornea. It results in a breakdown of the corneal epithelial layer allowing trauma, desiccation, oedema and infection and more rarely perforation. Causes include herpes simplex virus, herpes zoster, lattice dystrophy, corneal injury, fifth nerve lesion, diabetes mellitus and Riley–Day syndrome. Treatment mainly consists of tear substitute and intermittent or constant lid taping, but antiinfective regimen, punctal occlusion,

tarsorrhaphy or neurosurgical intervention may be necessary. *Syn.* neurotrophic keratitis. *See* **cornea.**

pseudophakic bullous k. *See* **keratopathy, bullous.**

keratophakia A surgical procedure on the cornea aimed at correcting ametropia. A donor corneal disc (or lenticule) that was previously frozen and reshaped is inserted into the host cornea to modify the anterior corneal curvature. There are many complications and technical difficulties associated with this procedure. *Syn.* refractive keratoplasty and keratorefractive surgery (both terms also include epikeratoplasty, keratomileusis and radial keratotomy). *See* **epikeratoplasty; Intacs; keratomileusis; keratectomy, photorefractive; LASIK; LASEK; lenticule.**

keratoplasty Excision of corneal tissue and its replacement by a cornea from a human donor. This can be done either over the entire cornea (**total keratoplasty**) or over a portion of it (**partial keratoplasty**). Two main techniques are used: (1) **penetrating keratoplasty** and (2) **lamellar keratoplasty.** *Syn.* corneal grafting; corneal transplant. *See* **ciclosporin; dystrophy, granular; eye bank; graft, corneal; immunosuppressants; trephine.**

endothelial k. *See* **keratoplasty, lamellar.**

lamellar k. Excision of a partial amount of the total thickness of the cornea (host button) and replaced by healthy tissue (donor button). There are two main types: (1) **Deep anterior lamellar keratoplasty** in which the anterior layers of the cornea are removed (almost 95%) leaving the healthy host endothelium and Descemet's membrane and replaced by a donor button without its endothelium/Descemet layers. This is performed in cases of keratoconus, stromal dystrophies, herpes simplex keratitis with corneal scarring or chronic inflammatory diseases such as atopic keratoconjunctivitis. There is much less risk of rejection than with penetrating keratoplasty because of the retention of the endothelium, but it takes longer to recover. (2) **Deep lamellar endothelial keratoplasty** (or **posterior lamellar keratoplasty**) in which the endothelium and Descemet's membrane are excised and replaced by a lamellar graft (donor button) without sutures. The button is inserted through a small scleral incision and placed against the host posterior stroma. This technique causes less risk of rupture with physical trauma, minimal induced astigmatism and usually more rapid visual recovery than with penetrating keratoplasty. The most common condition treated with this technique is Fuchs' endothelial dystrophy. Technical refinements have led to **Descemet's stripping endothelial keratoplasty** and **Descemet's stripping automated endothelial keratoplasty.**

penetrating k. Excision of the entire thickness of the cornea (host button) and replacement by a donor button and sutured. It is used for therapeutic reasons (e.g. keratoconus, Fuchs' endothelial dystrophy or other corneal dystrophies, pseudophakic/aphakic bullous keratopathy, perforation) or cosmetic (e.g. removing an unsightly opacity). Common complications include risk of rupture with physical trauma, immunological rejection and induced cornal astigmatism.

posterior lamellar k. *See* **keratoplasty, lamellar.**

keratoplasty, laser refractive; refractive *See* **keratectomy, photorefractive.**

keratoprosthesis An artificial implant, which is used to surgically replace a damaged or diseased cornea. The most common type is made of medical grade polymethylmethacrylate (PMMA). It is sutured to the peripheral cornea. It may achieve better therapy than a corneal graft in some cases (e.g. cicatricial pemphigoid, chemical burn, trachoma), which are unsuitable for keratoplasty.

keratoreformation The process of improving vision following photorefractive keratectomy by correcting a residual ametropia and an irregular corneal topography. This is usually accomplished with contact lenses.

keratorefractive surgery *See* **epikeratoplasty; Intacs; keratomileusis; keratophakia; keratectomy, photorefractive; LASEK; LASIK.**

keratoscleritis Inflammation of both the cornea and the sclera.

keratoscope Instrument for examining the front surface of the cornea. It consists of a pattern of alternately black and white concentric rings reflected by the cornea and seen through a convex lens mounted in an aperture at the centre of the pattern. Such an instrument gives a qualitative evaluation of large corneal astigmatism, and is useful in cases of irregular astigmatism as in keratoconus, for example (Fig. K4). *Syn.* Placido disc.
See **corneal topography; photokeratoscopy; videokeratoscope.**

keratosis nigricans *See* **acanthosis nigricans.**

keratosis, seborrhoeic Lesion of the skin appearing as brown or yellowish thickening of the skin of the face, eyelids and/or conjunctiva. It is common in the elderly and may be a precursor to squamous cell carcinoma. Management includes cryotherapy, local surgical excision or radiotherapy.

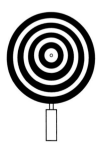

Fig. K4 Keratoscope.

keratotomy, radial A surgical procedure on the cornea aimed at correcting ametropia. It consists of making incisions in the anterior part of the cornea to flatten it and thereby produce a reduction of its power. The incisions are usually radial, extending from the limbus to about halfway towards the centre like the spokes of a wheel, but other patterns of incision are also used. In some cases, the procedure does not produce a perfect correction and vision is poor, especially in the dark. The use of the excimer laser provides greater accuracy and success. The technique is then called **laser refractive keratoplasty** or **photorefractive keratectomy**. *Syn.* refractive keratoplasty and keratorefractive surgery (both terms also include epikeratoplasty, keratomileusis and keratophakia).
See **epikeratoplasty; keratectomy, photorefractive; keratomileusis; keratophakia; keratoreformation; LASEK; LASIK.**

Kestenbaum's rule *See* **rule, Kestenbaum's.**

ketoconazole *See* **antifungal agent.**

ketotifen *See* **antihistamine.**

ketorolac *See* **antiinflammatory drug.**

keyhole bridge; pupil; visual field *See* under the nouns.

kinescope 1. An instrument for determining the refraction of the eye by having the subject observe the apparent 'with' or 'against' movement of a test object through a stenopaeic slit moved across the front of the eye. **2.** An instrument for recording television programmes.
See **disc, stenopaeic.**

kinetic depth effect *See* **effect, kinetic depth.**

kinetic perimetry *See* **perimetry, kinetic.**

Kirschmann's law *See* **law, Kirschmann's.**

Kjer-type optic atrophy *See* **atrophy, Kjer-type optic.**

Knapp's law *See* **law, Knapp's.**

Knapp procedure *See* **transposition.**

Koeppe lens; nodules *See* under the nouns.

Kollner's rule *See* **rule, Kollner's.**

König bars Target used to measure visual acuity consisting of two bars on a white background. The length of each bar is usually three times its width, but the space between the bars is always equal to the width of one bar. The smallest pair of bars that can be perceived as separate gives a measure of the acuity.

koniocellular system *See* **area, visual; geniculate body, lateral; system, koniocellular.**

Krause's end bulbs Corneal nerve endings enclosed by a capsule from 0.02 mm to 0.1 mm in length. They probably act as cold receptors. Their regular presence in the corneal limbus has been questioned.

Krause, glands of *See* **gland, of Krause.**

Krebs cycle A series of reactions in which the intermediate products of carbohydrate, fat and protein metabolism are converted to carbon dioxide and hydrogen atoms (electrons and hydrogen ions). This cycle can only operate in the presence of oxygen. Further oxidation yields carbon dioxide, water and adenosine triphosphate (ATP). This cycle occurs in the mitochondria that are found in the cytoplasm of cells of living organisms. It forms one of the processes in the metabolism of glucose providing energy (stored in ATP) to maintain the vital functions of the cells (e.g. mitosis). This cycle represents the principal energy pathway of the corneal endothelium. *Syn.* citric acid cycle; tricarboxylic acid cycle.
See **mitosis.**

Krimsky's test *See* test, Krimsky's.

Krukenberg's spindle A more or less vertical spindle-shaped deposition of brownish pigment on the corneal endothelium. It is often accompanied by pigment deposits on the lens, zonule, anterior surface of the iris and trabecular meshwork and may form part of the **pigment dispersion syndrome.** The pigment comes from the iris pigment epithelium, but the cause of its shedding is not established and may be strenuous exercise, mechanical rubbing by the zonules due to posterior bowing of part of the iris or degenerated pigment. It occurs in young to middle-aged myopic individuals and sometimes following uveitis.

krypton laser *See* laser, krypton.

Kuhnt, central meniscus of *See* membrane, Elschnig's inner limiting.

L

Labrador keratopathy *See* keratopathy, actinic.

lacquer cracks *See* spot, Fuchs'.

lacrimal Relating to tears.

lacrimal apparatus The system involved in the production and conduction of tears. It consists of the **lacrimal gland** and accessory lacrimal glands (glands of Krause and Wolfring), the **eyelid margins**, and the two **puncta lacrimale.** Each punctum is a small round or oval aperture situated on a slight elevation at the inner end of the upper and lower lid margin (**lacrimal papilla**) and forms the entrance to the **canaliculi.** Each canaliculus consists of a vertical portion of about 2 mm long, which dilates into a small sac, the **ampulla,** and then bends inward for some 8 mm, the upper one being slightly shorter. The canaliculi pierce the **lacrimal fascia** (i.e. the periorbita covering the **lacrimal sac** or **tear sac**) and unite (forming the **common canaliculus**) to enter a small diverticulum of the sac called the sinus of Maier. The **lacrimal sac** is closed above and open below where it is continuous with the **nasolacrimal duct** which extends over some 1.5 cm in length to **Hasner's valve** (or **Bianchi's valve** or **plica lacrimalis**) (folds of mucous membrane) at the inferior meatus of the nose. The inferior opening of the duct is called the **ostium lacrimale** (Fig. L1).
See canal, nasolacrimal; canaliculitis; dacryocystitis; dacryocystorhinostomy; dilation and irrigation; epiphora; fistula, lacrimal; fossa for the lacrimal sac; gland, lacrimal; syndrome, Sjögren's; tear duct; tear secretion; test, dye dilution; test, Jones II; test, Norn's; valve of Krause.

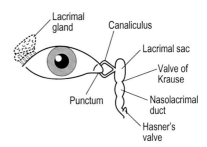

Fig. L1 Lacrimal apparatus.

lacrimal artery *See* artery, lacrimal.

lacrimal bone *See* orbit.

lacrimal canaliculi *See* lacrimal apparatus.

lacrimal caruncle A small pink fleshy structure situated in the inner canthus.

lacrimal crest, anterior The anterior margin of the fossa for the lacrimal sac located on the frontal process of the maxilla.
See fossa for the lacrimal sac.

lacrimal crest, posterior The posterior margin of the fossa for the lacrimal sac situated on the lacrimal bone.

lacrimal duct *See* tear duct.

lacrimal fascia *See* lacrimal apparatus.

lacrimal fluid *See* tears.

lacrimal gland *See* gland, lacrimal.

lacrimal gland, pleomorphic adenoma of the See gland, pleomorphic adenoma of the lacrimal.

lacrimal lake Accumulation of tears in the angle between the eyelids and the inner canthus prior to draining into the lacrimal puncta.
See epiphora; tear meniscus.

lacrimal layer See film, precorneal.

lacrimal lens See lens, liquid.

lacrimal nerve See nerve, ophthalmic.

lacrimal occlusion See occlusion, punctal.

lacrimal papilla A small elevation at the inner canthus of each eyelid containing a punctum lacrimale.

lacrimal prism See tear meniscus.

lacrimal pump See tear drainage.

lacrimal punctum A small round or oval opening of the lacrimal canaliculus (duct) on the margin of each eyelid near the inner canthus and situated in the middle of a small elevation of the **lacrimal papilla**. A lacrimal punctum is normally visible only if the lid is everted. *Plural*: lacrimal puncta. *Syn*. lacrimal point.

lacrimal reflex See reflex, lacrimal.

lacrimal sac See lacrimal apparatus.

lacrimal tubercle A small bump on the frontal process of the maxilla situated near the lower orbital and the anterior lacrimal crest, to which the medial palpebral ligament attaches. *Syn*. papilla lacrimalis.
See ligament, palpebral; lacrimal crest, anterior.

lacrimation 1. Secretion and flow of tears. **2.** Synonym for weeping.
See epiphora; reflex, lacrimal; tear secretion.

lacrimation, paradoxic See tears, crocodile.

lactoferrin One of the major proteins secreted by the lacrimal gland. The concentration of lactoferrin can be measured by several commercially available lactoferrin tests. It is significantly reduced in keratoconjunctivitis sicca.

laevoclination Rotation of the upper pole of an eye towards the subject's left. *Syn*. laevocycloduction; laevotorsion.

laevocycloduction See laevoclination.

laevocycloversion Rotation of the upper poles of the vertical meridians of both eyes towards the subject's left.
See dextrocycloversion.

laevodeorsumversion Movement of the eyes down and to the left.

laevoduction Rotation of one eye to the left.
See duction.

laevophoria A tendency of the visual axes of both eyes to deviate to the left in the absence of a stimulus to fusion.
See dextrophoria; heterophoria.

laevosursumversion Movement of the eyes up and to the left.

laevotorsion See laevoclination; torsion.

laevoversion Movement of both eyes to the left.
See version.

lag of accommodation See accommodation, lag of.

lagophthalmos Failure of the upper eyelid to close the eye completely. During sleep, about one-third of the population has a slight lagophthalmos.
See ectropion; keratopathy, exposure.

Lagrange's law See law, Lagrange's.

lambert Unit of luminance equal to 3183 candelas per m^2. *Symbol*: L.

Lambert's cosine law See diffusion.

lamella A thin plate or layer of tissue. The term is a diminutive of the Latin word lamina and implies a thinner structure.

lamellar keratoplasty See keratoplasty.

lamina Thin sheet or layer of tissue. It often refers to a flat surface. *Example*: the lamina vitrea of Bruch's membrane.

lamina cribrosa This is a part of the sclera which is situated at the site of attachment of the optic nerve, which is 3 mm to the inner side of and just above the posterior pole of the eye. There, the sclera is a thin sieve-like meshwork of cribriform plates or layers spanning the posterior foramen and through which pass bundles of ganglion cell axons and the central retinal vessels. The layers are composed of extracellular matrix components such as elastin with collagen types I, III and IV and laminin. The retinal axons become myelinated beyond the lamina cribrosa as they pass into the optic nerve. It is a relatively weak tissue, and an increase in intraocular pressure makes it bulge outward producing a cupped disc. In advanced glaucoma, it becomes distorted twisting the ganglion cell axons and possibly blocking the flow of molecules from cell body to axon terminal and eventually causing cell death and axonal degeneration. *Syn*. cribriform plate.
See disc, cupped; fibres, myelinated nerve; glaucoma.

lamina elastica See membrane, Bruch's.

lamina elastica anterior See layer, Bowman's.

lamina elastica posterior See membrane, Descemet's.

lamina fusca See choroid; sclera.

lamina papyracea A synonym for the orbital plate of the ethmoid bone, which forms part of the medial wall of the orbit. It is thus named because it is as thin as paper and this may contribute to an infection of an ethmoidal sinus spreading into the orbit and resulting in orbital cellulitis.
See cellulitis, orbital.

laminated lens See lens, laminated.

lamp Any device that produces light or heat.
Burton I. Ultraviolet lamp, including some short wavelengths from the visible spectrum (e.g. Wood's

light), mounted with a magnifying lens in a rectangular frame. Rarely used nowadays, it served in the evaluation of the fit of a hard contact lens in conjunction with the instillation of fluorescein into the eye, having been replaced by the slit-lamp. *See* **staining.**

filament l. Lamp in which light is produced by electrically heating a filament, usually of tungsten. The filament is contained in a bulb in which there is either a vacuum or an inert gas. The emitted spectrum is continuous. *See* **spectrum, continuous.**

fluorescent l. Discharge lamp in which most of the light is emitted by a layer of fluorescent material excited by the ultraviolet radiation from the discharge (CIE). *See* **fluorescence.**

halogen l. Tungsten filament lamp in which the glass envelope is made of quartz and is filled with gaseous halogens. This permits a higher filament temperature and consequently provides a higher luminance and a higher colour temperature as well as a longer operating life than a conventional filament lamp of the same input power. Halogen lamps are used in some ophthalmoscopes and retinoscopes and as very bright sources for people with low vision. *Syn.* tungsten-halogen lamp.

incandescent electric l. Lamp in which light is produced by means of a body (filament of carbon or metal) heated to incandescence by the passage of an electric current (CIE). *See* **incandescence; luminescence.**

Macbeth l. A lamp used in testing colour vision. It contains a powerful tungsten filament bulb with a blue filter of specific absorption properties such that it produces a source of a colour temperature of about 6800 K, thus approximating the spectral characteristics of natural sunlight. The lamp is also fitted with a stand to hold the colour vision booklet (Fig. L2). *Syn.* Macbeth illuminant C. *See* **illuminants, CIE standard; plates, pseudo-isochromatic; test, Farnsworth.**

tungsten-halogen l. *See* **lamp, halogen.**

Landolt ring A test object used for measuring visual acuity consisting of an incomplete ring resembling the letter C. The width of the break and that of the ring are each one-fifth of its overall diameter. The subject must indicate where the break is located, the break being positioned in any direction. The minimum angle of resolution corresponds to the angular subtense of the just noticeable break at the eye (Fig. L3). *Syn.* Landolt broken ring; Landolt C; Landolt test type. *See* **chart, Landolt broken ring.**

Lang stereotest *See* **stereotest, Lang.**

Langerhans' cells *See* **cell, Langerhans'.**

lantern test *See* **Edridge–Green lantern; test, lantern.**

Lanthony desaturated D-15 test *See* **test, Farnsworth.**

Lanthony tritan album *See* **plates, pseudoisochromatic.**

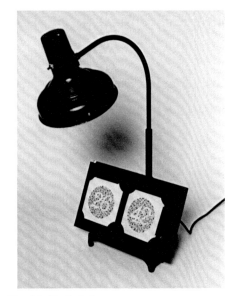

Fig. L2 Macbeth lamp.

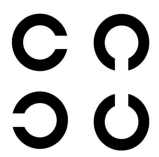

Fig. L3 Landolt ring.

LASEK A surgical procedure on the cornea aimed at correcting ametropia. An alcohol solution is applied to the cornea (usually for less than 30 seconds) to loosen the epithelium. A trephine is used to make an incision in the epithelium leaving a hinge of 2 to 3 clock hours of intact margin. The loosened edges of the epithelium are lifted along the trephine mark, and the epithelium is folded or rolled back exposing Bowman's layer. Excimer laser ablation is then performed on the anterior stromal surface, and Bowman's layer is ablated away over the treatment area. The epithelial flap is repositioned and a bandage soft contact lens is worn for 3 to 4 days to minimize discomfort and to protect the epithelium. The method is less invasive than LASIK and appears to give rise to fewer complications. LASEK is an acronym made from the following italic letters '*l*aser *a*ssisted *e*pithelial *k*eratomileusis'. *See* **keratectomy, photorefractive; pachometer.**

laser An intense luminous source of coherent and monochromatic light. The term is an acronym

for *l*ight *a*mplification by *s*timulated *e*mission of *r*adiation. Lasers are used in the treatment of a variety of ocular conditions, especially of the cornea, the retina (e.g. detached retina, diabetic retinopathy), glaucoma and refractive errors. They are also used to view different structures of the ocular fundus; a green laser images mainly the sensory retina and pigment epithelium, while a red laser images mainly the deeper structures of the ocular fundus, such as the choroid.
See cyclodiode; iridotomy; keratectomy, photorefractive; LASEK; LASIK; ophthalmo-scope, scanning laser; photocoagulation; trabeculoplasty.

argon *l*. Laser with ionized argon gas as the active medium, which emits a blue-green light beam with a wavelength of 514 nm. It may be used to perform iridectomy, iridoplasty, iridotomy, photocoagulation or trabeculoplasty.

excimer *l*. Gas laser that emits pulses of light in the ultraviolet region (at 193 nm). All the energy is absorbed by the superficial layers (e.g. the corneal epithelium), which are then exploded away or ablated without any change to the underlying or adjacent tissue or material.
See keratectomy, photorefractive; LASEK; LASIK.

***l*. interferometry** *See* maxwellian view system, clinical.

***l*. iridotomy** *See* iridotomy.

krypton *l*. A laser with krypton gas ionized by electric current as the active medium, which emits a light beam in the yellow-red region of the visible spectrum (521 nm, 568 nm or 647 nm). It may be used to perform photocoagulation or trabeculoplasty.

neodymium-YAG *l*. (Nd-YAG) A solid-state laser whose active medium is a crystal of yttrium, aluminium and garnet doped with neodymium ions. It emits an infrared light beam with a wavelength of 1064 nm. It is typically used with a slit-lamp and in conjunction with a helium-neon laser which produces a red beam of light (633 nm) to allow focusing. It may be used to perform capsulotomy, iridotomy or trabecular surgery. YAG is an acronym for *y*ttrium–*a*luminium–*g*arnet.

***l*. photocoagulation** *See* photocoagulation.

***l*. refraction** *See* refraction, laser.

***l*. refractive keratoplasty** *See* keratectomy, photorefractive; LASEK; LASIK.

***l*. trabeculoplasty** *See* trabeculoplasty, laser.

LASIK A surgical procedure on the cornea aimed at correcting ametropia. A suction ring is applied to the globe and an increase in intraocular pressure to approximately 65 mmHg is induced for a maximum of 2 minutes. During that time, an automated microkeratome advances across the cornea creating a corneal flap of about 8.5 mm in diameter, which contains the epithelium, Bowman's layer and a portion of the anterior stroma. The vacuum is then switched off and the suction ring removed. The corneal flap, which is hinged on one side of the cornea, is turned round onto the conjunctiva and the anterior part of the exposed stroma is ablated with the excimer laser. On completion of the laser ablation, the corneal flap is repositioned and left to adhere without sutures. (Fig. L4). LASIK is an acronym made from the following italic letters '*laser in situ keratomileusis*' or '*laser assisted intrastromal keratoplasty*'.
See ectasia, corneal; epikeratoplasty; Intacs; keratome; keratomileusis; keratophakia; keratectomy, photorefractive; LASEK.

latanoprost *See* prostaglandin analogues.

latent hyperopia *See* hyperopia, latent.

lateral geniculate body *See* geniculate body, lateral.

lateral inhibition *See* inhibition, lateral.

lateral rectus muscle *See* muscle, lateral rectus; muscles, extraocular.

lateral rectus paralysis *See* palsy, sixth nerve.

lathe-cut contact lens *See* lens, lathe-cut contact.

lattice degeneration of the retina *See* retina, lattice degeneration of the.

lattice dystrophy *See* dystrophy, lattice.

lattice theory *See* theory, Maurice's.

Laurence–Moon–Bardet–Biedl syndrome *See* syndrome, Bardet–Biedl.

law In science, a statement of facts or principles which is considered invariable under the given conditions having been tested and tried.

Abney's *l*. The total luminance of an area is equal to the sum of the luminances that compose it.

Alexander's *l*. An increase in the intensity of a jerk nystagmus which occurs when the eyes move in the direction of the fast phase.

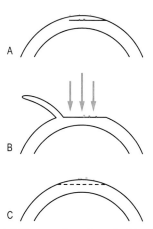

Fig. L4 LASIK procedure. A, an incision is made into the anterior part of the cornea leaving a hinge of intact margin (shown on the left). B, the corneal flap is rolled back leaving it attached at its hinge. Excimer laser ablation is performed on the exposed cornea. C, the flap is repositioned.

all or none l. The response in a nerve fibre to any stimulus, strong enough to produce a response, is always of the same amplitude. However, different nerve fibres have action potentials with different amplitudes. An increase in the intensity of the stimulus yields only an increase in the frequency of nerve impulses (or action potentials). *Syn.* all or nothing law.

Aubert–Förster l. *See* phenomenon, Aubert–Förster.

Bloch's l. The luminance L of a stimulus required to produce a threshold response is inversely proportional to the duration of exposure t of the stimulus, i.e.

$$Lt = C$$

where C is a constant. This law is only valid for exposure t below about 0.1 s.

Brewster's l. The maximum polarization (vibration in one plane) of a reflected ray of light incident on the surface of a transparent medium when it makes an angle of 90° with the refracted ray inside the medium. This occurs when the angle of incidence is equal to 56.7° (the polarizing angle or Brewster's angle).

See angle of polarization.

Bunsen–Roscoe l. In photochemistry, the product of the intensity of the light stimulus I and the duration of exposure t is a constant, i.e.

$$I \times t = C.$$

Syn. law of reciprocity.

cosine l. *See* diffusion.

Descartes' l. *See* law of refraction.

Donders' l. For any determinate position of the line of fixation with respect to the head, there corresponds a definite and invariable angle of torsion.

Draper's l. An effect is produced in a medium only by that portion of the spectrum which is absorbed by the medium. The effect may be thermal, chemical or the production of fluorescence. *Syn.* Grotthus' law.

Emmert's l. The apparent size of a projected after-image varies in proportion to the distance of the surface on which it is projected. The law can be expressed by the following relationship

$$h/H = d/D$$

where h is the linear size of the object, H the apparent size of the projected after-image, d the object's distance from the observer and D the distance between the observer and the surface on which the after-image is projected. It follows from the above expression that $H = hD/d$, i.e. the greater the distance of the projected image the larger its apparent size.

l. of equal innervation *See* law, Hering's of equal innervation.

Fechner's l. The intensity of a sensation S varies as the logarithm of the intensity I of the stimulus, i.e.

$$S = k \log I$$

where k is a constant. However, in some conditions this law is not valid and Stevens' law (or power law) is more appropriate. This stipulates that the intensity of a sensation S varies as the intensity of the stimulus I to the power of x, i.e.

$$S = k I^x$$

where x is a constant which depends on the stimulus.

See magnitude estimation.

Fermat's l. The path taken by a light ray in going from one point to another is that route which takes the least time. *Syn.* Fermat's principle.

Ferry–Porter l. The critical flicker frequency F is directly proportional to the logarithm of the luminance L of the stimulus, i.e.

$$F = a \log L + b$$

where a and b are constants.

See frequency, critical fusion.

Granit–Harper l. The critical fusion frequency F increases with the logarithm of the retinal area A stimulated, i.e.

$$F = c \log A$$

where c is a constant.

Grassmann's l's. Laws of colour mixture. **1.** The first law states that any colour C of the visible spectrum can be matched in appearance by a mixture of three primary colours, such as red R, green G and blue B, provided that none of these can be matched by a mixture of the other two, i.e.

$$C = \alpha R + \beta G + \gamma B$$

where α, β and γ are the relative proportions of the chosen primaries. **2. Additive property**: If a colour is added in an identical manner to two equivalent mixtures (or single colours), the two new mixtures will appear identical, i.e. if A + B = C + D, then A + B + X = C + D + X, or if A = B, then A + X = B + X. **3. Scalar property**: If the brightness of each of two equivalent mixtures is increased or decreased by the same factor, the two new mixtures will appear identical, i.e. if A + B = C + D, then k (A + B) = k (C + D). **4. Associative property**: If a colour is substituted in one of the mixtures by an equivalent colour, the two new mixtures will appear identical, i.e. if A + B = C + D and X = B, then A + X = C + D.

Grotthus' l. *See* law, Draper's.

Helmholtz's l. of magnification *See* law, Lagrange's.

Hering's l. of equal innervation Innervation to the extraocular muscles is equal to both eyes. Thus, all movements of the two eyes are equal and symmetrical. *Syn.* Hering's law; law of equal innervation.
See muscle, yoke.

l. of identical visual directions An object stimulating corresponding retinal points is localized in the same apparent monocular direction in each eye. *Syn.* law of oculocentric visual direction.
See line of direction; retinal corresponding points.

inverse square l. of illumination The illuminance E of a surface by a point source is directly proportional to the luminous intensity I of a point source and to the cosine of the angle θ of incidence and inversely proportional to the square of the distance d between the surface and the source, i.e.

$$E = I\cos(\theta)/d^2$$

Syn. law of illumination.
See illuminance.

Imbert–Fick l. Applied to applanation tonometry, this law states that the intraocular pressure IOP (in mmHg) is equal to the tonometer weight W (in g) divided by the applanated area A (in mm^2), hence,

$$IOP = W/A$$

This law is correct only for infinitely thin, dry, elastic, spherical membranes without resistance. Because the cornea has resistance due to its thickness and rigidity, the flattening must overcome this resistance R. The formula can be amended as

$$IOP = (W - R)/A$$

See rigidity, ocular.

Kirschmann's l. The greatest contrast in colour is seen when the luminosity difference is small.

Knapp's l. A correcting lens placed at the anterior focal plane of an axially ametropic eye forms an image equal in size to that formed in a standard emmetropic eye. Knapp's law applies to the relative spectacle magnification but not to the spectacle magnification. *Syn.* Knapp's rule.

Kollner's l. *See* rule, Kollner's.

Lagrange's l. In paraxial optics, the product of the index of refraction of image space n', the image size h' and the half-angle of the refracted cone in image space u' is equal to the product of the index of refraction of object space n, the object size h and the half-angle of the incident cone in object space u, i.e.

$$n'h'u' = nhu$$

Syn. Helmholtz's law of magnification; Lagrange's relation; Smith–Helmholtz law.
See sign convention.

Lambert's l. *See* diffusion.

Listing's l. When an eye moves to any position from the primary position, it may be considered to have made a single rotation about an axis that is perpendicular to both the initial and final lines of fixation at their point of intersection.

l. of oculocentric visual direction *See* law of identical visual directions.

Piéron's l. *See* law, Ricco's.

Piper's l. *See* law, Ricco's.

Planck's l. Law giving the energy distribution of a black body as a function of wavelength for a specified temperature.
See colour temperature.

power l. *See* law, Fechner's.

Prentice's l. The prismatic effect P in prism dioptres at a point on a lens is equal to the product of the distance c in centimetres of the point from the optical centre of the lens, and the dioptric power F of the lens, i.e.

$$P = cF$$

Syn. Prentice's rule (Table L1).
See effect, differential prismatic; power, prism; prism, induced.

l. of reciprocity *See* law, Bunsen–Roscoe.

l. of reflection The incident and reflected rays and the normal to the surface at the point of incidence lie in the same plane, and the angle of incidence is equal to the angle of reflection (Fig. L5).

l. of refraction The incident and refracted rays and the normal to the surface at the point of incidence lie in the same plane, and the ratio of the sine of the angle of incidence i to the sine of the angle of refraction i' is a constant for any two media, i.e.

$$\sin i/\sin i' = n'/n \text{ or } n\sin i = n'\sin i'$$

where n and n' are the refractive indices of the first and second medium, respectively. This constant (n'/n) is called the relative index of refraction for the two media. *Syn.* Descartes' law; Snell's law.
See index of refraction; sign convention.

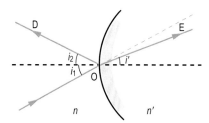

Fig. L5 Light ray incident at O on a surface separating two media of different refractive indices, n and n'. Some light is reflected along OD and most of the light is refracted along OE (i_1, angle of incidence = i_2, angle of reflection; i', angle of refraction; $n' > n$).

Table L1 The approximate amount of spectacle lens decentration (in mm) of its optical centre away from the pupillary centre of the eye to produce five prismatic effects (in prism dioptres) for distance vision and for various lens powers. The results ignore the effect of spherical aberration.

Lens power + or −	Prismatic effect required				
	1 Δ	2 Δ	3 Δ	4 Δ	5 Δ
20 D	0.5	1.0	1.5	2.0	2.5
16 D	0.6	1.3	1.9	2.5	3.1
14 D	0.7	1.4	2.1	2.9	3.6
12 D	0.8	1.7	2.5	3.3	4.2
10 D	1.0	2.0	3.0	4.0	5.0
9 D	1.1	2.2	3.3	4.4	5.6
8 D	1.3	2.5	3.8	5.0	6.3
7 D	1.4	2.9	4.3	5.7	7.1
6 D	1.7	3.3	5.0	6.7	8.3
5 D	2.0	4.0	6.0	8.0	10.0
4 D	2.5	5.0	7.5	10.0	12.5
3 D	3.3	6.7	10.0	13.3	16.7
2 D	5.0	10.0	15.0	20.0	25.0
1 D	10.0	20.0	30.0	40.0	50.0

Ricco's l. The product of the absolute threshold of luminance L and the image area A is a constant, i.e.

$$LA = C$$

This law is valid for small images subtending an angle of a few minutes of arc in the fovea and to one degree in the near macular region. For larger images in the macular area, **Piéron's law** applies; it states that the product of the luminance L of the image at threshold and the cube root of the retinal area A stimulated is a constant, i.e.

$$L\sqrt[3]{A} = C$$

In the peripheral retina, **Piper's law** becomes valid. This law states that the product of the luminance of the stimulus L and the square root of the area A is a constant, i.e.

$$L\sqrt{A} = C$$

In the far periphery of the retina, L tends to become independent of A.

Sherrington's l. of reciprocal innervation The contraction of a muscle is accompanied by simultaneous and proportional relaxation of its antagonist. For example, if the superior oblique muscle contracts, its antagonist, the inferior oblique muscle, relaxes. The validity of this law has been established by electromyography.

Smith–Helmholtz l. See law, Lagrange's.

Snell's l. See law of refraction.

square root l. See law, de Vries-Root.

Stevens' l. See law, Fechner's; magnitude estimation.

Talbot's l. See law, Talbot–Plateau.

Talbot–Plateau l. The brightness of a light source presented at short intervals above the critical fusion frequency is equal to that which would be produced by a constant light source of intensity equal to the mean value of the intermittent stimuli. *Syn.* Talbot's law.

de Vries-Rose l. The slope of the lower part of the scotopic portion of the light adaptation curve determined with an increment threshold ΔI as a function of background intensity I is equal to 0.5, so that

$$\Delta I = I^{0.5} = \sqrt{I}$$

Syn. square root law.

Weber's l. The just noticeable difference (or difference threshold) in intensity of a stimulus ΔI varies as a constant ratio of the initial intensity of the stimulus I, i.e.

$$\Delta I = kI$$

where $k = \Delta I / I$ is a constant called **Weber's fraction (Weber's constant)**. *Example*: If the initial stimulus was a light source of 1000 cd/m² and k = 0.01 (or 1%), ΔI = 0.01 × 1000 = 10 cd/m². The Weber's constant is also applicable to the slope of the main part of the scotopic portion of the light adaptation curve which is approximately equal to 1. The curve is determined with an increment threshold ΔI as a function of background intensity I, thus

$$\Delta I / I = k$$

Example: If Weber's constant k is equal to 0.14 and the background intensity is 100 units, the increment will be 14 units to be detected.

Syn. Weber–Fechner law.

See threshold, difference.

Weber–Fechner l. See law, Weber's.

layer A sheet of one thickness lying over or under another and distinguished from it by a difference in composition or colour.

Bowman's l. Thin layer of the cornea (about 12 μm) located between the anterior stratified epithelium and the stroma. This layer is acellular; it is a modified superficial stromal layer found only in primates. It is composed of a randomly orientated array of fine collagen fibrils, primarily of collagen types I, III and V. *Syn.* anterior limiting lamina; anterior limiting layer; Bowman's membrane; lamina elastic anterior.

l. of Chievitz, transient A temporary layer found in the developing embryonic retina lying between the inner neuroblastic layer (which will form the ganglion, amacrine and Mueller cells) and the outer neuroblastic layer (which will form the bipolar, horizontal and photoreceptor cells). It contains the inner processes of Mueller's fibres.

Haller's l. Outer layer of the choroid which lays between Sattler's layer and the suprachoroid. It contains connective tissue and large vessels, mainly veins.

l. of Henle, fibre Located in the macular region, it is formed by the inner fibres of the cones and rods which connect the cell body of the photoreceptors to the pedicles and spherules that run parallel to the retinal surface within the outer molecular layer of the retina. *Syn.* Henle's fibres. *See* Haidinger's brushes; macular star.

retinal l's. *See* retina.

Sattler's l. An inner layer of the choroid laying between the choriocapillaris and Haller's layer. It contains small blood vessels.

lazy eye *See* eye, amblyopic.

leaf room *See* room, leaf.

LEA acuity test *See* test, Lea-Hyvarinen acuity.

Leber's congenital amaurosis A hereditary, bilateral blindness present at birth or in early childhood. It is caused by mutation in many genes, the most common, being CEP290, CRB1, GUCY2D on chromosomes 12,1 and 17, respectively and for type 2 on the gene encoding the 65-kD protein specific to the retinal pigment epithelium (RPE65) on chromosome 1. Initially, the ocular fundus appears normal, although the ERG is markedly reduced. A salt and pepper fundus and optic atrophy appear later. The condition is often accompanied by nystagmus, keratoconus, photophobia and hyperopia.

Leber's disease *See* neuropathy, Leber's hereditary optic.

Leber's hereditary optic neuropathy *See* neuropathy, Leber's hereditary optic.

Leber's miliary aneurysms *See* disease, Coats'.

Lees screen *See* screen, Lees.

legibility Term referring to the difference in the ease of difficulty with which optotypes can be read. Some letters are easier to recognize (e.g. L, T, U, V, Z and C) than others (e.g. S, G, H, F, R and B). Test charts either mix these letters or use letters of similar difficulty; the latter facilitates standardization of charts.

length, equivalent focal In an optical system composed of more than one lens, it is the linear distance separating the principal focus from the corresponding principal point. It is usually the most important quantity in the specification of an optical system in objectives, eyepieces, etc. *See* focus, principal; power, equivalent.

length of the eye, axial The distance between the anterior and posterior poles of the eye. In vivo, it is measured either by **ultrasonography** or by **partial coherence interferometry**. These measurements represent the distance between the anterior pole and Bruch's membrane. (In young eyes in which there is a refractive index difference at the retina-vitreous interface, ultrasonography measures the distance between the anterior pole and the anterior surface of the retina.) The axial length of the eye at birth is approximately 17 mm and reaches approximately 24 mm in adulthood. It is typically longer than 24 mm in myopes and shorter than 24 mm in hyperopes. Each mm of change in axial length of the eye corresponds to approximately 2.7 D, depending on the power of the eye. *See* biometry of the eye; ultrasonography.

length, focal The linear distance separating the principal focal point (or focus) of an optical system from a point of reference (e.g. vertex, principal point, nodal point). The **first (anterior) focal length** is the distance from the lens (or first principal point) to the first principal focus. The **second (posterior) focal length** is the distance from the lens (or second principal point) to the second principal focus. *Symbol*: f.

In a spherical mirror, the focal length f (i.e. the distance between the focal point and the pole of the mirror) is equal to half its radius of curvature r.

$$f = r/2$$

Syn. focal distance. *See* focus, principal; mirror; points, cardinal; points, principal; power, equivalent; power, refractive; sign convention.

lens A piece of transparent glass, crystal, plastic or similar substance (e.g. liquid) having two opposite regular surfaces which can be plane or curved and which alter the vergence of pencils of light transmitted through it. *See* coquille; glass; moulding; surfacing.

absorptive l. Lens that absorbs a proportion of the incident radiation. Some lenses absorb mostly in the infrared region of the spectrum, others absorb mostly in the ultraviolet region and others absorb more or less equally throughout the visible spectrum. *See* CR-39; filter; lens, coated; pterygium.

accommodative intraocular l. *See* lens, intraocular.

achromatic l. A compound lens designed to reduce or eliminate chromatic aberration. The

most common type is called a doublet, also called achromatic doublet, and consists of a crown lens combined with a flint lens. *Syn.* achromat.
See **doublet; lens, apochromatic; lens, hyperchromatic.**

achromatizing l. Lens aimed at reducing or eliminating the chromatic aberration of the eye. It consists of either a doublet or a triplet that possesses longitudinal chromatic aberration opposite to that of the eye and thereby neutralizes it. Thus the lens system has negative power for short wavelengths and positive power for long wavelengths of an amount similar to that of the eye for those wavelengths.

l. adherence 1. A contact lens firmly attached to the cornea. **2.** Attachment of bacteria (e.g. pseudomonas, staphylococcus) to a contact lens, particularly soft lens materials (the amount and strength vary with the material). *Syn.* lens binding.
See **lens, silicone hydrogel; tear stasis.**

afocal l. A lens of zero power (Fig. L6). *Syn.* plano lens.
See **lens, aniseikonic.**

Alvarez l. A variable power lens composed of two elements that can be moved with respect to each other along two mutually perpendicular axes. When the two lenses are in exact register with each other, the Alvarez lens provides zero power. Moving one of the elements either laterally or vertically in relation to the other provides increasing spherical or cylindrical power. Moving both elements produces a combined spherocylindrical power.

anastigmatic l. 1. Lens that has a single focal point. **2.** A lens that is corrected for oblique astigmatism and minimum curvature of field. *Syn.* stigmatic lens.
See **lens, astigmatic; Petzval surface.**

aniseikonic l. Lens designed to correct aniseikonia. It can have power like a regular ophthalmic lens but also produces a magnification of the image. A lens which only produces magnification but has zero power is called an **overall size lens**, and if it magnifies in only one meridian it is called a **meridional size lens**. *Syn.* iseikonic lens; eikonic lens; size lens.
See **lens, afocal; magnification, shape.**

anterior chamber intraocular l. *See* **lens, intraocular.**

anti-actinic l. Lens that absorbs ultraviolet radiations to a much greater extent than a white spectacle lens.
See **actinic.**

anti-reflection coated l. *See* **lens, coated.**

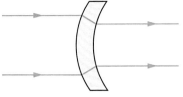

Fig. L6 Afocal size lens.

aphakic l. A lens used for the correction of aphakia. It is of high dioptric power, usually above +10 D. Due to their thickness, these lenses are usually made of plastic to reduce weight, and because of the aberrations, aspherical surfaces are used. Intraocular lenses have generally replaced these lenses.
See **lens, lenticular; phenomenon, jack-in-the-box.**

aplanatic l. A lens designed to correct for spherical aberration and coma.

apochromatic l. A compound lens designed to correct chromatic and spherical aberrations. It uses three or more kinds of glass. This lens corrects chromatic aberration more thoroughly than an achromatic lens.

aspheric l. Lens in which one or both surfaces are not spherical, so designed to minimize certain optical aberrations.

astigmatic l. Toric or cylindrical lens that produces two separate focal lines at right angles instead of a single focal point. Hence it has two principal powers. One of these powers may be zero (**cylindrical lens**).
See **axis, cylinder; lens, anastigmatic; lens, spherocylindrical; protractor; Sturm, interval of; transposition.**

back toric contact l. A contact lens used to correct corneal astigmatism in which the surface of the lens facing the cornea is not spherical but toroidal to obtain a good physical fit on the cornea. To create better stability of the lens on the eye, it usually incorporates a prism ballast.
See **ballast.**

Bagolini's l. *See* **glass, Bagolini's.**

balancing l. A lens fitted to a spectacle frame or mount to balance the weight and the appearance of the other lens, its power being unspecified or unimportant.

bandage l. *See* **lens, therapeutic contact.**

bent l. *See* **lens, meniscus.**

best-form l. Curved lens whose curvatures are calculated to eliminate or minimize aberrations when viewing through the peripheral portions of the lens. *Syn.* corrected lens; point-focal lens.
See **ellipse, Tscherning.**

biconcave l. Lens that has two concave surfaces.

biconvex l. Lens that has two convex surfaces.

bifocal contact l. Contact lenses consisting of two segments with different focal powers, which provide either **simultaneous** vision (light from both the distance and near portions enters the eye at the same time) or **alternating** vision (the lens must be moved to see through either portion). Other bifocal contact lenses have a zone of variable power between the two portions, and others are **diffractive** in which light from both distance and near objects can be focused on the retina (without moving the lens) owing to diffraction produced by a series of rings in the centre of the back surface of the lens (the higher the near addition, the greater the number of rings).

bifocal l. Lens having two portions of different focal power. Usually the upper portion is larger

and is used for distance vision while the lower portion is smaller and used for near vision. There are, however, many types of bifocals: those in which the use of the two portions is the opposite of that previously described, others in which the shape of the **near portion** (or **segment**) differs; in certain types, the near segment is fused onto the surface of the glass (**fused bifocal**); in others, the near portion is produced by grinding or moulding a different curvature on one surface (**solid bifocal** or **one-piece bifocal**). There is also a one-piece bifocal in which there is a gradual transitional zone between the two portions instead of a clear line of demarcation (**blended bifocal**). In addition, several other bifocals are known by their trade name (Fig. L7).
See **button; jump; lens, progressive; monocentric; segment height; segment of a bifocal lens; wafer.**
l. binding See **lens adherence.**
biomimetic contact l. A hydrogel contact lens made up of a material that imitates the chemistry of natural cell membranes to minimize changes in ocular physiology.
l. blank A moulded piece of ophthalmic glass before completion of the surfacing processes.
See **glass; lens, semi-finished.**
l. capsule See **capsule; lens, crystalline.**
l. carrier See **lens, lenticular; telescope, bioptic.**
cast-moulding contact l. A contact lens produced by pressing a concave female mould filled with liquid monomer against a male mould. The concave mould determines the front surface of the lens. The edge is formed when the two sides of the mould come together. The assembled moulds are irradiated with ultraviolet light to cause polymerization and a dry contact lens, which is then hydrated in saline water. Cast-moulding has been used to manufacture hard and soft lenses, especially mass production of the latter.
See **lens, lathe-cut contact; lens, spin-cast contact.**

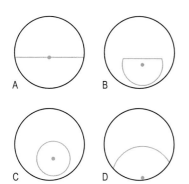

Fig. L7 Examples of bifocal lenses. In each case, the dot indicates the optical centre of the near portion (A, executive-type segment; B, flat-top segment; C, round segment; D, curved segment).

Chavasse l. A lens with an irregular surface used to depress the visual acuity while permitting the eye to be seen from the front (British Standard).
ChromaGen l. Trade name of a tinted soft contact lens worn with the aim of enhancing colour perception in individuals with colour vision deficiencies, especially red-green defects. It is fitted on either one or both eyes. The lenses exist in a variety of tints and are chosen by the patient by trial and error. Some patients with dyslexia or migraine have claimed to benefit from wearing these lenses.
See **lens, X-Chrom.**
l. clock See **lens measure.**
coated l. A lens upon which is deposited an evaporated film consisting of a metallic salt such as magnesium fluoride, about one-quarter as thick as a wavelength of light. This film reduces, by interference, the amount of light reflected by the surfaces and to some extent the amount of stray light reflected inside the lens. With **multilayer coating**, the lens can selectively reflect radiations and increase transmission. All coated lenses show some residual colour. *Syn.* anti-reflection (AR) coated lens; bloomed lens.
See **anti-reflection coating; coating; image, ghost.**
cobalt l. Lens that absorbs the central region of the visible spectrum and only transmits the red and blue ends of the spectrum. It is sometimes used in the testing of ametropia, because a light source located at 1.4 m from the eye will form, in an emmetropic eye viewing it through a cobalt lens, two equal circles superimposed on the retina, and the subject will report seeing a purple circle. A hyperope will see a blue spot surrounded by a red annulus, and a myope will see a red spot surrounded by a blue annulus. An appropriate spherical lens placed in front of the eye, which changes the appearance to a purple circle, represents the spherical refractive correction. *Syn.* cobalt-blue glass.
See **filter, cobalt blue; test, duochrome.**
collimating l. See **collimator.**
combination l. See **lens, hybrid contact.**
composite l. A contact lens composed of two or more different materials.
compound l. **1.** Lens that functions as a combination of a spherical lens and a cylindrical lens. *Example*: a spherocylindrical lens. **2.** A system composed of several refracting surfaces or lenses placed along the same axis. *Examples*: doublet; triplet.
See **lens, spherocylindrical.**
concave l. A lens that causes incident rays of light to diverge (Table L2). *Syn.* diverging lens; minus lens; negative lens.
condensing l. See **condenser.**
contact l. A small lens made of a plastic material, worn in contact with the cornea or sclera and used to correct refractive errors of the eye. There are many types of contact lenses. Lenses that rest on the sclera are called **scleral** (or **haptic**) contact lenses, whereas lenses that rest on the cornea are

Table L2   Relationship between object and image formed in a converging and in a diverging lens. The object is moved from left to right. *F* and *F'* are the first and second focal points, respectively.

Position of the object	Type of object	Type of image	Position of the image
Converging lens			
infinity	–	real (inverted)	*F'*
between infinity and *F*	real	real (inverted)	between *F'* and infinity
F	real	–	infinity
between *F* and lens	real	virtual (erect)	between infinity and lens
between lens and infinity	virtual	real (erect)	between lens and *F'*
Diverging lens			
infinity	–	virtual (erect)	*F'*
between infinity and lens	real	virtual (erect)	between *F'* and lens
between lens and *F*	virtual	real (erect)	between lens and infinity
F	virtual	–	infinity
between *F* and infinity	virtual	virtual (inverted)	between infinity and *F'*

called **corneal** contact lenses, or, more commonly, contact lenses. Lenses that are made of a hard plastic material used to be made of polymethyl methacrylate (PMMA), which is impermeable to oxygen. All rigid contact lenses nowadays transmit oxygen. They are called **gas permeable** contact lenses (GP, GPL, GPCL or RGP), or merely **rigid** contact lenses, and they usually contain silicone acrylate or fluorosilicone acrylate.

Other lenses made of a soft plastic material (e.g. polymers of hydroxyethyl methacrylate) which transmit a certain amount of oxygen are called **soft** (or **hydrophilic, hydrogel, gel** or **flexible**) contact lenses (SCL) whose water content varies; the greater the water content, the more oxygen is transmitted (for equal thickness). High water content lenses are used for **extended wear** (EW). There are also **toric** contact lenses in which the back optic surface is toroidal; they are used to improve the physical fit. **Bitoric** contact lenses are lenses in which both surfaces are toroidal; they are used to improve the physical fit and correct the induced astigmatism. **Disposable** contact lenses are worn for 1 day, 1 week, 2 weeks or more rarely 1 month, and then discarded.

See acidosis; hypercapnia; lens adherence; lens, back toric contact; lens, bifocal contact; lens, biomimetic contact; lens, cast-moulding; lens, combination; lens, cosmetic contact; lens, extended wear; lens, fenestrated; lens, flare; lens, flat; lens, flexure; lens, lathe-cut contact; lens, liquid; lens, ortho-k; lens, piggyback; lens, reverse-geometry contact; lens, scleral contact; lens, sealed scleral contact; lens, silicone hydrogel; lens, spin-cast contact; lens, steep; lens, therapeutic contact; lens, X-Chrom; modulus of elasticity; oxygen permeability; test, inside-out for soft contact lens; water content.

contact l. deposits *See* deposits, contact lens.
converging l. *See* lens, convex.
convex l. A lens that causes incident rays of light to converge (Table L2). *Syn.* convex lens; plus lens; positive lens.
corrected l. *See* lens, best-form.

l. cortex *See* **lens, crystalline.**
cosmetic contact l. A contact lens designed to improve the appearance of the eye, to conceal a disfigurement (e.g. a scar) or to change the colour of the eye. *Examples*: a tinted lens; an opaque lens with an artificial pupil and iris (**prosthetic contact lens**). *See* aniridia.
cross-cylinder l. An astigmatic lens consisting of a minus cylinder ground on one side and a plus cylinder ground on the other side, the two axes being located 90° apart. The dioptric power in the principal meridians is equal. Usual cross-cylinder lenses are provided in three powers: ±0.25 D, ±0.37 D and ±0.50 D (higher values are also available for use with low-vision patients). This lens is used in the subjective measurement of the power and axis of astigmatism, or to refine the cylindrical correction determined otherwise (Fig. L8). *Syn.* Jackson cross-cylinder lens. *See* **test for astigmatism, cross-cylinder.**
crystalline l. The biconvex, usually transparent body, situated between the iris and the vitreous

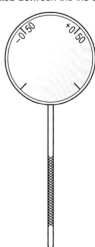

Fig. L8 Cross-cylinder lens.

body of the eye and suspended from the ciliary body by the zonular fibres (**zonule of Zinn**), which are attached to the equator of the lens. The diameter of the lens is equal to 9 to 10 mm and its thickness 3.6 mm, being greater when the eye accommodates. The radii of curvature of the anterior and posterior surfaces are 10.6 mm and −6.2 mm respectively in the unaccommodated eye, while maximum accommodation alters these values to about 6 mm and −5.3 mm respectively. The crystalline lens displays a complex gradient of refractive index (averaging 1.42) and a power of 21 D. It consists of the **capsule** which envelops the lens, the **epithelium** which consists of a single sheet of cells and lines the anterior and equatorial capsule and the **cortex** which surrounds the **nucleus**, the latter two containing the lens fibres. The lens has the highest protein content of any other tissue in the body. The most numerous proteins in the lens are the soluble proteins dominated by the crystallins followed by the insoluble proteins, especially cytoskeletal proteins. Light transparency is mainly caused by regular arrangement or packing of the crystallin molecules. With age, there is an increase in light scatter originating in the nucleus, as well as some light absorption and yellowing of the nucleus (Fig. L9). The equatorial diameter and lens thickness also increase with age mainly due to an increase in cortical thickness; consequently the volume increases. *Syn.* lens of the eye. *See* **capsule, crystalline lens; constants of the eye; disease, Wilson's; fibre, lens; fissure, optic; lens, intraocular; lens paradox; lens, prolapse of the; lens sutures; luxation of the lens; myopia, lenticular; phakic; shagreen; Zinn, zonule of.**

curved l. See **lens, meniscus.**

cylindrical l. Lens in which one of the principal meridians has zero refractive power. It usually consists of one plano surface and one cylindrical surface (Fig. L10). *See* **lens, astigmatic.**

l. dislocation See **lens, prolapse of the; luxation of the lens.**

disposable l. See **lens, contact.**

diverging l. See **lens, concave.**

eikonic l. See **lens, aniseikonic.**

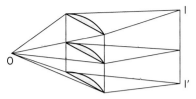

Fig. L10 Cylindrical lens (O, object; ll′, image).

equi-concave l. Lens having two concave surfaces of the same power.

equi-convex l. Lens having two convex surfaces of the same power.

equivalent l. See **equivalent, spherical.**

l. exfoliation See **exfoliation of the lens.**

extended wear l. A contact lens designed to be worn continuously for more than 1 day and, usually, no more than 7 days before cleaning and sterilization. It is, typically, a soft lens with high oxygen transmissibility. *See* **conjunctivitis, giant papillary; contact lens acute red eye; cornea guttata; corneal infiltrates; keratitis, microbial contact lens induced; lens, silicone hydrogel; microcysts, epithelial; microscope, specular; pannus; ulcer, corneal.**

fenestrated l. Hard contact lens having one or more small holes to aid tear exchange and corneal oxygenation. It was essential with PMMA scleral contact lenses, but with the advent of gas-permeable materials, fenestration is rarely necessary nowadays. *Syn.* ventilated lens.

finished l. A spectacle lens that has been surfaced on both sides to the required power and thickness and is still in uncut form. *Syn.* uncut lens. *See* **lens, semi-finished; surfacing.**

fisheye l. Camera lens with a very wide angle of view. The angle can be as wide as 220°. To achieve this, the lens has a large diameter that produces image distortion (especially barrel-shaped distortion); thus the image magnification varies across the picture causing some fishbowl effects. *See* **lens, wide-angle.**

l. flare Type of blur characterized by the presence of a secondary or ghost image. Flare may be caused by a contact lens with an optic zone diameter that is smaller than the pupil diameter or when the lens decentres so that part of the edge of the optic zone is within the pupil area. Flare is usually more apparent under conditions of reduced illumination as the pupil is larger. Management consists in refitting the patient with a lens with a larger optic zone diameter or with better centration. *See* **image, ghost.**

flat l. **1.** Any lens that is not of curved form. **2.** A contact lens in which the back optic zone radius is longer than the flattest meridian of the cornea. This definition may not be valid for a soft lens that may have a back optic zone radius longer than the flattest meridian of the cornea and yet not be flat fitting. *Syn.* loose lens (it is preferable to use this term for soft lenses).

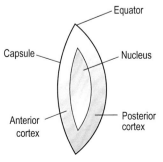

Fig. L9 Cross-section of the crystalline lens.

See fitted on K; lens, steep.

l. flexure Characteristic of a spherical contact lens to adopt a toroidal curvature when placed on an astigmatic cornea. Flexure depends upon the material and its thickness, being more common with thin lenses. As it occurs during blinking, it sometimes results in fluctuating vision.

l. flippers Two pairs of lenses mounted on a central bar, one pair on each side. One pair can be held in front of the patient's eyes and then quickly changed for the other pair by twisting the bar extension handle. The lenses may be one pair of minus lenses of equal power and the other pair of plus lenses of equal power. The most common pairs are ±2.00 D, although ±1.00 D, ±1.50 D and ±2.50 D are also available. These are used in the testing and training of accommodative facility. **Prisms** may also be used as, for example, base-in for one pair and base-out for the other. They are used in the testing and training of vergence facility (Fig. L11). *Syn.* flippers; flipper bar; flip lenses; flip prisms; prism flippers.

Fresnel l. A lens consisting of one surface on which there is a series of concentric prismatic rings or elements. A small central portion of the lens surface is either convex or flat, but the concentric prismatic rings make up the outer zone. The apical angles of these prismatic elements increase ring by ring towards the lens periphery. Thus, the Fresnel lens has the same power as a continuous spherical lens surface but without the thickness and the weight. However, owing to the imperfect surface of the lens a slight reduction in acuity is obtained. These lenses are usually made by fixing a translucent press-on plastic film (usually of polyvinyl chloride) of the concentric rings on one lens surface. They are called **Fresnel Press-On** lenses. They are used primarily for temporary correction in orthoptics therapy, following eye surgery and as condensers in overhead projectors, headlights, etc. (Fig. L12).
See prism, Fresnel Press-On.

frosted l. A lens made translucent by having one or both surfaces smoothed but not polished.

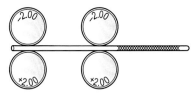

Fig. L11 Lens flippers.

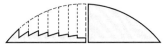

Fig. L12 Cross-section of a Fresnel lens of approximately the same refractive power as the planoconvex lens next to it.

See glass, ground; surfacing; translucent.

Goldmann three mirror l. *See* gonioscope; slit-lamp.

gonioscopic l. A lens placed in contact with the cornea for the purpose of viewing the angle of the anterior chamber. It may be a prismatic lens or a lens with mirrors, or merely a thick convex contact lens. Some, like the Goldmann three-mirror goniolens, enable visualization with a slit-lamp of the ciliary body and peripheral retina, as well as the angle of the anterior chamber. Other gonioscopic lenses (e.g. Zeiss) have four mirrors. *Syn.* goniolens. *See* biomicroscope; gonioscopy, indirect; lens, Koeppe; lens, Zeiss.

gradient-index l. A lens with an index of refraction that changes continuously through the whole material, or part of, thus providing an area of progressive power. They may have unwanted astigmatism.
See lens, progressive.

l. groove An indentation on the edge of a lens designed to accommodate a cord (usually a nylon thread), which retains the lens in a rimless mounting.
See rimless fitting; spectacles, rimless; spectacles, supra.

high index l. A specialized lens made with higher refractive material than crown glass. Included in these are flint and titanium glass in which the refractive index can be as high as 1.8. However, as the index increases, there is usually a decrease in the constringence. For example, Zenlite (a trade name) has a refractive index of 1.805 and a constringence of 25.4. Recently, technical advances have made it possible to manufacture high index progressive lenses. High index lenses are used for high prescriptions, as they can be made much thinner than crown glass lenses of equivalent power. As high index lenses have very reflective surfaces, it is valuable to have them coated.

high water content l. Contact lens whose water content is greater than 50%.

honey bee l. A compound magnifying lens consisting of three to six small telescopes mounted in the upper portion of a spectacle lens. The telescopes are so arranged as to resemble the multifaceted eye of the honey bee. They have their axes converging on the eye as well as prismatic objectives to provide an approximately continuous field of view.

Hruby l. A spherical diverging lens of −55 D mounted on a slit-lamp and biomicroscope in such a way that it can be placed very close to the patient's cornea. It is used, coupled with the microscope, to examine internal ocular structures including the retina.

hybrid contact l. A lens made from two different materials, usually a rigid centre portion made from gas-permeable material surrounded by a soft peripheral flange. It provides greater comfort and is used in the management of keratoconus irregular astigmatism and postsurgical intervention. *Syn.* combination lens.
See lens, piggyback.

hydrogel l. *See* **lens, contact; lens, silicone hydrogel.**

hyperchromatic l. A compound lens designed to have a large amount of chromatic aberration. It may be of use in the correction of presbyopia by extending the depth of focus of the eye; the eye receives a clear red image of distant objects and a clear blue image of near objects without having to change its focus. However, because of the reduced information in the retinal image, such a lens is more beneficial with high contrast objects. *See* **lens, achromatic.**

immersion l. Objective of a high-power microscope in which the space between its front lens and the cover plate of the microscope slide is filled with an immersion liquid (e.g. water, cedar wood oil, etc.).

l. implant *See* **lens intraocular.**

intraocular l. A lens inserted in the eye to replace the crystalline lens after cataract surgery. To obtain the correct lens power, it is necessary to measure corneal curvature and axial length of the eye. Several formulae exist to arrive at the power of the intraocular lens. Intraocular lenses are mostly made of silicone or acrylic (propenoic acid) and can be easily folded to be inserted into the eye through a very small opening. There are many types, including monofocal and multifocal ones. **Accommodative intraocular lenses** are monofocal lenses which are moved by the ciliary muscle, thus providing clear focus at a range of distances. **Anterior chamber intraocular lenses** are placed anterior to the iris. Fitting is usually carried out following intracapsular cataract extraction. **Posterior chamber intraocular lenses** are placed within the capsular bag or less commonly anchored into the ciliary sulcus. These lenses can be inserted through a larger incision made during extracapsular cataract extraction. **Multifocal intraocular lenses** have progressive change in power over the whole surface, thus providing clear focus at various distances. This is usually accomplished by a series of rings, using the principles of refraction and diffraction to change the direction of light propagation to focus at different distances. **Short-wavelength filtration intraocular lenses** absorb short wavelengths (ultraviolet and blue light). They may be valuable in preventing retinal damage (e.g. age-related macular degeneration). **Toric (astigmatism-correcting) intraocular lenses** are designed to correct astigmatism. They need to be perfectly positioned. *Syn.* intraocular lens implant. *See* **'bag' capsular; biometry of the eye; eye, pseudophakic; SRK formula; sulcus, ciliary; syndrome, UGH.**

Irlen l. *See* **syndrome, Meares–Irlen.**

iseikonic l. *See* **lens, aniseikonic.**

isochromatic l. Tinted lens which absorbs all radiations equally.

inverted l. *See* **test, inside-out for soft contact lens.**

Koeppe l. A diagnostic goniolens designed to be placed on the anaesthetized cornea for a direct view (without a mirror) of the angle of the anterior chamber. It consists of a high-plus (50 D) lens with a back concave surface and a flange that retains the lens in place. Like all goniolenses, its overall power more or less neutralizes the refractive power of the cornea. Its image magnification is about half that of goniolenses with mirrors but its field of view is wider. The lens is typically used with a hand-held biomicroscope, in surgery and with children in whom it can be used to examine the fundus as well. *Syn.* Koeppe contact lens; Koeppe gonioscopic lens. *See* **gonioscopy, direct; lens, gonioscopic.**

lacrimal l. *See* **lens, liquid.**

laminated l. A lens consisting of a thin layer of plastic (e.g. cellulose acetate) cemented between two layers of glass. Such a lens protects the eye because in case of breakage the glass pieces remain attached to the plastic layer. *See* **glass, safety; lens, safety.**

lathe-cut contact l. A contact lens in which the optic radii of the surfaces are cut to a block of plastic mounted in a lathe and then polished. Hydrophilic polymers are cut in a solid state with shorter radii and thinner centre thickness than is desired in the hydrated state, and they are polished with an oil-based compound, as water cannot be used. *See* **lens, cast-moulding contact; lens, spin-cast contact.**

lenticular l. An ophthalmic lens with a central zone finished to prescription surrounded by a supporting margin (carrier), generally made to reduce the weight of lenses of high power. They can be made either as one solid piece or the power element may be cemented on a plano carrier. *See* **aperture of a lenticular lens; lens, aphakic.**

l. liner *See* **lens washer.**

liquid l. The lens formed by the tear layer lying between the back surface of a rigid contact lens and the cornea. It must be taken into account when fitting contact lenses. If the back surface of the lens is steeper than the cornea, the liquid lens is positive and the eye is made more myopic. If the back surface of the lens is flatter than the cornea, the liquid lens is negative and the eye is made more hyperopic. (Fig. L13) *Syn.* fluid lens; lacrimal lens; tear lens.

loose l. *See* **lens, flat.**

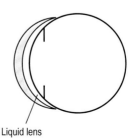

Fig. L13 Liquid lens between a contact lens and the cornea (it is positive in this diagram).

low water content l. Contact lens whose water content is less than 50%.

luxation of the l. See luxation.

magnifying l. A converging lens used to magnify an object without image inversion. *Syn.* magnifying glass.
See **magnifier**.

l. measure Instrument for determining the radius of curvature of a spherical or cylindrical surface based on measuring the sag of the curve. The instrument, which is shaped like a pocket watch, consists of two fixed pointed prongs attached to the edge and a movable one located halfway between the two. The sag of the surface in the meridian containing all three prongs is measured by the linear displacement of the central one. The instrument is calibrated to give a reading in dioptres of the surface power for that meridian which has been calculated, usually using the refractive index of crown glass ($n = 1.523$). If the material has a different refractive index, the true surface power, F_T, in dioptres, is given by the following formula

$$F_T = \frac{(n-1)}{0.523} \times F_{LM}$$

where n is the refractive index and F_{LM} is the reading, in dioptres, shown on the lens measure (Fig. L14). *Syn.* lens clock; spherometer (the old models had three outer fixed prongs instead of two).
See **focimeter; neutralization; vertex depth.**

meniscus l. Lens with one spherical convex surface and the other spherical concave. Meniscus lenses often have a base of 6 D for the surface of lesser curvature. *Syn.* curved lens; bent lens.
See **curve, base.**

meridional size l. See lens, aniseikonic.

microscopic l. See lens, telescopic.

mid-water content l. Contact lens whose water content is between 50% and 65%.

minus l. See lens, concave.

monocentric l. See monocentric.

multifocal l. Lens with various dioptric powers such as a bifocal, a trifocal or a progressive lens.

negative l. See lens, concave.

l. nucleus See lens, crystalline.

objective l. See objective.

L. Opacity Classification System (LOCS) See gradient scale.

ophthalmic l. Any lens used to correct refractive errors of the eye. Sometimes it also includes lenses used to measure the refractive error.

ortho-k l. A rigid gas permeable contact lens used temporarily to reshape the cornea and change its power resulting in a reduction of myopia or hyperopia. Most ortho-k lenses for myopia are based on a **reverse-geometry** design in which the central portion of the posterior surface of the lens is flatter than the average normal cornea and the peripheral portion is steeper. The design is the opposite if the ametropia is hyperopia. The lens is usually worn only at night. Significant improvement occurs within a month.
See **lens, reverse-geometry; orthokeratology.**

orthoscopic l. A lens corrected for peripheral aberrations.
See **ellipse, Tscherning.**

l. paradox A hypothetical decrease in the power of the crystalline lens due to a continuum of refractive index changes in the layers of the ageing crystalline lens, such that it compensates for an increase in lens power which would otherwise occur due to an increase in lens thickness and lens curvatures (and therefore myopia). This is proposed as an explanation for the fact that the refractive state of the eye actually shifts towards hyperopia (or less myopia) with age.

l. pattern See former.

periscopic l. A spherical lens in which the minus lenses have base curves of +1.25 D and the plus lenses have base curves of −1.25 D. Meniscus lenses are more curved.
See **curve, base.**

photochromatic l. See lens, photochromic.

photochromic l. A lens used either in sunglasses or as an ophthalmic lens. It is made up of glass or plastic material, which changes in colour and/or in light transmission as a result of changes in incident light intensity or heat. The changes are reversible and relatively rapid. There exist several types, which are known by their trade name. *Syn.* photochromatic lens.
See **vignetting.**

piggyback l. Combination of two contact lenses; usually a rigid contact lens over a hydrogel lens. The soft lens is used for comfort and the rigid lens for best visual results. Piggyback lenses can be used after corneal surgery, corneal scarring and in the management of severe keratoconus or irregular astigmatism, although hybrid contact lenses are usually preferred. *Syn.* combination system.
See **lens, hybrid contact; lens, therapeutic contact.**

plano l. See lens, afocal.

planoconcave l. Lens with one plane and one concave surface.

planoconvex l. Lens with one plane and one convex surface.

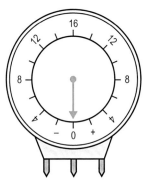

Fig. L14 Lens measure.

plastic l. Lens made of transparent plastic. It is approximately 50% lighter than a glass lens of equal power but more liable to scratching. Plastic lenses do not shatter like glass lenses and therefore give better protection. Practically all ophthalmic lenses are made of plastic.
See **CR-39; glass, safety; lens, safety.**

plus l. See **lens, convex.**

point-focal l. See **lens, best-form.**

polarizing l. A lens that transmits light waves vibrating in one direction only. In the other direction perpendicular to it, the light waves are absorbed. In this way, reflected glare is reduced. Common polarizing materials include herapathite crystal, calcite crystal or a stretched sheet of polyvinyl alcohol containing iodine.
See **light, polarized.**

positive l. See **lens, convex.**

posterior chamber intraocular l. See **lens, intraocular.**

prismatic l. Lens with prism power.

prism ballast l. See **ballast.**

prismatic effect of a l. See **convergence, correction induced; prism, induced.**

progressive addition l. A spectacle lens having a gradual and progressive change in power either over the whole lens or over a region intermediate between areas of uniform power. The **progression** is produced by a complex aspheric shape of one of the surfaces. This lens is used to correct presbyopia. (Fig. L15) Syn. varifocal lens.
See **distance, interpupillary; lens, gradient-index; lens, multifocal.**

prolapse of the l. A falling of the crystalline lens into the vitreous or less commonly into the anterior chamber as a result of a blunt trauma to the eye which resulted in a 360° rupture of the zonular fibres.
See **luxation of the lens.**

prosthetic contact l. See **lens, cosmetic.**

reading l. A lens prescribed for near vision (or a magnifying glass).

reverse-geometry contact l. A contact lens in which the back optic zone radius (BOZR) is flatter than the cornea. This zone is surrounded by a midperipheral curve, which is steeper than the cornea (some lenses omit this reverse curve); a peripheral curve, which is aligned with the peripheral cornea; and edge clearance. This lens design can be used in orthokeratology to control myopia, in the management of keratoconus, after keratoplasty or photorefractive surgery in which the corneal front surface is flatter than normal and there is partial alignment with the BOZR (Fig. L16).
See **lens, ortho-k; optic zone radius, back.**

rigid contact l. See **lens, contact.**

l. rim artefact An apparent reduction in the extent of the visual field when perimetry is carried out with the patient's correction. The greatest reduction is usually found with the standard trial case lens. It is even more noticeable in the elderly, possibly because many of them have deep-set eyes that increase the distance from the lens to the eye. With the patient's own spectacles, the artefact is less extensive. It is usually nonexistent when wearing contact lenses.

safety l. 1. A lens made of safety glass. **2.** A general term referring to any lens that protects the eyes against injury due to impact and which is more resistant to fracture and less likely to splinter than an ordinary glass lens. Examples: plastic lenses (especially polycarbonate); toughened lenses; laminated lenses. Plastic lenses have the greatest impact resistance of all these lenses.
See **glass, safety.**

scleral contact l. Contact lens that fits over both the cornea and the surrounding sclera. It is divided into an optical zone and a scleral (or haptic) zone. When made of PMMA material, it includes small holes (called fenestrations) to aid tear exchange and corneal oxygenation. Modern scleral contact lenses are made of gas-permeable material and do not require fenestration. Scleral contact lenses are used mainly therapeutically for corneal protection, tear retention and pain relief in ocular surface disorders, vision improvement as in keratoconus and after penetrating keratoplasty or occasionally for theatrical and sports purposes.

sealed scleral contact l. A scleral contact lens made up of gas-permeable material. The optic portion of the lens has a curvature such that there is no contact between the lens and the cornea and that a space (called corneal clearance) is filled with saline water forming a fluid precorneal reservoir. There is no tear exchange, and corneal oxygenation is essentially provided through the lens matrix, as there is no fenestration. This lens is used in patients with corneal ectasia, such as keratoconus, keratoglobus and pellucid marginal

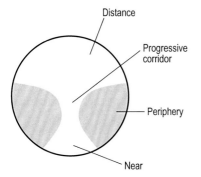

Fig. L15 Typical positions of the various portions of a progressive addition lens (PAL). The periphery has unwanted astigmatism and distortion.

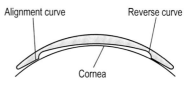

Fig. L16 A reverse-geometry contact lens design.

degeneration, dry eyes of various aetiologies (e.g. Stevens–Johnson syndrome), etc.

semi-finished l. Ophthalmic lens of which only one surface is completely polished. The other side can be surfaced to any required curvature. If it is a bifocal lens, the side with the segment is usually the one that is completely surfaced. *Syn.* semifinished lens blank.
See **lens blank; lens, finished.**

silicone hydrogel l. A contact lens made of elements of silicone and a hydrogel polymer to form a co-polymer that has the properties of both. A hydrogel-forming monomer such as HEMA is combined with a modified silicon-containing monomer such as TRIS [tris-(trimethylsilyloxy)silyl] propyl methacrylate or a derivative of TRIS. Such a lens has a high oxygen permeability, adequate wettability, good optical properties and acceptable lens movement on the eye (unlike basic silicone rubber material, which tends to adhere to the cornea). It can be used for extended wear as contact lens-induced oedema is virtually eliminated. Permeability (*Dk*) of such lenses exceeds 100.
See **lens, therapeutic contact; modulus of elasticity.**

single-vision l. An ophthalmic lens having only one power.

size l. *See* **lens, aniseikonic.**

slab-off l. A lens in which a portion of one surface has been ground with the same radius of curvature as the rest of the surface but with separated centres of curvature. That portion of the lens produces a prismatic effect. Slab-off lenses are used most commonly to correct an induced vertical imbalance as, for example, in a patient with anisometropia looking through the lower part of the spectacle lenses when reading.

soft contact l. *See* **lens, contact.**

spectacle l. Any lens used as a correction or protection and mounted a short distance from the eye, usually in a frame but also as a lorgnette, pince-nez, monocle, etc.
See **lens, ophthalmic.**

l. speed *See* **f number.**

spherical l. Lens in which the two surfaces are spherical.

spherocylindrical l. Lens with one surface spherical and the other cylindrical. It has two different refractive powers in its two principal meridians.
See **lens, astigmatic; lens, cylindrical; lens, toric.**

spin-cast contact l. A contact lens produced by placing a quantity of liquid mixture into a concave spinning mould with polymerization taking place during rotation. The curvature of the mould determines the front optic zone radius, whereas the speed of rotation and other factors determine the curvature of the back optic zone.
See **lens, cast-moulding contact; lens, lathe-cut contact; moulding.**

l. stalk *See* **cup, optic.**

steep l. Contact lens in which the back optic zone radius is shorter than the flattest meridian

of the cornea. This definition may not be valid for a soft lens, which may fit steeply even when its back optic zone radius is not shorter than the flattest meridian of the cornea. *Syn.* tight lens (it is preferable to use this term for soft lenses).
See **blanching, limbal; contact lens acute red eye; fitted on K; lens, flat.**

stigmatic l. *See* **lens, anastigmatic.**

Stokes l. A lens consisting of two planocylinders of equal and opposite power mounted with their flat surfaces almost in contact with each other in a cell and geared to rotate equally in opposite directions from a zero setting. At that setting, the two cylinder axes coincide and produce the minimum astigmatic value. When the lenses are rotated so that the two cylinder axes are at right angles to each other, the lens produces the maximum astigmatic value. Intermediate settings of the two cylinder axes result in intermediate astigmatic values. This lens is used in some ophthalmic instruments.

subluxation of the l. *See* **luxation of the lens.**

l. sutures Radiating lines in the crystalline lens formed by the meeting of lens fibres. Some of these systems of lens fibres form a Y in the fetus or infant, the arms of which are separated by angles of 120°. The anterior Y is upright and the posterior one is inverted. In the adult eye, the systems of lens fibres make up more complicated figures, but the Ys present at birth usually persist throughout life (Fig. L17).
See **fibre, lens; lens, crystalline.**

tear l. *See* **lens, liquid.**

telescopic l. A thick lens system forming a galilean telescope used to magnify the image. It is mounted in some form of frame and is lighter than an actual telescope. It is used to help low-vision patients for either distance or near vision, although for the latter the lens system (or sometimes a single lens) is often referred to as a **microscopic lens.**

therapeutic contact l. A contact lens, which acts as a protective device for the cornea, as in entropion, trichiasis or damage by application of a tonometer; as a pressure bandage to relieve pain, as in bullous keratopathy; to facilitate corneal healing, as in corneal erosion due to trauma; to improve vision during the healing process; and as a delivery mechanism for drugs, as soft contact lenses placed on the eye can slowly release a drug

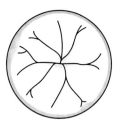

Fig. L17 Diagram of the anterior aspect of adult lens sutures showing a nine-point star.

which was previously absorbed. Silicone hydrogel lenses, which can be worn for up to 1 month at a time, are an efficient type of therapeutic contact lens. Gas permeable contact lenses are used therapeutically for extremely irregular corneas and some ocular surface disorders (e.g. keratoconus). Because of the risks associated with therapeutic lenses, it is important to follow the patient very assiduously. *Syn.* bandage lens.
See dystrophy, Cogan's microcystic epithelial; keratitis, Thygeson's superficial punctate; lens, hybrid contact; lens, ortho-k; lens, piggyback; lens, scleral.

thick l. *See* lens, thin.

l. thickness caliper *See* caliper.

thin l. A lens or combination of lenses in which the refracting surfaces are regarded as coincident, that is in which the separation between surfaces does not appreciably alter the total power of the system. Most ophthalmic lenses are thin lenses, but the crystalline lens of the eye is considered to be a **thick lens**. For optical purposes, contact lenses are also regarded as thick lenses.

Thorpe four mirror fundus l. *See* slit-lamp.

tight l. *See* lens, steep.

tinted l. An absorptive lens having a noticeable colour and which absorbs certain radiations more than others.
See bleaching; lens, absorptive; lens, cosmetic contact; photophobia; sunglasses; transmission curve.

toric l. This is usually a meniscus-type lens with a toroidal convex or concave surface. A toroidal surface is a surface with meridians of least and greatest curvature located at right angles to each other.
See lens, astigmatic; lens, meniscus; lens, spherocylindrical.

toughened l. A lens made of glass that has been either thermally or chemically strengthened and much less likely to fracture. When it does fracture, it breaks down into small fragments which are less harmful than large ones.
See glass, safety; lens, safety.

trial l. **1.** A lens used in a trial case. **2.** A trial contact lens.

trifield l. *See* field, visual expander.

trifocal l. Multifocal lens consisting of three portions of different focal power usually for distance, intermediate and near vision (Fig. L18).
See portion, intermediate.

uncut l. *See* lens, finished.

varifocal l. *See* lens, progressive.

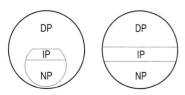

Fig. L18 Examples of trifocal lenses (DP, distance portion; IP, intermediate portion; NP, near portion).

ventilated l. *See* lens, fenestrated.

Volk l. *See* slit-lamp.

l. washer A plastic material which may be inserted between a loose lens and the eyewire of a frame to make the lens fit into the frame more securely. *Syn.* lens liner.

wide-angle l. Lens giving good resolution over a wide field of view, usually used in better quality cameras.
See lens, fisheye.

Wilson three mirror fundus l. *See* slit-lamp.

Wollaston l. Lens based on the values provided by Wollaston of the Tscherning ellipse.
See ellipse, Tscherning.

X-Chrom l. Trade name for a dyed hard corneal contact lens aimed at enhancing colour perception in red-green–deficient people. It is usually fitted on the non-dominant eye. The lens has maximum transmission above 575 nm with some additional transmission below 480 nm. Wearing this lens shifts the original absorption spectrum of the eye with the contact lens towards longer wavelengths. Objects may thus appear slightly different than with the other eye. This difference between the two eyes may, in certain conditions, improve colour discrimination.
See lens, ChromaGen.

Zeiss l. A type of goniolens, which when placed over the eye allows viewing of the anterior chamber angle. The Zeiss lens differs from other goniolenses in so much that it contains four mirrors, allowing visualization of the entire anterior chamber angle without the need to rotate the lens.
See gonioscopy, indirect; lens, gonioscopic.

zoom l. Lens in which the components can be adjusted to provide continuously variable magnification while the image remains constantly in focus.

lensectomy Surgical procedure performed to remove the crystalline lens of the eye.
See aphakia; cataract surgery.

lenscorometer *See* distometer.

lensometer *See* focimeter.

lenticele *See* phacocele.

lenticonus A rare congenital abnormality characterized by a conical projection of either the anterior or posterior (**posterior lenticonus**) surface of the crystalline lens of the eye The anterior lenticonus is the most common and most often associated with Alport's syndrome. If the bulging is spherical, instead of conical, the condition is referred to as **lentiglobus** and may be associated with polar cataract. It produces a decrease in visual acuity and irregular refraction that cannot be corrected by either spectacle or contact lenses.

lenticular astigmatism *See* astigmatism, lenticular.

lenticular fossa *See* fossa, hyaloid.

lenticular lens *See* lens, lenticular.

lenticular progressive degeneration *See* disease, Wilson's.

lenticular stereoscope *See* stereoscope, Brewster's.

lenticule A disc-shaped piece of corneal tissue or a piece of synthetic material manufactured to produce a given curvature and thickness. It is implanted into or on top of the cornea to change its anterior curvature.
See epikeratoplasty; keratophakia.

lentiglobus *See* lenticonus.

lentis ectopia *See* luxation of the lens.

lesion A localized pathological change in a tissue due to injury or disease.

letter acuity *See* acuity, visual.

leucocorea *See* leukocoria.

leucokeratosis *See* dyskeratosis.

leucoma *See* leukoma.

leucoplakia *See* dyskeratosis.

leukocoria A condition characterized by a whitish reflex within the pupil. It is secondary to cataract, Coats' disease, retinoblastoma, retrolental fibroplasia, persistent hyperplastic primary vitreous, toxocariasis, etc. *Syn.* white pupil; white pupillary reflex (Fig. L19). *Note*: also spelt leucocorea, leukocorea or leukokoria.
See disease, Norrie's.

leukoma A dense, white, corneal opacity caused by scar tissue. A localized leukoma appears as a whitish scar surrounded by normal cornea. A generalized leukoma involves the entire cornea, which appears white, often with blood vessels coursing over its surface. Visual impairment depends on the location and extent of the leukoma. If the opacity is faint, it is called a **nebula**. *Note*: also spelt leucoma.
See hyperacuity; ulcer, corneal.

levator aponeurosis; palpebrae superioris *See* muscle, levator palpebrae superioris.

levo Terms with this prefix can be found at laevo-.

levobunolol hydrochloride *See* beta-blocker.

levocabastine *See* antihistamine.

levofloxacin *See* antibiotic.

library spectacles *See* spectacles, library.

lid *See* eyelids.

lid eversion *See* eversion, lid.

lid laceration An injury to the eyelid caused by either a blunt or a sharp object. A thorough examination of the eye and orbit is needed as it may be associated with the laceration. It requires surgical intervention.

lid lag *See* disease, Graves'.

lid retraction *See* disease, Graves'; sign, Dalrymple's.

lid retractors Term used to refer to the muscles that open the eyelids. In the upper eyelid, it is the levator palpebrae muscle and its two divisions: the striated levator aponeurosis and the smooth Müller's muscle (or superior tarsal muscle). In the lower eyelid, it is the smooth fibre bundle derived from the inferior rectus muscle that forms the inferior tarsal muscle.
See muscle, levator palpebrae superioris; muscle, Müller's palpebral.

lidocaine hydrochloride (lignocaine hydrochloride) A local anaesthetic of the amide type used in eye surgery. It is used in 1% to 4% solution. Its action starts in less than 1 minute and lasts about 1 hour.

ligament A tough flexible band of white fibrous tissue that connects the articular extremities of bones or supports an organ in place.
check l. A strong band of connective tissue which leaves the surface of the sheath of the extraocular muscles and attaches to the surrounding tissues, so as to limit the action of the muscle. The medial rectus is attached to the lacrimal bone (**medial check ligament**) and the lateral rectus to the zygomatic bone (**lateral check ligament**). There are also check ligaments restricting the vertical movements, but the expansions of these muscles are thinner and less distinct than those of the horizontal recti muscles.
hyaloideocapsular l. *See* ligament of Wieger.
l. of Lockwood The lower part of the capsule of Tenon's capsule and parts of the tendons of the inferior rectus and oblique muscles which are thickened to form a hammock-like structure on which the eyeball rests.
palpebral l. Strong connective tissue attaching the extremities of the tarsal plates of the upper and lower eyelids to the orbital margin. There are two

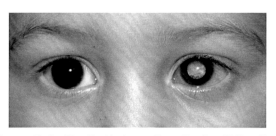

Fig. L19 Leukocoria in a patient with retinoblastoma. (From Bowling 2016, with permission of Elsevier. Courtesy of C Barry)

sets: (1) the **lateral palpebral ligament** (or **lateral canthal tendon**) about 7 mm long and 2.5 mm wide which constitutes the deeper portion of the lateral palpebral raphe of the orbicularis muscle and attaches the tarsal plates to the lateral orbital tubercle (**Whitnall's** tubercle) on the zygomatic bone and (2) the **medial palpebral ligament** (or **medial canthal tendon**) which attaches the medial ends of the tarsal plates to the frontal process of the maxilla and another insertion into the posterior lacrimal crest. It lies anterior to the canaliculi and the lacrimal sac.

superior transverse l. *See* **muscle, levator palpebrae superioris.**

suspensory l. Ligament whose principal function is to support another structure (e.g. ligament of Lockwood, the zonule of Zinn).

Whitnall's l. *See* **muscle, levator palpebrae superioris.**

l. of Wieger An attachment of the anterior surface of the vitreous humour to the posterior lens capsule in the shape of a ring about 8 to 9 mm in diameter. It forms a line called **Egger's line**. This adherence is strong in youth but weakens with age, enabling intracapsular cataract extraction without pulling the vitreous. *Syn.* hyaloideocapsular ligament.

light Electromagnetic vibrations which are capable of stimulating the receptors of the retina and of producing a visual sensation. The radiations that give rise to the sensation of vision are comprised within the wavelength band 380 to 780 nm. This band is called the **visible spectrum** or **visible light**. The borders of this band are not precise but beyond these radiations the visual efficacy of any wavelength becomes very low indeed (less than 10^{-5}).
See **coherent sources; infrared; lens, absorptive; spectroscope; spectrum, electromagnetic; spectrum, visible; Table C4, p. 64; theory, quantum; theory, wave; ultraviolet; wavelength.**

achromatic l. *See* **achromatic light stimulus.**

l. adaptation *See* **adaptation, light.**

artificial l. Light other than natural light.

beam of l. Collection of pencils arising from an extended source or object. *Syn.* bundle of light. *See* **light, pencil of.**

bundle of l. *See* **light, beam of.**

l. chaos *See* **light, idioretinal.**

cobalt blue l. Light which has passed through a cobalt blue filter.

cold l. Any visible light emitted by a process other than incandescence such as lasers, glow worms, certain chemical reactions, etc. Cold light is free of infrared.

compound l. Light composed of more than one wavelength.

diffuse l. Light coming from an extended source and having no predominant directional component. Illumination is thus relatively uniform with a minimum of shadows.
See **diffusion; source, extended.**

fluorescent l. Light emitted by fluorescence as in a fluorescent lamp. Electricity excites a gas that produces ultraviolet light, which in turn causes a phosphor coating on the inner surface of the fluorescent tube to fluoresce and emit visible light. *Examples*: mercury vapour lamp, neon and argon lamps, sodium vapour lamp, xenon flash lamp.

frequency of l. Number of vibrations of light waves per second. It is measured in hertz (Hz) and the symbol is the Greek letter ν (nu). The frequency of light, unlike its wavelength, is independent of the medium in which it passes.
See **hertz; spectrum, electromagnetic; Table C4, p. 64; wavelength.**

idioretinal l. Visual sensation occurring in total darkness that is attributed to spontaneous nervous impulses in the neurons of the visual pathway. *Syn.* intrinsic light; light chaos.

incandescent l. Light emitted by incandescence as in an incandescent lamp. An electrical current passes through a thin filament (e.g. tungsten) enclosed in a sealed oxygen-free glass bulb. The filament is heated and photons are released.
See **lamp, filament; lamp, halogen.**

infrared l. *See* **infrared.**

intrinsic l. *See* **light, idioretinal.**

monochromatic l. Light consisting of a single wavelength or, more usually, of a narrow band of wavelengths (a few nanometres).
See **light, polychromatic.**

natural l. Light received from the sun and the sky.

pencil of l. A narrow cone of light rays coming from a point source or from any one point on a broad source after passing through a limiting aperture. A pencil of light may be convergent, divergent or parallel. The ray passing through the centre of the aperture is the chief ray. *Syn.* homocentric bundle of rays; homocentric pencil of rays.
See **light, beam of.**

polarized l. Ordinary light is composed of transverse wave motions uniform in all directions in a plane perpendicular to its direction of propagation. Polarized light is composed of transverse wave motions in only one direction, called the **plane of vibration**. Polarized light can be obtained by using a polarizer (e.g. tourmaline crystals, polarizing material such as Polaroid, Nicol prism, etc.).
See **analyser; angle of polarization; crystal, dichroic; law, Brewster's; lens, polarizing; polarizer; prism, Wollaston; quartz; tourmaline; vectogram.**

polychromatic l. Light consisting of a mixture of wavelengths.
See **light, monochromatic.**

quantity of l. Product of luminous flux and its duration. *Unit*: lumen-second.
See **lumen.**

l. reflex *See* **reflex, corneal; reflex, pupil light.**

solar l. Light from the sun or having identical properties as the sun.
See **blindness, eclipse; light, white.**

l. source Any source of visible radiant energy such as natural light (e.g. daylight, moonlight, sunlight) or artificial light (e.g. a candle flame, an incandescent lamp, a discharge lamp, a fluorescent lamp).

See **coherent sources; illuminants, CIE standard.**

speed of l. The currently accepted figure is 299 792.5 km/s (in a vacuum). This velocity decreases, differentially with wavelength, when the radiation enters a medium.

See **index of refraction; spectrum, electromagnetic.**

l. stop *See* **diaphragm.**

stray l. Light reflected or passing through an optical system but not involved in the formation of the image such as that reflected by the surfaces of a correcting lens. *Syn.* parasitic light.

See **image, ghost.**

l. threshold *See* threshold, light absolute.

ultraviolet l. *See* ultraviolet; light, Wood's.

visible l. *See* light; spectrum, visible.

white l. Light perceived without any attribute of hue. Any light produced by a source having an equal energy spectrum will appear white after the eye is adapted. Some of the CIE illuminants are often used as a source of white light, e.g. B, C and D. Sunlight is a source of white light.

See **chromaticity diagram; illuminants, CIE standard; spectrum, equal energy.**

Wood's l. Ultraviolet light near the visible spectrum which, when used with certain dyes such as fluorescein, causes fluorescence. It is produced by a special type of glass (called **Wood's glass** or **Wood's filter**), which contains nickel oxide and transmits ultraviolet radiations near the visible spectrum. It is used to detect corneal abrasions and to evaluate the fit of hard contact lenses. It is available in a slit-lamp or in a Burton lamp.

See **fluorescein; fluorescence; slit-lamp.**

light-stress test *See* test, photostress.

lightness Attribute of visual sensation in accordance with which a body seems to transmit or reflect diffusely a greater or smaller fraction of the incident light. This attribute is the psychosensorial correlate, or nearly so, of the photometric quantity luminance (CIE).

See **luminance.**

lignocaine hydrochloride *See* lidocaine.

limbal furrow *See* furrow, limbal.

limbal relaxing incision A surgical procedure aimed at correcting astigmatism. It consists of performing one or, more commonly, two arcuate incisions, one on each side of the cornea near the limbus and along the steeper axis. It thus flattens that meridian. The length of the incision varies, usually between 6 and 10 mm depending on the amount of astigmatism to correct, the higher it is, the longer the incision. The procedure can be performed on its own but most frequently during cataract surgery.

limbus The transition zone, about 1.5 mm wide, between the conjunctiva and sclera on the one hand, and the cornea on the other. Anteriorly the corneo-limbal junction corresponds approximately to the termination of Bowman's layer and Descemet's membrane and to the separation between the transparent cornea and the opaque tissue of the limbus. Posteriorly the junction corresponds approximately to a thinning of the conjunctival epithelium. From the surface inwards it is comprised of the limbal conjunctiva, the episclera, the canal of Schlemm, the trabecular meshwork and the scleral spur. The limbal conjunctival epithelium contains stem cells that regulate and regenerate the basal cells of the corneal epithelium. *Syn.* corneoscleral junction.

See **corneal epithelium; blanching, limbal; stem cell deficiency, limbal; sulcus, scleral external; sulcus, scleral internal; Vogt's white limbal girdle.**

limen *See* threshold.

liminal Pertaining to a threshold.

limit of resolution *See* resolution, limit of.

Lindblom's method *See* method, Lindblom's.

line 1. The connection between two points. **2.** In anatomy, a long narrow band or streak that is distinct from the surrounding tissues by colour or texture.

base l. Line joining the centres of rotation of the two eyes. It is approximately equal to the interpupillary distance (Fig. L20).

See **distance, interocular.**

demand l. The line in Donders' diagram that represents the perfect amount of convergence required for each level of accommodation, for single binocular vision. *Syn.* orthophoria line; Donders' line.

l. of direction Line joining an object in space with its image on the retina (allowing for the optical properties of the eye). The line joining the fixation point to the fovea is called the **principal line of direction.** However, the object appears to lie along a **visual direction,** and that direction in visual space associated with the fovea is called the **principal visual direction.** All other visual

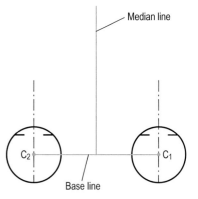

Fig. L20 Base line $C_1 C_2$ and median line. The base line is situated about 13.5 mm behind the vertex of the cornea in the straight-ahead position.

Table L3 Common spectral lines of the visible spectrum

Designation	Origin	Wavelength (nm)
A	oxygen	759.4
C	hydrogen	656.3
C′	cadmium	643.8
D	sodium	589.3
d	helium	587.6
e	mercury	546.1
F	hydrogen	486.1
F′	cadmium	480.0
G	calcium	430.8
h	hydrogen	410.2

directions associated with other retinal points are called **secondary visual directions**. The principal line of direction and the principal visual direction coincide, but the former indicates the direction towards the eye, while the latter indicates the direction away from the eye. *See* **law of identical visual directions**.

Donders' l. *See* **line, demand**.

Egger's l. *See* **ligament of Wieger**.

Ferry's line A line containing iron located in the corneal epithelium and adjacent to limbal filtering blebs. It may occur as a result of trabeculectomy.

l. of fixation *See* **axis, fixation**.

Fleischer's l. *See* **ring, Fleischer's**.

focal l. Any astigmatic optical system produces two mutually, usually perpendicular, focal lines of a point object. The focal lines are situated at different image distances. Each focal line lies parallel to its associated cylinder axis. *Syn.* image line; line focus; Sturm's line. *See* **circle of least confusion; Sturm, conoid of; Sturm, interval of**.

l. focus *See* **line, focal**.

Fraunhofer's l's. Fine dark lines distributed throughout the length of the solar spectrum due to the absorption of specific wavelengths by elements in the atmosphere of the sun and the earth. Fraunhofer observed about 600 of these lines and denoted the most prominent ones by letters from A in the extreme red to K in the violet. *Examples*: A corresponds to 759.4 nm, C to 656.3 nm, D to 589.3 nm, F to 486.1 nm, etc (Table L3). *See* **constringence; spectrum, solar**.

l. of Gennari A distinctive white stripe in the middle of the fourth layer of the visual cortex containing the termination of the optic radiation fibres, as well as intracortical connections. The stripe appears above and below the calcarine fissure except in the most anterior part of the fissure where it only appears below. *Syn.* area striata; stria of Gennari. *See* **area, visual; fissure, calcarine**.

Hudson–Stähli l. Yellowish-brown line, more or less horizontal, containing iron which runs across the cornea below the centre. It occurs in normal corneas, more frequently in the elderly or in association with corneal opacities.

iron l. Deposits of iron within the corneal epithelium appearing as a brown rust line. They often subside with time leaving a nebulous scar. Several eponymous types have been described depending on the cause and location. *See* **line, Hudson–Stähli; line, Stocker's; ring, Coat's white; ring, Fleischer's; siderosis bulbi**.

median l. Line formed by the intersection of the median plane and the plane of regard (Fig. L20). *Syn.* midline.

orthophoria l. *See* **line, demand**.

phoria l. On Donders' diagram, it is the line joining all the points representing the passive position of the eyes corresponding to various levels of accommodation.

principal l. of vision *See* **line of sight**.

pupillary l. *See* **axis, pupillary**.

retinal l. Operationally, the collection of retinal elements that are activated in response to a line stimulus.

Sampaolesi's l. Pigmented, wavy line anterior to Schwalbe's ring and found mainly in the periphery of the inferior cornea. It may be noted with gonioscopy in pigmentary dispersion syndrome and pseudoexfoliation syndrome.

l. of Schwalbe A bundle of connective tissue and elastic fibres forming the junction between the anterior termination of the trabecular meshwork and Descemet's membrane of the cornea. If it is unusually thickened or prominent, it is called **posterior embryotoxon**. *Syn.* anterior limiting ring of Schwalbe. *See* **gonioscopy, direct; syndrome, Axenfeld's; syndrome, Rieger's; trabecular meshwork**.

l. of sight Line joining the point of fixation to the centre of the entrance pupil. This line is more practical than the visual axis. *Syn.* principal line of vision.

l. spectrum *See* **spectrum, line**.

Stocker's l. An abnormal line containing iron located in the corneal epithelium which may appear in front of the advancing edge of a pterygium.

Sturm's l. *See* **line, focal**.

visual l. *See* **axis, visual**.

line-spread function *See* **function, line-spread**.

linear magnification *See* **magnification, lateral**.

linear perspective *See* **perspective, linear**.

lipid droplet degeneration; keratopathy *See* **keratopathy, lipid**.

lipid metabolism disorders Disorders caused by a lack of enzymes necessary to break down lipids (fats), hence a harmful amount of lipids accumulate in the body eventually causing damage to cells and tissues, especially in the brain, peripheral nervous system and liver. In the eye, they are mostly inherited. They include diseases such as those of Fabry's, Gaucher's, Niemann–Pick, Sandhoff's, Tay–Sachs and Refsum's syndrome.

lipofuscin Yellowish-brown pigment granules formed as a result of oxidation of protein and lipid residues, and found in various tissues (e.g.

liver, kidney, heart muscle, adrenals, nerve cells). It normally accumulates with age within the lysosomes of cells, and its accumulation in the retinal pigment epithelium (RPE) is a major risk factor of age-related macular degeneration and fundus flavimaculatus in Stargardt's disease as it may damage RPE cells and lead to the formation of drusen and RPE atrophy. In albinos, the pigment granules are immature and colourless.

liquid lens *See* **lens, liquid.**

liquid paraffin *See* **tears, artificial.**

Lisch nodule *See* **nodule, Lisch.**

lissamine green A vital stain with dyeing quality similar to that of rose bengal, but which causes less discomfort. It stains dead or degenerated epithelial cells green and is used to facilitate the diagnosis of keratoconjunctivitis sicca, xerophthalmia, etc. It has a molecular weight of 577.

Listing's law; plane; reduced eye *See* under the nouns.

lithiasis, conjunctival *See* **conjunctival, concretions.**

lobe, occipital *See* **occipital lobe.**

local sign *See* **direction, oculocentric.**

localization The perception of the location of an object in space with respect to either the eye (**oculocentric localization**) or the self (**egocentric localization**).
See **egocentre; oculocentre; pointing, past-.**

lock, binocular The part of the visual input that is common to both eyes and thus helps to maintain fusion. *Syn.* fusion lock.
See **prism, aligning.**

Lockwood's ligament *See* **ligament of Lockwood.**

lodoxamide *See* **mast cell stabilizers.**

logMAR chart *See* **chart, logMAR.**

logMAR crowded test *See* **Glasgow acuity cards.**

long ciliary nerve *See* **nerve, long ciliary.**

long sight *See* **hyperopia.**

loop A circular bend or fold in a vessel or a bundle of nerve or muscle fibres.
Archambault's l. *See* **loop, Meyer's.**
Axenfeld's nerve l. An anomalous nerve path of the long ciliary nerve, which after passing through the suprachoroidal space pierces the sclera a few millimetres behind the limbus, turns back on itself for a short distance and then resumes its normal course to the ciliary body. It is often accompanied by a branch of the anterior ciliary artery. The loop is usually pigmented giving rise to a 1- to 2-mm black dot on the sclera. It appears only in a small percentage of individuals (10% to 15%). Treatment is not necessary. *Syn.* Axenfeld's intrascleral nerve loop; Axenfeld's pigmented nerve loop.
Meyer's l. A bundle of inferior nerve fibres of the optic radiations that originate from the lateral portion of the lateral geniculate body, extend forward around the anterior tip of the temporal

horn of the lateral ventricle and then swing backward towards the occipital lobe. A lesion in this loop may cause a superior homonymous quadrantanopia. *Syn.* Archambault's loop.
See **radiations, optic.**

loratadine *See* **antihistamine.**

lorgnette Eyeglasses for occasional use, held before the eyes by a handle, into which the lenses may fold when not in use (British Standard).
See **lens, spectacle; spectacles.**

lorgnon A spectacle lens for occasional use, mounted on a handle (British Standard).

loteprednol etabonate *See* **antiinflammatory drug.**

Lotmar Visometer *See* **maxwellian view system, clinical.**

Lotze's local sign *See* **direction, oculocentric.**

loupe *See* **magnifier.**

loupe magnification *See* **magnification, apparent.**

loupe, Berger's A binocular loupe fitted with a headband.

Lowe's syndrome *See* **syndrome, Lowe's.**

low tension glaucoma *See* **glaucoma, normal-tension.**

low vision *See* **vision, low.**

lower-order aberration *See* **aberration, lower-order.**

lubricant, ocular *See* **tears, artificial.**

lug *See* **endpiece.**

lumen 1. SI unit of luminous flux. It is equal to the flux emitted within a unit solid angle of one steradian by a point source with a luminous intensity of one candela. *Symbol*: lm. 2. The space in the interior of a tubular organ, such as an artery.
See **light, quantity of; luminous flux; lux; SI unit.**

luminance A photometric term characterizing the way in which a surface emits or reflects light in a given direction. It is equal to the luminous intensity measured in a given direction divided by the area of this surface projected on a perpendicular to the direction considered. *Symbol*: L. *Units*: candela per square metre (SI unit); footlambert; lambert, etc (Table L4).
See **brightness; candela per square metre; footlambert; lambert; lightness; millilambert; nit; range of visible luminances; photometry; SI unit.**

luminaire A complete lighting unit consisting of a light source, a housing, enclosure, etc.

luminescence Emission of light by certain substances resulting from the absorption of energy (e.g. from electrical fields, chemical reaction, or other light), which is not due to a rise in temperature (unlike incandescence). The emitted radiation is characteristic of the particular substance. When the light emitted is due to exposure to a source of light, the process is usually called

Table L4 Approximate luminance (in cd/m² of some objects

sun	10^9
car headlight	10^7
incandescent lamp (tungsten)	10^6–10^7
fluorescent lamp	10^4–10^5
clear sky at noon	10^4
cloudy sky at noon	10^3
shady street by day	10^3–10^4
full moon	10^3
book print under artificial light	>10^2
photopic vision	>10
street illumination	1–10^{-1}
mesopic vision	10–10^{-3}
cloudless night sky with full moon	10^{-2}
scotopic vision	<10^{-3}
moonless and cloudless night sky	10^{-3}–10^{-6}

photoluminescence. When the light emitted is due to either a high-frequency discharge through a gas or to an electric field through certain solids such as **phosphor** which is used in fluorescent lamps, television picture tubes, etc., it is called **electroluminescence**.
See **bioluminescence; fluorescence; incandescence; lamp, fluorescent; phosphorescence.**

luminosity *See* **brightness.**

luminous 1. Emitting or reflecting light. **2.** Having the capacity of stimulating the photoreceptors.

luminous efficiency The amount of light emitted by a lamp for each watt of power consumed. It is expressed in lumens/watt.

luminous flux Flow of light which produces a visual sensation. It is measured in lumens. *Syn.* luminous power.
See **radiant flux.**

luminous intensity Quotient of the luminous flux leaving the source, propagated in an element of solid angle containing the given direction, divided by the element of solid angle. *Symbol*: I. *Unit*: candela (CIE).

luminous power *See* **luminous flux.**

luminosity curve *See* **efficiency, spectral luminous.**

Luneburg's theory *See* **theory, Luneburg's.**

lupus erythematosus, systemic *See* **keratitis, peripheral ulcerative; keratoconjunctivitis sicca; scleritis.**

lustre 1. The effect of one colour appearing to be situated behind and through another. This can occur when looking in a haploscope, it is then called binocular lustre. **2.** Appearance of glossiness on a metallic surface.

lux SI unit of illuminance. It is the illuminance produced by a luminous flux of one lumen uniformly distributed over a surface area of one square metre. *Symbol*: lx.

luxation of the lens A pathological and complete dislocation of the lens relative to the pupil. If the luxation is incomplete it is called **subluxation** of the lens (or **dislocation**), in which case the eye is rendered astigmatic and there is diplopia. Complete luxation results in high hyperopia and the eye is unable to accommodate as it is made aphakic. Luxation occurs in contusion of the globe, in many ocular (e.g. ciliary body tumour, high myopia, buphthalmos, hypermature cataract) or it can be inherited (e.g. the bilateral, symmetrical, superior subluxation commonly found in familial ectopia lentis, Marfan's syndrome, Weil–Marchesani syndrome or homocystinuria). It is sometimes associated with ectopic pupils and keratoconus. Anterior luxation may cause glaucoma. Treatment is surgical consisting of lens removal unless it is a partial dislocation, which is corrected optically (Fig. L21).
See **ectopia lentis; iridodonesis; pupillary block.**

luxometer *See* **photometer.**

lymphadenopathy An enlargement of a lymph gland. The preauricular lymph node located 1 cm in front of the external ear drains the orbital region and is sometimes involved with eyelid and conjunctival infection (e.g. adult inclusion conjunctivitis, follicular conjunctivitis).

lymphangioma A tumour of lymph vessels, which generally presents in childhood, progresses slowly and is usually benign. Superficial lesions affect the eyelids or conjunctiva. Deeper lesions affect the orbit. They often enlarge because of haemorrhages developing into large blood cysts called 'chocolate cysts', which may cause proptosis and diplopia. Blood-filled cysts may resolve spontaneously. If sight is threatened, drainage of blood may be required.

lymphoma A group of conditions characterized by proliferation of cells of the immune system, (called lymphocytes). There are two main types: Hodgkin (also called Hodgkin's disease) and non-Hodgkin lymphoma of which most are of B-cell (also called B lymphocyte) origin. The latter is the most common and strongly associated with primary central nervous system lymphoma, which

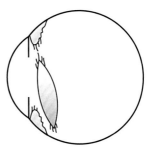

Fig. L21 Dislocation of the lens (usually in the vitreous humour).

arises from the brain or spinal cord and affects the orbit. Ocular features are diplopia and proptosis, while Hodgkin's lymphoma gives rise to anterior uveitis with keratic precipitates, vitritis and large multifocal subretinal infiltrates. Treatment is by radiotherapy and chemotherapy.

lysozyme An antibacterial enzyme present in the tears (as well as other tissues). It accomplishes this by breaking down the walls of bacterial cells (especially Gram-positive) and rendering them ineffective. In human tears, lysozyme makes up 21% to 25% of the total protein.

M

MacAdam ellipses *See* ellipses, MacAdam.

Mach bands When a light area is separated from a dark area by a transition zone in which the brightness increases or decreases regularly and rapidly, two bands are seen: one light band next to the dark area and another dark band next to the light area. The appearance of these two bands, known as Mach bands, is attributed to lateral inhibition processes occurring in the retina. The phenomenon is usually demonstrated with a rotating disc with black and white areas separated by a zone of brightness gradient. *Syn.* Mach rings. *See* inhibition, lateral.

macrophthalmia *See* megalophthalmos.

macrocornea *See* keratoglobus.

macropsia Anomaly of visual perception in which objects appear larger than they actually are. It may occur as a result of abnormal accommodation (less than required for the fixation distance), because of various retinal anomalies in which the visual receptors are crowded together or because of the recent wear of either base-in prisms or a presbyopic correction, etc. If it affects only one eye, the condition is related to aniseikonia. *Syn.* megalopsia.
See dysmegalopsia; micropsia; metamorphopsia.

macula *See* fovea centralis; macula lutea.

macula, ectopia of the An anomaly characterized by displacement of the macula, which can be either of acquired or congenital origin. It may follow some forms of retinal scarring, retinal detachment surgery, previous inflammation, etc. It may result in reduced acuity, metamorphopsia or strabismus. *Syn.* dystopia of the macula; heterotopia macula.

macula, false The retinal area of the deviating eye of a strabismic subject which corresponds to the fovea of the fixating eye.
See retinal correspondence, abnormal.

macula lutea An oval area of the retina 3 to 5 mm in diameter, with the foveal depression at its centre, slightly below the level of the optic disc and temporal to it (its centre lies 3.5 mm from the edge of the disc). The side walls of the depression slope gradually towards the centre where the fovea centralis is located and where the best photopic visual acuity is obtained. Around the fovea, the ganglion cells are much more numerous than elsewhere, being arranged in five to seven layers. The outer molecular layer is also thicker than elsewhere and forms the outer fibre layer of Henle and there is a progressive disappearance of rods so that at the foveola only cones are found. The area of the macula lutea is impregnated by a yellow-brown pigment (macular pigment) in the inner layers and for that reason is often called the **yellow spot.** *Syn.* area centralis (although that area is considered to be slightly larger, about 5.5 mm in diameter); punctum luteum.
See entoptoscope, blue field; fovea centralis; pigment, macular.

macula, sparing of the *See* macular sparing.

macular cyst A swelling in the macular area in which fluid has accumulated after injury to the eye or cystoid macular oedema. It may eventually burst into the vitreous producing a macular hole.

macular degeneration, age-related (AMD) A common, chronic, degenerative condition found in a large percentage of elderly patients (and sometimes middle-aged ones) characterized by loss of central vision. There are two main forms of the condition: **non-neovascular (dry, atrophic) AMD,** which is the most common (about 90%), and **exudative (wet, neovascular) AMD** in which the loss of vision is the most severe. The main features of **dry AMD** are the presence in the macular region of small yellowish-white spots (hard drusen) and large, poorly defined, coalescing soft drusen, focal hyperpigmentation of the retinal pigment epithelium (RPE) and, at a later stage, geographic atrophy of the RPE and depigmentation exposing choroidal vessels. Visual acuity becomes markedly reduced, there is metamorphopsia and the condition usually becomes bilateral over several years. The condition is managed essentially by the use of low vision aids.
Exudative AMD has a similar clinical picture initially but is followed by choroidal neovascularization (CNV), which gives rise to subretinal fluid, haemorrhages, exudation, RPE detachment and subretinal fibrosis in the macular region resulting

in severe loss of central vision. If detected early (usually with an Amsler chart), treatment with laser photocoagulation will reduce the risk of further visual loss. **Photodynamic therapy** (PDT) is another method of reducing the risk of visual loss. It allows selective destruction of the choroidal neovascularization with minimal damage to the overlying retinal tissue. It consists of injecting a photosensitizing agent (e.g. verteporfin) that is taken up by the abnormal vessels and, when activated by a laser light of a given wavelength (e.g. 689 nm), it damages and shrivels up the vessels. This method is less used nowadays. Recent drug therapies, such as the **anti-VEGF** ranibizumab, bevacizumab and aflibercept which are injected intravitreally at regular intervals and designed to stop the leakage and the growth of blood vessels, not only reduce loss of vision but improve visual acuity in a significant percentage of cases of wet AMD. There are various risk factors for AMD including older age, family history, smoking, hypertension, diabetes, alcohol consumption, blue irides and excessive exposure to sunlight. The risk of progression and even development of an advanced form of this condition may be decreased by dietary supplements of vitamin C and E, antioxidants (carotenoids such as lutein and zeaxanthin) and minerals (zinc and copper) in individuals with certain dry AMD features. *Syn.* senile macular degeneration.
See **disciform scar; drusen; dystrophy, macular; fluorescein angiography; lipofuscin; maculopathy, age-related; oxidative stress; pigment, macular; rule, Kollner's; test, photostress; VEGF.**

macular hole A condition in which there is a partial or full thickness absence of the retina in the macular area. It may occur as a result of trauma, degeneration, old age, preretinal macular fibrosis or pathological myopia. It appears ophthalmoscopically as a round or oval, well-defined, reddish spot at the macula. There is metamorphopsia, loss of visual acuity and a central scotoma. An operculum of retinal tissue may overlie the hole. The vitreous in front of the hole eventually condenses and separates from the retina. In partial macular hole, a layer of photoreceptors may still be attached to the retinal pigment epithelium (**lamellar hole**), as in cystoid macular oedema. Treatment usually consists of reattaching the retina, if detached, and possibly vitrectomy.
See **membrane, epiretinal; ophthalmoscope, confocal scanning laser; retinal break; retinopathy, solar; tomography, optical coherence.**

macular oedema *See* **oedema, cystoid macular; retinopathy, background diabetic.**

macular pigment *See* **pigment, macular.**

macular pucker *See* **membrane, epiretinal.**

macular sparing Retention of macular function in spite of losses in the adjacent visual field as, for example, in homonymous hemianopia due to a cortical lesion (e.g. an interference in the blood flow in the middle cerebral artery). This is due to the fact that most cortical lesions are not large enough to affect the whole extensive cortical area representing the macula, thus leaving some of the area unaffected.
See **magnification, cortical.**

macular star Deposits of hard exudates material, mainly lipids, in Henle's fibre layer radiating out in a star-like pattern. It can occur in neuroretinitis, hypertensive retinopathy, etc.

macular telangiectasia, idiopathic *See* **telangiectasia.**

maculopathy, age-related A condition in which there are large whitish-yellow soft drusen in the macular area and hyperpigmentation or depigmentation of the retinal pigment epithelium associated with the drusen. Small hard drusen may also be present. It occurs most commonly in individuals over 50 years of age and represents the early stage of age-related macular degeneration.
See **macular degeneration, age-related.**

maculopathy, bull's eye An ocular condition in which degeneration of the retinal pigment epithelium in the macular area causes alternating ring-like light and dark zones of pigmentation, as in a target. It may result from drug toxicity or hereditary conditions (e.g. cone dystrophy, Bardet–Biedl syndrome). The main symptoms are a loss of visual acuity, reduced colour vision and aversion to bright sunlight.

maculopathy, cellophane *See* **membrane, epiretinal.**

maculopathy, diabetic A pathological disorder of the macula which is frequently noted in diabetic patients. It is characterized by oedema, hard exudates, microaneurysms and ischaemia in the macular area. If the oedema is severe, visual acuity will be reduced, but a blue-yellow colour vision defect is usually noted before the loss of acuity. Management involves laser photocoagulation.
See **retinopathy, background diabetic; retinopathy, diabetic.**

madarosis A loss of either or both the eyebrows and the eyelashes. It may occur in blepharitis, in the presence of hair follicle mites, trauma from rubbing, in alopecia, in leprosy or as a complication of acquired syphilis.

Maddox cross A scale for measuring the angle of heterophoria and heterotropia consisting of one horizontal and one vertical line in the form of a cross with a light source placed at the centre of intersection. The lines are graduated in prism dioptres or degrees and calibrated for use at a given distance (usually 6 metres). *Syn.* Maddox tangent scale.

Maddox double prism *See* **Fresnel's bi-prism; test, double prism.**

Maddox rod This is not a rod but a series of cylindrical grooves ground usually into a coloured piece of glass and mounted in a rim. (Originally it consisted of a single cylindrical rod.) It is used to measure heterophoria by placing it in front of one eye of a subject viewing a spot of light binocularly. The Maddox rod and eye together form a long streak of light perpendicular to the axis of the grooves, and this retinal image is so unlike the image formed in the other eye that the fusion reflex is not stimulated. The eyes will then stay in the passive position. If there is a phoria, the streak of light will not intersect the spot of light. For horizontal phorias, the rod axis is placed horizontally and for vertical phorias, vertically. The amount and type of the phoria can be quantified by placing a prism of appropriate power and direction in front of either eye such that the streak appears superimposed on the spot of light. Alternatively, the angle of the phoria could be determined using a Maddox cross and placing a rod in front of one eye; the phoria can be read directly by the patient who indicates where the streak of light appears to cross the scale. The Maddox rod is also used to detect or measure cyclophoria (Fig. M1).

See **position, passive; test, Maddox rod; test, Thorington.**

Maddox wing Hand-held device used to measure heterophoria at near. It consists of a septum and two slit apertures, one for each eye. One eye sees a double tangent scale (vertical and horizontal) calibrated to read in prism dioptres, while the other eye sees a white arrow pointing upward and a red arrow pointing horizontally to the left. As the two retinal images are quite different, there is no attempt at fusion and the eyes stay in the passive position. The arrow which is seen by the left eye points to the numbers seen by the right eye. The numbers represent the vertical and horizontal components of the phoria, which can be read directly by the observer (Fig. M2).

magenta **1.** Hue produced by the additive mixture of red and blue. **2.** Hue evoked by any combination of wavelengths which act as the complement of a wavelength of 515 nm (green).

See **colour, complementary.**

magnetic resonance imaging (MRI) A non-invasive method of imaging part of the body to facilitate diagnosis and therapy. Unlike other radiological methods, this technique does not

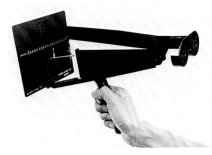

Fig. M2 Maddox wing.

expose the patient to ionizing radiations. It depends instead on a strong magnetic field which induces the spins of atomic nuclei within the body (e.g. hydrogen atoms) to align themselves along the axis of the magnetic field. When exposed to a pulse of electromagnetic energy at a specific radio frequency, the nuclear spins tilt momentarily then regain their original orientations thus re-emitting an electromagnetic signal at the same radio frequency, which can be detected and analyzed to generate a three-dimensional image. The rate at which the radio frequency signal decays can be used to characterize the properties of different tissues, both normal and abnormal. The rates are referred to as T1 and T2 and each yields different contrasts: T1-weighted images are best for ana-tomical details and T2-weighted images are best for pathological details. This technique provides better image contrast than X-ray computerized tomography in many instances (e.g. the patches of demyelination in the white matter of patients with multiple sclerosis), while the reverse is true in other instances (e.g. a meningioma in the posterior visual pathway). Usage includes the detection of optic nerve disease (e.g. glioma, optic neuropathy), retrobulbar neuritis, lesions in the chiasma and pituitary tumours. In general, this procedure takes longer than X-ray computerized tomography (Fig. M3).

functional MRI (fMRI) A non-invasive method used to map the various areas of the cortex, as well as brain tumour mapping, by observing brain activity in response to performing a task that engages a specific behaviour (e.g. tests of colour vision, face perception, motion perception, solving a mathematical problem). This is accomplished, within a conventional MRI scanner, by detecting changes in blood flow which has become more oxygenated in an area of the brain where neural activity has increased in the same area. This leads to a focal increase in MR image intensity, of around 1% to 5%, which can be detected using appropriate statistical methods.

See **area, visual association; radiology; tomography, positron emission.**

magnification **1.** An increase in the apparent size of an object. *Syn.* enlargement. **2.** Specification of a magnifying device to form an enlarged image.

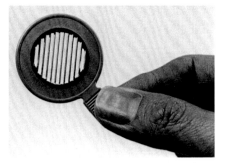

Fig. M1 Maddox rod.

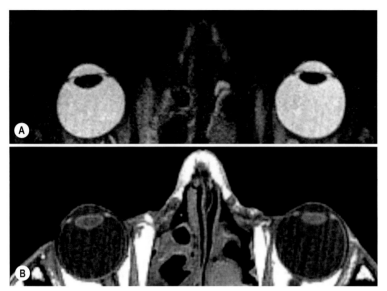

Fig. M3 MRI scans of the normal eyes of the same individual. A, a T2-weighted scan designed to show high contrast between the fluid-filled eyes and the surrounding tissues. B, a T1-weighted scan showing more tissue differentiation and darker fluid-filled eyes and the surrounding tissues. (Courtesy of Prof. K Singh, Cardiff University)

angular m. Magnification expressed as the ratio of the angle α' subtended at the eye by the image to the angle α subtended at the eye by the object (assuming small angles)

$$M = \tan\alpha'/\tan\alpha$$

Syn. angular enlargement. *Note:* Low vision practitioners consider this type of magnification in which no specific distance is specified as a synonym of apparent magnification.

apparent m. Magnification produced by a viewing instrument or lens expressed as the ratio of the angle w' subtended at the nodal point of the eye by the image, to the angle w subtended at the nodal point by the object, when placed at a standard (reference) distance called '**the least distance of distinct vision**' from the unaided eye. It is conventional to take this distance as 250 mm and to place the object in the anterior focal plane of the magnifying device. The magnification M is, then, equal to (assuming small angles)

$$M = \frac{\tan w'}{\tan w} = \frac{250}{f'} = \frac{F}{4}$$

where f' and F are the second focal length (in mm) and power (in dioptres) of the magnifying device, respectively (Fig. M4). In this object location, the magnification (and therefore the retinal image size) is constant and independent of the distance between the magnifier and the eye, but the field of view decreases as the distance between the

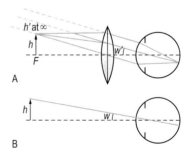

Fig. M4 Object *h* viewed, A, with a loupe and placed at its anterior principal focus F, and B, without.

eye and the magnifier increases (Table M1). *Syn.* conventional magnification; effective magnification; loupe magnification; nominal magnification; relative magnification; standard magnification.

If the object is closer to the magnifying device than its anterior focal plane so that its image is formed at the least distance of distinct vision (25 cm), and assuming that the eye is so close to the magnifier as to ignore the distance separating them and that the patient has an accommodation (or a near addition) of +4.00 D, the magnification M is then equal to

$$M = 1 + (F/4)$$

Example: a lens of +16.00 D provides, in these conditions, a magnification of 5×. *Syn.*

Table M1 Apparent magnification (or conventional magnification) of microscopic lenses of various powers used in the correction of low vision and their corresponding reading distance (assuming emmetropia or correction for distance and that no accommodation is exerted)

Magnification	Lens power (D)	Reading distance (cm)
1×	+4.00	25
1.5×	+6.00	16.7
2×	+8.00	12.5
2.5×	+10.00	10
3×	+12.00	8.3
4×	+16.00	6.25
5×	+20.00	5
6×	+24.00	4.2
8×	+32.00	3.12
10×	+40.00	2.5

Table M2 Approximate lateral magnification (in %) corresponding to various changes in spectacle lens distance and for various lens powers

Distance change	Lens power (D)					
	1	2	4	6	8	10
1 mm	0.1	0.2	0.4	0.6	0.8	1.0
2 mm	0.2	0.4	0.8	1.2	1.6	2.0
3 mm	0.3	0.6	1.2	1.8	2.4	3.0
4 mm	0.4	0.8	1.6	2.4	3.2	4.0
5 mm	0.5	1.0	2.0	3.0	4.0	5.0
10 mm	1.0	2.0	4.0	6.0	8.0	10.0

Minus lens: If moved closer to the eye, magnification increases; if moved further from the eye, magnification decreases. Plus lens: If moved closer to the eye, magnification decreases; if moved further from the eye, magnification increases.

magnifying power; maximum magnification; trade magnification.
See magnification, iso-accommodative; magnification, lateral; power, equivalent viewing.
axial m. Ratio of the distance *l′* along the optical axis between two points in image space to the distance *l* along the optical axis between the corresponding two points in object space, i.e. *l′/l*. The axial magnification is approximately equal to the square of the lateral magnification when the object is far away from the optical system. This magnification is useful when considering an image in its three dimensions. Clinically, it is important when assessing the thickness of a retinal lesion in indirect ophthalmoscopy. *Syn.* longitudinal magnification.
combined m. Product of the individual values of each type of magnification used in combination with each other. *Example*: If a patient uses a CCTV monitor to provide a magnification of 5× viewed at a distance of 50 cm, and then views the same screen at a distance of 25 cm, thus producing a relative distance magnification of 50/25 = 2×, the total magnification is 5 × 2 = 10×. *Syn.* total magnification.
conventional m. *See magnification, apparent.*
cortical m. Term referring to the fact that the amount of cortical area devoted to processing visual information from the central area of the retina far exceeds the amount devoted to the peripheral retina. It is estimated that about 25% of the cells in the visual cortex are devoted to processing the central 2.5° of the visual field. *Syn.* magnification factor.
See area, visual; macular sparing.
distance m. *See magnification, relative distance.*
effective m. *See magnification, apparent.*
electronic m. Magnification obtained using an electronic vision enhancement system (EVES), such as a closed-circuit television (CCTV). It is equal to

the ratio of the size of the image on the screen to the size of the original object being viewed. *Example*: An object 2 cm in height measures 6 cm on the screen, therefore the magnification is 6/2 = 3×. *Syn.* real image magnification; transverse magnification.
m. factor *See magnification, cortical.*
iso-accommodative m. The magnification of a lens (or lens system) when the distance of the image from the eye (or spectacle plane) formed by a magnifier is equal to the distance of the object from the eye viewed without the magnifier. Thus the same amount of accommodation (or near addition) is required with or without the magnifier. It is equal to

$$M = 1 + (F/D)$$

where *F* is the power of the magnifier (assumed to be so close to the eye as to ignore the distance separating them) and *D* is the object vergence. The special case in which the object distance from the eye is 25 cm (D = 4.00 D) is the **trade magnification**.
See magnification, apparent.
lateral m. Magnification of a lens or of an optical system, expressed as the ratio of the size of the image *h′* to the size of the object *h*. It is usually denoted by

$$M = h'/h = l'/l = L/L'$$

where *l′* and *l* are the distances of the image and object, respectively, from the principal plane of the lens (or lens system) and *L* and *L′* the object and image vergences, respectively. *Syn.* enlargement ratio; linear magnification; transverse magnification (Table M2). (*Note*: some authors consider this last term a synonym of electronic magnification.)
See enlargement; power, equivalent viewing.

linear m. *See* magnification, lateral.
longitudinal m. *See* magnification, axial.
loupe m. *See* magnification, apparent.
maximum m. *See* magnification, apparent.
negative m. *See* minification.
nominal m. *See* magnification, apparent.
m. power *See* magnification, spectacle.
real image m. *See* magnification, electronic.
relative m. *See* magnification, apparent.
relative distance m. Magnification that results from decreasing the distance between an object and the eye. It is expressed as

$$M_d = x/x'$$

where x and x' are the initial distance and the new distance, respectively. *Example*: If the viewing distance is decreased from 60 cm to 20 cm, $M_d = 60/20 = 3\times$. *Syn.* distance magnification; relative distance enlargement.
relative size m. The magnification which results from increasing the actual size of an object viewed. *Examples*: a larger TV screen; a larger print book than one used previously. It is expressed as

$$M_s = h_2/h_1$$

where h_2 and h_1 are the sizes of the enlarged object and the initial object, respectively. *Syn.* size magnification; relative size enlargement.
relative spectacle m. Ratio of the retinal image size in the corrected ametropic eye to that in a standard emmetropic eye.
See law, Knapp's.
shape m. Magnification resulting from a variation in the curvature of the front surface and thickness of an ophthalmic lens. In the treatment of aniseikonia, it may be necessary to alter the magnification of a lens while leaving its dioptric power unchanged. *Syn.* shape factor.
See lens, aniseikonic; magnification, spectacle.
size m. *See* magnification, relative size.
spectacle m. The ratio of the retinal image of a distant object in the corrected ametropic eye to the blurred or sharp image formed in the same eye when uncorrected. It is greater than unity in the hyperopic eye and less than unity in myopia. With a contact lens, though, this magnification is nearly equal to unity whatever the refractive error. Spectacle magnification SM depends both on the shape of the spectacle lens (i.e. the power of its front surface and its thickness) and on the power of the lens. Thus

$$SM = \left(\frac{1}{1 - (t/n)F_1}\right)\left(\frac{1}{1 - dF'_v}\right)$$

where F_1 is the power of the front surface, F'_v the back vertex power of the lens, t its thickness, n the index of refraction and d the distance from the back surface of the lens to the entrance pupil of the eye. The first term in the formula represents the **shape factor** (or **shape magnification**) and the second term the **power factor** (or **power magnification**). However, because the shape factor is very small for most common ophthalmic lenses (except for high plus lenses), it is often ignored in the above formula and thus

$$SM = \frac{1}{(1 - dF'_v)}$$

telescopic m. Magnification obtained with a telescope, such as a galilean telescope, which gives an erect image or an astronomical telescope in which an erecting system is used. The magnification is

$$M = \alpha'/\alpha = -F_e/F_o$$

where α' and α are the angles subtended at the eye by the image viewed through the telescope and the angle subtended at the eye by the object, respectively and F_e and F_o are the powers of the eyepiece and objective, respectively. Telescopes are used to magnify objects at distance (afocal) and placed over the spectacle correction. If the patient is uncorrected, the telescope can be adjusted but the magnification will change. They can be used for near and intermediate viewing by altering the distance between the objective and the eyepiece, or adding a plus lens in front of the objective, the result being a combined magnification, which is the product of the telescope magnification and the power of the plus lens magnification (Tables M3 and M4).
total m. *See* magnification, combined.
trade m. *See* magnification, apparent.
transverse m. *See* magnification, electronic; magnification, linear.

magnifier An optical device, commonly used for close viewing, which produces an apparent magnification. It can be monocular or binocular, held in the hand (**hand magnifier**) or mounted in front of the eye (**stand magnifier**). It rarely exceeds a magnification of 10× and does not produce an inversion of the image (Fig. M5). *Syn.* loupe. *See* distance of distinct vision; lens, magnifying; magnification, apparent; vision, low.

magnifying glass; lens *See* lens, magnifying.

magnifying power *See* magnification, apparent.

magnifying spectacles *See* spectacles, magnifying.

magnitude estimation A psychophysical method of evaluating stimuli above threshold. The subject assigns numbers according to the apparent magnitudes of the stimuli. The results relating the magnitude of sensation S and the stimulus intensity I usually follow a **power law** (or **Stevens' power law**), that is, $S = kI^n$ where k is a constant and n the exponent which depends on the sensory modality. *Example*: The magnitude perceived brightness of a 5 degrees target viewed by a dark-adapted subject follows the relation $S = kI^{0.33}$,

Table M3 Approximate spectacle magnification of lenses of various back vertex powers (F'_v in D) assuming d = 15 mm and the parameters of a typical spectacle lens of that power

F'_v	Shape factor (S)	Power factor (P)	Spectacle magnification (SM)	Percentage magnification
+12	1.08	1.22	1.32	32% increase
+10	1.06	1.18	1.25	25% "
+8	1.04	1.14	1.18	18% "
+6	1.03	1.10	1.13	13% "
+4	1.02	1.06	1.09	9% "
+2	1.01	1.03	1.04	4% "
0	1.01	1.00	1.01	1% "
−2	1.00	0.97	0.97	3% decrease
−4	1.00	0.94	0.94	6% "
−6	1.00	0.92	0.92	8% "
−8	1.00	0.89	0.89	11% "
−10	1.00	0.87	0.87	13% "
−12	1.00	0.85	0.85	15% "
−14	1.00	0.83	0.83	17% "
−16	1.00	0.81	0.81	19% "

Table M4 Approximate spectacle and contact lens magnification assuming d = 15 mm (vertex distance 12 mm plus 3 mm between cornea and entrance pupil) and negligible lens thickness. The percentage change in magnification going from spectacles to contact lenses was calculated using $(F_s/F_c - 1) \times 100$

Spectacle refraction (F_s)	Equivalent power of contact lens (F_c)	Percentage increased magnification spectacles	Percentage increased magnification contact lens	% change in magnification from specs. to contact lens
+12	+14.02	21.9	4.4	−14.4
+10	+11.36	17.6	3.5	−12
+8	+8.85	13.6	2.7	−9.6
+6	+6.47	9.9	2.0	−7.3
+4	+4.2	6.4	1.3	−4.8
+2	+2.05	3.1	0.6	−2.4
−2	−1.95	−2.9	−0.6	2.6
−4	−3.82	−5.7	−1.1	4.7
−6	−5.6	−8.3	−1.7	7.1
−8	−7.3	−10.7	−2.1	9.6
−10	−8.93	−13	−2.6	12
−12	−10.49	−15.3	−3	14.4
−14	−11.99	−17.3	−3.5	16.8
−16	−13.42	−19.3	−3.9	19.2

that is, the intensity of the light target needs to be increased some tenfold to see it twice as bright. *Syn.* direct scaling.

magno cells *See* cell, ganglion; geniculate body, lateral.

magnocellular layer *See* geniculate body, lateral.

magnocellular visual system *See* system, magnocellular visual.

Maier, sinus of *See* lacrimal apparatus.

major arterial circle of the iris *See* arterial circle of the iris, major.

malar bone *See* orbit.

malingering Feigning illness or disability (often for the purpose of gaining compensation or avoiding duty).
See test, optokinetic nystagmus; vision, tunnel.

Mallett fixation disparity unit Instrument used to measure the amount of aligning prism power required to eliminate fixation disparity. It consists of a small central fixation letter X surrounded by two letters O, one on each side of X, the three letters being seen binocularly, and two coloured polarized vertical bars in line with the centre of the X which are seen by each eye separately. The instrument can be swung through 90° to measure any vertical fixation disparity. The aligning prism

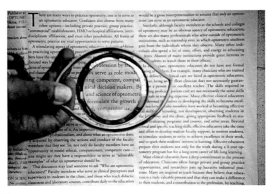

Fig. M5 A hand magnifier.

power is indicated by the misalignment of the two polarized bars when the subject fixates the X through cross-polarized filters in front of the eyes. The amount of aligning prism is given by the value of the base-in or base-out prism power necessary to produce alignment. The unit can also be used to detect suppression.
See **Disparometer; heterophoria, associated; heterophoria, uncompensated; prism, aligning.**

malprojection *See* **projection, false.**

Mandelbaum effect *See* **effect, Mandelbaum.**

mandibulofacial dysostosis *See* **syndrome, Treacher Collins.**

mannitol *See* **hyperosmotic agent.**

manometer An instrument for measuring the pressure of gases, vapour, blood or the intraocular pressure directly.
See **pressure, intraocular; tonometer.**

manoptoscope Apparatus for determining the dominant eye. It consists of a hollow truncated cone that subjects hold with the base against their face and over both eyes. The subject views a distant object through the hole at the end of the cone, using their dominant eye.
See **dominance, ocular.**

Marcus Gunn phenomenon *See* **phenomenon, Marcus Gunn jaw-winking.**

Marcus Gunn pupil *See* **pupil, Marcus Gunn.**

Marfan's syndrome *See* **syndrome, Marfan's.**

Mariotte's blind spot *See* **spot, blind.**

mask *See* **masking.**

masking A term describing any process whereby a detectable stimulus is made difficult or impossible to detect by the presentation of a second stimulus (called the **mask**). The main stimulus (typically called the **target**) may appear at the same time as the mask (**simultaneous masking**) as, for example, in the crowding phenomenon; or it may precede the mask (**backward masking**) as, for example, metacontrast or it may follow the mask (**forward masking**) as, for example,

paracontrast. Masking can also occur in the spatial domain as in **pattern masking** when the target and the mask appear in the same location and in metacontrast when the mask does not overlap with the target location.
See **metacontrast; phenomenon, crowding.**

masking, dichoptic The masking of the visual function of one eye by the view presented to the other, as for example in a haploscope.
See **dichoptic.**

mast cell stabilizers Prophylactic drugs used to treat allergic conjunctivitis, vernal conjunctivitis, giant papillary conjunctivitis, superior limbic keratoconjunctivitis. They act by stabilizing the membranes of mast cells thus preventing the release of histamine. Common agents are sodium cromoglicate (cromolyn sodium), lodoxamide, nedocromil sodium, olopatadine hydrochloride and pemirolast potassium.
See **antihistamine; cell, mast; hypersensitivity.**

matt surface A surface which reflects light diffusely. *Example*: a magnesium oxide surface. *Syn.* diffusing surface.
See **diffusion; gloss; reflection, diffuse.**

Maurice's theory *See* **theory, Maurice's.**

maximum plus *See* **best vision sphere; method, fogging; test, plus 1.00 D blur.**

Maxwell disc *See* **disc, Maxwell.**

maxwellian view Method of observation in which a converging lens forms an image in the plane of the entrance pupil of the observer. If the observer's eye is focused on the lens, the lens will appear as a disc filled with light of uniform intensity. This optical arrangement makes it possible to choose the point of incidence within the pupil, to minimize the effect of the optical aberrations of the eye and to avoid the effect of pupil size on the amount of light entering the eye (Fig. M6).
See **distance, conjugate.**

maxwellian view system, clinical Instrument designed to measure visual acuity by using a narrow beam or beams of light focused within

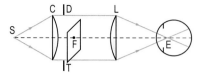

Fig. M6 Maxwellian view system (S, source of light; C, collimator; D, diaphragm; T, target situated in the focal plane of lens L; F, first focal point of lens L and conjugate of the retina of an unaccommodated emmetropic eye; E, centre of the entrance pupil of the eye and conjugate of S).

the entrance pupil of the eye. The location of the beam or beams within the pupil can be controlled by the clinician. Such an instrument is valuable to assess acuity when part of the pupil is obstructed by a cataract or other opacity as the beam or beams of light can be directed to enter the eye through an area of the pupil where there is no opacity, thus providing an estimate of the visual acuity unaffected by optical image degradation. The results can contribute to the decision as to whether removal of a cataract will be beneficial. There are several types of these instruments. The **Potential Acuity Meter** (PAM) focuses a single beam of light in the pupil and a letter chart onto the retina. Others focus two beams of light in the pupil and a grating which can be produced on the retina by interference (if the two sources are coherent). This method is called **laser interferometry**. Examples of these are the **Lotmar Visometer** and the **IRAS Randwal Interferometer**, which are referred to as **clinical interferometers**. They tend to penetrate dense cataracts better than the PAM.
See **coherent sources; entoptoscope, blue field; hyperacuity; interferometer.**

Maxwell's spot *See* **spot, Maxwell's.**

McCollough effect *See* **effect, McCollough.**

M cell *See* **cell, ganglion; cell, M.**

mean The most commonly used index of central tendency of a set of values. It is calculated by adding all the values *x* and dividing this sum by the number *n* of values in the set, that is

$$X = \frac{\Sigma x}{n}$$

See **median; mode; Student's t-test.**

Meares–Irlen syndrome *See* **syndrome, Meares–Irlen.**

measure, lens *See* **lens measure.**

media, ocular The transparent substances of the eye, i.e. the cornea, the aqueous humour, the crystalline lens and the vitreous humour.

medial Relating to the middle; nearer the median plane.

medial rectus muscle *See* **muscle, medial rectus.**

median One of the three indices of the central tendency of a set of values. It is the middle value of the set arranged from the smallest to the largest value. The median divides the values into two halves with an equal number of values above and below it. *Examples:* If n = 23 (**odd** number), the median is the (23 + 1) / 2 = 12th value of the ordered set. If n = 24 (**even** number), the median is calculated by the mean of the two middle values in the ordered set (i.e. (24/2) and (24/2 + 1)) and the median is equal to the mean of the 12th value (24/2) and the 13th value (24/2 +1).
See **mean; mode.**

median line; plane *See* under the nouns.

medium, optical Any material, substance or space through which light can be transmitted.

medullated nerve fibres *See* **fibres, myelinated nerve.**

Meesmann's dystrophy *See* **dystrophy, Meesmann's.**

megalocornea A non-progressive enlargement of the cornea (more than 13 mm in diameter) without significant change in corneal thickness and normal clarity and function. Intraocular pressure is normal and there is often high myopia and astigmatism. It is usually transmitted as an X-linked recessive trait. Some systemic associations include Marfan's syndrome, Apert's syndrome, Down's syndrome, Weil–Marchesani syndrome and osteogenesis imperfecta.
See **buphthalmos; cornea plana; keratoglobus; microcornea.**

megalophthalmos A congenital condition in which the eye is abnormally large, particularly the structures of the anterior segment. The condition is associated with megalocornea, Marfan's syndrome and Apert's syndrome. *Syn.* macrophthalmia.
See **buphthalmos; microphthalmos.**

megalopsia *See* **macropsia.**

meibography A method of observing the structures of the meibomian glands. It is used to facilitate the diagnosis of meibomian gland dysfunction in which the ducts are obstructed and the secretion is altered resulting in abnormality of the tear film lipid layer and dry eye. The most common methods are either non-contact using infrared illumination or transillumination of the everted eyelid.
See **gland, meibomian; transillumination.**

meibometry A method for quantifying the amount of lipids present in the tears. It may be used to facilitate the diagnosis of meibomian gland dysfunction.
See **gland, meibomian.**

meibomian cyst *See* **chalazion.**

meibomian gland dysfunction; glands *See* **gland, meibomian; meibography.**

meibomianitis Inflammation of the meibomian glands. It is characterized by the presence of a white frothy secretion or 'foam' on the eyelid margin. The posterior lid margin is hyperaemic

and the meibomian gland orifices are obstructed. Meibomianitis is often associated with blepharitis, conjunctivitis and chalazion. Symptoms include mild itching of the lids and occasionally blurred vision due to the oily secretion spreading over the cornea. This condition may also result from hard contact lens wear. Management of this disease consists of tarsal massage and removal of the secretion with a moist cotton-tipped applicator and antibiotic medication (e.g. tetracycline, erythromycin). *Syn.* meibomitis.
See **blepharitis, anterior or marginal; blepharitis, posterior; gland, meibomian; hordeolum, internal.**

meibomitis *See* **meibomianitis.**

melanin Dark brown to black pigment normally present in the skin, the hair, the choroid, the iris, the retina, the ciliary body, the cardiac tissue, the pia mater and the substantia nigra of the brain. It is absent in albinos.
See **albinism; fuscin; melanocyte; melanosis; naevus, choroidal; retinal pigment epithelium.**

melanocyte A pigment-bearing cell. It is found in the iris, the choroid, the retina, the sclera, the skin, etc.
See **melanin; naevus, choroidal; naevus, iris.**

melanocytoma A benign, usually bilateral, pigmented tumour which is most commonly found in the optic disc arising from dendritic uveal melanocytes in the lamina cribrosa of the optic nerve head but may occur anywhere throughout the uveal tract. The patient's visual field presents an enlarged blind spot. The condition is more frequent in dark-skinned people.

melanocytosis, ocular A congenital, usually unilateral lesion, characterized by slate grey areas of increased pigmentation. The pigment is curiously not found in the conjunctival epithelium, but is located in the uvea, sclera and episcleral tissues. It may predispose the individual to uveal melanoma. *Syn.* congenital melanosis oculi.
See **naevus of Ota.**

melanoma Tumour which originates from cells called melanocytes that form melanin and may lead to intraocular tumours. These tumours consist of spindle or epithelioid cells or both. Epithelioid cells are the most prone to spread to other tissues, such as the liver. *Plural*: melanomata.
choroidal m. The most common primary malignant tumour found in the eye of adults. It appears under ophthalmoscopic examination as a pigmented elevated mass, usually brown in colour and sometimes with orange pigment (lipofuscin). The tumour consists of spindle or epithelioid cells or more commonly both. It may cause a decrease in vision or brief **'balls of light'** moving across the visual field, or be asymptomatic, depending on its size or location. The condition is typically unilateral. Differential diagnosis with retinal detachment or choroidal naevus is essential. Treatment may include radiotherapy or photocoagulation, or enucleation if the melanoma is large and vision irreversibly lost. Episcleral plaque radiotherapy (brachytherapy) is effective as it delivers a highly concentrated radiation dose to the tumour with much less radiation to the surrounding healthy tissues. *Syn.* malignant melanoma of the choroid. *See* **radiotherapy, plaque; retinopathy, radiation.**
ciliary body m. A uveal melanoma which presents in older adults. It is often asymptomatic and may only be visible with pupillary dilatation as a ciliary mass overlaid with episcleral vessels. The lens may be dislocated and cataractous, which causes visual impairment. Treatment is by excision, radiotherapy and if the lesion is very large, enucleation.
conjunctival m. A rare lesion found on the episclera or limbus in older adults. It presents as a black or grey vascularized nodule. It is usually excised.
iris m. Pigmented lesion, which is easily seen on the surface of the iris. It alters the colour of the iris and may distort the shape of the pupil. A dilated episcleral vessel running towards the tumour may be present. There may be a localized cataract where the tumour is in contact with the lens, and secondary glaucoma may develop if the tumour has spread to the angle of the anterior chamber. The tumour arises from the iris stroma and is composed of epithelioid or more commonly only spindle cells, and occasionally a mixture of both. It is almost always unilateral and most commonly found in white patients with light irides. It is thought to originate from a previous pigmented naevus. If the tumour is found to enlarge, it will usually be excised surgically (Fig. M7).
See **naevus, iris.**
uveal m. Tumour which may be located in the choroid, the ciliary body or the iris. Choroidal melanomas make up about 80% of the total, ciliary body about 12% and iris about 8%. Although uveal melanomas can occur at any age, the majority of patients are beyond the age of 40 years. Uveal melanomas can metastasize, especially choroidal melanomas. Diagnosis is best achieved with a B-scan ultrasound examination. The patient must be referred to an ocular oncologist without delay.
See **radiotherapy, plaque; ultrasonography.**

melanopsin An opsin-like protein, sensitive to light with a peak sensitivity around 482 nm found in the very small proportion of retinal ganglion cells which are photosensitive. This retinal pigment synchronizes the circadian cycle to the day-night cycle as well as being involved in the control of pupil size. This neural circuit appears to be independent of the conventional retinal phototransduction in the rods and cones.
See **cell, photosensitive retinal ganglion; reflex, pupil light.**

melanosis An abnormal accumulation of melanin pigment in the skin or other tissues. If there is a larger quantity than normal of pigment in the tissues of the eye, the condition is referred to as **melanosis bulbi (melanosis oculi)** or **primary acquired melanosis** when on the conjunctival epithelium and limbus. It may extend onto the peripheral cornea. It may be benign or become

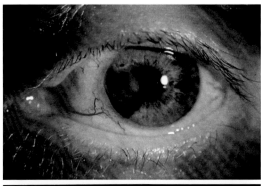

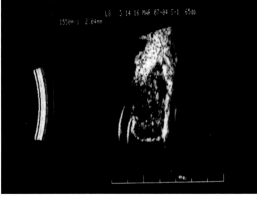

Fig. M7 Iris melanoma of the left eye. Note the dilated episcleral vessel in the nasal conjunctiva. Below is a B-scan of the melanoma showing a mass occupying the iris, filling the anterior chamber and touching the cornea. (From Millodot et al 2006, with permission of Blackwell Publishing)

malignant, in which case nodules appear and excision or cryotherapy is required. *Plural*: melanoses. *See* **naevus of Ota.**

melanosis bulbi; oculi *See* **melanosis.**

Melbourne Edge test *See* **test, Melbourne Edge.**

membrane A thin layer of tissue which covers a surface, separates cellular structures or organs, or connects adjacent structures.

basement m. of the corneal epithelium A very thin non-cellular layer adjacent to Bowman's layer and upon which the columnar basal cells of the corneal epithelium are bound by hemidesmosomes. It is composed of four primary components: collagens, laminins, heparin sulfate proteoglycans and nidogens. One likely function of the membrane is to act as a barrier to the penetration of cytokines from the epithelium to the stroma.
See **dystrophy, epithelial basement membrane.**

Bowman's m. *See* **layer, Bowman's.**

Bruch's m. Thin (about 2 µm), shiny, non-vascular layer of the choroid located on the inner side next to the retinal pigment epithelium and which extends forward into the pars plana of the ciliary body. It consists of five layers: the inner and outer layers are the basement membranes of the retinal pigment epithelium and choriocapillaris, respectively, and in between is the elastic lamina (lamina elastica) sandwiched between two layers of collagen fibres. It passes nutrients from the choriocapillaris to the photoreceptors and waste products back to the choroid. Bruch's membrane thickens with age due to accumulated waste material originating in the photoreceptors, and lipids. This may lead to the formation of drusen, slows the transport of metabolites, as well as allowing choroidal vessels into the membrane and beyond, and fragmentation of the membrane, which is commonly associated with choroidal neovascularization.
See **angioid streaks; drusen; retinal pigment epithelium.**

Descemet's m. Strong, resistant, thin (about 8 µm) layer of the cornea located between the endothelium (from which it is secreted) and the stroma. It is also elastic due to its composition of collagen fibrils. It is practically the last corneal structure to succumb to disease processes and it can regenerate after injury. *Syn.* lamina elastica posterior; posterior limiting layer.
See **descemetocele; ring, Kayser–Fleischer.**

Elschnig's inner limiting m. A thin layer of astrocytes covering the optic disc. It is in continuity with the inner limiting membrane of the retina. In some cases this layer is thickened in the central part of the disc to form the **central meniscus of Kuhnt**. It is transparent and not usually visible with the ophthalmoscope.

epiretinal m. Proliferation of fibroglial cells forming a sheet-like structure over the surface of the internal limiting membrane of the retina and its macular region. Ophthalmoscopically the retina presents a glinting reflex. The condition may be idiopathic or it may occur after trauma, retinal eye surgery, retinal vascular disease (e.g. branch retinal vein occlusion), retinal break, ocular inflammation or with any of the causes of retinitis proliferans and is most common in elderly patients. Initially the patient is asymptomatic or reports some distortion of vision. This stage is often called **cellophane maculopathy**. As the condition develops, with reduced visual acuity and metamorphopsia, there is retinal wrinkling and the epiretinal membrane becomes denser obscuring some retinal vessels in ophthalmoscopy. The condition is then called **macular pucker**. Some patients may also develop a macular hole and posterior vitreous detachment. If vision is significantly reduced, the main treatment is by vitreous surgery with removal of the layer of preretinal proliferative tissue. *Syn.* macular epiretinal membrane; preretinal macular fibrosis; preretinal membrane; preretinal vitreous membrane; surface wrinkling retinopathy.
See **retinopathy, proliferative.**

hyaloid m. This is not really a membrane, but a concentration of cells and fibres enclosing the vitreous body.
See **hyalitis.**

intermuscular m. A thin elastic membrane originating from the muscle sheath of each rectus muscle and connecting it to the neighbouring rectus muscle. The membrane fuses with the capsule of each muscle, as well as with Tenon's capsule.

nictitating m. A fold of the conjunctival mucous membrane that can be drawn over the whole cornea or only part of it in a winking-like action to clean and lubricate it. It is present in many birds, reptiles, fishes and some mammals and is normally hidden in the inner canthus. *Syn.* third eyelid.
See **plica semilunaris.**

m. of the retina, external limiting A membrane located between the photoreceptors and the outer nuclear layer of the retina. It has the form of a wire netting through which pass the processes of the rods and cones. It is believed to be formed by the fibres of Mueller.
See **cell, Mueller's; Fig. R8, p. 294.**

m. of the retina, internal limiting Glass-like membrane lying between the retina and the vitreous body and forming a boundary for both. For that reason it has sometimes also been considered to be the hyaloid membrane of the vitreous. The feet of the fibres of Mueller are attached to this membrane but do not form it. *Syn.* internal limiting layer of the retina.
See **cell, Mueller's; retina.**

preretinal m. *See* fibrosis, preretinal macular.

pupillary m. Embryonic mesodermal tissue which is present in the centre of the iris and normally disappears by the eighth foetal month to form the pupil. Some strands of the membrane may remain in adults; this is referred to as a **persistent pupillary membrane.**

meninges Membranes surrounding the brain and spinal cord. They are the dura mater, the arachnoid mater and the pia mater. All three meninges surround the optic nerve at the optic foramen, in the optic canal and in the orbit.
See **space, subarachnoid**

meniscus of Kuhnt *See* membrane, Elschnig's inner limiting.

meniscus, tear *See* tear meniscus.

meridional accommodation *See* accommodation, astigmatic.

meridional amblyopia *See* amblyopia, meridional.

meridional size lens *See* lens, aniseikonic.

meshwork, trabecular *See* trabecular meshwork.

mesoderm One of the three primary germinal layers of an embryo from which the eye is derived. It eventually forms the extraocular muscles and the orbital and ocular vasculature.
See **ectoderm.**

mesopic vision *See* vision, mesopic.

metacontrast This is an apparently paradoxical phenomenon because it consists of a reduction in subjective brightness of a flash of light which is caused by a second flash following shortly afterward in an adjacent region of the visual field. The effect depends upon the duration, intensity, surface areas of the two flashes, the retinal area stimulated and particularly the interval of time between the two flashes. The phenomenon appears most clearly with an interval of about 0.1 s and disappears when that interval reaches 0.3 to 0.4 s. *Syn.* backward masking (this term is used to indicate when the test stimulus and the masking stimulus overlap spatially).
A flash of light can also be made to appear slightly less bright when it is preceded by another flash in an adjacent region of the visual field and the interval of time is of the order of 0.05 s. This second phenomenon is called **paracontrast**. *Syn.* forward masking (this term is used when the test stimulus and the masking stimulus overlap spatially).
See **masking.**

metal spectacle frame *See* spectacle frame, metal.

metameric colour *See* colour, metameric.

metamers *See* colour, metameric.

metamorphopsia An anomaly of visual perception in which objects appear distorted in shape or of different size or in a different location than the actual object. It may be due to a displacement of the visual receptors as a result of inflammation, tumour or retinal detachment, it can be of central origin (e.g. migraine, drug intoxication, neurosis or brain injury), or it can be induced by recently prescribed myopic correction (e.g. micropsia) or presbyopic correction (e.g. macropsia), etc. Metamorphopsia can be detected with an Amsler chart. If it affects only one eye the condition is related to aniseikonia.

See **accommodation, spasm of; dysmegalopsia; macular hole; pelopsia; teleopsia.**

metastasis, choroidal *See* **choroidal metastasis.**

method A systematic procedure or process used for attaining a given objective; for example, doing an examination or an experiment.
See **procedure.**

Bruckner's m. *See* **test, Bruckner's.**

cross-cylinder m. *See* **test for astigmatism, cross-cylinder.**

Donders' m. *See* **method, push-up.**

Drysdale's m. Method that has been applied for the determination of the radius of curvature of hard contact lenses. The principle consists of placing a light source in a modified microscope in focus at the surface of the lens and at the centre of curvature of the surface, the distance between the two being recorded on a dial as the radius of curvature.
See **optic zone radius, back; Radiuscope.**

duochrome m. *See* **test, duochrome.**

fogging m. Method of relaxing accommodation during the subjective measurement of ametropia. This is achieved by placing enough plus lens power (or less minus lens power) in front of an eye to form an image in front of the retina. In this condition, any effort to accommodate will produce a poorer image and relaxation of accommodation is thus achieved (Fig. M8). Then, plus lens power is decreased (or minus lens power increased) until the patient reports no further improvement in visual acuity. This point represents the maximum positive lens power (or minimum negative lens power) and it is called the **best vision sphere**.
See **best vision sphere; refractive error; test, fan and block; test, plus 1.00 D blur.**

von Graefe's m. *See* **test, diplopia.**

van Herick, Shaffer and Schwartz m. Technique for estimating the angle of the anterior chamber. It is based on the fact that the width

of the angle of the anterior chamber is correlated to the distance between the posterior corneal surface and the anterior iris as viewed near the corneal limbus. This is done using a slit-lamp with a narrow slit beam perpendicular to the temporal or nasal corneal surface, viewing from the straight-ahead position and comparing the depth of the anterior chamber to the thickness of the cornea. If the AC depth is equal to or greater than the corneal thickness, the angle is considered to be **grade 4** (corresponding to a wide-open angle). If the AC depth is equal to one-half the corneal thickness, the angle is considered to be **grade 3**, moderately open (this is the most common angle width). If the AC depth is equal to one-fourth the corneal thickness, it is considered to be **grade 2**, moderately narrow, and if the AC depth is less than one-fourth the corneal thickness, it is considered to be **grade 1** (corresponding to a very narrow angle). **Grade 0** is considered to be a closed angle. The method is most useful for predicting the possibility of angle-closure glaucoma. The results of this method are in good agreement with those of the **Shaffer classification** in which, using a gonioscope the evaluation of the angle of the anterior chamber and its structures are visualized: grade 4 (40°) ciliary body, grade 3 (30°) scleral spur, grade 2 (20°) trabeculum meshwork, and grade 1 (10°) Schwalbe's line, and grade 0 (0°) cornea. *Syn.* van Herick's technique.
See **gonioscopy; test, shadow.**

Hirschberg's m. *See* **test, Hirschberg's.**

Humphriss m. Method of binocular subjective refraction in which one eye is blurred by means of a +0.75 D (or +1.0 D) spherical lens above the correcting lens. Visual acuity is thus reduced by three or four Snellen lines. This lens produces a suppression of foveal vision while allowing peripheral fusion to maintain binocular alignment of the two eyes during refinement of the correction to the other eye. This refinement is done using a +0.25 D sphere followed by a −0.25 D sphere until the minus lens is preferred. The +0.75 D (or +1.00 D) fogging lens is removed and placed in front of the eye just tested and the minus/plus procedure is repeated on the eye originally fogged. *Syn.* Humphriss immediate contrast test (HIC).
See **refractive error; test, balancing.**

Javal's m. Method for determining the objective angle of strabismus using a perimeter. The patient is seated before a perimeter arc with the deviating eye at the centre of the arc while the other eye fixates a distant point straight ahead. The examiner moves both a light source and his or her eye directly above it, until the corneal reflex appears centred in the entrance pupil of the deviating eye. The position of the source on the arc can be read to give the objective angle of strabismus. Angle lambda must be added in convergent and subtracted in divergent strabismus as the criterion used was the pupillary axis, which makes an angle with the line of sight. Strictly speaking, angle kappa, rather than lambda, should be taken into account.
See **angle of deviation.**

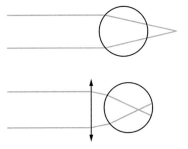

Fig. M8 Principle of the fogging method: The eye is rendered artificially myopic.

Krimsky's m. *See* test, Krimsky's.

Lindblom's m. A simple method performed to assess incomitant cyclovertical (vertical or torsional) deviations. It consists of using a 70-cm horizontal rod viewed at a distance of 1 metre. If the patient reports diplopia, as would happen in acquired cases, two lines will be seen, which are either parallel indicating a faulty rectus muscle (superior or inferior rectus) or tilted indicating a faulty oblique muscle, most commonly the superior oblique (fourth nerve palsy). In the latter, the patient perceives what resembles an arrow, the apex of which points to the eye with the paretic muscle. If the patient does not report any diplopia as happens in long-standing or congenital cases, two Maddox rods, one in front of each eye with axes at 90°, can produce two horizontal lines. The method is performed in up and down gaze and right and left gaze.

See palsy, fourth nerve.

minus lens m. Method of measuring the monocular amplitude of accommodation which consists in placing minus lenses in front of one eye while the subject fixates the smallest optotypes (usually subtending about one minute of arc, that is the 6/6 or 20/20 line or 0.00 logMAR). Progressively stronger lenses are used until the patient reports that the test appears blurred. The determination of the amplitude must take into account the vergence at the eye of the fixation point, and the test must be carried out with the patient's distance correction. If the minus lens to blur is −4 D and the fixation distance 40 cm, the amplitude will be equal to 6.5 D.

See accommodation, subjective.

Parks' m. *See* test, Parks three step.

preferential looking m. A method of assessing visual acuity in infants. It consists of presenting two stimuli on a uniform background, one of which contains a pattern (e.g. a checkerboard or a grating) and the other a plain field of equal shape, size and luminance, and observing the infant's eyes. If the infant can resolve the pattern, he or she tends to fixate on that stimulus for a larger percentage of time. By reducing the size of the detail in the pattern, a threshold can be obtained when the infant fixates at either stimulus for the same length of time.

See acuity, objective visual; acuity, Teller; test, Cardiff acuity.

push-out m. *See* method, push-up.

push-up m. Method of determining the near point of accommodation by moving a test object made up of small optotypes subtending one minute of arc (that is the 6/6 or 20/20 line or 0.00 logMAR) at the eye and uniformly illuminated, closer to the patient's eye. It is usually done monocularly and then binocularly. The near point is achieved when the small test object yields a sustained blur and not just begins to blur. Alternatively, the card is moved back after appearing blurred until the small test object just appears to clear again. This is often called the **push-out method**. In older patients, plus lenses may be needed to carry out the test and the power of the lens is subtracted from the reading. The amplitude of accommodation is deduced by taking into account the vergence at the eye of the far point (it is at infinity in emmetropes and corrected ametropes). *Examples:* The near point of an emmetrope or corrected ametrope is 20 cm, the amplitude is 1/0.20 = 5 D; a +1 D was added to the measured amplitude of 3.5 D, so the actual amplitude is 2.5 D. *Syn.* Donders' method.

See accommodation, amplitude of; rule, near point; test, Scheiner's.

Smith's m. Method performed to estimate the depth of the anterior chamber using a conventional slit-lamp. The angle between the illumination beam and the microscope, which is placed along the straight-ahead position, is set at 60°. To examine the patient's right eye, the examiner looks through the right eyepiece and through the left eyepiece to examine the left eye. A beam of moderate thickness is oriented horizontally and focused on the cornea. Two horizontal images of the slit will appear separated by a dark space, one sharply focused corresponding to the cornea and the other out of focus corresponding to the anterior lens surface. The slit is lengthened until the two separate reflections just touch. At this point, the length of the slit is measured and multiplied by a factor of 1.4 to arrive at an estimate of the depth of the anterior chamber. The method gives optimum results within the range of 1.4 mm and 3 mm. It is most useful in assessing shallow chambers as this could lead to angle-closure glaucoma.

See test, shadow.

m. of stabilizing the retinal image *See* stabilized retinal image.

methotrexate *See* immunosuppressants.

methylcellulose A highly viscous, water-soluble, non-irritating compound used as a thickening, lubricating and clinging agent in drugs such as artificial tears, wetting and contact lens solutions. *See* alacrima; keratoconjunctivitis sicca; tears, artificial.

methyl methacrylate *See* polymethyl methacrylate.

metipranolol hydrochloride *See* beta-blocker.

metre angle *See* angle, metre.

Michelson interferometer *See* interferometer.

miconazole *See* antifungal agent.

microaneurysm Tiny swelling in the wall of a blood vessel. It appears in the retinal capillaries as a small, round, red spot. It is commonly found in diabetic retinopathy, retinal vein occlusion or absolute glaucoma.

microbe Very minute living organisms, such as bacteria, protozoa, fungi or viruses.

microcoria Abnormally small pupils, usually congenital and due to an absence of the dilator pupillae muscle.

microcornea An abnormally small cornea with a horizontal diameter of less than 10 mm. The condition is usually inherited, either as an auto-somal dominant or autosomal recessive trait. It may be accompanied by hyperopia and glaucoma. *See* **cornea plana; megalocornea.**

microcysts, epithelial Very small round vesicles containing fluid and cellular debris observed on the surface of the cornea under slit-lamp examination in some types of corneal dystrophy (e.g. epithelial basement membrane dystrophy) and in wearers of extended wear contact lenses, due to chronic hypoxia. They appear to originate in the basal layer of the corneal epithelium as a result of cellular necrosis. They can be seen by slit-lamp examination using a magnification of at least 20×. If caused by extended wear contact lenses, the patient should be advised to change to daily wear contact lenses of high oxygen transmissibility. *Syn.* microepithelial cysts.

microfluctuations of accommodation *See* **accommodation, microfluctuations of.**

micrometre An SI unit of length equal to one-millionth of a metre (10^{-6} m). *Symbol*: μm. *Syn.* micron (obsolete term).
See **nanometre.**

micron *See* **micrometre.**

micronystagmus *See* **movement, fixation.**

micropachometer *See* **pachometer.**

microphakia *See* **microspherophakia.**

microphthalmos Congenital anomaly in which the eyeball is abnormally small and often deeply set in a small orbit. It is typically hyperopic with other features such as a coloboma or a cyst and associated with systemic abnormalities. *Syn.* microphthalmia; microphthalmus. When there is no other abnormality, the condition is called simple **microphthalmos** or **nanophthalmos** (Fig. M9). *See* **anophthalmos; megalophthalmos; monoph-thalmos; nanophthalmos; pseudoptosis; syn-drome, Patau's.**

micropsia Anomaly of visual perception in which objects appear smaller than they actually are. It may be due to a retinal disease in which the visual cells are spread apart, or to paresis of accommodation or to uncorrected presbyopia,

or to the recent wear of either base-out prisms or a correction for myopia, etc. If it affects only one eye, the condition is related to aniseikonia. *See* **dysmegalopsia; macropsia; metamorphopsia.**

microsaccades *See* **movement, fixation.**

microscope An optical instrument for magnifying small near objects. It can consist of a single converging lens such as a loupe (**simple microscope**) or of two or more lenses or lens systems (**compound microscope**) (Fig. M10). In this latter case, one lens or lens system serves as an objective to form real and magnified images of the object while the other lens or lens system serves as an eyepiece to examine the aerial image formed by the objective. The final image is inverted with respect to the object. It can use light or a beam of electrons (**electron microscope**) which produces magnification more than a 1000 times greater than with light. The magnification, M, of a light microscope, adjusted for a final image at infinity, is equal to

$$M = M_o \times M_e$$

where M_o is the lateral magnification of the objective, and M_e is the angular magnification of the eyepiece.
See **eyepiece; lens, immersion; objective; stage.**
confocal m. A microscope that provides viewing of cells, organisms (such as bacteria or fungi) and other structures within various tissues, in living patients. It allows each layer of a tissue to be viewed with much greater clarity than with a conventional microscope because signals from the viewed layer and the illumination beam have the same focus, while elements above or below the focal plane are out of focus and usually filtered out. The instrument has been used to investigate and diagnose corneal disease processes, including dystrophies and infec-tious keratitis, or to follow corneal healing after laser or traditional surgery. In addition, the instrument scans the object of interest by varying the plane of focus to form an image in three dimensions, of higher contrast and resolution than that provided by a specular microscope.
See **ophthalmoscope, confocal scanning laser.**

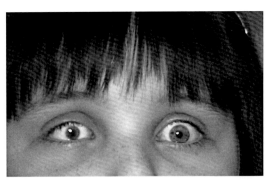

Fig. M9 Right eye microphthalmos. (From Kanski 2007, with permission of Butterworth-Heinemann)

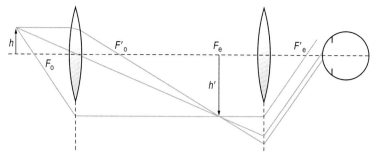

Fig. M10 Optical principle of a compound microscope (F_o, F'_o, first and second principal focus of the objective; F_e, F'_e, first and second principal focus of the eyepiece; h, h', object and image formed by the objective).

m. magnification *See* microscope.

slit-lamp m. Compound microscope used in conjunction with a slit-lamp. It is designed to have a working distance of about 90 to 125 mm to allow room for the clinician or for placing certain accessories such as a tonometer or pachometer. Slit-lamp microscopes have a magnification that varies usually within the range of 6× to 40×. *See* **distance, working; slit-lamp.**

specular m. Light microscope utilizing specular reflection to view the component layers of the cornea and particularly to observe and photograph the endothelium. It consists of an objective which is divided longitudinally. Light in the form of a slit beam is directed down one half and is reflected from the cornea-aqueous interface to the other half of the objective to form a visible and photographic image of the endothelium. The microscope is usually fitted with 40× water immersion objective which has a **working distance** of 1.6 mm. The cornea is covered with silicone fluid into which the objective tip is immersed. Good resolution is achieved provided that the width of the slit beam is kept small, to reduce the light scatter from the overlying corneal layers. This microscope allows examination of the corneal endothelium in vitro. For clinical measurements, the specular microscope is mounted horizontally using an objective with less magnification (usually 20×). The tip of the microscope has a glass-windowed, fluid-filled, screw-on cap, which applanates the cornea over a very small area. Photomicrography is accomplished with a flash unit, as otherwise eye movements make photography with long exposure impossible. However, corneal anaesthesia is necessary and clear images of the endothelium are not possible if the cornea is oedematous. For these reasons, new systems have been developed which fit on a slit-lamp and facilitate photography. Their magnification is greater than other slit-lamps, being 40× to 70×, and they do not require contact with the cornea as they have long working distances. Specular microscopy is used to monitor changes in corneal endothelium in contact lens wearers, especially those wearing extended wear lenses. *See* **distance, working; microscope, confocal; polymegethism, endothelial.**

microsperophakia A congenital, usually bilateral, condition in which the crystalline lens is smaller than normal and spherical in shape. It may give rise to lenticular myopia, subluxation or glaucoma. It may occur independently or it may be associated with the Weill–Marchesani syndrome or more rarely with Marfan's syndrome, Peter's anomaly or congenital rubella. If the lens is merely smaller than normal it is called **microphakia** and may be associated with Lowe's syndrome.

microsquint *See* microtropia.

microstrabismus *See* microtropia.

microtropia A small-angle (usually less than 6 to 8Δ in angle) inconspicuous strabismus which is not usually detected by cover test, either because the deviation is too small or because the angles of abnormal retinal correspondence and eccentric fixation coincide with the angle of deviation. There is usually amblyopia in the deviated eye and there may also be anisometropia. The patient with this condition displays nearly normal binocular vision without symptoms. Management usually consists of correcting the refractive error and occlusion for amblyopia. *Syn.* microsquint; microstrabismus; small angle strabismus. *See* **occlusion treatment; test, four prism dioptre base out.**

microvilli *See* corneal epithelium.

middle third technique *See* criterion, Percival.

midline 1. An imaginary line running along the surface of the brain (anterior to posterior), which separates the right and left hemispheres. **2.** *See* **line, median.**

migraine Intense and recurring pain, usually confined to one side of the head, which typically occurs in middle-aged adults. It is classified as **migraine without aura** (common migraine) which appears without ocular features, except photophobia and **migraine with aura** (classical migraine) which is accompanied by scotoma consisting of scintillating, flickering lights, tunnel vision and photophobia. The aura which does not usually exceed 60 minutes is typically followed by the headache with nausea and vomiting, but it may begin earlier or during the aura. Management includes resting in a quiet dark room and analgesics.

See **aura, visual; metamorphopsia; scotoma, scintillating.**

Mikulicz's syndrome *See* **syndrome, Mikulicz's.**

Millard–Gubler syndrome *See* **syndrome, Millard–Gubler.**

Miller–Nadler glare tester *See* **glare tester.**

millilambert Non-metric unit of luminance. It is equal to 3.183 cd/m^2.

millimicron *See* **nanometer.**

miner's nystagmus *See* **nystagmus.**

minification A reduction in the apparent size of an object. *Example*: viewing a distant object through the objective of a galilean telescope. *Syn.* negative magnification.

See **field, visual f. expander.**

minimum cognoscible The threshold of recognition of shapes or contours.

minimum legible The threshold for the recognition of letters or numbers.

minimum separable Perception of the least distance separating two objects, yet being still distinguished as two.

See **resolution, limit of.**

minimum visible Perception of the smallest area of light.

minus lens *See* **lens, diverging.**

minus lens method *See* **method, minus lens.**

miosis Contraction of the pupil or condition in which the pupil is very small (2 mm or less in diameter). It can be brought about by a spasm of the sphincter muscle or by the effect of a miotic drug (e.g. eserine, neostigmine, pilocarpine), or in certain spinal diseases or any stimulation of the parasympathetic supply to the eye. Miosis occurs naturally when doing close work or when stimulated by light. *Note*: also spelt myosis.

See **reflex, corneal; reflex, pupil light; spot, baring of the blind; syndrome, Horner's.**

miotics Drugs that constrict the pupil. They may be used in the treatment of glaucoma and accommodative esotropia and, sometimes, after a mydriatic examination. Miotics are either **parasympathomimetic (cholinergic-stimulating)** drugs which have a direct muscarinic action, such as pilocarpine and carbachol, or **anticholinesterase** drugs which block the effect of acetylcholinesterase thus letting acetylcholine produce its effect, such as physostigmine, neostigmine, echothiophate and demecarium. There are also some miotics which act by blocking α- or β-adrenergic receptors. For example, dapiprazole and thymoxamine block the α-adrenergic receptors and propranolol blocks the β-adrenergic receptors.

See **adrenergic receptors; glaucoma, open-angle; muscle, sphincter pupillae; mydriatic; parasympathomimetic drug.**

mire A pattern used in an optical instrument to guide the observer. *Examples*: the luminous pattern seen in a keratometer; the two half-circles seen in an applanation tonometer.

mirror A surface capable of reflecting light rays and forming optical images. Such surfaces are smooth or polished, made of highly polished metal, or a thin film of metal (e.g. aluminium) on glass, quartz or plastic (Fig. M11). Object distance *l* and image distance *l*′ relate to the focal distance *f* or the radius of curvature *r* of the mirror, as follows

$$\frac{2}{r} = \frac{1}{f} = \frac{1}{l'} + \frac{1}{l}$$

2/*r* represents the refractive power of the mirror, in air. If the medium that contains the incident and reflected rays is *n*, the power becomes $F = 2n/r$ and the focal length,

$$f = r/2n$$

See **length, focal; paraxial equation, fundamental; system, catadioptric.**

back surface m. Mirror which reflects from the back surface of a refracting layer, usually glass. *See* **mirror, front surface.**

concave m. Mirror with a spherical concave surface forming an erect, magnified, virtual image when the distance from the mirror is less than the

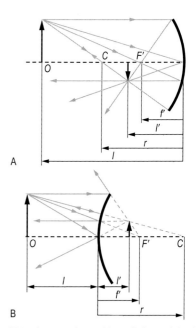

Fig. M11 Image of an object O formed in A, a concave mirror and B, a convex mirror. Four rays are drawn in each case for completeness, but two would suffice (C, centre of curvature; *F*′, focal point; *f*′, focal length; *l* and *l*′, object and image length; *r*, radius of curvature). Aberrations are ignored in this diagram.

focal distance and a demagnified inverted real image when the object distance is greater than the focal distance (Fig. M12).

convex m. Mirror with a spherical convex surface forming a virtual, erect and diminished image (Fig. M12).

front surface m. Mirror that reflects directly from its front surface. The advantages of this type are that, unlike back surface mirrors, there is no chromatic effect as the glass is not used optically; therefore, ultraviolet rays can be used which would otherwise be absorbed in the glass and there is no ghost reflection from the front surface. However, these mirrors can be easily scratched and the coating may tarnish. Often a coating of silicon monoxide is evaporated on top of the surface, but this causes a loss of reflectivity. *See* image, ghost; mirror, back surface.

plane m. Mirror whose surface is plane and forms a virtual image of the same size as the object. Object and image distances are equal.

semi-silvered m. See beam splitter.

m. writing Writing backward, Latin letters being written from right to left and the details of the letters reversed. The writing thus appears normal when viewed in a mirror. *Syn.* retrography.

mitochondrial inheritance *See* inheritance.

mitochondrion An organelle in the cytoplasm of cells, which produces most of the energy-rich molecule adenosine triphosphate (ATP) in cells. It is produced by using oxygen to break down nutrient molecules (e.g. glucose). The number of mitochondria in a cell varies; it is greater in active cells, such as muscle and liver cells which need more ATP. Mitochondria are involved in other processes (e.g. apoptosis, cellular proliferation). Each mitochondrion contains DNA, RNA, ribosomes and granules. The DNA is distinct from that of the cell nucleus. Mitochondrial DNA (mtDNA) is inherited only through the female. Mutations in mitochondrial DNA cause genetic disorders (e.g. Leber's hereditary optic neuropathy). *Plural*: mitochondria.

mitomycin C A chemotherapeutic agent that acts by inhibiting DNA synthesis. It is used in surgery, including glaucoma surgery such as trabeculectomy, to prevent scarring, in photorefractive surgery and LASIK to prevent haze and scar formation and in pterygium surgery to prevent recurrence.

mitosis Process by which a cell nucleus divides into two nuclei with chromosome numbers and genetic make-up identical to that of the parent cell. Mitosis is inhibited by anaesthetics and thus tissue repair is delayed. It is also slowed by hypoxia. *Examples*: the mitosis of the basal cells of the corneal epithelium; the mitosis of the epithelial cells of the crystalline lens adding new cells to it which eventually form new lens fibres. *See* apoptosis; chromosome; corneal abrasion; Krebs cycle.

Mittendorf's dot *See* hyaloid remnant.

mixed astigmatism *See* astigmatism, mixed.

Mizuo's phenomenon *See* phenomenon, Mizuo's.

Mobius syndrome *See* syndrome, Mobius.

modality One of the five types of sensation such as vision, the others being hearing, smell, taste and touch.

mode One of the three indices of the central tendency of a set of values. It is the value that occurs most frequently in a set of data. If there is more than one mode, it becomes ineffective as a descriptive statistic. *See* mean; median.

modulation transfer function *See* function, modulation transfer.

modulus of elasticity Ratio of a force applied to a material to the increment of change (e.g. increase in length; angular deformation) in that material. The modulus of elasticity is an indication of the stiffness of a material. Materials with low modulus of elasticity are less resistant to stress, while materials with high modulus of elasticity resist stress and hold their shape better. The SI unit of modulus of elasticity is the pascal (Pa). *Examples*: The modulus of elasticity of a PMMA contact lens is about 3000 MPa, is around 0.4 to 1.5 MPa for silicone hydrogel lenses and 0.3 to 0.5 MPa for hydrogel lenses. *Syn.* coefficient of elasticity; Young's modulus of elasticity.

Mohindra's technique of retinoscopy *See* retinoscopy, Mohindra's technique of.

moiré effect *See* effect, moiré.

Moll's glands *See* glands of Moll.

molluscum contagiosum A contagious disease of the skin caused by a double-stranded DNA virus of the poxvirus group. It is characterized by small, pinkish, pearly umbilicated nodules and mucoid discharge most commonly on the eyelid margins and brow area, and it may lead to conjunctivitis. It occurs most frequently in children and young adults, especially those with HIV infection. Treatment includes cauterization, cryotherapy or excision.

mondrian A complex visual display used in studies of colour perception. It consists of rectangles of various dimensions with all sides parallel or perpendicular to each other, and each rectangle of a colour or brightness different from the adjacent rectangles.

monoblepsia Condition in which monocular vision is more distinct than binocular vision.

monocentric Pertaining to a lens with only one optical centre. A **monocentric bifocal lens** is one in which the optical centres of the distance and near portions coincide and jump is eliminated. *See* jump; lens, bifocal.

monochromasia *See* achromatopsia.

monochromasy *See* achromatopsia.

monochromat A person who has a condition of monochromatism (total colour blindness). There are

two types of monochromats: the **cone monochromat** whose photopic luminosity curve resembles the normal and who has normal visual acuity and dark adaptation; and the **rod monochromat** whose retina does not contain functional cones and, therefore, has poor vision, photophobia and sometimes associated nystagmus and myopia. Monochromats are very rare: estimated at about three persons in 100 000.
See **achromatopsia; colour vision, defective; dystrophy, cone.**

monochromatic light *See* **light, monochromatic.**

monochromatism *See* **achromatism; achromatopsia; colour vision, defective; monochromat.**

monochromator A modified spectroscope for producing nearly monochromatic light.

monocle A single ophthalmic lens, with or without a frame, which is worn by holding it between the brow and the cheek.

monocular Pertaining to one eye. *Syn.* uniocular.

monocular cues to depth perception *See* **perception, depth.**

monocular estimation method *See* **retinoscopy, MEM.**

monocular diplopia; vision *See* under the nouns.

monofixation 1. Monocular fixation. 2. *See* **syndrome, monofixation.**

monophthalmos A rare abnormal development in which one eye is absent. The remaining eye is often microphthalmic. *Syn.* unilateral anophthalmos. *See* **anophthalmos; microphthalmos.**

monoptic Relating to the presentation of different stimuli to one eye.
See **dichoptic.**

monosomy *See* **chromosome.**

monovision Term referring to a method of correcting presbyopia by using a contact lens corrected for distance in one eye (usually the dominant one) and a contact lens corrected for near in the other eye. Binocular vision is impaired with this method, especially stereoscopic vision; however, it has been found to be relatively successful in many cases. It is assumed that at any time one eye is focused while the other is not and the cortical visual system suppresses this latter image (at least the central part of the image). Monovision may also occur without correction in a presbyopic patient who has emmetropia in one eye and myopia in the other eye.
modified m. A method of achieving monovision using bifocal contact lenses in which the powers, lens fit or other lens parameters are modified to emphasize distance vision for one eye and near vision for the other eye, while still retaining a reasonable level of binocular vision.

moon illusion *See* **illusion, moon.**

Mooren's ulcer *See* **ulcer, Mooren's.**

Morax–Axenfeld, diplobacillus of *See* conjunctivitis.

morgagnian cataract *See* cataract, morgagnian.

morning glory disc *See* disc, morning glory.

de Morsier syndrome *See* syndrome, de Morsier.

motility test *See* test, motility.

motion after-effect *See* after-effect, waterfall.

motion blindness; parallax *See* under the nouns.

motor cortex *See* cortex, motor.

motor end-plate *See* muscle, extraocular.

motor field *See* field of fixation.

motor fusion *See* fusion, motor.

motor neuron *See* neuron.

motor pathway A pathway from the cortex to the muscles that control the movements of the eyes enabling them to act as a unit.

motor unit A group of muscle fibres that respond to a stimulus from a single motor neuron. In the extraocular muscles, a motor unit consists of less than a dozen small fibres, considered to be a small unit. It produces a finer degree of neural control over contraction than a larger unit, which produces more powerful gross movements when activated. *See* neuron.

mouches volantes *See* image, entoptic; muscae volitantes.

mould *See* eye impression.

moulding A process for making a lens in which a hot piece of glass (called a parison or gob) or liquid polymer (for contact lenses) is pressed to a predetermined shape. Frames can also be manufactured by pouring a soft material (plastic or molten metal) into a mould which takes on the desired shape after cooling (or drying). The technique is useful for large volume production. *Note*: also spelt molding. *See* lens, spin-cast contact; surfacing.

mount Device (usually in metal or plastic) which holds the ophthalmic lenses before the eyes in rimless spectacles or in spectacles with rims, but which do not surround the lenses, the latter being held by holes, slots or grooves in their periphery. *Syn.* mounting.

mounting *See* mount.

movement 1. Change or apparent change in position. 2. The act of moving.
m. after-effect *See* after-effect, waterfall.
against m. 1. Apparent movement of an object seen through a lens in a direction opposite to that in which the lens is moved. This occurs when looking through a plus lens. 2. *See* retinoscope. *See* movement, with.
alpha m. A form of apparent movement perceived when different sizes of an object are presented in an alternating sequence with an interstimulus interval of about 60 ms, the object appears to expand and contract.
apparent m. Perception of movement induced by stationary separated objects, when the objects

are presented rapidly on and off, one after another with a brief time interval between the two stimuli. The illusion of apparent movement is generally attributed to the stimulation of motion-sensitive neurons in area MT (V5) of the visual cortex. *Examples*: alpha movement, beta movement, gamma movement, phi movement, stroboscopic movements. *Syn.* apparent motion.

autokinetic m. *See* illusion, autokinetic visual.

beta m. A form of apparent movement perceived when two or more separated stationary objects are presented in rapid sequence with an interstimulus interval of between 40 ms and 60 ms, the object appears to move continuously from one position to the other. Beta movement is the basis of smooth continuous motion perception in cinematography in which frames are commonly presented at a rate of 24 frames per second (or about 42-ms time interval). *Syn.* optimum movement. *See* movements, stroboscopic.

compensatory eye m's. *See* reflex, static eye.
conjugate eye m's. *See* version.
cyclofusional eye m's. *See* cyclofusion.
disjugate eye m's. *See* movement, disjunctive.
disjunctive eye m's. Movements of the two eyes in which the eyes move in opposite directions, as in convergence or divergence. *Syn.* disconjugate movements; disjugate eye movements. *See* vergence.

eye m's. The act or process of a change in position of the globe of the eye. Eye movements can be **rapid** such as saccades and the fast phase of optokinetic nystagmus or slow such as pursuit or vergence movements. The **horizontal** command or horizontal gaze centre is in the paramedian pontine reticular formation (PPRF), and the vertical gaze centre is in the midbrain in the rostral mesencephalic reticular formation from which impulses pass to the nuclei of the eye muscles. *See* brainstem; cerebellum; electrooculogram; fusion, motor; palsy, gaze; reflex, vestibulo-ocular; vergence; version.

fixation m's. Involuntary movements of the eye occurring when actually fixating an object. Three types of movements have been observed: the **drifts**, the **micronystagmus** (or **tremors**) and the **saccades** (or **microsaccades**). These movements are too subtle to be seen by direct observation. The drifts are characterized by small amplitude (1 to 7 minutes of arc) and a low frequency (2 to 5 Hz). The micronystagmus movements are characterized by very small amplitude (5 to 25 seconds of arc) and a higher frequency (30 to 100 Hz) and the saccadic movements by a small amplitude (1 to 20 minutes of arc) and low frequency (0.1 to 1 Hz). *Syn.* involuntary eye movements; miniature eye movements; physiological nystagmus (Fig. M12). *See* movement, saccadic eye; stabilized retinal image.

following m. *See* movement, pursuit.
fusional m's. *See* fusional movements.
gamma m. A form of apparent movement that is perceived when a single stimulus is presented in an alternating sequence with an interstimulus interval

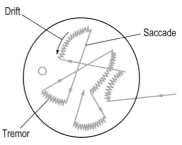

Fig. M12 Diagram of the movements of the optical image on the retina produced by the miniature involuntary eye movements of the eye (tremors, drifts and saccades) during fixation of a stationary object for a period of about 10 seconds. The large circle is 10 minutes of arc in diameter and the small circle represents the size of a cone (based on Pritchard 1961).

of about 60 ms under high and low illumination; the object appears to expand and contract.

optimum m. *See* movement, beta.
optokinetic m. *See* nystagmus.
phi m. *See* phenomenon, phi.
pursuit m. Movement of an eye fixating a moving object. The fixation can remain locked on the target as long as the movement is smooth and the velocity below about 40°/s. Abnormal pursuit eye movements could be due to ocular motor nerve palsy, cerebellar disease, internuclear ophthalmoplegia, systemic medication, etc. *Syn.* following movement. *See* test, motility.

rapid eye m's. **(REM)** Fast eye movements that occur periodically during sleep and are associated with dreaming.

saccadic eye m. A short rapid and abrupt movement of the eyes aimed at bringing onto the foveas the retinal images of an object in the peripheral visual field. It can be reflexive (e.g. while reading a line in a book) or the movement can be voluntary in which the person changes focus from one object to another. Saccades are generated by activity arising in the superior colliculi and the frontal motor cortex in response to a combined visual (via the visual cortical area) and non-visual (e.g. a sudden noise or a command) signal, which ultimately stimulate the abducens and oculomotor nerves. The peak velocity of a saccade of 10° amplitude can exceed 400°/s and be completed in 40 ms. *Syn.* saccade (Fig. M13). *See* antisaccade; hypermetria; movement, fixation; reading; reflex, fixation.

scissors m. 1. Apparent change in the angle made between two lines seen through a rotating astigmatic lens. 2. *See* retinoscope.
stroboscopic m's. Apparent movements as produced by a stroboscope. If the frequency of stroboscopic illumination is less than the rotation of a moving object, it appears to rotate slowly, but if the frequency is increased above that of the moving object, it appears to rotate slowly in the opposite direction to its real rotation. (If the moving

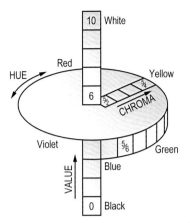

Fig. M13 Schematic representation of the three coordinates of the Munsell colour system.

object is rotating at *x* rotations per second when the frequency is a full multiple of *x*, one sees the object motionless.) Beta and phi movements are types of stroboscopic movements.
See **stroboscope.**
m. threshold   *See* **threshold, movement.**
torsional m.   *See* **torsion.**
vergence m's.   *See* **movements, disjunctive.**
with m.   **1.** Apparent movement of an object seen through a lens in the same direction as that in which the lens is moved. This occurs when looking through a minus lens. **2.** *See* **retinoscope.**
See **movement, against.**

moxifloxacin   *See* **antibiotic.**

moxisylyte (thymoxamine)   *See* **alpha-adrenergic antagonist.**

mucin   Glycoprotein, rich in carbohydrates, produced by the goblet cells and the subsurface vesicles of the conjunctiva which forms the basis of the mucous layer of the precorneal film. Mucin and the secreted **glycocalyx** (which consists of glycoproteins) are adsorbed by the epithelium of the cornea to convert it from a hydrophobic into a wettable hydrophilic surface. A deficiency in the production of mucin leads to an abnormally short precorneal film break-up time and to desiccation of the ocular surface. In addition, the mucous layer prevents microbial invasion of the cornea. In some contact lens wearers (especially of silicone hydrogel lenses) collapsed mucin, as well as lipids and tear proteins, accumulate behind the lens and form small, discrete spheres (called **mucin balls** or **mucin plugs**). These mucin balls cause neither discomfort nor loss of vision.
See **keratoconjunctivitis sicca; tear film; test, break-up time; vitamin A deficiency; xerophthalmia.**

mucocele   A slowly expanding accumulation of mucoid secretions due to a blockage of the nasolacrimal passage. The obstruction may occur as a result of infection, allergy, trauma or tumour, or it may cause the infection as is often the case with dacryocystitis. The patient may present with epiphora, proptosis, diplopia, eyelid or periorbital swelling, but rarely pain unless there is an infection. Treatment involves removal of the mucocele and perhaps construction of a new drainage channel.

mucolipidosis   An autosomal recessive neurodegenerative disorder due to the absence or malfunction of a protein, normally present in cell lysosomes, which cannot break down lipids and carbohydrates and transport them in the body thus accumulating in the cells of many tissue (e.g. nerve, muscle, liver) and leading to this lysosomal storage disease. Patients present with motor and mental deficiencies, corneal clouding, photophobia, esotropia and retinal degeneration.

mucolytic agent   *See* **tears, artificial.**

mucopolysaccharidosis type 1   *See* **syndrome, Hurler's.**

mucous   Adjective referring to membranes or layers which line many hollow organs of the body (e.g. conjunctiva, mouth, nose, digestive tract) and are lubricated with mucus generally secreted by glands beneath the membranes.

mucus   A clear viscous secretion of mucous membranes consisting mainly of mucin, as well as inorganic salts suspended in water.

Mueller's cells   *See* **cell, Mueller's.**

Müller–Lyer illusion   *See* **illusion, Müller–Lyer.**

Müller's muscle   *See* **muscle, ciliary.**

Müller's palpebral muscles   *See* **muscle, Müller's palpebral.**

multifocal electroretinography; lens; visual evoked potential   *See* under the nouns.

multiple sclerosis   *See* **sclerosis, multiple.**

multiple vision   *See* **polyopia.**

M units   *See* **acuity, near visual.**

Munsell colour system   A system of classification of colours composed of about 1000 colour samples, each designated by a letter and number system. The letter and number of each sample indicate its hue, saturation (called **chroma** in this system) and brightness (called **value**). They are represented by a three-dimensional polar coordinate system in which the hue is represented along the circumference, the value along the vertical axis and the chroma along a radius (Fig. M13).
See **colorimetry; test, Farnsworth.**

Munson's sign   *See* **sign, Munson's.**

muscae volitantes   An entoptic phenomenon produced by the presence of remnants of embryonic structures floating within the vitreous humour. They appear like floating spots on a bright uniform background. As they are lighter than the vitreous body they tend to float upward but appear to the patient to move downward because of the reversal of the retinal image. *Syn.* mouches volantes.
See **floaters; image, entoptic; myiodesopsia; opacity.**

muscarine *See* acetylcholine; mydriatic.

muscle A contractile organ of the body which produces movements of the various parts or organs. Typically it is a mass of fleshy tissue, attached at each extremity by means of a tendon to a bone or other structure. Muscles are classified according to structure as non-striated (or unstriated or unstriped or smooth) or striated (or striped), by control as voluntary or involuntary, or by location as cardiac, skeletal or visceral.

abducens m. *See* muscle, lateral rectus.

adducens m. *See* muscle, medial rectus.

agonistic m. Muscle that performs the desired movement, or does the opposite to an antagonistic muscle. *Example*: The left lateral rectus is the agonistic muscle when the left eye turns to the left (Table M5).
See muscle, antagonistic.

antagonistic m. Muscle that opposes the action of another. *Example*: The right superior rectus muscle is the contralateral antagonist of the left superior oblique (Table M5).
See muscle, agonistic; muscle, synergistic.

Brücke's m. *See* muscle, ciliary.

ciliary m. Smooth (unstriated and involuntary) muscle of the ciliary body. In a meridional section of the eye, it has the form of a right-angled triangle, the right angle being internal and facing the ciliary processes. The posterior angle is acute and points to the choroid, and the hypotenuse runs parallel with the sclera. Some of its fibres have their origin in the scleral spur at the angle of the anterior chamber, while other fibres take origin in the trabecular meshwork. The fibres radiate backward in three directions: (1) Fibres coursing **meridionally** or **longitudinally** more or less parallel to the sclera and can be traced posteriorly into the suprachoroid to the equator or even beyond. They end usually in branched stellate figures known as muscle stars with three or more rays to each. These fibres represent **Brücke's muscle**. (2) Other fibres course **radially**. These fibres lie deep in the longitudinal fibres from which they are distinguished by the reticular character of their stroma but are often very difficult to separate from the circular fibres. (3) The **circular** fibres (**Müller's muscle**) occupy the anterior and inner portion of the ciliary body and run parallel to the limbus. As a whole, these fibres form a ring. **Innervation** to the ciliary muscle (mainly parasympathetic fibres derived from the oculomotor nerve) is provided through the short ciliary nerves and stimulation causes a contraction of the muscle. However, a small amount of sympathetic supply is also believed to act and relax the muscle. Blood supply to the ciliary muscle is provided by the anterior and long posterior ciliary arteries. Contraction of the ciliary muscle causes a reduction in its length thus causing the whole muscle to move forward and inward. Consequently the zonule of Zinn, which suspends the lens, relaxes. This leads to a decrease in the tension in the capsule of the lens allowing it to become more convex and thereby providing accommodation. *Syn.* Bowman's muscle.
See accommodation, mechanism of; adrenergic receptors; ciliary body; scleral spur; theory, Helmholtz's of accommodation; Zinn, zonule of.

m. cone A structure formed by the sheath of the four recti muscles as they pass forward from their common origin at the apex of the orbit in the fibrous ring called the annulus of Zinn (and around the optic nerve) to be inserted into the sclera around the eyeball. Some authors consider the muscle cone to include the superior oblique muscle. *Syn.* muscular funnel.
See annulus of Zinn.

cyclovertical m's Extraocular muscles that rotate, elevate or depress the eye. They are the inferior rectus (depression and extorsion), the superior rectus (elevation and intorsion), the inferior oblique (extorsion and elevation) and the superior oblique (intorsion and depression) muscles (Table M6).
See method, Lindblom's; method, Parks'; torsion.

depressor m. The muscle that depresses the lower eyelid. It is the inferior tarsal muscle of Müller's palpebral muscle.

dilator pupillae m. Smooth (unstriated and involuntary) muscle whose fibres constitute the posterior membrane of the iris. This muscle extends from the ciliary body close to the margin of the iris where it fuses with the sphincter pupillae muscle. Contraction of the dilator pupillae muscle draws the pupillary margin towards the ciliary body and therefore dilates the pupil. This muscle is supplied by the sympathetic fibres in the long ciliary nerves and by a few parasympathetic fibres.
See adrenergic receptors; muscle, sphincter pupillae; mydriatic.

Table M5	Agonistic, antagonistic and synergistic extraocular muscles		
Agonist	**Ipsilateral antagonist**	**Ipsilateral synergist(s)**	**Contralateral synergist**
lateral rectus	medial rectus	superior oblique inferior oblique	medial rectus
medial rectus	lateral rectus	superior rectus inferior rectus	lateral rectus
superior rectus	inferior rectus	inferior oblique	inferior oblique
inferior rectus	superior rectus	superior oblique	superior oblique
superior oblique	inferior oblique	superior rectus	inferior rectus
inferior oblique	superior oblique	inferior rectus	superior rectus

Table M6 Innervation and action of the six extraocular muscles

Muscle	Innervation	Action in the primary position
medial rectus	oculomotor (III)	adduction
lateral rectus	abducens (VI)	abduction
inferior rectus	oculomotor (III)	**depression*** adduction extorsion
superior rectus	oculomotor (III)	**elevation** adduction intorsion
inferior oblique	oculomotor (III)	**extorsion** elevation abduction
superior oblique	trochlear (IV)	**intorsion** depression abduction

*Bold characters indicate primary action. The actions below each are the subsidiary actions.

elevator m's. *See* muscle, inferior oblique; muscle, superior rectus.

external rectus m. *See* muscle, lateral rectus.

extraocular m's. Striated (voluntary) muscles that control the movements of the eyes. There are six such muscles: four recti muscles (lateral rectus, medial rectus, superior rectus and inferior rectus) which move the eye more or less around the transverse and vertical axes, and two oblique muscles (inferior oblique and superior oblique) which move the eyes obliquely. The muscles are composed of striated fibres of varying length, mostly running parallel to the direction of the muscle and united by fibrous connective tissue. They have a greater ratio of nerve fibres to muscle fibres than other striated muscles of the body. The fibre thickness varies from 3 to 50 µm, although functionally there seem to be two main types of fibres, the fast and the slow fibres. The former are the thickest and probably responsible for the fast movements of the eyes (saccades) and the latter consist of thin fibres. The **tendons** (bands of connective tissue) at one end of each extraocular muscle are attached to bones. This is the origin of the muscle. At the other end of the muscle, the tendon is attached to the eye and this area is called the **insertion**. The substance proper of the muscle is called the **belly**. Contraction of a muscle occurs in the direction of its constituent fibres and causes a shortening of the muscle. Consequently the eye turns in a given direction depending upon which extraocular muscle is contracting. Contraction results from nervous impulses arriving at the **motor end-plate** (the neuromuscular junction between an axon and a striated muscle fibre)

of the muscle through one of the ocular motor nerves. This causes a neurotransmitter substance to be discharged in the microscopic gap (the cleft) between the end-plate and a muscle fibre. These muscles also possess specialized receptors called **muscle spindles**, which are small groups of muscle fibres that are provided with both a sensory and a motor nerve supply. There are between 12 and 50 in each muscle. The muscle spindles provide a constant and continuous monitoring of the degree of tension of the muscle itself (Table M6). *Syn.* extrinsic muscles; oculorotary muscles. *See* cholinergic; fibres, feldestruktur; fibrosis of the extraocular muscles; motor unit; ophthalmoplegia; position, diagnostic of gaze; strabismus surgery; test, motility; test, three-step.

extrinsic m's. *See* muscle, extraocular.

eyelid retractor m's. *See* muscle, levator palpebrae superioris; muscle, Müller's palpebral.

frontalis m. A striated muscle with fibres attached to the orbital portion of the orbicularis oculi muscle and thus to the skin of the eyebrow. It is innervated by the facial nerve and causes horizontal wrinkling of the forehead as it lifts the eyebrow.

Horner's m. Thin layer of fibres that originates from the upper part of the **posterior lacrimal crest**, (a ridge on the lacrimal bone which borders the fossa of the lacrimal sac), just behind the lacrimal sac. The muscle passes outward and forward and divides into two slips surrounding the canaliculi. It then becomes continuous with the pretarsal portions of the orbicularis muscle of the upper and lower lids and with the muscle of Riolan. Horner's muscle may be involved in tear drainage through squeezing the lacrimal sac. *Syn.* pars lacrimalis muscle; tensor tarsi muscle. *See* **muscle of Riolan.**

inferior oblique m. One of the extraocular muscles, it takes its origin at the antero-medial corner of the floor of the orbit. It passes underneath the inferior rectus in a backward direction (making an angle of about 50° with the sagittal plane of the eye), then under the lateral rectus to be inserted by the shortest tendon of all extraocular muscles on the posterior, temporal portion of the eyeball, for the most part below the horizontal meridian, some 5 mm away from the optic nerve. It is innervated by the oculomotor nerve and it extorts (main action), elevates and abducts the eyeball when the eye is in the primary position. Combined with the action of the superior rectus muscle, it directs the eye upward (Fig. M14). *See* **test, Bielschowsky's head tilt; test, three-step.**

inferior rectus m. This is the shortest of the four recti muscles. It arises from the lower part of the annulus of Zinn, runs forward, downward and outward (making an angle of about 23° with the sagittal plane) and inserts into the inferior portion of the sclera about 6.5 mm from the corneal limbus. It is innervated by the inferior division of the oculomotor nerve and it depresses (main action), adducts and extorts the eyeball when

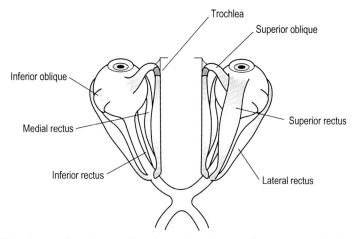

Fig. M14 Extraocular muscles of the eye (the left superior rectus muscle is not shown to allow a clearer view of the muscles underneath). (After Millodot 1976, with permission of Aquila Communications Inc)

Table M7 Intraocular muscles of the eyeball (unstriated muscles)		
Name of muscle	**Nerve supply**	**Action**
sphincter pupillae	parasympathetic via oculomotor nerve	constricts pupil
dilator pupillae	sympathetic via trigeminal nerve	dilates pupil
ciliary	parasympathetic via oculomotor nerve	controls shape of lens in accommodation

the eye is in the primary position (Fig. M14 and Table M9).

See annulus of Zinn; muscle, Müller's palpebral; test, Bielschowsky's head tilt.

inferior tarsal m. See muscle, Müller's palpebral.

internal rectus m. See muscle, medial rectus.

intraocular m's. The smooth (unstriated and involuntary) muscles found within the eye. They are the ciliary, the dilator pupillae and the sphincter pupillae muscles (Table M7). *Syn.* intrinsic muscles. *See* cholinergic.

lateral rectus m. One of the extraocular muscles, it arises from both the lower and upper parts of the annulus of Zinn which bridge the superior orbital fissure. The muscle passes forward along the lateral wall of the orbit, crosses the tendon of the inferior oblique muscle and inserts into the sclera about 6.9 mm from the corneal limbus. It is innervated by the abducens nerve and it abducts the eyeball when the eye is in the primary position (Fig. M14 and Table M9). *Syn.* external rectus muscle; abducens muscle. *See* annulus of Zinn; ligament, check.

levator m's. Muscles that elevate the upper eyelid. They are the levator aponeurosis of the

levator palpebrae superioris muscle and thesuperior tarsal muscle of Müller's palpebral muscle.

levator palpebrae superioris m. Striated muscle that arises from the undersurface of the lesser wing of the sphenoid bone above and in front of the optic canal. It passes forward below the roof of the orbit and above the superior rectus muscle and terminates in a tendinous expansion or **aponeurosis** (also called **levator aponeurosis**), which spreads out in a fan-shaped manner so as to occupy the whole breadth of the orbit and thus gives the whole muscle the form of an isosceles triangle. The aponeurosis is attached to the orbital roof by a connective tissue, the **superior transverse ligament** (or **Whitnall's ligament**). From the inferior surface of the aponeurosis arises a thin sheet of smooth muscle fibres called **Müller's palpebral muscle** (or **superior tarsal muscle**) which inserts into the superior margin of the superior tarsal plate and into the superior fornix of the conjunctiva while some fibres fuse with bundles of the orbicularis oculi muscle to attach to the skin. These latter sets of fibres produce the horizontal skin crease of the upper eyelid. These smooth muscle fibres are innervated by sympathetic nerves from the superior cervical sympathetic ganglion and assist in elevating the upper eyelid. The striated levator aponeurosis is innervated by the superior division of the oculomotor nerve and elevates the upper eyelid. Its antagonist is the orbicularis muscle.

See muscle, Müller's palpebral; muscle, orbicularis; myokymia.

medial rectus m. One of the extraocular muscles, it arises from the medial part of the annulus of Zinn. It passes forward along the medial wall of the orbit and is inserted into the sclera about 5.5 mm from the corneal limbus. It is innervated by the inferior division of the oculomotor nerve and it adducts the eyeball when the eye is in the primary position (Fig. M14 and Table M9). *Syn.* internal rectus muscle; adducens muscle.

See **annulus of Zinn; ligament, check**.

Müller's m. *See* **muscle, ciliary**.

Müller's palpebral m's. Smooth muscles of the eyelids. The superior one (also called **superior tarsal muscle**) originates from the undersurface of the levator palpebrae superioris muscle and passes below to insert into the upper margin of the tarsal plate of the upper eyelid. The inferior one (also called **inferior tarsal muscle** or **inferior tarsal aponeurosis**) originates from the muscular fascia covering the inferior rectus muscle. It extends upward and inserts into the bulbar conjunctiva and the lower margin of the tarsal plate of the lower eyelid. Müller's palpebral muscles are innervated by sympathetic fibres and help in lifting the upper eyelid and depressing the lower eyelid. They are sometimes referred to as the **eyelid retractors**. *See* **myokymia**.

oculorotary m's. *See* **muscle, extraocular**.

orbicularis m. A thin oval sheet of striated muscle that surrounds the palpebral fissure, covers the eyelids and spreads out for some distance onto the temple, forehead and cheek. It consists of three portions: (1) The **marginal** or **ciliary** portion (muscle of Riolan). (2) The **palpebral portion** (also called the **pars palpebralis muscle**) which is the essential part of the muscle and is confined to the lids and may itself be divided into **pretarsal** portion whose fibres lie in front of the tarsal plates, and the **preseptal** portion whose fibres extend from the tarsal plates to the orbital margin. The palpebral portion is used in closing the eye without effort and in reflex and spontaneous blinking. (3) The **orbital portion** (also called the **pars orbitalis muscle**) which is found in the eyebrow, the temple, the forehead and the cheek. This portion of the muscle is used to close the eye tightly, and the skin of the forehead, temple and cheek is drawn towards the inner side of the orbit. The orbicularis muscle is innervated by the facial nerve. *Syn.* orbicularis oculi muscle; sphincter oculi muscle. *See* **ectropion; muscle, Horner's; muscle, levator palpebrae superiotis; muscle of Riolan; myokymia; tear drainage**.

orbicularis oculi m. *See* **muscle, orbicularis**.

pars ciliaris m. *See* **muscle of Riolan**.

pars lacrimalis m. *See* **muscle, Horner's**.

pars orbitalis m. *See* **muscle, orbicularis**.

pars palpebralis m. *See* **muscle, orbicularis**.

pupillary m's. The dilator pupillae and the sphincter pupillae muscles.

m. of Riolan The ciliary portion of the orbicularis muscle, it consists of very fine striated muscle fibres which lie in the dense tissue of the eyelids near their margin. It is continuous with Horner's muscle and encircles the eyelid margins mainly between the tarsal glands and the eyelash follicles. Its action is to bring the eyelid margins together when the eyes are closed. *Syn.* pars ciliaris muscle. *See* **muscle, Horner's; muscle, orbicularis**.

sphincter oculi m. *See* **muscle, orbicularis**.

sphincter pupillae m. Smooth circular muscle about 1 mm broad, forming a ring all around the pupillary margin near the posterior surface of the iris. It is innervated by parasympathetic fibres of the oculomotor nerve that synapse in the ciliary ganglion and by a few sympathetic fibres. Its contraction produces a reduction in the diameter of the pupil. *See* **miotics; muscle, dilator pupillae; reflex, pupil light**.

m. spindle *See* **muscles, extraocular**.

superior oblique m. This is the longest and thinnest of the extraocular muscles. It arises above and medial to the optic foramen on the small wing of the sphenoid bone. It passes forward between the roof and medial wall of the orbit to the **trochlea** (which is in the form of a pulley made of fibrocartilage) located at the front of the orbit where it loops over and turns sharply backward, downward and outward (making an angle of about 55° with the sagittal plane), passes under the superior rectus and inserts into the sclera just behind the equator on the superior temporal portion of the eyeball. It is innervated by the trochlear nerve and it intorts (main action), depresses, and also abducts the eyeball when the eye is in the primary position (Fig. M14). *See* **fossa, trochlear; test, Bielschowsky's head tilt; test, three-step**.

superior rectus m. One of the extraocular muscles, it arises from the upper part of the annulus of Zinn. It passes forward and outward (making an angle of about 23° with the sagittal plane) and inserts into the sclera about 7.7 mm from the corneal limbus. It is innervated by the superior division of the oculomotor nerve and elevates (main action), adducts, and also intorts the eyeball when the eye is in the primary position (Fig. M14 and Table M9). *See* **annulus of Zinn; test, Bielschowsky's head tilt**.

synergistic m's. Muscles which have a similar and mutually helpful action as for example, the inferior rectus and superior oblique muscles in depressing the eyeball. *See* **Table M5, p. 219**.

superior tarsal m. *See* **muscle, Müller's palpebral**.

tarsal m's. *See* **muscle, Müller's palpebral**.

tensor tarsi m. *See* **muscle, Horner's**.

yoke m's. Muscles of the two eyes which simultaneously contract to turn the eyes in a given direction. *Example*: the medial rectus of the right eye and the lateral rectus of the left eye when turning the eyes to the left (Table M8). *See* **law of equal innervation, Hering's; test, motility; version**.

muscular imbalance *See* **imbalance, muscular**.

mutation A permanent transmissible change in the nucleotide sequence of the DNA within a gene, or a change in the physical structure of a chromosome. It can occur by **substitution** (one base or nucleotide is replaced by another), **transition** (a purine (adenine or guanine) is replaced by another purine or one pyrimidine (cytosine or thymine) is replaced by another pyrimidine), **transversion** (a pyrimidine is replaced by a purine or vice versa),

deletion or insertion of one or more bases. Mutations can also occur in a chromosome as a result of inversion (a segment of chromosome is inserted in reverse order), deletion (a loss of a piece of chromosome) or translocation (a piece of chromosome attaches to another). Mutations result in the formation of a protein with an abnormal amino acid or an absence of the protein and these may result in disease, but some mutations may be beneficial in allowing us to adapt to changes in the environment. Mutations may be caused by copying errors in the genetic material during cell division, by exposure to ultraviolet or ionizing radiation (X-rays, gamma rays), carcinogens, viruses or spontaneously.
See chromosome; gene.

'mutton fat' *See* keratic precipitates.

myasthenia gravis An autoimmune disease affecting neuromuscular junctions characterized by muscle weakness and fatigability. It is due to a destruction of acetylcholine receptors in the postsynaptic membrane of the neuromuscular junction. In the eye, it may result in ptosis, diplopia, improper blinking and consequent dryness of the cornea, and eyelid twitch and defects of ocular motility due to a paresis of the extraocular muscles. Drugs that inhibit acetylcholinesterase (e.g. pyridostigmine) and prolong the excitatory action of acetylcholine usually combined with steroids and immunosuppressants are used in the treatment of this disease.
See dysmetria, ocular; ophthalmoplegia, chronic progressive external; sign, Cogan's lid twitch.

Table M8 Yoke muscles		
Right eye	**Left eye**	**Version***
lateral rectus	medial rectus	to the right
medial rectus	lateral rectus	to the left
superior rectus	inferior oblique	up and to the right
inferior rectus	superior oblique	down and to the right
superior oblique	inferior rectus	down and to the left
inferior oblique	superior rectus	up and to the left

*The directions refer to those of the patient.

Table M9 Dimensions of the four recti muscles			
	Muscle length (mm)	**Insertion distance from limbus (mm)**	**Tendon length (mm)**
lateral rectus	48	6.9	8.8
medial rectus	40	5.5	3.7
inferior rectus	40	6.5	5.5
superior rectus	42	7.7	5.8

mycophthalmia A conjunctivitis caused by a fungus. The term is sometimes used to refer to inflammation of the whole eye.
See keratitis, fungal; uveitis, fungal.

mydriasis 1. Dilatation of the pupil. 2. The condition of an eye having an abnormally large pupil diameter (5 mm in daylight). The condition may be due to a paralysis of the sphincter pupillae muscle, to an irritation of the sympathetic pathway, to a drug (e.g. atropine, homatropine), or to adaptation to darkness.
See miosis; muscle, dilator pupillae; mydriatic; pupil.

mydriasis, traumatic A dilated pupil, temporary or permanent, with a sluggish pupillary reaction to light caused by a blunt injury to the globe. It is usually associated with a tear in the iris sphincter muscle. Cycloplegics may be beneficial to prevent posterior synechia.

mydriatic 1. Causing mydriasis of the pupil. 2. A drug which produces mydriasis. Mydriatics are used to carry out a thorough inspection of the fundus and lens, especially in elderly patients in whom the pupils are usually smaller. However, in older people it must be ascertained that the patient does not have glaucoma. There are two classes of mydriatics: (1) antimuscarinic (or parasympatholytic, anticholinergic, atropine-like) drugs which antagonize the action of acetylcholine at muscarinic receptors in the ciliary muscle, such as atropine, cyclopentolate, homatropine, hyoscine (scopolamine) and tropicamide. Antimuscarinic drugs produce cycloplegia as well. (2) sympathomimetic (or adrenergic stimulating) drugs which directly or indirectly stimulate the dilator pupillae muscle which is innervated by the sympathetic division of the autonomic nervous system. These include cocaine, ephedrine hydrochloride, adrenaline (epinephrine), naphazoline and phenylephrine hydrochloride.
See adrenergic receptors; cholinergic; cycloplegia; miotics; muscle, dilator pupillae; mydriasis; reflex, pupil light; sympathomimetic.

myectomy The detachment of a portion of a muscle from its insertion without reattachment. It is done to decrease the effective action of an extraocular muscle in strabismus surgery. *Syn.* disinsertion.
See myotomy; strabismus surgery.

myelinated nerve fibres *See* fibres, myelinated nerve.

myiasis An infection or infestation of tissues or cavities by larvae of flies. In the eye (called ophthalmomyiasis or ocular myiasis), the larvae may affect the ocular surface, the conjunctival sac, the intraocular tissues or occasionally the deeper orbital tissues. Treatment consists of the mechanical removal of the larvae following topical anaesthesia.

myoclonus, ocular Bursts of pendular eye movements normally associated with lesions in the midbrain.
See flutter, ocular; opsoclonus.

myodesopsia The perception of spots passing across the visual field, such as muscae volitantes or floaters. *Note:* also spelt myiodeopsia, myodesopsia.

myodioptre The contractile power of the ciliary muscle, such that it induces an increase in the accommodation of the eye of 1 D.
See **dioptre.**

myoid *See* **ellipsoid.**

myokymia Twitching of a few bundles of fibres of the eyelid muscles. It occurs most commonly when fatigued, sometimes on exposure to cold, and in some pathological cases (e.g. multiple sclerosis) in which case the entire muscle is involved. **Superior oblique myokymia** can often be diagnosed by noting fine torsional nystagmus of the affected eye on slit-lamp examination. In cases where no nystagmus is noted, a patient's history of monocular episodic oscillopsia, associated with vertical diplopia, may be sufficient to make a diagnosis. The use of carbamazepine or propranolol has been suggested as possible treatments in stopping the myokymia.
See **muscle, levator palpebrae superioris; muscle, Müller palpebral; muscle, orbicularis; sclerosis, multiple.**

myopathy Any abnormality or disease of a muscle or muscle tissue.
See **ophthalmoplegia.**

myopathy, ocular *See* **ophthalmoplegia.**

myopathy, restrictive *See* **disease, Graves'.**

myope A person who has myopia.

myopia The refractive condition of the eye in which the images of distant objects are focused in front of the retina when accommodation is relaxed. Thus distance vision is blurred. In myopia, the point conjugate with the retina, that is, the far point of the eye, is located at some finite point in front of the eye (Fig. M15). The percentage of myopes in Caucasian populations is about 25% to 30%, and it is much higher among Chinese (70% to 85%). *Syn.* near sight; short sight.
See **crescent, myopic; gene-environment interaction; keratectomy, photorefractive; orthokeratology; pseudomyopia; retina, lattice degeneration of the; syndrome, Marfan's; theory, use-abuse.**
acquired m. Myopia appearing after infancy or in adulthood when almost all myopias are acquired. Those myopias developing in the late teens and adulthood are usually referred to as **late-onset myopia** (or **adult-onset myopia**), whereas those

occurring earlier are often referred to as **early-onset myopia** (or **juvenile-onset myopia**).
axial m. Myopia due to an elongation of the length of the eye such that it exceeds its posterior focal length. The elongation occurs mainly in the posterior segment of the eye. Almost all childhood myopias which do not result from a disease are axial.
See **myopia, lenticular.**
m. control Term used to encompass the various methods aimed at slowing or arresting the progression of myopia. They include bifocals, contact lenses, pharmaceutical agents (e.g. atropine), incorrect single vision lenses (undercorrection, overcorrection), vision therapy and feedback strategies. None has yet been found to be reliably effective, although atropine appears to reduce myopia progression by about 0.5 D per year in many children.
dark-focus m. *See* **myopia, night.**
degenerative m. *See* **myopia, pathological.**
early-onset m. *See* **myopia, acquired.**
empty-field m. *See* **myopia, space.**
false m. *See* **accommodation, spasm of.**
form-deprivation m. Myopia developing in children when the retina is stimulated by a blurred image during the critical period of development. It may occur as a result of a pathological condition, such as cataract, vitreous haemorrhage, ptosis, eyelid closure or in inordinately long occlusion therapeutic sessions.
See **period, critical; occlusion therapy.**
high m. Myopias above 6.0 D or more are usually considered as high myopias. They are believed to be partly the result of genetic influence with very early onset. It is often associated with ocular problems (e.g. retinal dystrophies, lenticular abnormalities and amblyopia) as well as systemic disorders (e.g. Marfan's syndrome, Stickler's syndrome, Down's syndrome and homocystinuria).
See **glaucoma, open-angle; lens, high index; myopia, pathological.**
hypertonic m. *See* **accommodation, spasm of.**
index m. *See* **myopia, lenticular.**
instrument m. Temporary or permanent increase in accommodation induced by looking through an optical instrument.

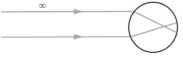

Fig. M15 A myopic eye looking at a distant axial point.

Table M10 Approximate relationship between uncorrected myopia and visual acuity		
	Snellen visual acuity	
Myopia	**(m)**	**(ft)**
−10.0 D	6/600	20/2000
−6.00 D	6/232	20/775
−5.00 D	6/170	20/565
−4.00 D	6/126	20/420
−3.00 D	6/85	20/285
−2.50 D	6/68	20/225
−2.00 D	6/50	20/165
−1.50 D	6/33	20/110
−1.00 D	6/20	20/65
−0.50 D	6/9	20/30

Table M11 Common ocular and systemic diseases with myopia as an associated sign

Marfan's syndrome	retinopathy of prematurity
Ehlers–Danlos syndrome	Stargardt's disease
Down's syndrome	homocystinuria
Cornelia de Lange syndrome	choroideraemia
Weil–Marchesani syndrome	gyrate atrophy
Laurence–Moon–Bardet–Biedl syndrome	rod monochromat
Riley–Day syndrome	ectopia lentis
Turner's syndrome	Fabry's disease
congenital stationary night blindness	buphthalmos
Stickler's syndrome	Wagner's syndrome
pigment dispersion syndrome	

See accommodation, resting state of.

juvenile-onset m.; late-onset m. See myopia, acquired.

lenticular m. Myopia attributed to an increase in the index of refraction of the lens. As a result, there is an increase in refractive power. Such a change usually accompanies the development of some cataracts. This type of myopia may also accompany or follow an increase in blood sugar level, in which case it is usually of a transient nature, i.e. the power of the crystalline lens diminishes after the blood sugar level returns to normal. *Syn.* index myopia.
See cataract, nuclear; diabetes; microspherophakia; myopia, refractive.

low m. Myopias of 3.0 D or less are usually considered as low myopias.

malignant m. See myopia, pathological.

medium m. Myopias between 3.0 and 6.0 D are usually considered as medium myopias.

night m. An increase in ocular refraction (essentially accommodation) occurring at low levels of illumination. *Syn.* dark focus myopia.
See accommodation, resting state of.

pathological m. Myopia attributed to retinal and choroidal degeneration resulting from excessive elongation of the eye. The myopia usually exceeds −6 D, tends to increase rapidly during adolescence and continues to increase during adulthood. Visual acuity is usually subnormal after correction and the fundus appears tessellated with areas of chorioretinal atrophy peripherally and around the optic disc (myopic crescent), tilted disc, breaks in

Bruch's membrane (lacquer cracks) and macular haemorrhage and subsequent pigmented scar (Fuchs' spot), staphyloma, with possible risk of retinal detachment, choroidal neovascularization and even blindness. *Syn.* degenerative myopia; malignant myopia; progressive myopia.
See choroideremia; crescent, myopic; macular hole; retinal detachment; sclerochoroiditis; spot, Fuchs'; staphyloma, anterior; vitreous detachment.

physiological m. This is the most common type of myopia. It is believed that high myopia is influenced by genetic factors whereas low myopia is more likely due to environmental influences. It occurs because of a failure in correlation of the refractive power of lens and cornea, and the length of the eye. Thus, the power of the eye is too great for its length. Unlike pathological myopia, this myopia usually stabilizes when the growth process has been completed. It is associated with normal visual acuity after correction. *Syn.* simple myopia; typical myopia.

progressive m. See myopia, pathological.

refractive m. Myopia due to an abnormally small focal length compared to the axial length of the eye. This may occur with an increase in power of the cornea as in keratoconus, or of the lens as in developing cataract, or with diabetes mellitus. *See* myopia, lenticular.

senile lenticular m. See sight, second.

simple m. See myopia, physiological.

space m. An increase in accommodation which occurs when viewing a field without any stimuli to accommodation as, for example, a clear sky. *Syn.* empty-field myopia.
See accommodation, resting state of.

spurious m. See accommodation, spasm of.

typical m. See myopia, physiological.

myopic conus; crescent *See* crescent, myopic.

myopic defocus *See* defocus, myopic.

myopigenic Pertains to factors causing myopia. They are genetic predisposition which includes ethnicity and a family history of high myopia; visual experiences, such as prolonged reading and extensive near work and possibly accommodative lag; and diseases such as congenital cataract, congenital ptosis and haemangiomas of the eyelids and orbit.

myosis *See* miosis.

myotomy The surgical division or dissection of a muscle. It is done to reduce the pull of an extraocular muscle in strabismus surgery.
See myectomy; strabismus surgery.

myotonic dystrophy; pupil *See* under the nouns.

N

naevus Any localized area of pigmentation or vascularization of the skin or eye tissues, usually benign and congenital. It may occasionally transform into a malignant melanoma (1 in 4300 to 8800 naevi cases). *Note*: also spelt nevus. *Plural*: naevi.

choroidal n. Benign accumulation of melanocytes in the choroid. It affects some 10% of the population. Ophthalmoscopically, it appears as a slate-grey lesion, flat or minimally elevated, oval or circular. It is asymptomatic. With time, drusen may also appear.
See melanocyte; melanoma, choroidal.

conjunctival n. A naevus located on the conjunctiva, most often near the limbus. It appears as a yellowish-red area or deeply pigmented mass usually before the age of 20. A pigmented conjunctival naevus must be distinguished from an acquired melanoma of the conjunctiva which occurs later in life (after the third decade, it is typically unilateral and may become malignant). A conjunctival naevus rarely becomes malignant. It can be excised if cosmetically undesirable or has enlarged to such a degree as to irritate the eye.

flammeus n. *See* syndrome, Sturge–Weber.

iris n. Pigmented spot of variable size on the surface of the iris. It is composed of an accumulation of melanocytes in the iris stroma. It is usually benign but occasionally it may transform itself into a malignant melanoma.
See melanocyte; melanoma, iris; syndrome, ICE.

n. of Ota A benign, congenital, usually unilateral accumulation of melanocytes on the cheek, eyelids, forehead, nose or sclera. Some naevi may become malignant melanoma. *Syn.* oculocutaneous melanosis; oculodermal melanocytosis.
See melanocytosis, ocular; melanosis.

strawberry n. *See* haemangioma, capillary orbital.

Nagel anomaloscope *See* anomaloscope.

nanometre (nm) SI unit of length equal to one-millionth of a millimetre (or 10 ångströms or 10^{-9} m). *Syn.* millimicron (obsolete).
See ångström; micrometre.

nanophthalmos An eye that is congenitally small but has no structural abnormality. It is hyperopic and may develop angle-closure glaucoma. *Syn.* simple microphthalmos.
See microphthalmos.

naphazoline hydrochloride A sympathomimetic vasoconstrictor, which may be used as a topical decongestant in 0.1% eyedrops. It causes slight mydriasis. It also comes as naphazoline nitrate.
See adrenaline (epinephrine); decongestant, ocular.

narrow-angle glaucoma *See* glaucoma, angle-closure.

nasal step *See* Roenne's nasal step.

nasolacrimal blockage *See* epiphora; test, dye dilution; test, Jones.

nasolacrimal canal *See* fossa of the lacrimal sac.

nasolacrimal duct *See* lacrimal apparatus.

nasotemporal overlap A vertical strip passing through the fovea and above and below it, within which retinal ganglion cells may send their axons either ipsilaterally or contralaterally. The width of this strip is less than 1° in the central retina and increases to several degrees in the upper and lower areas. Therefore, information from the fovea and a small area around it is projected to both sides of the visual cortex and this may have some involvement with stereopsis. *Syn.* bilateral strip.

natamycin *See* antifungal agent.

nativism The belief that knowledge or behaviour is inborn.
See empiricism.

nativist theory *See* theory, nativist.

Nd-Yag laser *See* laser, neodymium-yag.

near addition *See* addition, near.

near point of accommodation; convergence *See* under the nouns.

near point retinoscopy *See* retinoscopy, dynamic.

near point rule; point sphere *See* under the nouns.

near point stress *See* asthenopia; stress.

near reflex *See* accommodation, reflex; reflex, near.

near sight *See* myopia.

near triad *See* reflex, accommodative.

near vision; visual acuity *See* under the nouns.

nearsightedness *See* myopia.

nebula *See* leukoma.

Necker cube Perspective drawing of the outline of a cube that can induce two perceptions, either a three-dimensional cube orientated upward or a three-dimensional cube orientated downward (Fig. N1).
See figure, Blivet; Rubin's vase; Schroeder's staircase.

necrosis Death of some or all cells in an organ or tissue. The process involves swelling of the nucleus (pyknosis), fragmentation of the nucleus (karyorrhexis) and complete dissolution of the nuclear chromatin (karyolysis). Necrosis is caused by disease, trauma or interference with blood supply. There are many sequelae to ocular necrosis (e.g. inflammation, reduction in aqueous humour production following ciliary epithelium necrosis, corneal opacity following necrosis of corneal epithelial cells and visual loss and floaters as well as pain following retinal necrosis).
See apoptosis.

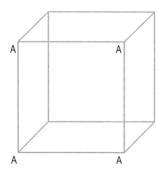

Fig. N1 Necker cube. This ambiguous figure can appear with the plane AAAA either in front or at the back.

necrosis, retinal *See* retinal necrosis, acute; retinal necrosis, progressive.

necrotizing stromal keratitis *See* keratitis, necrotizing stromal.

necrotizing scleritis *See* scleritis, anterior.

nedocromil sodium *See* mast cell stabilizers.

negative A response to a test indicating the absence of an abnormality or of a reaction.
See false negative; true negative.

negative convergence *See* divergence.

negative eyepiece *See* eyepiece, negative.

negative relative accommodation *See* accommodation, relative amplitude of.

negative relative convergence *See* convergence, relative.

negative scotoma *See* scotoma, negative.

spherical aberration *See* aberration, spherical.

neglect, visual A rare phenomenon in which a patient can see all of the visual field binocularly but somehow ignores objects on one side (e.g. patient may draw a diagram omitting one side or shave only one side of the face). It is due to a lesion of the brain (e.g. a stroke), most often in the right cortex and the patient, although conscious of objects in the left visual field, does not pay attention to them. The lesion occurs in the posterior parietal lobe, which receives projections from the primary visual cortex. A confrontation visual field test in which objects are presented to both sides simultaneously often facilitates detection of the condition. Yoke prisms have been found beneficial in those patients.
See phenomenon, extinction.

neodymium-YAG laser *See* laser, neodymium-YAG.

neomycin sulfate A broad-spectrum antibiotic agent effective against gram-negative and gram-positive organisms, although it is not effective against *Pseudomonas aeruginosa*. It may be applied topically as eyedrops or eye ointment, but it is most commonly combined with bacitracin and polymyxin B. *Syn.* framycetin (a mixture of neomycin A, neomycin B and neomycin C).

neonatal conjunctivitis *See* ophthalmia neonatorum.

neoplasm A new abnormal growth of cells forming a tumour, which may be either benign or malignant.

neostigmine A reversible anticholinesterase drug, which neutralizes the effect of acetylcholinesterase and thereby allows the prolonged action of acetylcholine on the iris and ciliary muscle. Its action is similar to physostigmine, but it is not so irritating a miotic. Both are occasionally used in the treatment of glaucoma.
See acetylcholine; parasympathomimetic; physostigmine; miosis; miotics.

neovascular glaucoma *See* glaucoma, neovascular.

neovascularization Development of new blood vessels, especially in tissues where circulation has been impaired by disease or trauma.
choroidal n. Abnormal growth of blood vessels, originating in the choriocapillaris, which pass through Bruch's membrane and then proliferate under the retinal pigment epithelium (type 1) and/or under the retina (type 2). It may occur as a result of a rupture of Bruch's membrane, release of cytokines (e.g. VEGF), inflammation, oxidative stress to the retinal pigment epithelium or vascular insufficiency. The condition is the main cause of exudative (wet) age-related macular degeneration, and it may be associated with various disorders including angioid streaks, choroidal rupture, pathological myopia, chorioretinal scars and birdshot retinochoroidopathy.
See macular degeneration, age-related.
corneal n. *See* pannus.
iris n. Abnormal formation of new blood vessels on the anterior surface of the iris. It is commonly associated with many conditions that have led to retinal ischaemia, such as diabetic retinopathy, occlusion of the central retinal vein, carotid arterial disease, uveal melanoma, long-standing retinal detachment, etc. The neovascularization begins at the pupil margin and often at the same time in the angle of the anterior chamber and spreads over the whole surface. New vessels are associated with fibrous tissue membranes, which may block the passage of aqueous humour through the trabecular meshwork (neovascular glaucoma) and ectropion uveae near the pupillary margin. Treatment typically includes photocoagulation to prevent the formation of new blood vessels.

nepafenac *See* antiinflammatory drug.

nerve A whitish cord made up of myelinated or unmyelinated nerve fibres held together by connective tissue sheath in bundles and through which stimuli are transmitted from the central nervous system to the periphery or vice versa.
abducens n. Sixth cranial nerve. It has its origin from the abducens nucleus at the lower border of the pons and at the lateral part of the pyramid of the medulla. It passes through the cavernous

sinus and enters the orbit through the superior orbital fissure. It supplies motor innervation to the ipsilateral lateral rectus muscle. Additionally, interneurons leave the abducens nucleus and project to the contralateral medial rectus subnucleus to allow conjugate gaze. A lesion in the nuclear region will cause gaze palsy, whereas an abducens nerve lesion will produce only an abduction deficit.
See **nucleus, abducens; palsy, sixth nerve.**

cranial n's. Twelve pairs of nerves, one set on each side of the brain, that emerge or enter the cranium. They carry sensory information from the sense organs, the muscles of the head, neck, shoulders, heart, viscera and vocal tract. The motor neurons with axons in the cranial nerves control pupil diameter, accommodation, movements of the eyes and eyelids, mastication, facial expression and head movements, as well as cardiorespiratory and digestive functions (Table N1).

facial n. Seventh cranial nerve. It is classified as a mixed nerve. It arises from the lower border of the pons and gives rise to many branches which are distributed to the facial musculature, including the orbicularis muscle and muscles of the nose, upper lip, tongue and mandible and to the lacrimal gland. A palsy of the muscle can cause facial nerve palsy with ectropion of the lower lid or Bell's palsy.
See **syndrome, Millard–Gubler.**

n. fibre layer *See* **retina.**

fifth cranial n. *See* **nerve, trigeminal.**

fourth cranial n. *See* **nerve, trochlear.**

frontal n. *See* **nerve, ophthalmic.**

n. growth factor (NGF) A neuropeptide involved in the regulation of growth and differentiation of a number of sympathetic and sensory neurons. Corneal and retinal cells produce and express NGF. NGF may prevent the degeneration of brain and ocular cells, stimulate recovery following trauma and play a role in neuroprotection. A decrease in NGF may result in apoptosis.

n. impulse *See* **potential, action.**

infratrochlear n. *See* **nerve, ophthalmic.**

lacrimal n. *See* **nerve, ophthalmic.**

long ciliary n. One of a pair of nerves that comes off the nasociliary nerve and runs with the short ciliaries, pierces the sclera, travels in the suprachoroidal space and supplies sensory fibres to the iris, cornea and ciliary muscle, and sympathetic motor fibres to the dilator pupillae muscle (Fig. N2).
See **nerve, ophthalmic; reflex, pupil light.**

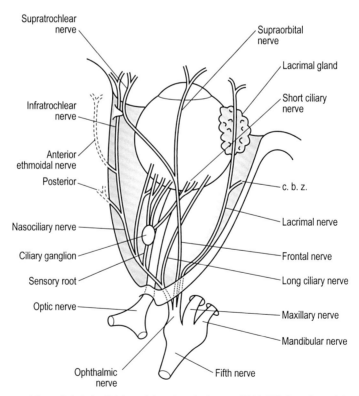

Fig. N2 Diagram of the ophthalmic division of the trigeminal nerve (fifth). This is a view of the right eye from above (c.b.z, communicating branch to the zygomatic nerve). *Note*: The ciliary ganglion is usually situated lateral to the optic nerve.

Table N1 Cranial nerves

Nerve		Type	Function (sensory is in italic, the rest is motor)
I	olfactory	sensory	*smell*
II	optic	sensory	*vision*
III	oculomotor	mixed, primarily motor	movement of eye and eyelids, regulation of pupil size, accommodation, *proprioception*
IV	trochlear	mixed, primarily motor	eye movements, *proprioception*
V	trigeminal	mixed	chewing movements, *sensations from head and face, proprioception*
VI	abducens	mixed, primarily motor	abduction, *proprioception*
VII	facial	mixed	facial expression, secretion of saliva and tears, taste, *proprioception*
VIII	vestibulo-cochlear 1. auditory (or cochlear) branch 2. vestibular branch	sensory	*hearing* *sense of balance*
IX	glossopharyngeal	mixed	secretion of saliva, *taste, control of blood pressure and respiration, proprioception*
X	vagus	mixed	smooth muscle contraction and relaxation (e.g. heart) *sensations from organs supplied, proprioception*
XI	accessory	mixed, primarily motor	movements of head, swallowing movements and voice production, *proprioception*
XII	hypoglossal	mixed, primarily motor	tongue movements, *proprioception*

nasociliary n. *See* nerve, ophthalmic.

oculomotor n. Third cranial nerve. It is classified as a motor nerve. Its origin lies in the tegmentum of the midbrain. It passes through the cavernous sinus and, just before it enters the orbit, it divides into a small superior and a larger inferior division. Both divisions penetrate into the orbit through the superior orbital fissure. In the orbit, the superior division passes inward above the optic nerve to supply the superior rectus and the levator palpebrae superioris muscles. The inferior division sends branches to the medial rectus, the inferior rectus and inferior oblique muscles, as well as providing parasympathetic fibres to the sphincter pupillae and ciliary muscles via a branch to the ciliary ganglion.
See **nucleus, oculomotor; palsy, third nerve.**

ophthalmic n. This is the smallest of the three divisions of the trigeminal nerve, the other two being the maxillary and mandibular branches. It comes off the medial and upper part of the convex anterior border of the gasserian ganglion (trigeminal ganglion), passes through the cavernous sinus and, just behind the superior orbital fissure, it divides into three branches, the **lacrimal, frontal** and **nasociliary**, which pass through the fissure to enter the orbit. (1) The smallest of the three, the **lacrimal** nerve, supplies sensory fibres to the lacrimal gland, the skin of the upper eyelid and the conjunctiva. Just before reaching the gland, the nerve communicates with the zygomaticotemporal nerve (itself a branch of the zygomatic nerve). This branch contains parasympathetic fibres from the facial nerve that pass to the lacrimal gland.

(2) The **frontal nerve**, which is the largest of the three divisions, divides into the **supratrochlear** and **supraorbital** nerves. The supratrochlear nerve further anastomoses with the **infratrochlear** nerve and supplies the lower part of the forehead, the upper eyelid and the conjunctiva. The infratrochlear nerve supplies sensory fibres to the skin and conjunctiva around the inner angle of the eye, the root of the nose, the lacrimal sac and canaliculi and caruncle. The supraorbital nerve sends sensory fibres to the forehead, the upper eyelid and conjunctiva. (3) The **nasociliary** nerve gives origin to several nerves: the long ciliary nerves, the long or sensory root (ramus communicans) to the ciliary ganglion, the posterior ethmoidal nerve and the infratrochlear nerve (Fig. N2).

optic n. Second cranial nerve. It forms a link in the visual pathway. It takes its origin at the retina and is made up of nearly 1.2 million axons from the ganglion cells and some efferent fibres that end in the retina. Over 80% of the axons are of small diameter originating from the ganglion cells associated with the cones; the rest are of large diameter coming from ganglion cells associated with the rods. The nerve runs backward from the eyeball and emerges from the orbit through the optic canal and then forms the optic chiasma. The total length of the optic nerve is 5 cm; the portion before the chiasma called **intracranial** being about 1.0 to 1.6 cm, the **intracanalicular** about 6 mm, the **intraorbital** about 2.8 cm and the **intraocular** about 1 mm. The optic nerve is more often divided into only two portions: the **intraocular** (**bulbar**) portion and the **orbital** (**retrobulbar**) portion.

Surrounding the optic nerve is a subarachnoid space, which is covered with pia mater, arachnoid mater and dura mater. The central retinal artery and vein are found in the intraocular portion of the nerve (Fig. N2).
See **atrophy, optic; fibre, pupillary; glioma, optic nerve; hypoplasia, optic nerve; lamina cribrosa; neuritis, optic; neuropathy, anterior ischaemic optic; papilloedema.**

short ciliary n. One of six to ten branches from the ciliary ganglion that enters the eye around the optic nerve, travels in the suprachoroidal space and innervates the ciliary muscle, the sphincter pupillae muscle and the cornea.
See **rami oculares; reflex, pupil light.**

sixth cranial n. *See* **nerve, abducens.**

supraorbital n.; supratrochlear n. *See* **nerve, ophthalmic.**

third cranial n. *See* **nerve, oculomotor.**

trigeminal n. Fifth cranial nerve. It is the largest of the cranial nerves. It originates above the middle of the lateral surface of the pons as two divisions, a larger sensory root and a motor root. The sensory root passes to the gasserian ganglion (trigeminal ganglion) and from that ganglion the three divisions of the fifth nerve are given off: the **ophthalmic, maxillary** and **mandibular** nerves. The fifth nerve is sensory to the face, the eyeball, the conjunctiva, the eyebrow, the teeth and the mucous membranes in the mouth and nose. The motor root of the nerve has no connection with the ganglion. It joins the mandibular nerve and is motor to the muscles of mastication.

trochlear n. Fourth cranial nerve. It is the most slender of the cranial nerves but with the longest intracranial course (75 mm). It is the only motor nerve that originates from the dorsal surface of the brain between the midbrain and the cerebellum. It passes through the cavernous sinus and then enters the orbit through the superior orbital fissure and supplies motor fibres to the superior oblique muscle.
See **nucleus, trochlear; palsy, fourth nerve.**

zygomatic n. A branch of the maxillary division of the trigeminal nerve, it enters the orbit by the inferior orbital fissure and soon divides into the **zygomaticotemporal** and **zygomaticofacial** branches. The former gives a twig to the lacrimal nerve and is thought to conduct autonomic fibres to the lacrimal gland and the latter supplies the skin over the zygomatic bone.

neural crest *See* **ectoderm.**

neural rim *See* **neuroretinal rim.**

neuritis, optic Inflammation of the optic nerve, which can occur anywhere along its course from the ganglion cells in the retina to the synapse of these cell fibres in the lateral geniculate body. If the inflammation is restricted to the optic nerve head the condition is called **papillitis** (or **intraocular optic neuritis**) and if it is located in the orbital portion of the nerve, it is called **retrobulbar optic neuritis** (or **orbital optic neuritis**) and **neuroretinitis** if associated with retinal involvement.

In **papillitis**, the optic nerve head is hyperaemic with blurred margins and slightly oedematous. Haemorrhages and exudates may also appear. In **retrobulbar optic neuritis**, there are usually no visible signs in the fundus of the eye until the disease has advanced and optic atrophy may appear. However, both types are accompanied by a loss of visual acuity along with a central scotoma and impairment of colour vision. The loss of vision may occur abruptly over a few hours and recovery may be equally rapid, but in some patients the loss may be slow. In retrobulbar optic neuritis, there is also pain on movement of the eyes and sometimes tenderness on palpation. The disease is usually unilateral although the second eye may become involved later. It is usually transient, and full or partial recovery takes place within weeks. The main causes of optic neuritis are demyelination (the most common), viral infection, sarcoidosis, meningitis or syphilis.
See **disease, Devic's; papilloedema; neuroretinitis; pupil, Marcus Gunn; rule, Kollner's; test, photostress.**

neuritis, demyelinating optic A condition characterized by loss of the myelin sheath of nerve fibres. It occurs in the brain and spinal cord and fibres of the optic nerve, particularly in retrobulbar optic neuritis. It is associated with multiple sclerosis in many cases and Devic's disease and, in other cases, with optic neuritis but without clinical evidence of demyelination. Clinical features include rapid monocular reduction of visual acuity, impaired colour vision, pain especially worse with eye movements and relative afferent pupillary defect in patients aged between 20 and 50 years. Most patients do recover to some extent but may need steroids.

neuroectoderm *See* **ectoderm.**

neurofibromatosis type 1 An autosomal dominant inherited disease caused by mutation in the neurofibromin gene (NF1) on chromosome 17q11. It is characterized by tumours in the central nervous system and in cranial nerves, enlarged head, 'café au lait' spots on the skin, choroidal naevi, optic nerve glioma, peripheral neurofibromas (e.g. on the eyelid) and Lisch nodules. Glaucoma may occur because of thickening of the ciliary body causing angle closure. *Syn.* von Recklinghausen disease.
See **phakomatoses; retinal pigment epithelium hyperplasia.**

neurofibromatosis type 2 An autosomal dominant inherited disease with a gene (NF2) locus at 22q12 characterized by bilateral acoustic neuromas, meningioma, glioma and Schwannoma. Ocular manifestations are juvenile cataract and hamartoma (benign tumour-like nodules) of the retina and retinal pigment epithelium. It is much less common than neurofibromatosis type 1.
See **retinal pigment epithelium, congenital hypertrophy of the.**

neuroglia *See* **cell, glial.**

neuroimaging, functional Methods used to detect structural abnormalities in the central nervous system and localized brain neural activity in response to performing specific sensory, motor and cognitive tasks. Two common methods are **functional MRI** and **positron emission tomography**. These techniques can be used to detect tumours, strokes, focal cerebral lesions and to map the cortex in healthy individuals.

See **magnetic resonance imaging; tomography, optical coherence; tomography, positron emission**.

neuromuscular junction *See* **muscle, extraocular.**

neuromyelitis optica *See* **disease, Devic's.**

neuron Structural unit of the nervous system consisting of a nerve cell body and its various processes, the dendrites, the axon and the ending (also called bouton, end foot or axon terminal). There are many types of neurons within the nervous system; some transmit **afferent** nerve impulses to the brain (e.g. those carrying information from the photoreceptors to the visual cortex) or to the spinal cord (e.g. those carrying information from the receptors in the skin to the spinal cord). They are called **sensory neurons**. Others transmit **efferent** motor nerve impulses to a muscle (e.g. those carrying information from the Edinger–Westphal nucleus to the sphincter pupillae and ciliary muscles). These are called **motor neurons**. Other neurons carry nerve impulses from one neuron to another (**interneurons**). *Note*: also spelt neurone.

See **potential, action; synapse.**

neuroparalytic keratitis *See* **keratitis, neuroparalytic.**

neuropathy Any abnormal or pathological change in the peripheral nervous system or nerves.

arteritic anterior ischaemic optic n. A disorder caused by giant cell arteritis in which an inflammation of several arteries including the ophthalmic artery and the short posterior ciliary arteries leads to ischaemic necrosis of various vessels. Affected patients, usually aged over 50 years, present with headache, scalp and joint tenderness, weight loss and sudden and severe visual loss (amaurosis fugax) often accompanied by periocular pain and jaw claudication. The disc is pale and swollen, and severe optic atrophy eventually ensues. Ischaemia is due either to inflammation of the arterioles (posterior ciliary arteries) supplying blood to the anterior portion of the optic nerve (i.e. arteritic) or to an idiopathic aetiology (i.e. non-arteritic). Rapid diagnosis and treatment (usually topical and systemic corticosteroids) are crucial to avoid permanent visual loss as well as systemic complications.

See **retinopathy, non-arteritic anterior ischaemic optic.**

Leber's hereditary optic n. A mitochondrial inherited bilateral condition, which appears suddenly in healthy people, primarily young adult males, of about the age of 20 years and results in a marked loss of vision and ultimately optic disc atrophy and blurred disc margins. The disease has been associated with mutations in many genes encoded by the mitochondrial DNA (mtDNA). A very small percentage of people recover some visual acuity spontaneously in one or both eyes after the disease has run its course (Fig. N3). *Syn.* Leber's disease; Leber's hereditary optic atrophy.

See **atrophy, optic; inheritance; mitochondrion.**

non-arteritic anterior ischaemic n. A disorder caused by occlusion of the short posterior ciliary arteries resulting in partial or total obstruction of the blood supply to the optic nerve head. Risk factors include hypertension, diabetes, an optic disc with a very small physiological cup, hyperlipidaemia and hypotensive episodes as happen at night. Patients, aged over 50 years, present with a sudden visual loss, visual field defects (typically inferior altitudinal hemianopia), swollen hyperaemic optic disc and dyschromatopsia. No

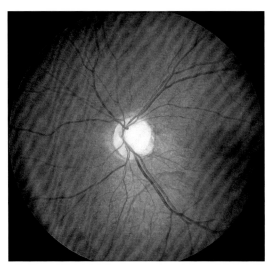

Fig. N3 Leber's hereditary optic atrophy. (From Kanski 2007, with permission of Butterworth-Heinemann)

specific treatment has been identified, although aspirin is often prescribed.
See arteriosclerosis; hemianopia, altitudinal.

nutritional optic n. An uncommon acquired neuropathy believed to be due to a deficiency of mitochondrial function. It mainly occurs in patients who have a history of high alcohol and tobacco consumption combined with a poor diet lacking vitamin B complex, especially cobalamin (B-12) and thiamine (B-1), as well as riboflavin (B-2), niacin (B-3) and pyridoxine (B-6). Patients present with painless bilateral reduction of visual acuity, centrocaecal scotoma and reduced colour vision, and the optic disc may show pallor and slight oedema. Management includes healthy diet, vitamin supplements and abstinence or drastic reduction of alcohol and tobacco.

optic n. A non-inflammatory or degenerative disease of the optic nerve. There will be reduced visual acuity, visual field defects, light sensitivity, relative afferent pupillary defect and optic disc abnormalities. It may be caused by inflammation (e.g. optic neuritis), ischaemia, heredity, drug toxicity, excessive alcohol and tobacco consumption with vitamin B deficiency, compression by a tumour or associated with a systemic disease (e.g. sarcoidosis, rheumatoid arthritis, multiple sclerosis, tuberculosis) or trauma (**traumatic optic neuropathy**). Treatment depends on the primary cause.
See atrophy, Kjer-type optic; glaucoma; neuritis, optic; neuropathy, nutritional; ophthalmopathy; pupil, Marcus Gunn.

posterior ischaemic optic n. A rare condition characterized by ischaemia of the retrolaminar (behind the lamina cribrosa) portion of the optic nerve possibly caused by obstruction of blood supply from the surrounding pial arteries, most of these being branches of the short posterior ciliary arteries. It may be associated with hypotension or following some surgical interventions (e.g. to the spine). There is sudden visual loss but a normal disc. Treatment must not be delayed and may include corticosteroid medication.

neuroprotection A therapeutic strategy aimed at preventing the ultimate result of a neurodegenerative disease process. *Example*: In current glaucoma therapy, the principal objective is to lower the intraocular pressure, but that is only one of the risk factors that lead ultimately to shrinkage and/or death of retinal ganglion cells and visual field loss. Visual field losses occur even after the intraocular pressure is returned to within the normal range in some patients. Neuroprotection is aimed at preventing that secondary ganglion cell degeneration in glaucomatous eyes, which may have been caused as a result of inflammatory or toxic mediators released by the primary degenerative event. Neuroprotective strategies presently being evaluated include glutamate antagonists, calcium channel blockers, nitric oxide synthase inhibitors and neurotrophins.

neuroretina *See* retina, neurosensory.

neuroretinal rim A term used in describing the area of the optic disc which contains the neural elements and is located between the edge of the disc and the physiological cup. When describing the neuroretinal rim, as is often done in cases of glaucoma, one must include its colour, size, slope and uniformity. *Syn.* neural rim.

neuroretinitis Inflammation of the optic nerve head and adjacent retina. It is characterized by optic disc oedema, loss of vision, macular exudates, which frequently form a star-like pattern, and whitish lesions scattered throughout the fundus. A common cause is cat-scratch disease; others appear as a complication of syphilis, Lyme disease and others are idiopathic.
See neuritis, optic.

neurosensory retina *See* retina, neurosensory.

neurotransmitter A substance stored in the synaptic vesicles that is released when the axon terminal is excited by a nervous impulse. The substance then travels across the synaptic cleft to either excite or inhibit another neuron. This is accomplished by either decreasing the negativity of postsynaptic potentials (excitation) or increasing the negativity of postsynaptic potentials (inhibition). Common neurotransmitters include acetylcholine (ACh), dopamine, endorphins, adrenaline (epinephrine), gamma-aminobutyric acid (GABA), amino acids such as glutamate and glycine, noradrenaline (norepinephrine), serotonin and substance P. Common neurotransmitters in the retina are glutamate (the primary excitatory neurotransmitter), GABA (inhibitory), glycine (inhibitory), dopamine (excitatory) and acetylcholine (excitatory).
See neuron; synapse.

neurotrophic keratitis; keratopathy *See* keratopathy, neurotrophic.

neutral density filter *See* filter.

neutral point *See* point, neutral.

neutralization 1. A technique for determining the power of an ophthalmic lens. It is accomplished by placing a lens of known power and opposite sign in contact with the unknown lens and moved back and forth in a plane perpendicular to the line of sight until the observation of movement (against or with) of the distant image seen through the lenses disappear. The unknown lens will have the opposite power to that which neutralizes this apparent movement. 2. A method of breaking down hydrogen peroxide from a contact lens (mostly soft) following contact lens disinfection to avoid possible irritation to ocular tissues. This can be achieved by rinsing and dilution with saline, by using a solution with an enzyme catalase or a platinum disc incorporated into the lens case or with a chemical agent such as sodium pyruvate or sodium thiosulfate.
See disinfection; focimeter.

nevus *See* naevus.

New Aniseikonia Test *See* test, New Aniseikonia.

Newton's formula An expression relating the focal lengths of an optical system (*f* and *f*′) and the object x and image x' distances measured from the respective focal points. Thus,

$$ff' = xx'$$

If the optical system is a lens in air $-f = f'$ the formula becomes

$$-f^2 = xx'$$

Syn. Newton's equation; Newton's relation. *See* paraxial equation, fundamental; sign convention; theory, gaussian.

Newton's rings; theory *See* under the nouns.

newtonian telescope *See* telescope.

nicking, AV *See* AV crossing.

Nicol prism *See* prism, Nicol.

nicotine An alkaloid with pharmacological actions similar to those of acetylcholine at autonomic ganglia and skeletal neuromuscular junctions. *See* acetylcholine; cholinergic.

nictitating membrane *See* membrane, nictitating.

Niemann–Pick   disease *See   disease*, Niemann–Pick.

night blindness, congenital *See* achromatopsia; disease, Oguchi's; fundus albipunctatus; hemeralopia.

night vision *See* vision, scotopic.

nit *See* candela per square metre.

nocturnal vision *See* vision, scotopic.

nodal plane; points *See* under the nouns.

nodes of Ranvier *See* cell, Schwann.

nodule A small circumscribed mass of tissue or an aggregation of cells.
 Busacca's n's. Nodules often found in the iris stroma of an eye affected by granulomatous uveitis (up to about 30% of cases). *Syn.* floccules of Busacca.
 See nodules, iris; uveitis, acute anterior.
 Dalen–Fuchs n's. Multiple, small, yellow-white mounds consisting mainly of epithelial cells protruding through the retinal pigment epithelium. They are seen in the fundus of an eye with sympathetic ophthalmia, Vogt–Koyanagi–Harada syndrome or some other granulomatous inflammations.
 iris n's. Small solid elevations found on the iris and epithelial cells and lymphocytes. They are usually whitish or grey, depending on their location. *See* nodule, Busacca's; nodule, Koeppe's; nodule, Lisch.
 Koeppe's n's. Small nodules frequently found on the iris around the pupillary margin of an eye affected by both granulomatous and non-granulomatous anterior uveitis.
 See nodule, iris; uveitis, acute anterior.
 Lisch n. Small, abnormal, lightly pigmented swelling, which develops on the surface of the iris in almost all patients with neurofibromatosis type 1 during the second or third decade of life. *See* neurofibromatosis type 1.

nomogram *See* tonography.

non-concomitance *See* incomitance.

non-contact   tonometer *See   tonometer*, non-contact.

non-invasive break-up time test *See* test, non-invasive break-up time.

non-steroidal antiinflammatory drug *See* antiinflammatory drug.

noniceptor A sensory receptor which detects noxious stimuli, generally perceived as pain.

nonius horopter *See* horopter, nonius.

noradrenaline (norepinephrine) A neurohumoral transmitter for most postganglionic sympathetic fibres. It is produced with adrenaline (epinephrine) in the adrenal medulla. It is a powerful excitator of α-adrenergic receptors.
 See adrenaline (epinephrine); adrenergic receptors; mydriatic; neurotransmitter.

norepinephrine *See* noradrenaline.

norfloxacin *See* antibiotic.

normal retinal correspondence *See* retinal corresponding points.

normal saline *See* saline, physiological.

Norn's test *See* test, Norn's.

Norrie's disease *See* disease, Norrie's.

nose pad *See* pad.

N notation *See* acuity, near visual.

Nott retinoscopy *See* retinoscopy, Nott.

NSAID *See* antiinflammatory drug.

nuclear layer, inner retinal *See* retina.

nucleus 1. A mass of grey matter composed of nerve cell bodies in any part of the brain or spinal cord and dealing with a common function. **2.** Core or central portion of the cell body of a neuron, containing cellular DNA in particular. *Plural*: nuclei.
 abducens n. Nucleus of the abducens nerve (sixth cranial nerve) located in the lower part of the pons and whose axons supply the lateral rectus muscle.
 accessory oculomotor n. *See* nucleus, Edinger–Westphal.
 n. of the crystalline lens *See* lens, crystalline.
 Edinger–Westphal n. Part of the oculomotor nucleus, it is situated posterior to the main nucleus and contains the parasympathetic component of the complex. Axons from the Edinger–Westphal pass out along the third (or oculomotor) nerve to synapse in the ciliary ganglion. Postganglionic fibres pass through the short ciliary nerves to the sphincter pupillae and ciliary muscles. The nucleus also receives fibres concerned with accommodation and fibres from the pretectal nucleus dealing with pupil light reflexes. *Syn.* accessory oculomotor nucleus; accessory parasympathetic nucleus. *See* nucleus, pretectal; reflex, pupil light.
 lateral n. Part of the oculomotor nucleus which supplies, via the oculomotor nerve, all the extraocular muscles except the superior oblique and the lateral rectus muscles.

lateral geniculate n. See geniculate body, lateral.

oculomotor n. This is the nucleus of the oculomotor nerve (third cranial nerve). It is a complex mass of cells located in the midbrain at the level of the superior colliculus and beneath the cerebral aqueduct (of Sylvius) which connects the third and fourth ventricles. It is divided into several subnuclei. A subnucleus innervates both levator palpebrae superioris muscles, and separate subnuclei innervate the respective contralateral superior rectus, the ipsilateral medial rectus, inferior rectus and inferior oblique muscles. *See* nerve, oculomotor; nucleus, Edinger–Westphal; nucleus, Perlia's; nucleus, trochlear.

olivary n. *See* pretectum; reflex, pupil light.

Perlia's n. Midline part of the oculomotor nucleus. It is rudimentary in man and primates and may provide part of the innervation of the superior rectus muscle.

pretectal n. Complex group of nerve cells in the midbrain anterior to the superior colliculi. One of these, the pretectal olivary nucleus receives retinal inputs via the optic tract and superior brachium and sends axons to both Edinger–Westphal nuclei. It constitutes a centre of the pupil light reflex. Another, the nucleus of the optic tract, may be involved in the control of reflex eye movements. Other fibres from the pretectal nucleus innervate the cornea, the iris, the ciliary muscle and the extraocular muscles (except the lateral rectus and superior oblique muscles), as well as the levator palpebrae muscle. *See* brainstem; pretectum.

suprachiasmatic n. Small cluster of cells in the hypothalamus located just above the optic chiasma. It receives input from retinal axons. It is involved in the light-dark circadian rhythm. *See* rhythm, circadian.

trochlear n. A nucleus of the trochlear nerve (fourth cranial nerve) located at the level of the inferior colliculus and below the posterior end of the oculomotor nerve nucleus; it sends fibres to the contralateral superior oblique muscle.

null point *See* nystagmus.

nyctalopia *See* blindness, congenital stationary night; hemeralopia.

nystagmograph Instrument for recording the movements of the eyes in nystagmus.

nystagmoid Resembling nystagmus.

nystagmus A regular, repetitive, involuntary movement of the eye whose direction, amplitude and frequency are variable. Nystagmus can be induced, acquired or congenital. (In a very small percentage of people, it can even be induced voluntarily.) These eye movements typically appear as one of two types: **jerk nystagmus** or **pendular nystagmus** (Fig. N4). **Jerk nystagmus** is one in which there is a slow and fast phase, the nystagmus being conventionally defined by the direction of the fast phase, which aims to return the eye to the fixation point. A feature of jerk nystagmus is the **null zone**

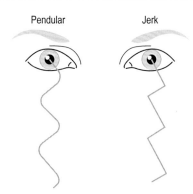

Fig. N4 The two main types of nystagmus, jerk and pendular. The jerk nystagmus has a slow phase to the right (nasalward) and a fast phase to the left (templeward). (After Huber 1976, with permission of Mosby)

(or **null point**) which represents the direction of gaze at which the nystagmus has the smallest amplitude. A jerk nystagmus is usually due to a motor defect that may be induced by brainstem or cerebellar lesions, drug intoxication (**upbeat nystagmus** in which the fast phase is in the upward direction or **downbeat nystagmus** in which the fast phase is downward), associated with a lesion of the central nervous system or the vestibular nerve or nuclei (**central nystagmus** and **vestibular nystagmus**) or to disease or injury to the labyrinth (**labyrinth nystagmus**), or to multiple sclerosis. Jerk nystagmus can also be induced physiologically as, for example, **optokinetic nystagmus** (OKN) or **train nystagmus**, which occurs when watching objects that traverse the visual field rapidly, as a result of thermal stimulation of the labyrinth of the inner ear by cold or hot water (**caloric nystagmus** or **Barany's nystagmus**), when the eyes of a fatigued person are turned into an extreme position of gaze (**end-point nystagmus**) or when a person who had been spinning round is stopped (**vestibular nystagmus**).

The other type, **pendular nystagmus** is characterized by movements of equal velocity in each direction. A pendular nystagmus usually occurs as a result of poor central vision (**sensory deprivation nystagmus**) as in bilateral chorioretinitis, total colour blindness, albinism, congenital cataract, corneal scarring, amblyopia (**amblyopic nystagmus**) or in coal miners after many years of working in the dark (**miner's nystagmus**). In some cases, one eye rotates upward and intorts while the other rotates downward and extorts (**see-saw nystagmus** as a result of brainstem stroke, chiasmal lesion or multiple sclerosis). In some cases, there is a mixture of the two main types: pendular in the primary position and jerk on lateral gaze (**mixed nystagmus**). The movements of the eyes are usually the same in both eyes (**conjugate nystagmus**) but in other cases they may be unrelated as a result of brainstem and cerebellar disease or tumour (**disconjugate, dissociated nystagmus**). Examples of the latter are

end-gaze nystagmus, **convergence-retraction nystagmus** and **see-saw nystagmus**. Or the eye movements are of equal amplitude and type but in opposite or different directions (**disjunctive nystagmus**), also commonly associated with internuclear ophthalmoplegia. There are also cases of unknown origin (**idiopathic nystagmus**). Treatment of nystagmus includes medication (e.g. GABA-ergic, an inhibitory neurotransmitter such as gabapentin), optical correction such as high plus spectacle with high minus contact lenses, botulinum toxin injection or surgery.
See **ataxia, hereditary spinal; brainstem; disease, Wernicke's; foveation period; law, Alexander's; monochromat; ophthalmoplegia, internuclear; oscillopsia; prism; yoke; procedure, Faden; reflex, vestibulo-ocular; sign, Bard's; spasmus nutans; syndrome, Down's; test, optokinetic nystagmus.**
Barany's n. See **caloric testing.**
n. **blockage syndrome** *See* **syndrome, nystagmus blockage.**
caloric n. See **caloric testing.**
congenital n. A motor nystagmus that is present at birth or soon after. It may be inherited as X-linked recessive or autosomal dominant, or induced in the uterus, and results in decreased vision due to corneal opacity, cataract, albinism, aniridia, macular disease or optic atrophy. Initially it is typically pendular but eventually turns into a horizontal jerk nystagmus, and it may be associated with abnormal head movement and decreases in intensity with convergence. The visual prognosis is reasonably good, but if the head turn is excessive, extraocular muscle surgery may be needed.
See **sign, Bard's; spasmus nutans.**
convergence-retraction n. A jerk nystagmus which appears on attempted upward gaze and in which the fast phase brings the two eyes towards each other in a convergent movement with retraction of the globes into the orbit. It may result from a lesion affecting the tectum or dorsal midbrain or a pineal tumour, or form part of Parinaud's syndrome.
See **brainstem; pinealoma.**
gaze-evoked n. An acquired form of horizontal nystagmus characterized by a jerk nystagmus on eccentric gaze in with the fast phase occurs towards the direction of gaze. This type of nystagmus

is believed to be due to cerebellar or brainstem disease affecting the conjugate gaze centres.
occlusion n. A form of nystagmus which occurs when one eye is covered, or which increases in intensity when one eye is covered. The nystagmus is typically of the horizontal, jerk variety, with the fast phase occurring in the direction of the occluded eye.
optokinetic n. A physiological jerk nystagmus induced by the attempt to fixate objects moving rapidly across the visual field. It consists of a smooth pursuit movement followed by a saccade in the opposite direction.
See **test, optokinetic nystagmus.**
physiological n. See **movements, fixation.**
rotary n. Very rare form of nystagmus in which the eyeball makes a movement about the visual axis. It may result from a lesion to the vestibular nerve.
See **nystagmus, vestibular.**
sensory n. A form of nystagmus thought to be due to an abnormality in the afferent mechanism. It is most often due to inadequate image stimulation of the macula, leading to abnormal development of the ocular fixation reflex. Causes include congenital cataracts, optic nerve hypoplasia, aniridia, albinism, achromatopsia, as well as Leber's congenital amaurosis.
vestibular n. There are two main types of vestibular nystagmus: **peripheral vestibular nystagmus** results from stimulation, injury or disease (e.g. Menière's disease) of the labyrinth or of the vestibulo-cochlear nerve (VIII). It presents as a jerk, mainly horizontal, nystagmus with a torsional component. It may be accompanied by vertigo, tinnitus and hearing loss. Fixation inhibits the nystagmus. **Central vestibular nystagmus** results from stimulation, injury, disease of the central vestibular pathways of the brainstem or the cerebellum or lesion of the vestibular nuclei. It may be elicited by irrigating the ear with either hot or cold water; if it is hot, the nystagmus is towards the stimulated ear, and if it is cold, it is away from the stimulated ear. It is typically a jerk nystagmus, which can be purely horizontal, vertical or torsional. It is not inhibited by fixation.
See **test, caloric.**

nystatin *See* **antifungal agent.**

O

object 1. Something that has a fixed shape or form that you can touch or see. **2.** Anything from which an image is formed by an optical system.
extended o. An object consisting of many point objects separated laterally to form a certain shape (e.g. trees, people).

See **light, beam of; light, pencil of; source, extended.**
o. plane See **plane, object.**
point o. Small component of an extended object in relation to an optical system. If the point object is situated on the axis of an optical system, it

gives rise to the axial ray and it is referred to as the axial point object.

real o. Object from which emergent rays diverge.

o. of regard See fixation, point of.

o. space See space, image.

virtual o. One towards which incident rays are converging after refraction or reflection. *Example*: A positive lens forms an image of an object placed beyond its anterior focal point. Introducing a mirror between the lens and the image makes that image become a virtual object.
See image, virtual.

objective An optical system or a lens used to provide a real image of an object. In cameras, this image is situated on the film but in viewing instruments (telescopes, microscopes, etc.), this image is seen through an eyepiece. *Syn.* objective lens.
See aperture, numerical.

objective refraction See optometer; refraction, objective; retinoscopy.

oblique astigmatism; effect See under the nouns.

oblique illumination shadow test See test, shadow.

oblique muscles See muscle, superior oblique; muscle, inferior oblique.

obliquely crossed cylinders See crossed cylinders, obliquely.

occipital Relating to the back of the head or the skull.

occipital cortex See cortex, occipital.

occipital lobe Portion of each cerebral hemisphere posterior to the parietal lobe where visual information is received and processing begins.
See area, visual.

occluder A device placed before an eye to block vision or to partially obscure vision. *Syn.* eye shield.

occluder, Bangerter See Bangerter foils.

occlusion The act of blocking or the state of being blocked. *Examples*: vision with an occluder, a vessel with an embolus.

o. amblyopia See amblyopia; occlusion treatment.

o nystagmus See nystagmus; occlusion.

punctal o. Sealing of the lacrimal punctum, temporarily (e.g. with a plastic plug) or permanently (e.g. by heat cauterization), to retain the natural tears or prolong the effect of artificial tears. This method is commonly used in the management of keratoconjunctivitis sicca. Occasionally, a plug made of collagen is used prior to insertion of a more permanent type of punctal plug, because it dissolves within a week. This is done to determine whether permanent or semipermanent occlusion (as with a silicone plug) is likely to succeed.
See keratopathy, neurotrophic.

retinal arterial o. See retinal artery occlusion.

retinal vein o. See retinal vein occlusion.

o. test See test, cover.

o. treatment A method of treating amblyopia or strabismus by covering the good eye. Such a method is most effective below the age of 4 years and with little effect after the age of 9 years, which is beyond the critical period of development. However, this technique must be used with caution as prolonged occlusion in very young children can lead to a reversal of eye dominance in which the previously good eye becomes amblyopic (called **occlusion amblyopia**). Moreover, it has been shown that the effect of occlusion does not improve beyond 6 hours at a time. Alternate occlusion is preferred as both eyes are thus stimulated. *Syn.* patching.
See myopia, form-deprivation; penalization; period, critical; pleoptics.

octave The interval between two frequencies having a ratio of two to one. *Example*: from 4 to 8 c/deg. Two octaves is a quadrupling of frequencies, and so on. Octaves are commonly used in specifying the bandwidth of the frequencies (e.g. spatial frequencies) to which cells in the visual pathway respond.
See cycle per degree.

ocular 1. See eyepiece. **2.** Appertains to eye.

ocular adnexa See appendages of the eye.

ocular albinism; appendages; apraxia; bobbing; column; cup; decongestant; dominance; dysmetria; ferning test; flutter; fundus; headache; hypertension; hypotonia; impression; media; myoclonus; pathology; pemphigoid; prosthesis See under the nouns.

ocular lubricant See tears, artificial.

ocular mucous membrane pemphigoid See pemphigoid, cicatricial.

ocular myopathy See ophthalmoplegia.

ocular refraction See power, effective; refractive error.

ocular tension See pressure, intraocular.

ocular tremors of fixation See movement, fixation.

ocularist One who designs and fits artificial eyes. *Syn.* orbital prosthetist.
See eye, artificial.

oculist See ophthalmologist.

oculoauriculovertebral dysplasia See syndrome, Goldenhar's.

oculocardiac reflex See reflex, oculocardiac.

oculocentre Pertains to the eye as a centre of reference.
See direction, oculocentric; egocentre; localization.

oculocentric direction; localization See under the nouns.

oculocerebrorenal syndrome See syndrome, Low.

oculocutaneous albinism See albinism.

oculocutaneous melanosis; melanocytosis See naevus of Ota.

oculogyric Pertaining to movement of the eye about the anteroposterior axis.

oculogyric crisis Sudden involuntary contractions of some eye muscles resulting in repetitive conjugate ocular deviations, usually, though not always, in an upward direction. The attack or crisis may last from seconds to minutes. It occurs most frequently after the use of neuroleptic medication, but it may be precipitated or accompany emotional stress, alcohol or general fatigue.

oculomandibulofacial syndrome *See* syndrome, Hallermann-Streiff-Francois.

oculomotor Pertaining to movement of the eyes or to the oculomotor nerve.

oculomotor nerve; nucleus *See* under the nouns.

oculomotor paralysis A general term referring to abnormal eye movements caused by a partial paralysis (palsy) of the third (oculomotor), fourth (trochlear) and/or sixth (abducens) cranial nerves to the extraocular muscles.

oculomycosis Any disease of the eye caused by a fungus.
See antifungal agent; keratitis; keratomycosis.

oculorotary muscles *See* muscles, extraocular.

oculus Latin for eye. *Plural*: oculi.

oculus dexter (OD) Latin for right eye.

oculus sinister (OS) Latin for left eye.

oculus uterque (OU) Latin for both eyes.

oedema The presence of an excessive amount of fluid in or around cells, tissues or serous cavities of the body. In the eye, oedema can occur in the cornea, the conjunctiva, the uvea, the retina, the choroid, and the ciliary body.

oedema, corneal Oedema which usually accompanies eye diseases or contact lens wear with low oxygen transmissibility. Corneal oedema is easily seen with a slit-lamp using retroillumination or sclerotic scatter illumination. Quantitatively, it can be assessed with the addition of a pachometer that measures corneal swelling. Beyond about 4% swelling, there appear **striae** (wispy greyish-white lines usually vertical) in the stroma. Beyond about 8% swelling, there appear **folds** (dark lines) believed to represent physical buckling of the posterior corneal layers. Corneal swelling of 15% or greater, which indicates a gross separation of the collagen fibres of the stroma, results in a hazy or cloudy appearance of the cornea. There is a physiological oedema occurring during sleep in every human cornea amounting to an increase in thickness of about 4%. Corneal oedema gives rise to the appearance of haloes around lights, photophobia, spectacle blur, losses in corneal transparency and sometimes stinging. Management depends on the cause and tissue involved. If due to contact lenses, refitting with daily wear lenses of higher oxygen transmissibility and reducing wearing time usually solve the problem. Hypertonic ophthalmic solutions of sodium chloride 5% reduce corneal oedema. *Note*: also spelt edema.
See blebs, endothelial; corneal clouding, central; hypoxia; lens, silicone hydrogel; oxygen permeability; oxygen requirement, critical; pachometer; syndrome, overwear.

oedema, cystoid macular Oedema and cyst formation of the macular area of the retina. Fluid accumulates in the outer plexiform and inner nuclear layers forming cystoid spaces. It may occur as a result of, or be associated with, systemic vascular disease, retinal vein occlusion, diabetic retinopathy, uveitis, hypertensive retinopathy, retinitis pigmentosa and following some ocular surgery such as vitreoretinal, photocoagulation, glaucoma procedures and especially cataract surgery. When cystoid macular oedema follows cataract surgery, it is called the **Irvine–Gass syndrome** and it is sometimes accompanied by intraoperative vitreous loss or vitreous adhesion to the iris or to the corneoscleral wound. There may be blurring and metamorphopsia. In some cases, antiinflammatory therapy may help in restoring visual acuity and in other cases the vitreous adhesion may be disrupted with a Nd-YAG laser.

ofloxacin *See* antibiotic.

Oguchi's disease *See* disease, Oguchi's.

ointment A semisolid preparation of one or more medicinal substances applied to the skin or mucous membrane as local drug administration.

olopatadine hydrochloride *See* antihistamine; mast cell stabilizers.

ommatidium One of the visual elements of the compound eye of arthropods. It is hexagonal in shape and about 10 times longer than its diameter. It consists of a corneal facet below which is a crystalline cone which collects light and a sensory area called the **rhabdom**, all of it being enclosed in a dark pigment.

onchocerciasis A disease caused by infestation with the filarial worm (*Onchocerca volvulus*) spread by blackflies. It is common in tropical Africa and Central America, especially in areas near rivers. Large numbers of microfilariae are present on the skin and often enter the eye. The patient initially complains of itching with signs of anterior uveitis, sclerosing keratitis, chorioretinitis and optic neuritis. The disease is treated effectively with ivermectin. *Syn.* onchocercosis; river blindness.

'one and a half' syndrome *See* syndrome, 'one and a half'.

onset The beginning of symptoms.

opacity The condition of a tissue or structure which is not transparent or being opaque. The location of an opacity within the eye can be determined with a slit-lamp. It can also be determined using an ophthalmoscope and asking the patient to look in various directions. If the opacity moves very little or not at all, it is situated in the lens. If the opacity moves in the same direction as the eye, it is situated in front of the lens, and if it moves in the opposite direction, it is situated in the vitreous humour.
See cataract; muscae volitantes; ulcer, corneal.

opaque Impervious to the passage of light. *See* **transparent**.

operculum A flap of detached retina which projects forward or is totally free in the vitreous. It can happen as a result of a retinal tear (break).

ophryosis Spasmodic twitching in the region of the eyebrow.

ophthalmagra A sudden pain in the eye.

ophthalmia Severe inflammation of the eye, especially, but not exclusively, one involving the conjunctiva. *See* **conjunctivitis**.
o. neonatorum An acute conjunctivitis that occurs in the first month of life as a result of infection acquired in the birth canal. The most common causes are *Chlamydia trachomatis*, *Streptococcus pneumoniae*, *Neisseria gonorrhoeae*, *Staphylococcus aureus* and herpes simplex virus. The eyelids are swollen and stuck together by purulent discharge. If the cause is gonococcal, loss of the eye is a real and immediate threat. A gonococcal infection develops within 2 to 4 days after birth, whereas a chlamydial infection normally appears 5 to 14 days after birth. Differential diagnosis is facilitated by laboratory tests (e.g. Gram staining of conjunctival scrapings). Management depends on the cause: systemic erythromycin and topical tetracycline for chlamydial infection, ceftriaxone or cefotaxime for gonococcal infection and eye irrigation with saline solution. *Syn.* blennorrhoea neonatorum; gonococcal ophthalmia; neonatal conjunctivitis. *See* **conjunctivitis, acute; conjunctivitis, adult inclusion**.
sympathetic o. A rare bilateral granulomatous inflammation of the uveal tract that usually follows perforation of one eye due to trauma or, more rarely, intraocular surgery. The inflammation occurs first in the injured eye (called the **exciting eye**) and follows in the other eye (called the **sympathetic eye**). It usually occurs within 2 to 12 weeks after the incident, although some cases may appear later. The condition is believed to be a T-lymphocyte-mediated delayed hypersensitivity. Treatment usually involves enucleation of the exciting eye and high doses of systemic and topical corticosteroids in the sympathetic eye. *Syn.* sympathetic ophthalmitis. *See* **immunosuppressants; uveitis**.

ophthalmic Pertaining to the visual apparatus and its function.

ophthalmic crown *See* **glass, crown**.

ophthalmic cup *See* **cup, optic**.

ophthalmic Graves' disease *See* **disease, Graves'**.

ophthalmic lens; nerve *See* under the nouns.

ophthalmic optician *See* **optician; optometrist**.

ophthalmic optics *See* **optics, ophthalmic**.

ophthalmic zoster *See* **herpes zoster ophthalmicus**.

ophthalmitis, sympathetic *See* **ophthalmia, sympathetic**.

ophthalmodynamometer 1. Instrument used to measure the near point of convergence of the eyes. 2. Instrument for measuring the blood pressure of the central retinal artery. There are two types: the compression type (e.g. Bailliart's ophthalmodynamometer) in which the pressure is raised by pressing on the eye, the force being produced by a spring-loaded plunger resting on the temporal bulbar conjunctiva of the anaesthetized eye, while the examiner observes the optic nerve through an ophthalmoscope. The other type is by suction in which negative pressure is applied to the eye using a scleral vacuum cup near the limbus (e.g. Doppler's ophthalmodynamometer). The diastolic pressure is read from the gauge provided with the instrument when the central retinal artery is seen to pulsate on the optic disc, and the systolic pressure is read when all arterial pulsations just cease (the instrument should be removed immediately afterwards). A low systolic pressure is indicative of an occlusive disease of the carotid artery (a comparison between the two eyes is also very informative) as such disorders are responsible for a significant percentage of ocular symptoms and strokes. *See* **amaurosis fugax; artery, internal carotid; plaques, Hollenhorst's**.

ophthalmologist A medical specialist who practises ophthalmology. *Syn.* oculist (this term is rarely used nowadays); ophthalmic surgeon.

ophthalmology Part of medical science concerned with the medical and surgical care of the eye and its appendages.

ophthalmometer *See* **keratometer**.

ophthalmopathy Any eye disease. **External ophthalmopathy** refers to any disease of the conjunctiva, cornea, eyelids or the appendages of the eye. **Internal ophthalmopathy** refers to any disease of the lens, retina or other internal structures of the eye.

ophthalmopathy, thyroid *See* **disease, Graves'**.

ophthalmophakometer Optical instrument used to measure the curvatures of the crystalline lens. It was designed by Tscherning in 1892. *See* **phakometer**.

ophthalmoplegia Paralysis of the ocular muscles. **External ophthalmoplegia** refers to paralysis of one or more extraocular muscles. If the levator palpebrae muscle is also involved, the condition is usually referred to as **ocular myopathy**. **Internal ophthalmoplegia** refers to a paralysis of the muscles of the iris and the ciliary muscle. **Total ophthalmoplegia** refers to a paralysis of all the muscles in the eye, which results in ptosis, immobility of the eye and pupil and loss of accommodation. *See* **disease, Graves'; palsy, third nerve**.
chronic progressive external o. (CPEO) A rare disorder characterized by a progressive bilateral ptosis and a loss of ocular motility. It is

associated with mutation of mitochondrial DNA, which results in abnormalities in highly oxidative tissues such as the muscles and the brain. The initial sign is bilateral ptosis, followed later by strabismus. A related mitochondrial myopathy is the **Kearns–Sayre syndrome** in which there is CPEO, pigmentary retinopathy characterized by coarse pigment clumping which principally affects the central retina and cardiac conduction defects. This syndrome presents before age 20 years. *See* **myasthenia gravis.**

internuclear o. An eye movement disorder which results from a lesion in the medial longitudinal fasciculus, disrupting the coordination between the oculomotor nucleus and the abducens nucleus. It is characterized by a limited adduction by the eye on the same side of the body as the lesion and a jerky horizontal nystagmus and overshoot by the other eye on abduction, when moving the eyes towards the side of the body opposite to that of the lesion. Convergence is usually intact, unless the lesion is widespread. Vertical gaze gives rise to nystagmus and oscillopsia. Surgery may be needed for persistent diplopia. The condition is associated with multiple sclerosis, vascular disease, tumour of the brainstem or encephalitis. *See* **brainstem; dysmetria, ocular; palsy, supranuclear gaze; syndrome, 'one and a half'.**

ophthalmorrhagia Ocular haemorrhage.

ophthalmorrhoea A discharge of mucus, pus or blood from the eye. *Note*: also spelt ophthalmorrhea.

ophthalmoscope An instrument for viewing the media and fundus of the eye. It consists essentially of (1) a light source (a halogen or tungsten bulb), a condenser system, a lens and a reflector (a prism, mirror or metallic plate) to illuminate the interior of the eye and (2) a viewing system comprising a sight hole and focusing system (usually a rack of lenses of different powers) to compensate for the combined errors of refraction of the patient and practitioner. *See* **transillumination; Visuscope.**

binocular indirect o. An indirect ophthalmoscope with a binocular viewing system used to obtain a magnified, inverted, stereoscopic image of the fundus. It consists of a light source mounted above and between the examiner's eyes on a headset. This illuminates a hand-held condensing lens of high positive power close to the patient's eyes, which forms an image of the patient's pupil in both of the examiner's pupils. An aerial image of the patient's fundus is formed between the condensing lens and the examiner (if the patient is emmetropic the image will be formed in the focal plane of the condensing lens). It appears inverted and stereoscopically through the oculars attached to the headset. Stereopsis is obtained by reducing the interpupillary distance by means of mirrors or prisms within the headset of the instrument. This ophthalmoscope allows examination of a wide area of fundus and perception of depressed and raised areas (Fig. O1).

confocal scanning laser o. An instrument using a confocal laser system to provide and analyse a three-dimensional image of the optic nerve head, peripapillary retina and macular region. The instrument uses a 670-nm diode laser and measures the amount of light reflected from a series of 16 to 64 optical sections in depth and reconstructs them. Image contrast is increased because light scattered from areas in front and behind the plane of focus is filtered out. *Abbreviated*: **confocal SLO. Adaptive optics** has been applied to the instrument to provide a spot of light which is focused on the retina free of aberrations. *Abbreviated*: **confocal AOSLO.** This

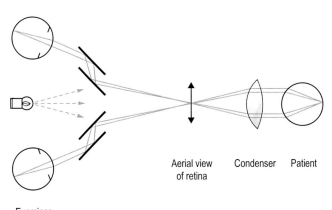

Examiner   Aerial view   Condenser   Patient
            of retina

Fig. O1 Binocular indirect ophthalmoscope. The light source mounted above and between the examiner's eyes illuminates the condenser, which images the source at the periphery of the patient's pupil. The illumination does not overlap the observation beam. The condenser lens is hand-held; it forms an inverted aerial image of the retina. The patient's pupil and the examiner's pupils are conjugate and the patient's ocular fundus is viewed stereoscopically.

method allows visualization of the retinal fibre layer, retinal blood flow, cone photoreceptor mosaic in normal and diseased retina (e.g. age-related macular degeneration, diabetic retinopathy, retinitis pigmentosa, choroideremia). *Syn.* confocal scanning laser tomograph.
See **glaucoma detection; microscope, confocal; ophthalmoscope, scanning laser; optics, adaptive.**

direct o. An ophthalmoscope that provides a virtual erect image with a magnification of about 15× of the fundus formed by the patient's eye in combination with whatever focusing lenses are needed to correct for the refractive errors of the observer and patient. The instrument is held at close range to the patient's eye and the field of view is small (less than 10°) (Fig. O2). The magnification M of a direct ophthalmoscope is equal to

$$M = F_e/4$$

where F_e is the power of the eye (Table O1). *Example*: The magnification of the fundus of an aphakic eye of +40.00 D is equal to 40/4 = 10×.

indirect o. An ophthalmoscope that provides an aerial image of the fundus (and not the fundus itself as with a direct ophthalmoscope), which is real, inverted, with a magnification of 5× to 7× and formed at approximately arm's length from the practitioner. This aerial image is usually produced by a strong positive lens ranging in power from +13 D to +30 D that is held in front of the patient's eye. The practitioner views this aerial image through a sight hole with a focusing lens to compensate for ametropia and accommodation. This instrument provides a large field of view (25° to 40°) and allows easier examination of the periphery of the retina. This instrument has been supplanted by the binocular indirect

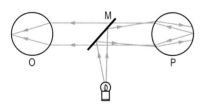

Fig. O2 Optical principle of the simplest form of direct ophthalmoscope. (O, observer's eye; P, patient's eye; M, semisilvered mirror)

ophthalmoscope. The magnification of an indirect ophthalmoscope M is equal to

$$M = F_e/F_c$$

where F_e and F_c are the powers of the eye and of the condensing lens, respectively (Table O1). *Example*: Using a condensing lens of +15.00 D to view the fundus of an emmetropic eye yields a magnification of 60/15 = 4×.
See **camera, fundus.**

scanning laser o. Ophthalmoscope that provides a continuous image of the ocular fundus on a TV monitor. It consists of a narrow laser beam, which is scanned horizontally and vertically to produce a rectangular area (called a raster) on the retina. A small beam of light is reflected back out of the eye to a light detector, which monitors the brightness of each point on the raster and relays the information to the corresponding element on a TV monitor where the image can be viewed and/or stored. Low illumination is used to make this procedure more comfortable than conventional photography, and mydriatics are usually unnecessary. The field of view extends up to 60 degrees, although some newer models can scan a much wider field. The instrument has been especially valuable in diagnosing glaucoma and in research.
See **ophthalmoscope, confocal scanning laser.**

ophthalmoscopy Method of examination of the interior of the eye with an ophthalmoscope.

ophthalmoscopy, red-free Method of ophthalmoscopy using a blue-green filter in the illumination system. This gives a better contrast between the retinal vessels and the background and helps to differentiate more easily between retinal and choroidal lesions; retinal lesions appear black while choroidal ones appear grey. Green light illumination of the fundus images mainly the sensory retina and pigment epithelium, whereas red illumination gives an image of the deeper layers such as the choroid.

Oppel–Kundt visual illusion *See* **illusion, Oppel–Kundt visual.**

opponent-colour cells *See* **cell, colour-opponent.**

opponent-colour theory *See* **theory, Hering's of colour vision.**

opsin *See* **rhodopsin.**

opsoclonus Involuntary chaotic movements of both eyes in horizontal and vertical directions. It may be a sign of cerebellar disease.
See **flutter, ocular; myoclonus, ocular.**

Table O1 Comparison between direct and indirect ophthalmoscopes

Ophthalmoscope	Form	Image	Field of view (in degrees)	Magnification
direct	monocular	erect	8	15×
indirect	monocular	inverted	20–40*	5× to 7×
indirect	binocular	inverted	40–75	1.5× to 4.5×*

*Varies according to the power of the condensing lens.

optic Pertaining to light or to vision.

optic atrophy; canal; chiasma; cup; disc; disc coloboma; disc drusen See under the nouns.

optic disc pit See disc, optic d. pit.

optic fibre See optics, fibre.

optic foramen See canal, optic.

optic nerve head See disc, optic.

optic nerve; nerve hypoplasia; neuritis; neuropathy; neuropathy, anterior ischaemic; pit See under the nouns.

optic portion of a scleral lens See transition.

optic radiations See radiations, optic.

optic stalk See cup, optic.

optic sulcus See pit, optic.

optic tectum See tectum of the mesencephalon.

optic tracts; vesicle See under the nouns.

optic zone, central Central region of a contact lens that has a prescribed optical effect where there is a peripheral optic zone or zones (British Standard).
See diameter, total.

optic zone diameter Diameter of the optic zone (front or back) of a contact lens measured to the surrounding junction. It is commonly specified in millimetres. Specifically, there are the **back optic zone diameter** (BOZD), formerly called back central optic diameter (BCOD), and the **front optic zone diameter** (FOZD). It is often difficult to measure these dimensions due to the blending of the line separating the zones, especially for the back optic zone diameter. The region surrounding the central optic zone is the **peripheral zone**. If there is more than one, the zones will be numbered first, second, etc., beginning with the zone immediately surrounding the central optic zone. The diameter of each peripheral zone is referred to as the **back** (or front) **peripheral zone diameter** (BPZD).
See blending; diameter, total; edge lift.

optic zone radius, back (BOZR) Radius of curvature of the back optic zone of a contact lens. (It was formerly called the back central optic radius (BCOR or BC) or posterior central curve radius (PCCR).) If the optic zone is surrounded by a peripheral zone, there will be a radius of curvature of a back peripheral zone (BPR). If there are several zones, there will be BPR$_1$, BPR$_2$, etc., beginning with the zone immediately surrounding the central optic zone.
See method, Drysdale's; radiuscope; Toposcope.

optical aid See appliance, optical.

optical anisotropy; axis; centre See under the nouns.

optical biopsy Any technique that provides imaging of tissue morphology without the need for excision of the tissue. Example: optical coherence tomography (OCT).

optical centre position, standard See centre, standard optical position.

optical coherence tomography; density; dispensing; illusion; interface; medium See under the nouns.

optical microspherometer See radiuscope.

optical surface; system; system, compound; wedge See under the nouns.

optical zone of cornea A theoretical zone of about 4 mm in diameter in the centre of the cornea. It is assumed to be spherical for clinical purposes. Syn. corneal cap.
See apex, corneal.

optician 1. One who designs and makes optical instruments or lenses. **2.** Dispensing optician. **3.** Ophthalmic optician.

optician, dispensing One who fits and adapts spectacles and contact lenses on the basis of a prescription by an ophthalmologist or optometrist (or ophthalmic optician). In many countries, dispensing opticians cut and edge lenses and fit them into a frame.
See dispensing, optical; glazing.

optician, manufacturing One who makes optical or ophthalmic instruments, lenses, prisms or spectacles.

optician–optometrist See optometrist.

opticin An extracellular matrix glycoprotein secreted by the non-pigmented epithelium of the ciliary body into the vitreous cavity where it associates with vitreous collagen and adjacent basement membranes (e.g. retinal internal limiting membrane and posterior lens capsule). It is believed to bind growth hormone in the vitreous and to regulate growth factor activity thus producing antiangiogenic properties. Opticin also binds glycosaminoglycans including heparin and chondroitin sulfates thus stabilising the structure of the vitreous and possibly maintaining vitreoretinal adhesion.
See VEGF.

optics 1. The branch of physics which deals with the phenomena of light. **2.** The elements and/or design of an optical instrument, including the eye (optics of the eye).
See theory, gaussian; theory, Newton's; theory, quantum; theory, wave.
adaptive o. The design of ophthalmic instruments or lenses such that they compensate for the subject's aberrations, based on an analysis of the wavefront aberrations of the eye. The method can be applied to various instruments used to view the retina, to lenses including intraocular lenses and to the correction of ametropia.
See ophthalmoscope, confocal scanning laser.
dispensing o. See optics, ophthalmic.
fibre o. Fine flexible glass or plastic rod, which transmits light longitudinally by repeated total internal reflection. By using a bundle of such fibres in a fixed array, a complete image can be transmitted. As total internal reflection can occur even if the fibres are curved, the system is of great

Table O2	Common optical symbols
f, f'	primary and secondary focal lengths
h, h'	object and image sizes
i, i'	angles of incidence or reflection and refraction
k, k'	distances from the corneal pole to the far point and to the retina, respectively
l, l'	distances of object and image from the optical system
n, n'	refractive indices of object and image space
u, u' or w, w' or α, α'	angular size of object and image
x, x'	distances between object and first focal point, and image and second focal point, respectively
r	radius of curvature
c	centre of curvature
A	ocular accommodation
A_s	spectacle accommodation
Amp	amplitude of accommodation
Add	addition for near vision
B	dioptric distance to near point of accommodation, measured from the eye
D	dioptre
d	vertex distance
d or dec	decentration
F	power
F_c	power of a contact lens correction
F_e	equivalent power; power of the eye
F_{sp}	power of a spectacle lens correction
F_v, F'_v	front and back vertex power
K	ocular correction
K'	vergence of the retina or dioptric length of the eye
E, E'	centres of entrance and exit pupils
L, L'	object and image vergences
M or m	magnification
F, F'	first and second focal points
N, N'	first and second nodal points
P, P'	first and second principal points
RSM	relative spectacle magnification
SM	spectacle magnification
ε or P	refractive power of a prism
Δ	prism dioptre

value for viewing or photographing inaccessible objects, such as internal organs of the body. *Syn.* fibre optic (although strictly this term is an adjective, e.g. a fibre optic cable, whereas the term fibre optics is a noun).
See angle, critical; endoscope.
first-order o. *See* optics, paraxial.
gaussian o. *See* optics, paraxial.
geometrical o. Branch of optics that deals with the tracing of light rays through optical systems (Table O2).

See sign convention; theory, gaussian.
mechanical o. *See* optics, ophthalmic.
ophthalmic o. **1.** The branch of optics which deals with the design, measurement, assembly and fitting of lenses, spectacles, contact lenses, as well as optical aids for low vision patients. *Syn.* dispensing optics; mechanical optics. **2.** In the UK and the Republic of Ireland it was used as a synonym for optometry.
See dispensing, optical; optometry.
o. of the eye The eye considered as an optical system composed of several elements, the two aspherical surfaces of the cornea (total power about +42 D), the two aspherical surfaces of the lens (total power +21 D), the depth of the anterior chamber (a change of 1 mm in depth corresponds to a change of about 0.7 D in the total power of the eye) and the refractive indices of the various media (it is a gradient in the lens) and their role in the formation of a retinal image. The total power of the eye is about +60 D (Table O2). *Syn.* dioptric system of the eye.
See constants of the eye; Table P5, p. 271.
paraxial o. A simplified representation of geometrical optics which deals only with paraxial rays and in which the law of refraction and the fundamental paraxial equation are applicable. *Syn.* first-order optics; gaussian optics.
See law, Lagrange's; law of refraction; paraxial equation, fundamental; ray, paraxial.
physical o. Branch of optics that deals with the nature of light and with the phenomena of diffraction, interference, polarization and velocity of light.
See theory, quantum; theory, wave.
physiological o. The branch of optics concerned with physiological, psychological and optical aspects of visual perception.
visual o. Branch of optics and optometry which deals with the dioptric system of the eye and its correction.
See optics of the eye.

optogenetics The combination of optics (e.g. light stimulation) and genetics to target specific proteins or cells that are light-sensitive (e.g. photoreceptors) to express their effect to observe or control neuronal function or to be used in therapeutics. This is currently being tested in the treatment of retinitis pigmentosa and age-related macular degeneration.

optogram Trace left on the retina by a retinal image due to the bleaching of rhodopsin.

optokinetic Term referring to movements of the eyes in response to the movement of objects across the visual field. *Example*: optokinetic nystagmus.
See nystagmus, optokinetic; reflex, vestibulo-ocular.

optokinetic drum; nystagmus test *See* test, optokinetic nystagmus.

optokinetic reflex *See* reflex, vestibuloocular.

optokinetoscope *See* test, optokinetic nystagmus.

optometer Instrument for measuring the refractive state of the eye. There are two main types of optometers: subjective and objective. **Subjective** optometers rely upon the subject's judgment of sharpness or blurredness of a test object while **objective** ones contain an optical system which determines the vergence of light reflected from the subject's retina. Electronic optometers in which all data appear digitally within a brief period of time after the operator has activated a signal can be of either type. Optometers are based on various principles including Scheiner, Scheiner combined with vernier alignment, retinoscopy, Badal and fundus ray reflection. Some instruments referred to as **aberrometers** measure aberrations as well as refraction. Objective types (also called **autore-fractors** or **autorefractometers**) have become very popular, and several of these autorefractors are now providing both objective and subjective systems within the same instrument. Objective instruments may contain either an internal fixation target (closed-view) or an external target (open-view). *Syn.* refractometer.
See **accommodation, objective; autorefraction; optometer, infrared; photorefraction; refractive error.**

Badal's o. Simple subjective optometer consisting of a single positive lens and a movable target. The vergence of light from the target, after refraction through the lens, depends upon the position of the target. The patient is instructed to move the target towards the lens from a position where it appears blurred until it becomes clear. That point distance (converted in dioptric value) represents the refraction of the patient's eye. This is a crude and inaccurate instrument, in which the measurement is marred by accommodation, variation in retinal image size with target distance, large depth of focus, non-linearity of the scale, etc. Badal's improvement was to place the lens so that its focal point coincides with either the nodal point of the eye or the anterior focal point of the eye or the entrance pupil of the eye, thus overcoming the problems of the non-linear scale and the changing retinal image size (Fig. O3).

coincidence o. An optometer based on the vernier alignment principle. The target, usually three lines, is divided into two and the light from each half is passed into the eye through different parts of the pupil. The vergence of the light is adjusted until the two targets are aligned subjectively at which point the eye is focused correctly and a measure of ametropia is obtained.

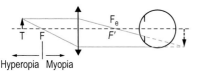

Fig. O3 Optical principle of the Badal optometer. (*F*, *F'*, first and second principal focus of the lens; *F*e, anterior focal point of the eye; T, target)

infrared o. Optometer that uses infrared light rather than visible light. This is done so that the target used in the optometer is invisible to the patient. Otherwise when it is altered, it tends to become a stimulus to accommodation. However, the instrument must be corrected for the chromatic aberration of the eye. Modern automated objective optometers use infrared light. They are based on one of several principles: (1) retinoscopy, (2) Scheiner's experiment, (3) a Badal lens system in which its focal point is conjugate with the anterior focal point of the eye and (4) Scheiner combined with ray reflection of two small regions of the pupil.
objective o.; subjective o. *See* **optometer.**
Young's o. Simple optometer consisting of a single positive lens and based on the Scheiner's disc principle. The target is either a single point of light or a thread, which is moved back and forth until it is seen singly by the observer. When the target is out of focus, it is seen double and slightly blurred.
See **experiment, Scheiner's.**

optometric physician *See* **optometrist.**

optometrist A person trained in the practice of optometry. The **World Council of Optometry** defines optometrists as 'the primary health care practitioners of the eye and visual system who provide comprehensive eye and vision care, which includes refraction and dispensing, the detection/diagnosis and management of diseases in the eye, and the rehabilitation of conditions of the visual system'. *Syn.* ophthalmic optician (term which was used principally in the UK and the Republic of Ireland); optician-optometrist (term used in some European countries); optometric physician (term used in some U.S. states, especially where therapeutic drugs are used).

optometry An autonomous healthcare profession involved in the services and care of the eye and visual system, and the enhancement of visual performance. *Syn.* ophthalmic optics (term which was used principally in the UK and the Republic of Ireland).
See **optometry, primary care.**
behavioural o. A branch of optometry concerned with the diagnosis and treatment of visual problems taking into account not only the ocular history, signs and symptoms but also the whole person and his or her environment.
experimental o. The branch of optometry concerned with the scientific investigation of optometric problems by experimentation upon humans or animals, or by clinical research.
See **psychophysics.**
geriatric o. A branch of optometry concerned with the prevention, diagnosis and treatment of visual problems in old age.
paediatric o. A branch of optometry concerned with the prevention, development, diagnosis and treatment of visual problems in children.
primary care o. Term referring to the basic field of optometry to which patients usually come directly and are not usually referred by

other professionals. Primary care optometric practitioners may refer some of their patients to other practitioners (secondary care) such as ophthalmologists, neurologists or to other optometric specialists for specialized services such as paediatric optometry, low vision aids or highly specialized aspects of contact lens fitting. The patient may have to be referred to a tertiary care practitioner as for example a retinal surgeon who depends on referrals from ophthalmologists or optometrists.

optophysiology The use of optical imaging techniques (e.g. optical coherence tomography) to study the function and processing of living tissue (e.g. retinal neurons).

optotype Test type used for measuring visual acuity. *See* **acuity, monotype visual; chart, Snellen; Jaeger test types; König bars; Landolt ring.**

ora serrata The serrated anterior boundary of the retina located some 8 mm from the limbus. At the ora serrata, the retina firmly adheres to the choroid, which is the reason why a retinal detachment ends here. *See* **ciliary body; retinal dialysis; stria.**

orange Hue corresponding to wavelengths between 590 and 630 nm. *See* **colour; light.**

orbicularis muscle *See* **muscle, orbicularis.**

orbicularis ciliaris *See* **ciliary body.**

orbit A rigid bony cavity in the skull which contains the eyeball, orbital fat, the extraocular muscles, the optic nerve, nerves and blood vessels, lacrimal system and fibrous tissue of various kinds. This packing serves to keep the eyeball reasonably well fixed in place as it rotates. The orbital cavity has the approximate form of a pyramid. The walls of the orbital cavity are formed by seven bones. The *medial* wall of the orbit consists of (1) the frontal process of the **maxilla (maxillary)**; (2) the **lacrimal bone**; (3) the lamina papyracea of the **ethmoid** and (4) a small part of the body of the **sphenoid**. The *floor* of the orbit consists of (1) the orbital plate of the maxilla; (2) the orbital surface of the **zygomatic (malar)** bone and (3) the orbital process of the **palatine** bone. The *lateral* wall of the orbit consists of (1) the orbital surface of the greater wing of the **sphenoid** and (2) the orbital surface of the **zygomatic**. The *roof* of the orbit is made up mainly by the **frontal** bone and behind this by the lesser wing of the **sphenoid**. The orbit is lined with a **periorbita**. The bones are much thicker at the margin (rim) than they are along the walls of the orbital cavity. There are many apertures and gaps in the orbit through which blood vessels and nerves pass (Tables O3 and O4). *See* **axis, orbital; canal, optic; fissure, inferior orbital; fissure, superior orbital; fracture, orbital; haemangioma, capillary; haemangioma, cavernous; lamina papyracea; periorbital; skull.**

orbital cellulitis *See* **cellulitis, orbital.**

orbital decompression A surgical technique used to decrease pressure within the orbit, usually performed in thyroid eye disease when there is progressive optic neuropathy or excessive proptosis. It commonly involves removal of one or two of the orbital walls (excluding the orbital roof).

orbital fat Fat (e.g. adipose tissue) which fills all the space not occupied by the other structures of the orbit (eyeball, optic nerve, muscles, vessels, etc.). It extends from the optic nerve to the orbital wall and from the apex of the orbit to the septum orbitale.

orbital fissure *See* **fissure, inferior orbital; fissure, superior orbital; syndrome, orbital fissure.**

orbital fracture A term relating to any break in the bony integrity of the orbital walls, most commonly occurring in the orbital floor or less frequently in the medial wall (called '**blow-out**' fracture). Although most frequently resulting from blunt trauma, it may also result as a necessary step in surgical treatment (e.g. orbital decompression). There is periorbital bruising, oedema, haemorrhage or enophthalmos. Diplopia and limited upward movement are present usually as a result of a muscle or its fascia being entrapped in the break. There may be concomitant intraocular injury if caused by trauma (e.g. tennis ball). Fractures in the orbital apex or roof are less common. The lateral wall of the orbit is very tough and more solid than the others and acts as a protective shield to the globe and it is only involved in very severe maxillofacial trauma.

orbital implant A biocompatible ball made up of hydroxyapatite, polyethylene or silicone placed in the orbit after enucleation or evisceration to maintain the volume of the eye socket. It is covered with Tenon's capsule and attached to the four recti muscles and covered anteriorly with stitched conjunctiva. Placed in front of the implant is a clear plastic scleral shell (called a **conformer**), which is replaced several weeks later by an artificial eye. *See* **eye, artificial; conformer.**

orbital inflammatory syndrome *See* **syndrome, orbital inflammatory.**

orbital margin *See* **orbit.**

orbital optic neuritis *See* **neuritis, optic.**

orbital prosthetist *See* **ocularist.**

Table O3 Bones forming the walls of the orbit	
Roof	**Medial wall**
1. frontal	1. maxilla
2. lesser wing of sphenoid	2. lacrimal
	3. ethmoid
	4. sphenoid
Floor	**Lateral wall**
1. maxilla	1. greater wing of sphenoid
2. zygomatic	2. zygomatic
3. palatine	

Table O4 Orbital apertures

Aperture	Location	Contents
optic canal	at the apex (in lesser sphenoid)	optic nerve ophthalmic artery sympathetic nerve fibres
superior orbital fissure	at the apex (gap between greater and lesser sphenoid)	III, IV, V, VI nerves sympathetic nerve fibres ophthalmic vein recurrent lacrimal artery
inferior orbital fissure	between lateral wall and posterior part of the floor	infraorbital nerve zygomatic nerve branch of inferior ophthalmic vein nerve fibres from the pterygopalatine (sphenopalatine) ganglion to orbital periosteum
ethmoidal foramina (anterior and post.)	medial wall (frontal/ethmoidal suture)	ethmoidal vessels ethmoidal nerve/external nasal nerve
zygomatic foramen	lateral wall	zygomatic nerve and vessels
nasolacrimal canal	medial wall (maxilla/lacrimal)	nasolacrimal duct

orbital septum A thin membrane containing collagenous and elastic fibres which is attached to the orbital margin at a thickening called the **arcus marginale**. It is continuous with the tarsal plates of the upper and lower eyelids except where it is pierced by the fibres of the levator aponeurosis of the levator palpebrae superioris muscle in the upper lid and the expansion from the inferior rectus in the lower lid. *Syn.* palpebral fascia; septum orbitale.
See **dermatochalasis; tarsus.**

orbital tubercle A small elevation on the orbital surface of the zygomatic bone, which serves as a point of attachment to the cheek ligament of the lateral rectus muscle, the ligament of Lockwood, the lateral palpebral ligament and aponeurosis of the levator palpebrae muscle.

orbitotomy A surgical incision made into the orbit to allow the removal of a tumour or foreign body, to treat a lesion or to drain an abscess.

ordinary ray *See* **birefringence.**

organ of sight; organ, visual *See* **eye.**

organic Pertaining to a disorder in which there is a lesion within the body.
See **functional.**

organic amblyopia *See* **amblyopia.**

orientation column *See* **column, cortical.**

orthokeratology Programmed application of contact lens fitting for the purpose of altering the curvature of the cornea, especially to reduce the eye's refractive power in myopia.
See **lens, ortho-k.**

orthophoria The case when the two visual axes are directed towards the point of binocular fixation in the absence of an adequate stimulus to fusion. It represents a perfect balance of the oculomotor system, and the active and passive positions coincide, unlike in heterophoria. *Syn.* phoria.

See **orthophorization; position, active; position, passive.**

orthophorization A process that is presumed to operate to produce a greater frequency of nearly orthophoric conditions (in distance vision) than would otherwise occur on the basis of chance. This process may also operate after prolonged occlusion of one eye or after the introduction of prisms in front of one eye or both eyes.
See **adaptation, vergence; emmetropization.**

orthopic fusion *See* **fusion, orthopic.**

orthoptics The study, diagnosis and nonoperative treatment of anomalies of binocular vision, strabismus and monocular functional amblyopia.
See **training, visual.**

orthoptist A person who practises orthoptics.

orthoscope A device by which water is held in contact with the cornea and thereby neutralizes the refractive power of the front surface of the cornea.

orthoscopic eyepiece *See* **eyepiece, orthoscopic.**

orthoscopic lens *See* **lens, orthoscopic.**

orthotropia 1. Absence of strabismus. 2. The term is sometimes used following successful surgery or prism compensation of a strabismus or when there is a vertical deviation with no deviation in the horizontal plane.

oscillation, saccadic *See* **flutter, ocular; myoclonus, ocular; opsoclonus.**

oscillopsia Vision in which objects appear to oscillate. It may be due to acquired nystagmus, loss of vestibular function, neurosis, multiple sclerosis, superior oblique myokymia, etc.
See **myokymia.**

osmosis A passive process of movement of water through a semipermeable membrane in response to a concentration gradient, from an area of low solute (e.g. glucose molecules) concentration (i.e. high water concentration) to one of high solute concentration (i.e. low water concentration). The process ends when the concentration on both sides of the membrane is equalized. It is one of the three mechanisms that create aqueous humour, the others being ultrafiltration and active transport. A semipermeable membrane is permeable to water but relatively impermeable to solutes. *See* **pressure, osmotic; solution, hypertonic.**

osmotic pressure *See* **pressure, osmotic.**

osteogenesis imperfecta *See* **keratoconus; sclera, blue.**

ostium lacrimale *See* **lacrimal apparatus.**

Ostwalt curve *See* **ellipse, Tscherning.**

Ota's naevus *See* **naevus of Ota.**

otitis media *See* **syndrome, Gradenigo's.**

outer segment *See* **cell, cone; cell, rod.**

outflow, aqueous *See* **pathway, uveoscleral.**

out of phase *See* **phase.**

overaction Term referring to the excessive action of an extraocular muscle as a consequence of palsy or limitation to the ipsilateral antagonist or the contralateral synergist. *See* **Table M5, p. 219.**

overcorrection A term applied to a corrective prescription of slightly higher power than required. It has occasionally been suggested as an attempt to slow the progression of myopia. *See* **myopia control.**

over-refraction Determination of a residual error of refraction of the eye while the patient is wearing spectacles or contact lenses.

overall size lens *See* **lens, aniseikonic.**

overcorrected spherical aberration *See* **aberration, spherical.**

overcorrection, postoperative *See* **strabismus, consecutive.**

overwear syndrome *See* **syndrome, overwear.**

oxidative stress A term used to describe the effect of oxidation in which an abnormal level of **reactive oxygen species (ROS)**, such as the free radicals (e.g. hydroxyl, nitric acid, superoxide) or the non-radicals (e.g. hydrogen peroxide, lipid peroxide) lead to damage (called **oxidative damage**) to specific molecules with consequential injury to cells or tissue. Increased production of ROS occurs as a result of fungal or viral infection, inflammation, ageing, UV radiation, pollution, excessive alcohol consumption, cigarette smoking, etc. Removal or neutralization of ROS is achieved with **antioxidants**, endogenous (e.g. catalase, glutathione reductase, peroxidase, superoxide dismutase) or exogenous (e.g. vitamins A, C, E, bioflavonoids, carotenoids). Oxidative damage to the eye, particularly the retina and the lens, is a contributing factor to age-related macular degeneration and cataract.

oxyblepsia *See* **oxyopia.**

oxybuprocaine hydrochloride A topical corneal anaesthetic, generally used in 0.4% solution. It may be used to perform tonometry, gonioscopy, to remove a foreign body, etc. *Syn.* benoxinate hydrochloride. When used for applanation tonometry, it is combined with 0.25% sodium fluorescein.

oxygen permeability The degree to which a polymer allows the passage of a gas or fluid. *Symbol*: Dk. Oxygen permeability (Dk) of a material is a function of the **diffusivity** (D) (that is, the speed at which oxygen molecules traverse the material) and the **solubility** (k) (or the amount of oxygen molecules absorbed, per volume, in the material). Values of oxygen permeability (Dk) in contact lenses typically fall within the range $10–150 \times 10^{-11}$ (cm^2/sec) $(ml\ O_2\ /\ ml \times mmHg)$. A semi-logarithmic relationship has been demonstrated between hydrogel water content and oxygen permeability. *Unit*: Barrer.

The International Organization for Standardization (ISO) has specified the permeability of contact lenses using the SI unit hectopascal (hPa) for pressure. Hence $Dk = 10^{-11}$ $(cm^2\ ml\ O_2)/(s\ ml\ hPa)$. The former unit can be converted to this new SI unit by multiplying it by the constant 0.75. The **ISO** has established a classification of contact lens materials based on a range of values of oxygen permeability Dk. Group 1: 1 to 15; group 2: 16 to 30; group 3: 31 to 60; group 4: 61 to 100; group 5: 101 to 150; group 6: 151 to 200; group 7: 201 to 250; higher codes can be added in bands of 50.
See **Barrer; oedema; oxygen pressure, equivalent; oxygen requirement, critical.**

oxygen pressure, equivalent (EOP) A percentage value of the assumed oxygen pressure existing behind a contact lens. The rate of corneal oxygen uptake behind a lens is compared to that following exposure to an environment of known oxygen content. The oxygen pressure in the air corresponds to about 20.9% (or about 159 mmHg; that value is actually close to 155 mmHg because of the presence of water vapour) and each percentage point is equal to a pressure of about 7.4 mmHg.

oxygen requirement, critical (COR) The minimum oxygen pressure at the epithelial surface required to prevent corneal swelling during the day. This value was initially assumed to be between 11 and 19 mmHg but it is nowadays considered to be at least 74 mmHg near the centre of the cornea (or 10% EOP or a Dk/L of about 25×10^{-9} $(cm^2\ /\ sec)$ $(ml\ O_2\ /\ ml \times mmHg)$ at 25°C for daily wear. This figure increases to at least 90×10^{-9} for overnight wear. *Syn.* critical oxygen tension. *See* **hypoxia.**

oxygen tension, critical *See* **oxygen requirement, critical.**

oxygen toxicity *See* **retinopathy of prematurity.**

oxygen transmissibility The degree to which oxygen may pass through a particular material of a given thickness. It is equal to the oxygen permeability divided by the thickness of the measured

sample under specific conditions. *Symbol*: *Dk/t*. *Unit*: Barrer/cm.
See **hypercapnia; oedema; oxygen permeability; syndrome, corneal exhaustion.**

oxyopia Extreme acuteness of vision. *Syn.* oxyblepsia.

oxyphenbutazone eye ointment A non-steroidal antiinflammatory agent usually used in 10% concentration for non-purulent inflammatory anterior eye conditions. It does not have the side effects of topical steroid therapy.

P

pachometer A device, mounted on a slit-lamp, that is used for measuring corneal thickness (or the depth of the anterior chamber). It consists of an optical system that provides two half-fields by means of two glass plates with parallel sides placed in front of one objective of the microscope, the other being occluded. These plates rest one on top of the other with the junction between them situated so as to horizontally bisect the objective. The top plate can be rotated while the bottom one is fixed. The observer viewing through the microscope sees two corneal optical sections and adjusts the top plate until the outer surface of the epithelium appears aligned with the inner surface of the endothelium (Fig. P1). The corneal thickness is then read directly from a scale attached to the pachometer and calibrated in millimetres. The measurement of the depth of the anterior chamber is made with a similar device but with a different scale. *Note*: also spelt pachymeter.
Pachometry can also be carried out using **slit-scanning topography** in which a computerized system integrates a series of slit-beam images to produce a map of the curvature and elevation of the anterior and posterior surfaces as well as corneal thickness. An instrument with greater magnification (called a **micropachometer**) has been devised, principally for research purposes, using a projection system which incorporates variable doubling plates and forms two slit images on the cornea in conjunction with the viewing system of a slit-lamp and a magnification of up to ×100, mounted on another arm. This instrument allows the measurement of the thickness of the corneal epithelium alone with a precision that can reach ±1 μm. The previously described pachometers are referred to as **optical pachometers** to differentiate them from **ultrasonic pachometers**, which use high-frequency ultrasound waves, reflected from the anterior and posterior corneal surfaces and a transducer probe placed against the cornea. Ultrasound and slit-scanning pachometers have higher reproducibility and less interobserver variation than subjective optical pachometers. Usage of pachometers (pachymeters) includes evaluation of contact lens wear, pre- and post-refractive surgery (e.g. PRK, LASEK, LASIK), glaucoma detection and monitoring corneal oedema.
See **ultrasonography**.

pad arm An extension of a spectacle frame either integral with the bridge or as a separate attachment to which a pad is fitted.

pad, nose One of a pair of protuberances attached to the bridge of a spectacle frame or mounting that rests against the side of the nose. *Syn.* nose pad.
See **bridge, pad; pince-nez; spectacle frame, metal.**

Paget's disease *See* **disease, Paget's.**

palinopsia Visual persistence of the image of an object noticed in the absence of its original stimulus. There is usually a latent period, which may amount to several minutes between the visual stimulation and the corresponding mental image. The latter typically disappears within seconds, although it may persist in some cases for several minutes. The subsequent mental image is quite faithful to the original stimulus. It is usually associated with a lesion in the parieto-occipital or temporal-occipital areas as a result of a cerebral infarction, epilepsy, tumour or brain injury. *Syn.* visual perseveration.

palisades of Vogt The crests of epithelium folds that run radially towards the cornea, at the limbus, from the bulbar conjunctiva. They are often seen

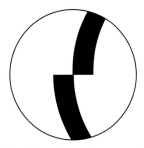

Fig. P1 View through a pachometer after having rotated the top corneal section to align its back with the front of the bottom section. At this point, the exact corneal thickness is read from the scale of the optical pachometer.

in slit-lamp examination, especially in pigmented individuals, and clearly in fluorescein angiography. They may contain stem cells, which play a role in the regeneration of corneal epithelium cells. *See* **corneal epithelium.**

palpebrae *See* **eyelids.**

palpebrae muscle, levator *See* **muscle, levator palpebrae.**

palpebral aperture; conjunctiva *See* under the nouns.

palpebral, elephantiasis *See* **elephantiasis oculi.**

palpebral fissure *See* **aperture, palpebral.**

palpebral furrow *See* **sulcus, inferior palpebral; sulcus, superior palpebral.**

palpebral ligament *See* **ligament, palpebral.**

palsy Synonym for paralysis, although it often implies both paralysis and paresis. *See* **paralysis; paresis.**

   abducens nerve p. *See* **palsy, sixth nerve; syndrome, Millard–Gubler.**

   Bell's p. A paralysis of the upper and lower muscles of the face on one side due to a facial nerve dysfunction. It is an idiopathic condition, although a viral link is a possibility. Symptoms usually begin suddenly and the condition ranges from mild weakness to total paralysis with an inability to close the eye on the affected side. It results in a wider palpebral aperture and drying of the cornea. Mild cases usually subside within about 2 or 3 weeks. Immediate management with corticosteroids may help reduce the severity of the disease. *See* **sign, Bell's; tears, artificial; tears, crocodile.**

   double elevator p. A condition characterized by limited or complete inhibition of the upward rotation of an eye, due either to paresis of its superior rectus and inferior oblique muscles or to entrapment of the inferior orbital tissues. It may be congenital or acquired (e.g. a lesion in the pretectum). Treatment is principally surgical.

   fourth nerve p. (trochlear) A condition characterized by a hypertropia of the eye with the affected superior oblique muscle. It may be congenital, although symptoms may not be present until adulthood or due to a lesion of the fourth cranial nerve or its nucleus as a result of injury (the most common cause), vascular lesions, aneurysm or tumour. The patient usually presents with an abnormal head posture to avoid diplopia. If the condition does not recover by itself following therapy of the underlying cause, surgery is usually the only alternative treatment. *Syn.* trochlear paralysis. *See* **head posture, abnormal; nerve, trochlear; strabismus, paralytic; test, Parks three-step.**

   gaze p. Inability of the eyes to make conjugate movements due to a lesion in the cortical or subcortical oculomotor centres. In **horizontal** gaze palsy, the two eyes are unable to move beyond the midline to the side of the lesion if the lesion is in the paramedian pontine reticular formation (horizontal gaze centre). In **vertical** gaze palsy, following lesions in the midbrain in the rostral mesencephalic reticular formation (vertical gaze centre) movements above and/or below the horizontal plane are limited. *See* **brainstem; movement, eye; ophthalmoplegia, internuclear; palsy, fourth nerve; palsy, sixth nerve; palsy, third nerve; palsy, supranuclear; syndrome. Parinaud's.**

   sixth nerve p. (abducens) A condition characterized by an esotropia of the eye with the affected lateral rectus muscle and limitation of abduction on the affected side. It may be due to a lesion of the sixth cranial nerve or its nucleus as a result of a vascular disease (e.g. diabetes, hypertension), injury, multiple sclerosis or tumour. The patient presents with an abnormal head turn to avoid diplopia. If the condition does not recover by itself following therapy with temporary occlusion and prismatic correction and frequently botulinum toxin injection into the ipsilateral medial rectus, surgery may be needed (Fig. P2). *Syn.* abducens paralysis; lateral rectus palsy. *See* **brainstem; head posture, abnormal; nerve, abducens; strabismus, paralytic; syndrome, Foville's; syndrome, Gradenigo's; syndrome, Millard-Gubler; transposition.**

   oculomotor p. *See* **palsy, third nerve.**

   progressive supranuclear p. A progressive neurodegenerative disease caused by a gradual deterioration of neurons in the brainstem and basal ganglia. It is characterized by ocular, motor (e.g. loss of balance and falls) and mental (e.g. cognitive dysfunction) features. Its onset is in the sixth decade of life, and ocular manifestations include an inability to move the eyes, especially downward and subsequently upward and to converge, as well blinking impediment. *Syn.* Steele–Richardson–Olszewski syndrome.

   supranuclear gaze p. Disturbance of the conjugate movements of the eye. Horizontal eye movements are generated in the paramedian pontine reticular formation (PPRF) from where fibres connect to the abducens and oculomotor nuclei. A PPRF lesion results in **horizontal gaze palsy**. In bilateral lesion, the patient is unable to turn the eyes voluntarily beyond the midline in the direction of the lesion but is able to maintain fixation and perform pursuit movements although unable to converge. If the lesion is in the midbrain, it produces Parinaud's syndrome, while a lesion in the medial longitudinal fasciculus produces internuclear ophthalmoplegia. *Syn.* Steele-Richardson-Olszewski syndrome. *See* **brainstem; ophthalmoplegia, internuclear; palsy, gaze; syndrome, one and a half; syndrome, Parinaud's.**

   third nerve p. (oculomotor) A condition that leads to a wide impairment of motor function, as this nerve innervates most of the muscles of the eye. It may be due to a vascular disease (e.g. diabetes, hypertension), aneurysm (especially of the internal carotid artery), injury or tumour. In total paralysis, only the lateral rectus and the superior

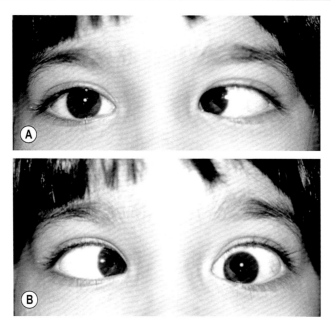

Fig. P2 Sixth nerve palsy in a child. A, left esotropia in the primary position. B, marked limitation of left abduction. (From Bowling 2016, with permission of Elsevier)

oblique muscles will be spared and the eye will be in a position of abduction, slight depression and intorsion. Ptosis will also be present and the pupil will be dilated and non-reactive, and there will also be paralysis of accommodation and diplopia. If the condition does not recover by itself following therapy of the underlying cause, surgery is usually the only alternative. *Syn.* oculomotor paralysis. *See* **brainstem; circle of Willis; nerve, oculomotor; ophthalmoplegia; strabismus, paralytic; syndrome, Benedikt's; syndrome, Weber's; test, forced duction; transposition.**
trochlear p. See **palsy, fourth nerve.**

pannus Abnormal superficial vascularization of the cornea covering the upper half or sometimes the entire cornea. It is characterized by a thick plexus of vessels. It is found in some cases of contact lens wear, mainly soft lenses. Pannus following contact lens wear is referred to as **corneal vascularization**. If induced by soft lenses, it can be reduced by changing to lenses of high oxygen transmissibility or ceasing contact lens wear. Deep corneal vascularization involving the stroma is usually the result of a disease process (e.g. interstitial keratitis, phlyctenular keratitis, severe long-standing trichiasis, trachoma).

panophthalmitis Acute inflammation of the eyeball involving all its structures and extending into the orbit. The disease develops very rapidly. The eyelids are red and swollen and there is severe chemosis of the conjunctiva. The cornea is often a whitish mass of necrotic tissue and there may be severe ocular pain.
See **endophthalmitis.**

pantoscopic angle *See* angle, pantoscopic.

Panum's area; fusional space *See* under the nouns.

panuveitis *See* uveitis.

papilla Any small elevation shaped like a nipple with a vascular core. They appear in various forms of conjunctivitis such as bacterial, allergic, giant papillary conjunctivitis and floppy eyelid syndrome. *Plural*: papillae.
See **follicle, conjunctival.**
Bergmeister's p. A cone-shaped sheath of glial cells (astrocytes) and connective tissue covering the hyaloid artery formed during embryonic development over the optic disc and projecting into the vitreous humour. It usually atrophies before term but, in some individuals, it persists and a proliferation of glial cells forms a **glial veil**. It may obscure the full view, or usually only part, of the optic disc and may sometimes suggest a disc tumour but it is in fact benign, stable and does not interfere with vision.
See **hyaloid remnant.**
lacrimal p. See lacrimal papilla.
p. lacrimalis See lacrimal tubercle.
optic p. See disc, optic.

papillary conjunctivitis, giant *See* conjunctivitis, giant papillary.

papillitis *See* neuritis, optic; pseudopapilloedema.

papilloedema A non-inflammatory oedema of the optic nerve head produced by intracranial hypertension, which may be caused by a cerebral tumour, subarachnoid haemorrhage, head injury or is idiopathic. The optic disc appears raised above

Table P1   Differential diagnosis between papilloedema and papillitis

	Papilloedema	Papillitis
Signs		
disc elevation	raised	slightly raised
disc hyperaemia	present	present
disc margins	blurred	blurred
retinal veins	congested	congested
haemorrhages	near disc	some in late stage
pupil light reflex	normal	impaired
venous pulsation	absent	present
secondary optic atrophy	present in late stage	may appear in late stage
Symptoms		
visual acuity	normal, except in late stage	reduced
visual field	enlarged blind spot	central scotoma
diplopia	present	absent
colour vision	normal	impaired
pain	absent	present on moving the eyes
headache	present	absent

the level of the retina and its margins are blurred, the central vessels on the surface of the disc are displaced forward, the retinal veins are dilated and there is nearly always a loss of induced venous pulsation. The swollen disc displaces the retina and this causes an enlargement of the blind spot on visual field measurement. In the early stages, visual acuity is not affected (unlike in papillitis), although if the condition persists there will be some loss. In advanced stages, there may be haemorrhages around the disc, secondary optic atrophy, exudates, as well as headaches and vomiting. The condition is usually bilateral. Urgent neuroimaging (e.g. MRI) is advised and treatment depends on the underlying cause. *Note*: also spelt papilledema (Table P1). *Syn.* choked disc. *See* **atrophy, optic; neuritis, optic; pseudopapilloedema; syndrome, Foster Kennedy; venous pulsation.**

papilloma A tumour most commonly found on the conjunctiva, the limbus or the lid margins. It is usually benign. It should be excised, but it is likely to recur.

papillomacular bundle; fibres *See* **fibre, papillomacular.**

paracontrast *See* **metacontrast.**

paradoxical ARC *See* **retinal correspondence, abnormal.**

paradoxical diplopia *See* **diplopia, incongruous.**

paraffin *See* **tears, artificial.**

parallax Apparent displacement of an object viewed from two different points not on a straight line with the object.
  binocular p. The difference in angle subtended at each eye by an object that is viewed first with one eye and then with the other.
  chromatic p. Apparent lateral displacement of two monochromatic sources (e.g. a blue object and a red object) when observed through a disc

with a pinhole placed near the edge of the pupil. When the pupil is centred on the achromatic axis (in some people, the pinhole may have to be placed away from the centre of the pupil), the two images appear superimposed. The relative displacement of the two images becomes reversed when the pinhole is on the other side of that axis. This phenomenon is attributed to the chromatic aberration of the eye. *See* **chromstereopsis; aberration, longitudinal chromatic.**
  monocular p. Apparent change in the relative position of an object noticed when the eye is moved from one position to another.
  motion p. Apparent difference in the direction of movement or speed produced when the subject moves relative to his or her environment (Fig. P3).

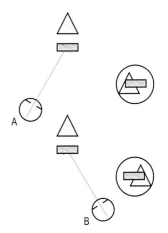

Fig. P3 An example of motion parallax. As the eye moves from A to B, the more distant object (triangle) appears to move in the same direction while the near object (rectangle) appears to move in the opposite direction, as shown in the circles on the right.

Example: When viewing the landscape through the window of a moving train, near objects appear to move much more quickly than distant objects. *See* perception, depth; stereopsis.

relative binocular p. *See* acuity, stereoscopic visual.

paralysis Loss of action of a muscle caused by injury or disease of that muscle or its nerve supply. *See* palsy; paresis.

p. of accommodation *See* accommodation, paralysis of.

p. of convergence A condition characterized by an inability of the eyes to converge while all other monocular eye movements are unaffected. The patient notices diplopia in near vision, which usually occurs suddenly. It is presumably due to some lesion in the nuclei responsible for convergence, as may happen in tabes dorsalis or Parkinson's disease.

divergence p. A condition characterized by an inability of the eyes to diverge while all other monocular eye movements are unaffected. It is characterized by a sudden development of diplopia with marked esotropia at distance and sometimes headaches. The key difference with divergence insufficiency is the sudden onset of symptoms. Its association includes encephalitis, multiple sclerosis, head trauma, cerebral haemorrhage, brain tumour and vascular lesions of the brainstem.

p. of the fourth nerve *See* palsy, fourth nerve.

p. of the sixth nerve *See* palsy, sixth nerve.

p. of the third nerve *See* palsy, third nerve.

paralytic ectropion *See* ectropion.

paraoptometric Individual trained to assist an optometrist in various functions (e.g. autorefractometry, contact lens instruction, frame fitting). Certificate programs have been established to train paraoptometric personnel.

parastriate area *See* area, visual association.

parasympathetic nervous system *See* system, autonomic nervous.

parasympatholytic Pertains to a drug that blocks the effects of acetylcholine at muscarinic receptors. *Examples*: atropine, homatropine, cyclopentolate and tropicamide. *Syn.* antimuscarinic, anticholinergic, atropine-like. *See* acetylcholine; cycloplegia; mydriatic.

parasympathomimetic drug A drug with an action resembling that caused by the effects of acetylcholine. *Example*: a miotic of which there are two types: a direct-acting cholinergic, such as pilocarpine or carbachol, and the other, indirect-acting anticholinesterase, such as physostigmine, neostigmine, echothiophate iodide or demecarium bromide. *Syn.* cholinergic drug. *See* acetylcholine; miotics.

paraxial Pertains to light rays situated near enough to the axis of an optical system for the gaussian theory to apply. *See* theory, gaussian.

paraxial approximation *See* ray, paraxial.

paraxial equation, fundamental Equation based on gaussian theory and dealing with refraction at a spherical surface:

$$\frac{n'}{l'} - \frac{n}{l} = \frac{n'-n}{r} \text{ (or) } L' - L = \frac{n'-n}{r}$$

where n and n' are the refractive indices of the media on each side of the spherical surface, r is the radius of curvature of the surface and l and l' the distances of the object and the image from the surface, respectively. n/l and n'/l' are the **vergences** (or **reduced vergences**) of the incident and refracted light rays respectively. $L'-L$ corresponds to the change produced by the surface in the vergence of the light and is called the **focal power** or **vergence power**, or **refractive power** F of the surface. Thus

$$L' - L = F$$

Focal power is usually expressed in dioptres and can be either positive or negative.

At a **reflecting** surface or a **mirror,** the equation becomes

$$L' - L = 2/r$$

where r is the radius of curvature of the surface or mirror. *Syn.* general refraction formula. *See* distance, image; distance, object; sign convention; theory, gaussian; vergence.

paraxial optics; ray *See* under the nouns.

paraxial region The hypothetical cylindrical narrow space surrounding the optical axis within which rays of light are still considered paraxial. *Syn.* gaussian space. *See* ray, paraxial; theory, gaussian.

paraxial theory *See* theory, gaussian.

paresis Slight or partial paralysis. *See* palsy; paralysis.

parietal cortex *See* area, visual association.

Parinaud's oculoglandular syndrome *See* syndrome, Parinaud's oculoglandular.

Parinaud's syndrome *See* syndrome, Parinaud's.

Parks' three-step test *See* test, Parks' three-step.

pars An anatomical part.

pars ciliaris muscle *See* muscle of Riolan.

pars plana; plicata *See* ciliary body.

pars planitis *See* uveitis, intermediate.

partial sight *See* vision, low.

parvo cells *See* cell, ganglion; geniculate body, lateral.

parvocellular layer *See* geniculate body, lateral.

parvocellular visual system *See* system, parvocellular visual.

past-pointing *See* pointing, past-.

Patau's syndrome *See* syndrome, Patau's.

patching The act of occluding or protecting the eye (e.g. after eye surgery).
See amblyopia; occlusion treatment.

patellar fossa *See* fossa, patellar.

pathological myopia *See* myopia, pathological.

pathology, ocular The discipline which deals with the nature of diseases of the eye and its surrounding structures, their effect on the ocular tissues and on ocular functions, as well as the causes and management.

pathway 1. A course made up of nerve fibres (axons) along which nervous impulses travel. 2. A path or a route.

centrifugal p. Pathway in which impulses travel from the visual cortex to the lateral geniculate bodies and onward to the retina and from ganglion cells to the photoreceptors. It is not known what function this feedback pathway has. It also refers to the pathway from the visual cortex to the extraocular muscles.
See pathway, centripetal.

centripetal p. Pathway in which impulses travel from the photoreceptors to the bipolar cells, ganglion cells, lateral geniculate bodies and visual cortex.
See pathway, centrifugal.

geniculocalcarine p. *See* radiations, optic; tract, geniculocalcarine.

geniculostriate p. 1. *See* radiations, optic. 2. Some authors consider this term to be a synonym of visual pathway.

magnocellular p. *See* system, magnocellular visual.

motor p. Pathway from the cortex to the muscles that control the movements of the eyes enabling them to act as a unit.

parvocellular p. *See* system, parvocellular visual.

retinocortical p. *See* pathway, visual.

retinohypothalamic p. Neural pathway consisting of the axons of the photosensitive retinal ganglion cells which leave the main visual pathway from the upper (dorsal) surface of the optic chiasma. They then enter several nuclei of the hypothalamus, such as the suprachiasmatic and paraventricular nuclei.
See cell, photosensitive retinal ganglion; nucleus, suprachiasmatic.

retinotectal p. 1. The nervous pathway that connects the retina to the pretectal region (anterior to the superior colliculi) and from there to the Edinger–Westphal nucleus. It is involved in the pupillary light reflexes. 2. The nervous pathway between the retina and the superior colliculus. It is involved in the involuntary blink reflex to a dazzling light and in the eye movements occurring in response to the sudden appearance of a novel or a threatening stimulus.
See blind sight; fibre, pupillary; reflex, pupil light; pretectum.

uveoscleral p. Unconventional route through which the aqueous humour drains out of the eye. The aqueous passes from the anterior chamber across the iris root through small spaces between the ciliary muscle fibres into the supraciliary space and suprachoroid space. The fluid is believed to escape the eye via veins in the ciliary muscle and anterior choroid. The amount of aqueous outflow through this route amounts to between 10% and 15%, the rest flows out through the conventional pathway via the trabecular meshwork and into Schlemm's canal. Prostaglandin drugs reduce the intraocular pressure by increasing the outflow through the uveoscleral pathway. This pathway is occasionally made use of in cyclodialysis.

visual p. Neural path starting in the photoreceptors of the retina and travelling through the following structures: the optic nerve, the optic chiasma, the optic tract, the lateral geniculate body, the optic radiations and the visual cortex where the pathway ends. The fibres of the optic nerve of one eye meet with the fibres from the other eye at the optic chiasma, where approximately half of them (the nasal half of the retina) cross over to the other side. Thus, there is semidecussation in the visual pathway. *Syn.* retinocortical pathway (Fig. P4 and Table P2).
See area, visual; decussation; magnification, cortical; retinotopic map.

patient Term originating from the Latin *patior* meaning to suffer; one who suffers or is ill and requires treatment.

pattern A combination of acts or parts, forming a consistent or characteristic arrangement or behaviour.
A p. *See* pattern, alphabet.

alphabet p. Anomalies of binocular vision in which there is a marked difference in the angle of deviation when upward gaze is compared to downward or straight-ahead gaze. There are several patterns: A, V, X, Y, λ. The most common is V pattern. In **A pattern (A syndrome)**, there is an increase in convergence on upgaze and an increase in divergence on downgaze. In **V pattern (V syndrome)**, there is an increase in divergence on upgaze and an increase in convergence on downgaze. (The difference between up- and downgaze must be at least 10Δ.) In **X pattern,** there is an increase in divergence in both up- and downgaze. In **Y pattern,** there is an increase in divergence on upgaze and no significant difference between the primary position and downgaze. In **λ pattern,** there is no significant difference between the primary position and upgaze and an increase in divergence on downgaze. These patterns are common in patients with strabismus and much less frequent in patients with heterophoria. They are caused by either overaction or underaction of some extraocular muscles, especially the oblique muscles, as a result of innervational dysfunction or abnormal insertions or trauma or part of a syndrome (e.g. Brown's syndrome). Management may be necessary if there are symptoms and may include prisms, visual training or extraocular muscle surgery.
See incomitance.

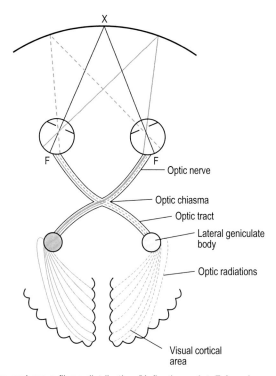

Fig. P4 Visual pathway and nerve fibres distribution (X, fixation point; F, fovea).

---

checkerboard p. A square set of equal size black and white squares placed adjacent to one another. It is used to test visual acuity and as a stimulus in pattern ERG and visual evoked potentials. The common way of using this pattern in acuity testing is to present it in the form of a square diamond made up of four smaller diamonds. Three of these are composed of a pattern of much smaller squares than the fourth. Resolution of the pattern with larger squares consists in indicating where it is located (top, bottom, right or left) while the other three squares appear as a uniform grey. This acuity test is less dependent on cognitive factors than letters (Fig. P5).
See **acuity, visual; alternating checkerboard stimulus; test type.**
V p. *See* **pattern, alphabet.**
X p. *See* **pattern, alphabet.**
Y p. *See* **pattern, alphabet.**

paving-stone degeneration *See* **degeneration, paving-stone.**

P cell *See* **cell, ganglion; cell, P.**

PD Abbreviation for interpupillary distance and also, but more rarely, for prism dioptre.

PD gauge; meter *See* **pupillometer.**

PD rule *See* **rule, PD.**

pearls, Elschnig's *See* **Elschnig's pearls.**

pedicle, cone *See* **cone pedicle.**

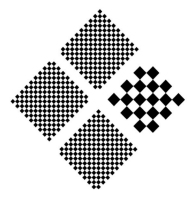

Fig. P5 Checkerboard pattern.

pedigree A chart or diagram of the ancestral history of a family or of an extended family (**kindred**), or of individual family members, their relationships and their status regarding a trait or condition. It is used in genetics to analyze inheritance. The analysis often begins with an affected family member (called a **proband** or **propositus**) through whom the family is ascertained (Fig. P6).
See **gene; inheritance.**

pegaptanib sodium *See* **anti-VEGF drugs.**

Pelli–Robson chart *See* **chart, Pelli–Robson.**

Table P2 Clinical manifestations of lesions in the visual pathway

Site of lesion	Clinical manifestations
macula	central scotoma
papillomacular bundle	central or centrocaecal scotoma
other part of the retina	scotoma on the opposite side of the central fixation point
complete section of one optic nerve	total blindness of that eye
	absence of direct light reflex
	presence of consensual light reflex
	other eye: normal pupil reaction, direct but not consensual
pituitary enlargement pressing on inferior part of chiasma	bitemporal hemianopia or bitemporal superior quadrantanopia
aneurysm pressing on lateral part of the chiasma	binasal hemianopia
sagittal section in the middle of the chiasma	bitemporal hemianopia normal pupil reflexes if light falls on temporal retina
optic tract	contralateral incongruous homonymous hemianopia Wernicke's pupillary reflex
lateral geniculate body	contralateral incongruous homonymous hemianopia normal pupil reflexes
anterior optic radiations on one side	contralateral incongruous homonymous hemianopia often sparing of the macula normal pupil reflexes
visual cortex on one side	contralateral congruous homonymous hemianopia often sparing of the macula normal pupil reflexes

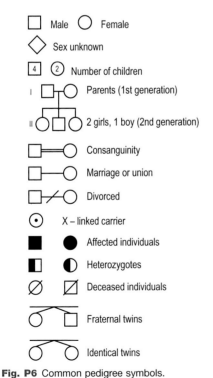

Fig. P6 Common pedigree symbols.

pellucid Allowing maximum passage of light.

pellucid marginal corneal degeneration *See* degeneration, pellucid marginal corneal.

pelopsia Anomaly of visual perception in which objects appear to be much nearer than they actually are. It may be due to vision in a very clear atmosphere, recent wear of an optical correction, neurosis, etc.
See **metamorphopsia**.

pemirolast potassium *See* **mast cell stabilizers**.

pemphigoid, cicatricial A rare autoimmune systemic disease found most commonly in the elderly and characterized by recurrent blisters and bullae of the skin and mucous membranes, with subsequent scarring and shrinkage. It is believed to be a type 2 hypersensitivity with deposition of immunoglobin and complement at the basement membrane of mucosal surfaces leading to a loss of adhesion and bullae formation eventually resulting in cicarization. The disease may affect only the conjunctiva (**ocular pemphigoid**). In this case, the clinical picture is conjunctivitis with hyperaemia, mucous discharge and small vesicles which, upon bursting, result in ulceration, pseudomembranes, conjunctival subepithelial fibrosis and conjunctival shrinkage. The disease may give rise to adhesion between the palpebral and bulbar conjunctiva (symblepharon), ankyloblepharon, xerophthalmia, keratoconjunctivitis sicca, entropion, trichiasis

and dry eye with corneal ulcer. There is pain or irritation and blurred vision. Management includes systemic and local treatments with artificial tears, corticosteroids, surgery for entropion and trichiasis, and keratoprosthesis if vision is affected. *Syn.* ocular mucous membrane pemphigoid.
See **conjunctivitis, pseudomembranous; hypersensitivity; syndrome, Stevens–Johnson; test, ocular ferning.**

pemphigoid, ocular *See* **pemphigoid, cicatricial.**

penalization A clinical method of treating amblyopia and eccentric fixation in which vision by the fixating eye is decreased by various means (optical overcorrection, atropinization for near vision especially, and neutral density filters) to compel the amblyopic eye to fixate. Sometimes the treatment consists of using the amblyopic eye for near vision and the fixating eye for distance vision.
See **attenuation; Bangerter foils; occlusion treatment; pleoptics.**

pencil of light *See* **light, pencil of.**

pencil push-up *See* **convergence insufficiency.**

pencil-to-nose   exercise *See* **convergence insufficiency.**

penetrance The frequency with which the characteristics transmitted by a gene appear in individuals possessing it. Penetrance is represented as the ratio of individuals who carry the gene and express its effects, over the total number of carriers of the gene in a population. Few of the genes in the genome have a high penetrance because environmental factors play a role in development. There is incomplete penetrance when some individuals with the gene show very mild or no manifestation of the disease or trait. *Examples*: Familial exudative vitreoretinopathy and neurofibromatosis (type 1 and type 2), which are both inherited as autosomal dominant, have 100% penetrance; about 90% of the children who carry the retinoblastoma gene develop the disease while the gene remains non-penetrant in the remaining 10% of the children.
See **expressivity; vitreoretinopathy, familial exudative.**

penetrating keratoplasty *See* **keratoplasty.**

pendular nystagmus *See* **nystagmus.**

penicillin *See* **antibiotic.**

penumbra 1. Region of low illumination on a dark background. 2. An area surrounding the region of complete darkness or shadow (called **umbra**) in which the brightness varies from about zero at the edge of the umbra to illumination beyond the outer edge of the penumbra. It is caused by an opaque object intercepting light from an extended light source. When the source is smaller than the object, the umbra is large and the penumbra small. When the source is larger than the object, the umbra disappears at a certain distance from the object and the shadow is completely penumbral (Fig. P7). *Example*: When the moon passes

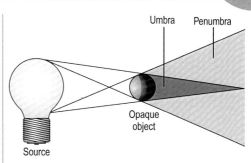

Fig. P7 Umbra and penumbra caused by a source larger than the opaque object. If a screen is placed away from the opaque object, a large circular patch of penumbra will be noticed, but if it is placed near the opaque object, one will notice a central dark patch (the umbra) surrounded by a light grey patch (the penumbra).

between the sun and the Earth, and because the Earth is situated near the point where the umbra disappears, people in a part of the Earth can see a total eclipse whereas others in the penumbra see a partial eclipse.

Pepper test *See* **test, Pepper.**

percept The complete mental image of an object obtained in response to sensory stimuli.

perception The mental process of recognizing and interpreting an object through one or more of the senses stimulated by a physical object. Thus one recognizes the shape, colour, location and differentiation of an object from its background.
See **sensation; integration, visual.**
anorthoscopic p. See **anorthoscope.**
binocular   p. Perception obtained through simultaneous use of both eyes.
contour p. See **contour.**
depth p. Perception of the distance of an object from the observer (**absolute distance**) or of the distance between two objects (**relative distance**). Our ability to judge the latter is much more precise than for the former. Many factors contribute to depth perception. Most important is the existence on the two retinae of different images of the same object (called **binocular disparity** or **retinal disparity**). There are also many other contributing factors, such as the characteristics of the stimulus (called cues), binocular parallax and, to a smaller extent, the muscular proprioceptive information due to the efforts of accommodation and convergence. Depth perception is more precise in binocular vision but is possible in monocular vision using the following **cues**: interposition (superposition), relative position, relative size, linear perspective, textural gradient, aerial perspective, light and shade, shadow and motion parallax (Fig. P8). Syn. spatial vision.
See **acuity, stereoscopic visual; cell, binocular; cliff, visual; disparity, retinal; illusion, moon; perspective, aerial; perspective, linear; relief; room, Ames; room, leaf; stereo-blindness; stereopsis.**

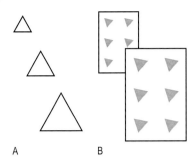

A   B

Fig. P8 Examples of monocular cues to depth perception: A, relative size; B, interposition and relative size.

dermo-optical p. *See* perception, extrasensory.

extrasensory p. Perception obtained by means other than through the ordinary senses as, for example, telepathy (mind reading) or reading by moving a finger over a printed text (dermo-optical perception).

light p. Term used to indicate a barely seeing eye that can just see light but not the form of objects. Loss of light perception represents blindness.

subliminal p. Stimuli below the threshold of sensation (i.e. subliminal) may, in rare circumstances (e.g. exposure of 40-ms duration masked by another stimulus), unconsciously arouse perception. The effect is then of extremely short duration (less than 200 ms).

visual p. Perception obtained through the sense of vision.

perceptual learning The practice of acquiring a facility with certain visual tasks in an attempt to improve visual performance. It can be used in amblyopes to better recognize certain feature of a visual stimulus.

perceptual span *See* reading.

Percival criterion *See* criterion, Percival.

peribulbar block *See* injection, peribulbar.

perichoroidal space *See* space, suprachoroidal.

pericorneal plexus *See* plexus, pericorneal.

perimeter An instrument for measuring the angular extent and the characteristics (e.g. presence of scotoma) of the visual field.
See campimeter; field, visual; isopter; screen, tangent.

arc p. Perimeter consisting of a semicircular arc, the inside surface of which is painted matt black or grey. The patient's head is placed such that the eye under investigation is located at the centre of curvature of the arc. The visual field is determined by moving a target along the black surface of the perimeter until the patient either just sees it or just no longer sees it. The targets are small discs of varying colour and size attached to the end of black wands or may be projected on the arc, which can be rotated around the fixation point located at its centre. Thus the visual field can be tested along any meridian.

automated p. An instrument to test the visual field in which the presentation of the stimuli and the recording are carried out electronically and under the control of a built-in computer. There exist many commercial types. Computerized perimeters have the following advantages: the examination strategy is reproducible; they can be operated by non-specialists; the testing routine (e.g. number of stimuli or their location) can be altered by modifying the program; each instrument can contain several examination routines aimed at testing various pathologies (e.g. one for glaucoma and another for hemianopic defects) or the computer capacity can be used for quantifying the results in which the visual fields can be classified as normal, suspect or defective on the basis of a software included in the instrument (Fig. P9). *Syn.* computerized perimetry.
See **Algorithm, Swedish Interactive Thresholding; perimetry, frequency doubling; perimetry, short wavelength automated; test, Esterman.**

bowl p. *See* perimeter, Goldmann.

Goldmann p. Perimeter consisting of a hemispherical bowl, the inside radius of which is 30 cm. Targets of varying intensity and size are projected onto the inside white surface. The background luminance of the bowl is also controlled. In addition, there is a telescope attached to the back of the bowl through which the practitioner can verify that the patient maintains fixation. Goldmann perimeter can be used either for kinetic or static perimetry, although it is more appropriately designed for the former. *Syn.* bowl perimeter.
See **perimetry, kinetic; perimetry, static.**

projection p. A perimeter in which the target is projected either onto an arc or a bowl such as the Goldmann perimeter.

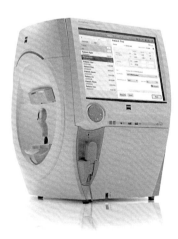

Fig. P9 Humphrey Field Analyzer HFA3. (Courtesy of ZEISS Medical Technology)

perimetry The determination of the extent of the visual field, usually for the purpose of detecting anomalies in the visual pathway.
See **glaucoma; lens rim artifact; perimeter.**

frequency doubling p. A method of testing the visual field based on the frequency doubling illusion and thus assessing the functional integrity of the large-diameter retinal ganglion M cells, which are very susceptible to early glaucomatous damage. It is usually a computerized perimeter in which the stimulus display consists of a low spatial frequency (0.25 c/deg) sinusoidal grating which flickers in a counterphase fashion (i.e. light bars become dark and vice versa) at a rate of 25 Hz. The grating is presented in many locations throughout the visual field, and the patient's task is to detect it.
See **glaucoma, open-angle; illusion, frequency doubling.**

kinetic p. Measurement of the visual field with a moving target of fixed luminance.

short wavelength automated p. A valuable procedure used for detecting and monitoring visual defects in patients with ocular hypertension and patients with early glaucomatous visual field losses. It uses a blue stimulus on a yellow background, as may be arranged in an automated perimeter. It is a more sensitive and efficient method of detecting and monitoring early visual field losses than standard white-on-white automated perimetry (white stimulus on a white background).
See **glaucoma, open-angle.**

static p. Measurement of the visual field with a target that can be varied in dimension and luminance. The target can be presented in any part of the visual field.

period, critical A time after birth during which neural connections can still be modified by interference with normal visual experience or lesion of the visual pathway. If a person has an anomaly (e.g. amblyopia), the treatment is most likely to be effective during the earliest part of the critical period. In man, it lasts up to about 7 to 8 years of age. If neural connections are impaired permanently during this period, it will usually be impossible to repair later, and the younger the child, the more damaging it is. *Example*: Binocularly sensitive cortical cells (stimulated by normal binocular vision) may never develop in uncorrected strabismus, or prolonged occlusion occurring during the critical period, especially before the age of 3 years, and therefore the patient will not have binocular vision. *Syn.* plastic period. (however, this term relates more specifically to the time course during which the visual system is still responsive to treatment; this may differ from the critical period of development); sensitive period.
See **myopia, form-deprivation; occlusion treatment.**

periocular Situated around the eye.

perioptometry The measurement of the extent of the visual field or of peripheral visual acuity.

periorbita A membrane of tough connective tissue which extends to the **orbital margin** (anterior rim of the orbit) where it becomes continuous with the periosteum covering the facial bones. The periorbita is also continuous with the dura mater surrounding the optic nerve at the optic foramen. It is loosely attached to the bones except at sutures, foramina and the orbital margin where it is firmly attached. *Syn.* orbital periosteum.
See **orbit.**

peripapillary Pertains to the area surrounding the optic nerve head.
See **atrophy, peripapillary.**

peripheral clearance *See* **edge lift.**

peripheral fundus examination *See* **ophthalmoscopy, indirect.**

peripheral vision; visual acuity *See* under the nouns.

peripheral zone *See* **optic zone diameter.**

periphoria *See* **cyclophoria.**

periscope An optical instrument using two right angle reflectors to allow observation of an object from behind a shield or around an obstruction where direct vision is impossible. It has many applications, especially in the military forces (e.g. in tanks, submarines).
See **lens, periscopic.**

peristriate area *See* **area, visual association.**

Perkins tonometer *See* **tonometer, applanation.**

Perlia's nucleus *See* **nucleus, Perlia's.**

persistence of vision *See* **after-image.**

persistent hyaloid artery *See* **hyaloid remnant.**

persistent hyperplastic primary vitreous *See* **vitreous, persistent hyperplastic primary.**

persistent pupillary membrane *See* **membrane, pupillary.**

perspective One of the cues to perception of the third dimension induced by a graphic representation on a plane, as in a drawing, or as a monocular cue, such as aerial perspective or linear perspective (Fig. P10).
See **perception, depth.**

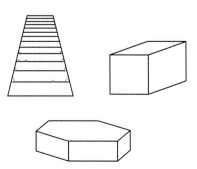

Fig. P10 Examples of perspective drawings.

aerial p. Perspective influenced by the state of clarity of the atmosphere. Far away objects appear less distinct and desaturated in colour due to the diffusion of light by the air in between the object and the eye. However, a very pure atmosphere may lead to underestimation of the distance of objects as they retain their distinctness and colour in this case. Aerial perspective is used by artists who soften and blur the colour and outlines of objects that they wish to appear as far away. *See* **shadow.**

geometrical p. See **perspective, linear.**

linear p. Perspective conveyed by drawing images in different sizes. For example, parallel lines receding into the distance are made to converge (Fig. P10). *Syn.* geometrical perspective.

Peter's anomaly A rare congenital anomaly of the anterior segment of the eye which occurs during fetal development in which there is an incomplete separation of the cornea from the iris or the lens. It is characterized by a central corneal opacity, usually accompanied by the adhesion of strands of iris tissue to the margins of the opacity, thinning of the stroma and attenuation or absence of Descemet's membrane (type 1). A variant of Peter's anomaly (called **type 2**) presents in addition to the previously described, either a displacement or a lack of transparency of the lens, which may become adherent to the posterior surface of the cornea. It is frequently associated with glaucoma. *Syn.* anterior chamber cleavage syndrome. *See* **Axenfeld's anomaly; syndrome, Axenfeld–Rieger; syndrome, Rieger's.**

Petit, canal of *See* **canal of Petit.**

Petzval surface The imaginary curved surface upon which images would be formed if curvature of field were the only aberration present. It is the curved surface in which the tangential and sagittal image shells of a point-focal lens coincide. *See* **astigmatism, oblique; curvature of field; lens, anastigmatic.**

pH Symbol for the logarithm to base 10 of the reciprocal of the hydrogen (H) ion concentration measured in gram molecular weight in an aqueous solution. A solution with a pH 7.0 is neutral, one with a pH of more than 7.0 is alkaline and one with a pH lower than 7.0 is acid. It is a convenient way of expressing the acidity or alkalinity of solutions, particularly of contact lens buffer solutions. Alkaline ophthalmic solutions generally cause less discomfort than acidic ones. *Note*: pH stands for *power* (or *potency*) of *H*. *See* **acidosis.**

phacoanaphylactic uveitis *See* **uveitis, phacoanaphylactic.**

phacocele A hernia of the crystalline lens through a rupture of the sclera near the limbus. It lodges underneath the conjunctiva. *Syn.* lenticele.

phacodonesis A tremulous condition of the crystalline lens. It usually results from an injury to the eye in which some or most of the zonular fibres are broken. *See* **iridodonesis.**

phacoemulsification Procedure for removal of the crystalline lens in cataract surgery, which consists of emulsifying and aspirating the contents of the lens with the use of a low-frequency ultrasonic needle inserted into the eye near the limbus. This technique usually produces rapid wound healing and early stabilization of refractive error with less astigmatism, due to the small incision. Following injection of a viscoelastic substance (e.g. sodium hyaluronate) into the anterior chamber for protection, especially of the corneal epithelium, the lens cortex and nucleus are removed and an intraocular lens is typically implanted within the remaining lens capsule. The lens is folded and inserted through a small incision (e.g. 2.8 mm) using a special injector. This procedure is preferred over other cataract extraction techniques due to both the rapid wound healing (no suture needed) and the lower incidence of potentially vision-threatening side effects (e.g. retinal detachment). *See* **after-cataract; biometry of the eye; cataract extraction; iodine-povidone; lens, intraocular; iridectomy.**

phacolytic glaucoma *See* **glaucoma, phacolytic.**

phacoscope Instrument for observing the crystalline lens and measuring accommodative changes using the Purkinje–Sanson images, as in the ophthalmophakometer. *See* **phakometer.**

phagocytosis The process of ingestion of solid substances (e.g. cells, bacteria, parts of necrosed tissue) by cells and transported to a site within the cell where it is broken down by lysosomal enzymes. *Example*: The discs that are shed from the tip of the outer segment of the rods and cones form membrane-bound spherules, which are engulfed into the cells of the retinal pigment epithelium (called **phagosomes**). *See* **cell, cone; cell, rod; retinal pigment epithelium.**

phagosome *See* **phagocytosis.**

phakic Refers to an eye possessing its crystalline lens or an intraocular lens implant. *See* **aphakia; eye, pseudophakic; lens, intraocular.**

phakomatoses A group of diseases characterized by ocular, skin and central nervous system hamartomas (non-malignant tumours). The main conditions are neurofibromatosis, tuberous sclerosis, von Hippel–Lindau, Sturge–Weber and Wyburn–Mason syndromes. *Note*: also spelt phacomatosis (singular), phacomatoses (plural).

phakometer Optical instrument designed to measure the radii of curvature of the crystalline lens. The method is based on a comparison of the sizes of the third h'_3 and fourth h_4' Purkinje images (typically determined by photography) with that of the first image h'_1, that is the anterior corneal surface, the characteristics of which are easily measured. The radius of curvature of, say, the fourth Purkinje image r'_4 can be calculated using the approximate equation

$$r'_4 = r_1(h'_4/h'_1)$$

where r_1 is the radius of curvature of the front surface of the cornea. If the test object is near the eye, a correction factor is necessary.
See image, Purkinje–Sanson; ophthalmophakometer; phacoscope.

phase The state of vibration of a light wave at a particular time. Light waves vibrating with the same frequency are said to be **in phase** if their peaks and troughs occur at the same time (angle difference 0° or 360°); otherwise they are said to be **out of phase** (angle difference 180° or π radians). One wave may lag or precede another by a **phase difference** (e.g. a fraction of a wavelength, or one wavelength, or a number of wavelengths). For waves exactly out of phase, the phase difference is half a wavelength, and for waves exactly in phase, it is zero.
See interference; wavelength.

phenol red cotton thread test *See* test, phenol red cotton thread.

phenomenon 1. A remarkable event or appearance. 2. A fact or an occurrence that can be described or explained. *Plural*: phenomena.
Abney's p. Slight change in hue resulting from a change in saturation. This is especially noticeable when white light is added to a monochromatic blue or green light.
Aubert's p. If, in the dark, the head is tilted slowly to one side while looking at a bright vertical line, this line will appear to tilt in the opposite direction. This phenomenon is due to the absence of compensatory postural changes. *Syn.* Aubert's effect.
Aubert–Förster p. When targets (e.g. letters) of different sizes are placed peripheral to the foveal region and at different distances from the observer, visual acuity is better for the smaller targets nearer the observer than for the larger targets farther than the observer, although they subtend the same visual angle. *Syn.* Aubert–Förster law.
Behr's pupillary p. In patients with hemianopia caused by optic tract lesions (homonymous hemianopia), light stimulation of the eye with the functioning nasal retina causes more vigorous pupillary responses than stimulation of the eye with the functioning temporal retina. This is possibly due to the fact that the density of ganglion cells is higher in the nasal than in the temporal retina.
Bell's p. An outward and upward rolling of the eyes when closing, or attempting to close, the eyelids.
See sign, Bell's.
Bezold–Brücke p. Change in perceived hue of some spectral colours which occurs with a change in intensity. However, some wavelengths, such as 478, 503 and 578 nm, remain a constant hue with varying intensity. These are called **invariant wavelengths** or **unique hues**. *Syn.* Bezold–Brücke effect.

Bielschowsky's p. In alternating hypertropia, occluding one eye leads to its rotation upward, and then placing a neutral density filter in front of the other eye gives rise to a downward movement of the occluded eye.
See test, Bielschowsky's phenomenon
Broca–Sulzer p. *See* effect, Broca–Sulzer.
Brücke–Bartley p. *See* effect, Brücke–Bartley.
crowding p. A difficulty or inability to discriminate small visual acuity tests when they are presented next to each other in a row, thus inducing **contour interaction**, whereas the same-sized acuity symbols presented singly against a uniform background are resolved. Although this phenomenon may be experienced by normal patients, it is most often characteristic of amblyopic eyes (especially strabismic amblyopia) and of people with reading difficulties. *Syn.* crowding effect.
See acuity, morphoscopic visual; amblyopia; masking.
doll's head p. Reflex movement of the eyes in a direction opposite to the direction of a rapid head turn, followed by a return towards the original position. These vestibular-elicited eye movements are aimed at maintaining fixation. The phenomenon can be used to assess the integrity of the vestibulo-ocular response system (**doll's head test**). If the eye movements do not accord with the above description, it may indicate a brainstem defect. *Syn.* doll's eye sign.
See reflex, vestibulo-ocular.
entoptic p. *See* image, entoptic.
extinction p. A condition in which individual stimuli placed in the visual field are seen, but when the nasal field of one eye and the temporal field of the other eye are stimulated simultaneously, the subject fails to see one of the stimuli. This condition is common following a stroke. *Syn.* pseudo-hemianopia.
See neglect, visual.
Fick's p. *See* Sattler's veil.
jack-in-the-box p. When wearing very high positive lenses (e.g. in aphakia), there exists an area in the periphery situated between the outer extent of the field seen through the lens and the field beyond the edge of the lens, which is not seen (**ring scotoma**). This phenomenon refers to the disappearance and sudden reappearance of an object when the eye moves from the periphery to the centre passing over the ring scotoma. This phenomenon can be avoided by turning the head rather than the eye for peripheral viewing or by correcting with contact lenses. Modern aspheric lenses minimize this phenomenon as they have reduced peripheral power.
See field of view, real; scotoma, ring.
Marcus Gunn jaw-winking p. An abnormal condition associated with congenital ptosis, characterized by the elevation of the ptotic eyelid when the mouth is opened or the jaw is moved laterally to the side opposite to the ptosis. The eyelid droops again if the jaw maintains its new position or is closed. The condition often diminishes spontaneously, otherwise surgery is

the main treatment (levator palbebrae superioris resection). *Syn.* Marcus Gunn phenomenon; Marcus Gunn jaw-winking syndrome.

Mizuo's p. The appearance of a golden brown colour of the retina as it adapts to light in Oguchi's disease. When adapted to darkness, the fundus has the normal red appearance. *Syn.* Mizuo's sign.

phi p. Illusion of movement created when one object disappears and an identical object appears in a neighbouring region of the same plane. If the time interval between the two sources is between 0.06 s and 0.2 s, the observer will see an apparent movement of the source, which appears to jump from the first to the second position without the perception of continuity. Hence, it is considered as a partial illusion of movement. Some observers also see each source flickering depending on the rate of alternation. The phi phenomenon has been applied to test patients with convergent and divergent strabismus. This is the **phi phenomenon test of Verhoeff:** two light sources, separated by the angle of strabismus, are placed in front of the patient, as in a major amblyoscope. The two foveas are stimulated with a short time interval between stimulations and patients with normal retinal correspondence do not see a movement whereas those with abnormal retinal correspondence do. *Syn.* phi movement. *See* movement, stroboscopic; retinal correspondence, abnormal; threshold, movement.

Pulfrich p. *See* stereophenomenon, Pulfrich.

Purkinje's p. *See* Purkinje shift.

Riddoch p. Ability to perceive the motion of an object while being unable to detect any other features of that object, such as its colour or its form. This may occur in a scotomatous area of the visual field caused by a lesion somewhere in the visual pathway from the lateral geniculate body to the occipital and temporal cortex.

Troxler's p. An image in the periphery of the retina tends to fade or disappear during steady fixation of another object. This phenomenon is rarely noticed due to the involuntary eye movements. When these are neutralized optically, as in stabilized retinal imagery, the phenomenon occurs readily even in central vision. *See* movement, fixation; stabilized retinal image.

Uhthoff's p. *See* Uhthoff's symptom.

phenotype The observable characteristics (e.g. eye colour, height) of an individual that are the result of an interaction between the genes and the environment. *See* expressivity; gene-environment interaction; genotype

phenylephrine hydrochloride *See* alpha-adrenergic agonist; alpha-adrenergic antagonist; mydriatic; sympathomimetic drugs.

phi movement *See* phenomenon, phi.

phlyctenulosis *See* keratoconjunctivitis, phlyctenular.

phoria Synonym for heterophoria as well as orthophoria.

phoria line *See* line, phoria.

phorometer An instrument for measuring heterophoria consisting usually of Maddox rods and rotary prisms mounted on a phoropter or trial frame.

phoropter An instrument for measuring the ametropias, phorias and the amplitude of accommodation of the eyes. It consists of a large unit placed in front of the patient's head in which there are three rotating discs containing convex and concave spherical and cylindrical lenses, as well as occluders, Maddox rods, pinholes, Polaroids, prisms and coloured filters. An attachment on the instrument allows sets of rotary prisms and cross-cylinders to be swung in front of each sight hole (Fig. P11). *Syn.* refracting unit; refractor; refractor head. *See* Simultantest; trial case.

phosphene A visual sensation arising from stimulation of the retina by something other than light. The stimulation can be either electrical, mechanical (e.g. a blow to the head or pressure on the eyeball) or some electromagnetic waves such as X-rays. *See* image, entoptic; photopsia; stimulus, adequate.

phosphorescence Luminescence that persists for some time after the exciting stimulus has ceased.

photic Pertaining to light or the production of light.

photoablation The use of radiant energy (e.g. UV light) to destroy tissues. *Example*: the use of excimer laser light to ablate the anterior surface of the cornea in LASIK.

photocell Physical receptor that produces electric current when light is incident upon it. *Syn.* photoelectric cell.

photochemical Relating to a chemical change as a result of the absorption of light. *Example*: the action of light on rhodopsin in the photoreceptors of the retina. *See* rhodopsin.

photochromatic interval; lens *See* under the nouns.

photocoagulation Process of changing blood and tissue from a fluid to a clotted state produced by

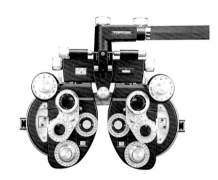

Fig. P11 Phoropter. (Courtesy of Topcon)

the heat of an intense beam of light (e.g. laser), as used in the treatment or prophylactic treatment of retinal diseases (e.g. diabetic retinopathy, retinal detachments, retinal breaks, haemorrhages).
See laser; macular degeneration, age-related; retinal break; retinal detachment; retinopathy, diabetic.

photodynamic therapy See macular degeneration, age-related.

photoelectric Pertains to the interaction between radiation and matter, resulting in the absorption of photons and the consequent emission of electrons.

photokeratitis See keratoconjunctivitis, actinic.

photokeratoconjunctivitis See keratoconjunctivitis, actinic.

photokeratoscopy Determination of corneal curvatures and topography by photographing the corneal image of a target (usually black and white concentric rings) provided with the instrument. Measuring the size of the image and knowing the size of the object, it is possible to calculate the topography of the cornea. The theory is the same as that of the keratometer. A permanent photographic record is given with this method. The area of the cornea that is evaluated is much larger than with a keratometer.
See corneal topography; keratoscope; videokeratoscope.

photoluminescence See luminescence.

photometer An instrument for measuring the luminous intensity of a light source or a surface by comparing it with a standard source. The comparison can be done either with the human eye (as in the Lummer–Brodhun or SEI exposure photometers) or with a photoelectric cell (as in the Pritchard photometer). Syn. illuminometer; luxometer.
See illuminance; luminance.

flicker p. Visual photometer in which the observer sees a field illuminated alternately by two sources to be compared. When the sensation of flicker disappears, the intensity of the test source can be deduced by reading that of the reference standard source to which it is compared. For luminance difference, the frequency of alternation is chosen to be below the critical fusion frequency, but for colour difference (**heterochromatic flicker photometry**) it is chosen above it. Note: Although the adjective heterochromic is commonly used, heterochromatic is the correct word.
See frequency, critical fusion; photometry, heterochromatic flicker.

Lummer–Brodhun p. A cube in which two adjacent or concentric portions are compared, each projected from a different light source. One source is the standard source and the other the comparison one, the brightness of which is thus determined when equal brightness is achieved. The instrument gives quite accurate readings when the two sources are of identical colour.

Macbeth p. A photometer using a Lummer–Brodhun cube, an eyepiece and a movable

standard source illuminating a diffusing surface which is seen as an annulus by reflection within the cube. The portion of the source to be measured is seen through the cube as a spot within the annulus. The brightness of the annulus is adjusted until it matches that of the spot.

objective p. See photometer, physical.

physical p. Photometer employing a radiant energy sensitive element (e.g. a photoelectric cell, a thermopile) and an intensity indicator. Example: Pritchard photometer. Syn. objective photometer.

Pritchard p. See photometer, physical.

SEI exposure p.; subjective p. See photometer, visual.

visual p. Photometer in which the equality of brightness of a light source or a surface with a standard source is made by visual observation. Examples: flicker photometer; Lummer–Brodhun photometer; Macbeth photometer; SEI photometer. Syn. subjective photometer.

photometry The measurement of visible light with a photometer (Table P3).
See candela per square metre; flux, luminous; footcandle; footlambert; illuminance; lambert; luminance; luminous intensity; millilambert; photometer; radiometry.

photometry, heterochromatic flicker The measurement of a coloured light source with a flicker photometer, which alternates temporally above the critical fusion frequency. The observer adjusts the intensity of one of the two sources until the perception of flicker disappears. Heterochromatic flicker photometry is used in instruments measuring macular pigment absorption. Syn. heterochromic flicker photometry.
See photometer, flicker.

photon The basic unit of radiant energy defined by the equation

$$E = h\nu$$

Table P3	Common photometric units
luminous flux	
lumens	
luminous intensity (I)	
candela = lumens/steradian	
illuminance (E)	
lux = lumens/m^2	
footcandle = lumens/ft^2	
luminance (L)	
candela/m^2	
candela/ft^2	
footlambert	
lambert	
millilambert	
1 footlambert (fL) = 3.426 cd/m^2	
1 lambert = 3183 cd/m^2	
1 millilambert = 3.183 cd/m^2	
1 candela/m^2 = 0.2919 fL	
1 candela/ft^2 = 3.142 fL	

where h is **Planck's constant** (6.623×10^{-34} joule $\times$ second), ν the frequency of the light and E the energy difference carried away by the emission of a single photon of light. The energy of light of wavelength 507 nm (light frequency 5.9×10^{14}) is equal 3.9×10^{-19} joules ($6.623 \times 10^{-34} \times 5.9 \times 10^{14}$). The absorption of a single photon can produce a rod photoreceptor excitation. The term photon usually refers to visible light whereas the term **quantum** refers to other electromagnetic radiations.

See **isomerization; spectrum. electromagnetic; theory, quantum; theory, wave; threshold, absolute; transduction; troland.**

photonics Term referring to all the methods, procedures and systems used to measure, transmit or utilize light.

photophobia Abnormal fear or intolerance of light. It can be physiological, although it often accompanies inflammations of the anterior segment of the eye, especially anterior uveitis. It is also noted in patients with cone degeneration. Management is usually aimed at treating the primary cause (e.g. keratitis, uveitis), but in other cases (e.g. albinism, drug-induced mydriasis, recent aphakes, fear of light), tinted lenses will give relief.

See **albinism; corneal abrasion; corneal erosion, recurrent; cystinosis; iritis; keratitis; monochromat; uveitis.**

photophthalmia *See* **keratoconjunctivitis, actinic.**

photopia *See* **vision, photopic.**

photopic eye *See* **eye, light-adapted.**

photopic vision *See* **vision, photopic.**

photopigment Any pigment, such as the visual pigment found in the photoreceptors of the retina, which is altered by the absorption of light energy. Each retinal photopigment is made up of two elements: the protein *opsin* and a small attached molecule *retinal*, which is vitamin A aldehyde (one of many forms of vitamin A). *Retinal* is the portion of the photopigment first altered by light absorption. The *opsin* differs in each photopigment, and it absorbs different wavelength depending on the photopigment, while the same *retinal* is found in all photopigments.

See **carotene; pigment, visual; rhodopsin; vitamin A deficiency.**

photopsia Perceptions such as sparks, lights or colours arising as a result of diseases of the optic nerve, retina (e.g. retinal and vitreous detachment) or the brain; migraine; or they can also occur with pressure upon the closed eye.

See **floaters; flashes; retinitis, cytomegalovirus; spot, Fuchs'.**

photoreceptor A receptor capable of reacting when stimulated by light, such as the rods and cones of the retina.

See **cell, cone; cell, rod.**

photorefraction A family of photographic techniques that provide a rapid, objective method of measuring the refractive error and accommodative response of the eye. Light emitted from a small flash source placed close to a camera lens is reflected from the eye and returned to the camera. Three methods have been developed: **orthogonal, isotropic** and **eccentric** (also called **photoretinoscopy**). The optical design of each method results in a specific photographic pattern, which varies with the degree to which the eye is defocused with respect to the plane of the camera. Photorefractive methods are not as accurate as retinoscopy but as they are entirely objective, much quicker and do not require prolonged fixation on the part of the patient, they are highly suited for testing infants and young children.

See **optometer; refractive error; retinoscope.**

photorefractive keratectomy *See* **keratectomy, photorefractive.**

photoretinoscopy *See* **photorefraction.**

photostress test *See* **test, photostress.**

phototransduction *See* **transduction.**

phototropism The reaction of certain plants and animals to move towards (positive phototropism) or away from (negative phototropism) a source of light.

phthiriasis Infestation of the eyelid margin by the crab louse (*Phthirus pubis*). It causes itching along the eyelid margin. Removal of the parasites is relatively easy either with forceps or by **cryotherapy** (removal under cold or freezing conditions). Chemical options (e.g. organophosphate insecticide malathion, mercuric oxide 1%, or shampoo containing 1% gamma-benzene hexachloride) may also be used.

phthisis bulbi A shrinkage and atrophy of the eyeball following a severe inflammation (e.g. uveitis), absolute glaucoma or trauma.

phthisis corneae A shrinkage and atrophy of the cornea following a severe inflammation of the cornea or trauma. It is associated with shrinkage of the globe.

phycomycosis A fungal infection caused by various microorganisms. These fungi may spread from the sinuses or the nasal tissue into the orbit, particularly in patients with diabetes, renal failure, malignant tumour or on steroid therapy. Therapy is aimed at the underlying disease, often accompanied by antifungal agents. *Syn.* zygomycosis.

physical optics *See* **optics, physical.**

physiological astigmatism; blind spot; cup; diplopia; optics; position of rest; saline *See* under the nouns.

physostigmine A reversible anticholinesterase drug used as a parasympathomimetic which, when used in the eye constricts the pupil. It may be used in solution of 0.25% to 1% or ointment 0.25% to 0.50% in the treatment of glaucoma, but because of its side effects, its usage is rare nowadays. It is sometimes combined with pilocarpine. *Syn.* eserine.

See **miotics; neostigmine; parasympathomimetic drug.**

pia mater A delicate fibrous membrane closely enveloping the brain, spinal cord and the optic nerve. It terminates at the eye.

Pickford–Nicholson anomaloscope *See* anomaloscope.

'pie on the floor' *See* quadrantanopia, inferior.

'pie in the sky' *See* quadrantanopia, superior.

Piéron's law *See* law, Ricco's.

Pigeon–Cantonnet stereoscope *See* stereoscope, Pigeon–Cantonnet.

piggyback lens *See* lens, piggyback.

pigment A coloured substance (e.g. haemoglobin, melanin) found in cells or tissue.
> **p. dispersion syndrome** *See* syndrome, pigment dispersion.
> **p. epithelium** *See* retinal pigment epithelium.
> **macular p.** Yellow-brown pigment, insensitive to light with a maximum absorption around 460 nm, and located in the inner layers of the macular area of the retina. It extends over an area of about 12° in diameter. Its density declines markedly with eccentricity. The major components of this pigment are the carotenoids: lutein and zeaxanthin. These yellow pigments absorb blue light maximally. The macular pigment has been thought to mitigate the effect of chromatic aberration and to protect the retina against short wavelength radiations. Moreover, lutein and zeaxanthin are antioxidants, which help protect the macula from oxidative stress, and larger plasma concentrations of these pigments may lower the risk of age-related macular degeneration.
> *See* filter, red; macula lutea; oxidative stress; photometry, heterochromatic flicker.
> **retinal p.** *See* melanopsin; pigment, visual.
> **visual p.** Photosensitive pigment contained in the outer segments of both rods and cones. It contains a large protein *opsin* and a small attached molecule called *retinal*. The chemical composition of the pigment in both cells is almost the same, there is only a slight difference in the protein *opsin* but the *retinal* molecule is the same in all pigments. The pigment in the rods is called rhodopsin and it has a maximum spectral absorption around 498 nm. The cones contain three other types of pigments (one in each cone), which have spectral absorption curves with a maximum around 420 to 440 nm (S cone), 530 to 545 nm (M cone) and 560 to 580 nm (L cone). These three pigments form the basis of normal trichromatic colour vision. Absorption of light by the visual pigments and the subsequent chemical changes that result in photoreceptor potentials represent the first stage in the visual process. *Syn.* for cone visual pigments: **cyanolabe** (blue pigment), **chlorolabe** (green pigment) and **erythrolabe** (red pigment) names sometimes used for the short-wave (S), middle-wave (M) and long-wave (L) sensitive cone pigments, respectively. *Note*: Erythrolabe, meaning red pigment, has, in fact, its maximum spectral absorption around 560 to 580 nm, which is in the greenish-yellow portion of the visible spectrum (Table P4).

See bleaching; cell, cone; cell, rod; colour vision, defective; densitometry, retinal; iodopsin; porphyropsin; rhodopsin; test, photostress; trichromatism; theory, Young–Helmholtz; transduction.

pigment dispersion syndrome *See* syndrome, pigment dispersion.

pigmentary glaucoma *See* glaucoma, pigmentary; syndrome, pigment dispersion.

pigmentary reaction of the retina *See* albinism; atrophy, gyrate; choroideremia; disease, Batten–Mayou; disease, Best's; disease, Stargardt's; dystrophy, cone; dystrophy, cone-rod; dystrophy, macular; dystrophy, pattern; fundus albipunctatus; fundus flavimaculatus; Leber's congenital amaurosis; retinitis pigmentosa; syndrome, Bassen–Kornzweig; syndrome, Laurence–Moon–Bardet–Biedl; syndrome, Refsum's; syndrome, Stickler's; syndrome, Usher's.

pilocarpine An alkaloid obtained from the leaves of *Pilocarpus microphyllus* and other species of *Pilocarpus*. It is a **parasympathomimetic (direct-acting cholinergic) drug**, which mimics the effect of acetylcholine causing miosis and accommodation. It counteracts sympathomimetic mydriatics. It is used in the treatment of glaucoma. Pilocarpine hydrochloride is most commonly applied to the eye as a 1% solution. Carbachol and bethanechol chloride are other parasympathomimetic drugs with similar effects to pilocarpine.
See parasympathomimetic drug; physostigmine.

pince-nez Eyeglasses without sides, held on the nose by tension from springs attached to the nose pads.
See lens, spectacle; pad nose.

pincushion distortion *See* distortion.

pineal body *See* pinealoma.

pinealoma A tumour of the pineal body, a small glandular structure that lies between the two superior colliculi in a depression below the splenium of the corpus callosum. It may result in a loss of the pupil light reflex, vertical gaze palsy (especially in children), diplopia, hydrocephalus, as well as a disturbance of the secretion of melatonin, which is related to the diurnal dark-light cycles. *Syn.* pineoblastoma. *See* nystagmus, convergence-retraction; syndrome, Parinaud's.

pinguecula A benign degenerative tumour of the bulbar conjunctiva that appears as a slightly raised, yellowish-white, oval-shaped thickening on either side of the cornea, but usually the nasal side. Histologically, it shows elastotic degeneration of vascularized collagen. It becomes more common in elderly people, especially those exposed to high levels of ultraviolet radiation, wind and dust. Although benign and ocular lubrication is sufficient, surgical excision may be requested for cosmetic reasons (Fig. P12). *Note:* also spelt pinguicula. *Plural*: pingueculae.
See pterygium.

Table P4 Cone pigments in normal and congenital dichromatic colour vision defects (excluding cases due to anomalies of the central visual pathway)

Colour vision	Long-wave sensitive (560–580 nm)	Middle-wave sensitive (530–545 nm)	Short-wave sensitive (420–440 nm)
normal	present	present	present
protanope	absent or abnormal	present	present
deuteranope	present	absent or abnormal	present
tritanope	present	present	absent or abnormal

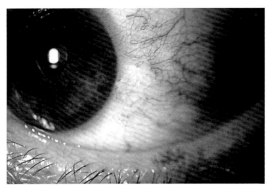

Fig. P12 Pinguecula. (From Kanski 2003, with permission of Butterworth-Heinemann)

pingueculitis A non-bacterial inflammatory response of a pinguecula which results in swelling, vascularization and irritation of the eye. It is found typically in people of middle age. It may be caused by excessive exposure to sun, wind or mechanical irritation, which leads to tear film disruption and dryness. Symptoms can be alleviated with artificial tears, temporary use of antiinflammatory drugs and constant use of sunglasses. Excision may be necessary in some cases.

pinhole disc; spectacles *See* under the nouns.

pinhole test *See* disc, pinhole.

pink eye *See* conjunctivitis, contagious.

Piper's law *See* law, Ricco's.

pit, optic A depression that is present on each side of the end of the neural ectoderm (or neural tube) of the embryo. The pit deepens to form the optic vesicle. *Syn.* optic sulcus.
See vesicle, optic.

pit, optic disc *See* disc, optic disc.

pituitary adenoma; gland *See* under the nouns.

placebo A substance or a prescription (e.g. plano lenses) devoid of any physiological effect that is given merely to satisfy a patient. It is also used in research as a control against which the real effect of another product (similar in appearance) can be established.
See study, single-blind; trial, randomized controlled.

Placido disc *See* keratoscope.

Planck's constant *See* photon.

Planck's law *See* law, Planck's.

plane A flat surface.
aperture p. Plane that passes through the aperture of an optical system.
apparent frontoparallel p. Plane passing through the fixation point and containing all other points judged to appear in the same frontal plane. At about 1 metre from the eye, it more or less coincides with a frontal plane; this is the **abathic distance**. Closer to 1 metre, it is often a concave surface with its concavity turned towards the observer, and beyond 1 metre, it is a convex surface with its convexity turned towards the observer.
See deviation, Hering–Hillebrand; horopter.
cardinal p's. Planes, normal to the optical axis, which pass through the cardinal points of a lens or optical system. They are the focal planes, the nodal planes and the principal planes. (Sometimes, this definition also includes the object and image planes.)
See point, cardinal.
equatorial p. Vertical plane passing through the centre of curvature of the large circle of the eyeball, perpendicular to the optical axis and which divides the eyeball into anterior and posterior halves.
See anterior segment of the eye; plane, Listing's.
p. of fixation *See* plane of regard.
focal p. Plane, perpendicular to the optical axis, which passes through one of the focal points of an optical system.

See **focus, principal.**

frontal p. Vertical plane which is perpendicular to the median plane. When this plane passes through the centre of rotation of the eye, it is called Listing's plane.

frontoparallel p. Frontal plane passing through the fixation point.

horizontal p. of the eye Plane, such as the *xy* plane, passing through the centre of rotation of the eye and dividing it into superior and inferior halves. When the eye is looking straight ahead, this plane is horizontal.

See **plane, subjective horizontal; plane, xy.**

image p. Plane which is perpendicular to the optical axis at any axial image point of an optical system.

p. of incidence The plane containing the incident and reflected rays, and the normal to the surface at the point of incidence.

Listing's p. A frontal plane passing through the centre of rotation of the eye, which corresponds to the equatorial plane when it is looking in the straight-ahead position (Fig. P13).

median p. Vertical plane that divides the head into right and left halves.

p. mirror *See* **mirror, plane.**

nodal p. Plane which is perpendicular to the optical axis, and passes through one of the nodal points of an optical system (Fig. P14).

object p. Plane perpendicular to the optical axis at any axial object point of an optical system.

principal p. A plane perpendicular to the optical axis of an optical system at the point where the incident rays parallel to the optical axis intersect the refracted rays converging to the secondary focal point (**secondary principal plane**); or in which the refracted rays parallel to the optical axis intersect the incident rays coming from the primary focal point (**primary principal plane**). Each plane is an erect image of the other, and of the same size. For this reason, they are sometimes also referred to as **unit planes** as they are conjugate planes in which the magnification is 1. In a thin lens, these planes coincide at the lens (Fig. P14).

See **distance, image; distance, object; length, focal; lens, thin; point, nodal; point, principal; power, equivalent.**

p. of regard Plane containing the fixation point, the axes of fixation from the two eyes and the base line. *Syn.* plane of fixation.

sagittal p. Vertical plane parallel to the median plane as, for example, the *yz* plane.

spectacle p. Plane representing the orientation of the spectacle lenses relative to the eyes and passing through the posterior vertices of the two lenses.

See **angle, pantoscopic; angle, retroscopic; vertex distance.**

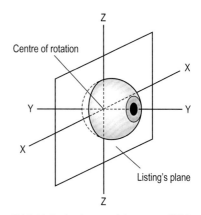

Fig. P13 Listing's plane and the axes of Fick.

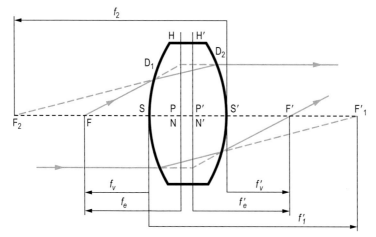

Fig. P14 Primary and secondary principal planes HP and H′P′ of a thick lens in air (PF, anterior focal length; P′F′, posterior focal length; SF, front vertex focal length; S′F′, back vertex focal length; SF′₁, back focal length of the first surface D₁; S′F₂, front focal length of the second surface D₂; N and N′, nodal points).

subjective horizontal p. Plane fixed with respect to the eye (i.e. horizontal when the eye is in the primary position).
See **plane, horizontal p. of the eye; position, primary.**
unit p's. See **plane, principal.**
p. of vibration See **light, polarized.**
visual p. Plane containing the two visual axes.
xy p. Horizontal plane of the eye containing both the *x*- and *y*-axes (Fig. P13).
See **axis, anteroposterior; axis, transverse.**
yz p. Vertical plane of the eye containing both the *y*- and *z*-axes (Fig. P13).
See **axis, anteroposterior; axis, vertical.**

plano lens *See* **lens, afocal.**

planoconcave lens *See* **lens, planoconcave.**

planoconvex lens *See* **lens, planoconvex.**

plaques, Hollenhorst's Orange-yellow spots usually found at branching sites of retinal arterioles. They are due to necrosis and ulceration of atheromatous, cholesterine-containing emboli in the carotid arteries which discharge into the circulation. They do not usually obstruct the retinal arterioles and, as such, do not cause visual symptoms. However, they indicate the possible development of larger emboli (**fibrinoplatelets**) that may temporarily obstruct the retinal circulation and cause amaurosis fugax, and may even presage a myocardial infarction or stroke.
See **atheroma; corneal arcus; xanthelasma.**

plaque radiotherapy *See* **radiotherapy, plaque.**

plastic Various organic or synthetic materials (e.g. CR-39, HEMA, polymethyl methacrylate, polycarbonate, etc.) that can be transformed into solid shapes to make spectacle frames, contact lenses, ophthalmic lenses, etc. and can be made to have good optical surfaces, high light transmission and refractive indices and dispersions similar to that of crown or flint glass.
See **acetone; index of refraction; spectacle frame, plastic.**

plastic period *See* **period, critical.**

plastic spectacle frame *See* **spectacle frame, plastic.**

plateau iris; iris syndrome *See* **iris, plateau.**

Plateau's spiral A white disc on which there is a black band, which winds around and around with each curve outside the previous one and with its origin at the centre of the disc. When the spiral is rotated and fixated at its centre, the circular bands appear to move in and out. When rotation is stopped a motion after-effect (or **motion after-image**) appears, i.e. the circular bands now seem to move in the opposite direction, and if another stationary object is fixated, it will appear to swell or shrink in size in a direction opposite to that seen when fixating the rotating disc. *Syn.* Archimedes spiral; Talbot-Plateau spiral.
See **after-effect, waterfall.**

plates, pseudoisochromatic Charts for testing colour vision on which are printed dots of various colours, brightness, saturation and sizes, arranged so that the dots of similar colour form a figure (a letter, a numeral, a geometrical shape or winding path) among a background of dots of another colour. The colours of the figure and the background correspond to the confusion colours of the various types of anomalous colour vision. A dichromat or an anomalous trichromat has difficulty in perceiving the pattern because it is distinguishable from the background only by its difference in hue. There are many different sets of such plates, some using figures (circles, crosses or triangles) such as the **AO**, **HRR** plates, or numbers or lines such as those of **Ishihara** (Fig. P15) and **Dvorine**, or five spots such as the **City University colour vision test**, or the **Lanthony tritan album**, which consists of a square matrix of grey dots in which one corner on each plate contains blue-purple dots of different saturation and the subject has to identify the corner.
See **colour, confusion; colour vision, defective; lamp, Macbeth; test, Farnsworth; test, City University colour vision.**

pleochroism The property of an optically anisotropic medium (e.g. certain crystals) to exhibit different brightness and/or colour when the light transmitted through it is viewed from different directions. (A particular case of pleochroism is dichroism.) *Syn.* polychroism.
See **anisotropic; dichroism.**

pleomorphic adenoma of the lacrimal gland *See* **gland, pleomorphic adenoma of the lacrimal.**

pleomorphism, endothelial *See* **polymorphism, endothelial.**

pleoptics A method of treating amblyopia with eccentric fixation, which consists of dazzling the eccentrically fixating retinal area with high illumination while protecting the fovea with a disc projected onto the fundus and thereby rendering the fovea more responsive to fixation stimuli. There

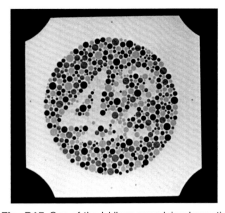

Fig. P15 One of the Ishihara pseudoisochromatic plates.

exist several variations of this procedure, but the therapy is very fastidious.
See occlusion treatment; orthoptics; Visuscope.

plexiform layer *See* retina.

plexus A network of interweaving nerves, blood vessels or lymphatic vessels.

cavernous p. A network of nerve fibres derived from the internal carotid nerve and located on the inferomedial aspect of the internal carotid artery in the cavernous sinus. It supplies sympathetic innervation via the ciliary and gasserian ganglia to almost all the tissues of the orbit, including fibres to the dilator pupillae muscle, Müller's superior palpebral muscle, the ciliary muscle and vasoconstrictor fibres for the blood vessels of the eye.
See sinus, cavernous; syndrome, Horner's.

ciliary venous p. A network of vessels situated in the outer portion of the ciliary body. It receives blood from the ciliary muscle and drains into anterior ciliary vein. It also communicates with the intrascleral venous plexus. *Syn.* ciliary plexus.

deep episcleral p. See plexus, pericorneal.

episcleral p. Network of vessels near the limbus which receives blood from the anterior ciliary arteries and drains into the anterior ciliary veins. It also receives blood from the conjunctival veins and drains the perilimbal conjunctiva. *Syn.* superficial episcleral plexus.

internal carotid p. A network of nerve fibres derived from the internal carotid nerve and located on the lateral side of the internal carotid artery near the apex of the petrous bone. It sends sympathetic axons to the abducens, ophthalmic and nasociliary nerves, the deep petrosal nerve, the caroticotympanic nerve (which supplies the eardrum) and the ophthalmic and lacrimal arteries.
See ganglion, superior cervical.

pericorneal p. A network of vessels situated around the limbus and formed by the anastomosing of the episcleral arteries (branches of the anterior ciliary arteries) and the conjunctival arteries. It forms a series of arcades parallel to the corneal margin. This plexus is arranged in two layers: (1) a **superficial conjunctival pericorneal plexus** liable to injection in inflammation of the superficial cornea or conjunctiva (conjunctival injection) and (2) a **deep episcleral plexus** liable to injection in diseases of the iris, ciliary body or deep portion of the cornea, or angle-closure glaucoma (ciliary injection).
See artery, ciliary; vein, anterior ciliary.

scleral p. A network of vessels situated in the deep layers of the sclera near the limbus. It is made up of the deep- and mid-scleral plexuses. It receives aqueous humour from the canal of Schlemm via collector channels, as well as blood from the ciliary venous plexus. It drains into the anterior ciliary veins.

superficial episcleral p. See plexus, episcleral.

plica A fold of tissue.

plica lacrimalis *See* lacrimal apparatus.

plica lunata *See* plica semilunaris.

plica semilunaris A crescent-shaped fold of conjunctiva located at the inner canthus lateral to the caruncle. It is a vestigial structure that represents the third eyelid or **nictitating membrane** of lower vertebrates. *Syn.* plica lunata; semilunar fold.

plus lens *See* lens, converging.

plus 1.00 D blur test *See* test, plus 1.00 D blur.

pneumatic retinopexy *See* retinal detachment, rhegmatogenous.

Poggendorff's visual illusion *See* illusion, Poggendorff's visual.

point A small spot, considered only as to its position.

aplanatic p's. See focus, aplanatic.

blur p. 1. The point at which the fixation target appears blurred on the introduction of increasing prisms and/or lens power, as for example in a test for relative convergence. 2. A point on a graph representing the limit of clear, single, binocular vision.
See convergence, relative; zone of clear, single, binocular vision.

break p. The point at which diplopia occurs when increasing prism or lens power during binocular fixation.
See blur point; convergence, relative.

cardinal p's. Six points on the optical axis of a lens system or thick lens: the two principal foci, the two principal points and the two nodal points. (Sometimes, this definition also includes the axial object and image points.) (Fig. P16) *Syn.* gaussian points (some authors consider this term synonymous, although it does not include the two nodal points).
See plane, cardinal.

centration p. The point at which the optical centre (of a lens) is to be located in the absence of a prescribed prism or after any prescribed prism has been neutralized. If the centration point is not specified, it is located at the standard optical centre position (British Standard).
See centre, standard optical position; decentration.

conjugate p's. See distance, conjugate.

p. of convergence 1. The point of intersection of the lines of sight. 2. The point to which rays of light converge.

corresponding retinal p's. See retinal corresponding points.

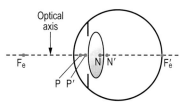

Fig. P16 Cardinal points of the eye. F_e and F'_e, first and second principal foci; P and P', first and second principal points; N and N', first and second nodal points. Note that $F_eP = N'F'_e = f'$ and $NN' = PP'$.

distance visual p. An assumed position of the visual point on a lens used for distance vision under given conditions, when the eyes are normally in the primary position.

p. of divergence The point from which rays of light diverge.

equivalent p's. See point, nodal.

far p. of accommodation See accommodation, far point of.

far p. of convergence See convergence, far point of.

p. of fixation See fixation, point of.

focal p. See focus, principal.

gaussian p's. The two principal points, the two nodal points and the two focal points situated on the optical axis of a lens system.
See **point, cardinal.**

image p. Point at which an object point is formed by an optical system (Fig. P16).

p. of incidence The point at which a ray of light intersects a refracting or reflecting surface.

lacrimal p. See lacrimal punctum.

near p. of accommodation See accommodation, near point of.

near p. of convergence See convergence, near point of.

near visual p. An assumed position of the visual point on a lens used for near vision under given conditions.
See **point, visual.**

neutral p. 1. In retinoscopy, it is the point at which the sight hole of the retinoscope is conjugate with the patient's retina. At this point, no reflex motion can be seen by the examiner and the entire pupil is illuminated completely or is completely dark. This is obtained in a myopic eye when the retinoscope is placed at the far point of accommodation. When testing emmetropes and hyperopes, this neutral point is reached when sufficient converging lens power has been added to displace the far point (artificially) to the sight hole of the retinoscope. See **distance, conjugate.** 2. In dichromats, it is a region of the spectrum that appears colourless.
See **deuteranopia; protanopia; tritanopia.**

nodal p's. In a centred optical system, they are a pair of conjugate points on the axis which have the property that any incident ray which passes through the first nodal point leaves the system as though from the second nodal point and parallel to the incident ray. Thus, the refracted ray is unchanged in direction, although displaced. The distance between the two nodal points is equal to the distance between the two principal points. When the refractive indices on each side of an optical system are equal, as is the case of a thick lens in air, the principal and nodal points coincide. They are then called **equivalent points.** In a single refracting surface, the nodal points coincide with the centre of curvature, while the principal points coincide with the vertex of the surface (Figs. P14 and P16).
See **centre, optical; plane, principal; vertex.**

null p. See nystagmus.

p. object See object, point.

principal p's. The points of intersection of the principal planes with the optical axis. The principal points are the usual reference points from which the focal lengths and the object and image distances are measured (Figs. P14 and P16).
See **plane, principal; power, equivalent.**

recovery p. The point at which fusion is regained on decreasing the prism or lens power which originally induced diplopia in investigation of relative accommodation and convergence.
See **convergence, relative.**

p. of regard Usually a synonym of point of fixation. However, in some circumstances, it may be a peripheral point in space upon which visual attention is directed, while the eye is looking foveally at a point of fixation.
See **fixation, point of.**

p. source See source, point.

visual p. The point of intersection of the visual axis with the back surface of a spectacle lens (British Standard).
See **point, distance visual; point, near visual.**

p. zero A point on the retina of a strabismic eye which has acquired the same visual direction, under binocular conditions, as the fovea of the fixating eye.

Points See acuity, near visual.

point-spread function See function, point-spread.

pointing, past- Misjudging the location of an object and pointing too far in the same direction in which the object was displaced when presented monocularly in the direction of action of a recently paralysed extraocular muscle. *Example:* If the left lateral rectus is paralysed and the left eye attempts (the right eye being occluded) to look at an object to the left, that object will be thought to be located further to the side than it actually is, as shown, for example, by the patient pointing a finger.
See **localization; projection, false; strabismus, incomitant.**

pointing, short- Opposite reaction to past-pointing in which the location of an object fixated monocularly appears to be located less peripherally than it actually is. This happens when the affected muscle is in spasm.

polarimetry, scanning laser An instrument using polarized laser light (780 nm) to determine the thickness of the retinal nerve fibre layer (RNFL) in the peripapillary area. It utilizes the birefringent properties of the RNFL, which produces a change in polarization (called **retardation**) of the light reflected by the RNFL. The degree of retardation is assumed to be proportional to the thickness of the RNFL. The instrument includes a means of neutralizing the birefringence of the anterior segment of the eye. A comparison of the retardation values of the RNFL is made with an age-matched normative database. The instrument is used to detect RNFL defects and progressive changes over time in glaucomatous eyes.
See **glaucoma detection.**

polariscope An instrument for examining substances in polarized light. It consists of a polarizer and an analyser with their planes of polarization at right angles to each other. In the regions where the material is strained (such as an ophthalmic lens tightly mounted in a metal frame), it becomes birefringent and the observer sees a system of dark fringes in that region. When used to detect strain in glass or plastic, it is called a **strain tester**. Safety glass (except the chemically strengthened type) displays a characteristic strain pattern when viewed in a polariscope.
See **glass, safety; strain.**

polarization *See* **light, polarized.**

polarizer 1. An optical element or a device that produces polarized light from incident unpolarized light. *Examples*: Nicol prism, Polaroid sheet, tourmaline crystal. To see that light is polarized, another device called an analyzer is necessary. **2.** In a polariscope, the first of the two polarizing elements, the second being the analyzer.
See **light, polarized; polariscope; prism, Nicol.**

Polaroid *See* **light, polarized.**

poles of the eyeball They are (1) The point on the anterior surface of the cornea which constitutes the summit. It is located at the intersection of the cornea with the geometrical axis of the eye (this is the **anterior pole**). (2) The point of intersection of the sclera with the geometrical axis (this is the **posterior pole**).
See **axis, anteroposterior; length of the eye, axial.**

poliosis A condition in which there is a lack of pigment in the hair, eyebrows and eyelashes, which appear whitish or grey. The condition normally occurs in patches. It is often associated with vitiligo, alopecia and forms part of the **Vogt–Koyanagi–Harada syndrome.**

polishing The final stage in the surfacing process in which the lens is made smooth and provides regular (instead of random) transmission and specular (instead of diffuse) reflection. It is accomplished by rubbing the lens over a tool covered with felt cloth, a plastic sheet or with pitch (which produces the best results) sprayed with water containing finely powdered cerium oxide or rouge. The curvatures of the lens remain unaltered in this procedure. Polishing of spectacle frames is referred to as **buffing**, **mop polishing** or **barreling** (if the polishing is done using a drum).
See **cerium oxide; grinding; rouge; roughing; smoothing; surfacing.**

poloxamine *See* **surfactant.**

polyarteritis nodosa *See* **keratitis, peripheral ulcerative; scleritis.**

polycarbonate *See* **lens, plastic; plastic.**

polychroism *See* **pleochroism.**

polycoria An anomaly characterized by the presence of two or more pupils in one iris. This condition may be produced by hypoplasia, hyperplasia of the iris stroma or by surgical or accidental trauma.

Depending upon the location of the extra pupil, vision may be affected.
See **corectopia; diplopia, monocular.**

polymegethism, endothelial Variation in the size of the endothelial cells of the cornea as a result of disturbed metabolism. It may be induced by contact lens wear, surgery, trauma or disease processes. Endothelial polymegethism is detected by observation with a specular microscope or a high magnification slit-lamp. If the condition is caused by contact lens wear, management consists of refitting the patient with daily wear contact lenses of higher oxygen transmissibility.
See **acidosis; corneal endothelium; microscope, specular; polymorphism, endothelial.**

polymethyl methacrylate Polymerized methyl methacrylate forming a light transparent thermoplastic material used in the manufacture of some spectacle lenses and formerly hard contact lenses. It is commonly referred to by its abbreviation PMMA.
See **modulus of elasticity; spectacle frame, plastic.**

polychromatic *See* **light, polychromatic.**

polymorphism, endothelial The presence of many cell shapes that accompanies polymegethism. *Syn.* endothelial pleomorphism.
See **polymegethism, endothelial.**

polymyxin B sulphate An antibiotic solution effective against many gram-negative organisms and particularly *Pseudomonas aeruginosa*, but not *Proteus*. It is used topically in combination with either bacitracin as an ointment, trimethoprim as drops or ointment or neomycin plus gramicidin as drops. These combinations render polymyxin B active against a wide range of bacteria.

polyopia A condition in which more than one image of a single object is perceived. It may be double vision but more commonly it is multiple vision. Irregular ocular refraction as in some cataracts may sometimes be the cause. *Syn.* multiple vision.
See **diplopia; triplopia.**

polystichia A condition in which there are two or more rows of eyelashes in a single eyelid.
See **distichiasis.**

polyvinyl alcohol *See* **tears, artificial.**

pons A mass of nerve cells and fibres found on the anterior part of the brainstem between the midbrain (above) and the medulla oblongata (below) and which relays impulses. It contains the abducens and facial nuclei, the reticular formation and ascending and descending tracts such as the medial longitudinal fasciculus. *Syn.* pons cerebelli; pons varolii.
See **brainstem; movement, eye; palsy, gaze.**

Ponzo visual illusion *See* **illusion, Ponzo visual.**

porphyropsin A visual pigment found in the retinas of freshwater fish. It differs from rhodopsin in having its maximum absorption at about 522 nm.
See **pigment, visual.**

Porro prism *See* **prism, Porro.**

port-wine stain *See* syndrome, Sturge–Weber.

portion *See* lens, bifocal; segment of a bifocal lens.

portion, intermediate The portion of a trifocal or progressive addition lens that has the correction for vision of an area situated between distance and near.

position The way in which the eyes are placed.
   active p. Position of the eyes characterized by foveal fixation of an object by both eyes. Thus, they are under the control of postural, fixation and fusion reflexes.
   See esophoria; exophoria; position, passive; reflex.
   cardinal p's. of gaze These are the following six version movements of the eyes: dextroversion (to the right), laevoversion (to the left), dextroelevation (up to the right), laevoelevation (up to the left), dextrodepression (down to the right) and laevodepression (down to the left).
   See test, motility; version.
   diagnostic p's. of gaze Method of evaluating the integrity of the extraocular muscles by testing the primary, the four secondary and the four tertiary positions of gaze, monocularly or binocularly.
   See palsy, gaze; test, motility; version.
   dissociated p. *See* dissociation.
   passive p. Position of the eyes when they are only under the control of the postural and fixation reflexes, but not the fusion reflex, as, for example, when one eye is covered and the other is fixating an object.
   See heterophoria.
   primary p. Position of an eye in relation to the head from which a pure vertical and a pure horizontal movement is not associated with any degree of torsion. The eye is usually, but not necessarily, in the **straight-ahead (straightforward)** position.
   See centre of rotation of the eye; torsion.
   p. of rest, anatomical Position of the eyes when they are completely devoid of tonus, as in death.
   p. of rest, physiological Position of the eyes when they are only under the control of the postural reflexes, but completely free from any visual stimuli.
   See accommodation, resting state of; convergence, initial; tonus; vergence, tonic.
   secondary p. Movement of an eye represented by a horizontal or vertical rotation away from the primary position.
   See version.
   straight ahead p.; straightforward p. *See* centre of rotation of the eye; position, primary.
   tertiary p. Movement of an eye to an oblique position, as, for example, 'up and in'.
   See version.

positive A response to a test indicating an abnormality or a reaction.
   See false positive; true positive.

positive eyepiece *See* eyepiece, positive.

positive lens *See* lens, convex.

positive spherical aberration *See* aberration, spherical.

positron emission tomography *See* tomography, positron emission.

Posner–Schlossman syndrome *See* syndrome, Posner–Schlossman.

posterior chamber; ciliary artery *See* under the nouns.

posterior embryotoxon *See* ring, anterior limiting of Schwalbe.

posterior pole *See* poles of the eyeball.

posterior polymorphous dystrophy *See* dystrophy, posterior polymorphous.

posterior segment of the eye; synechia; uveitis *See* under the nouns.

posterior vitreous detachment *See* vitreous detachment.

postlenticular space, Berger's *See* space, Berger's postenticular.

postoperative overcorrection *See* strabismus, consecutive.

potential The amount of energy required to transfer a unit of positive charge from one point in an electrical field to another (potential difference). It is typically measured in volts.
   action p. The electric current generated in an axon of a nerve cell in response to a stimulus. The stimulus must be above a certain threshold value to have an effect. The **sodium pump** (or **sodium/potassium pump**), which transports most sodium ions outside the cell and potassium ions inside the cell, ceases to function and the sodium ions rush in making the interior of the axon a positive voltage with respect to the outside. The voltage changes from about -70 mV to $+40$ mV and then falls rapidly back to the resting membrane potential as the sodium pump regains its effect. The whole process takes less than 1 millisecond and its amplitude is always the same (all or none law) for a given axon, whatever the magnitude of the stimulus (only the frequency changes). The action potential is followed by an inexcitable period called the **refractory period**, which usually lasts one or two milliseconds. The action potential travels as a wave in both directions from the point of stimulation and the speed is faster in myelinated than in unmyelinated nerve fibres. Ganglion cells are the only retinal neurons that generate an action potential. *Syn.* nerve impulse.
   See adaptation; cell, Schwann; neuron; potential, receptor; potential, resting membrane; synapse.
   dark p. of the eye *See* potential, resting p. of the eye.
   early receptor p. This is an early rapid response that can be detected when the retina is stimulated with an intense flash of light, approximately 10^6 times brighter than that required to elicit the electroretinogram (ERG). It is completed within 1.5 ms and is followed by the a-wave of the ERG. It is primarily, in man, a cone-generated potential.
   See electroretinogram.

graded p. A depolarization or a hyperpolarization (e.g. in the photoreceptors) generated by a neuron in response to a stimulus. The amplitude of the response varies with the intensity of the stimulus. If the neuron becomes depolarized to threshold an action potential is triggered in its axon.

membrane p. *See* **potential, resting membrane.**

oscillatory p's. Subwaves of low amplitude but high frequency (70 to 140 Hz) superimposed on the b-wave of the electroretinogram. The amplitude of these oscillatory responses is usually enhanced by a filtering technique. These potentials are presumed to originate from the vicinity of the inner plexiform layer of the retina (probably the amacrine cells and bipolar cells) and may reflect disturbances of that part of the retina.

receptor p. Difference in potential occurring in a receptor in response to a stimulus. This is a graded type of response with an amplitude proportional to the intensity of the stimulus (**graded potential**). The photoreceptors produce a receptor potential but, surprisingly, it is a hyperpolarization, i.e. the inside of the membrane becomes more negative with respect to the outside. Some bipolar cells hyperpolarize but others such as the rod bipolar cells depolarize. The ganglion cells respond with action potentials.
See **potential, action; rhodopsin.**

resting membrane p. Difference in direct current potential between the inside and outside of a living cell. The inside of the cell is usually about −70 mV compared to the outside, but this value depends on the quantity of potassium (mainly), sodium and chloride ions on both sides of the membrane, and the permeability to these ions of the membrane itself. *Syn.* membrane potential; transmembrane potential.
See **depolarization; hyperpolarization; potential, action; tonus.**

resting p. of the eye A direct current potential which exists between the anterior and posterior poles of the eye, the cornea being positive relative to the back of the eye. It is of the order of several mV in humans. This potential is used in recording the electrooculogram. *Syn.* dark potential of the eye; standing potential of the eye.
See **electrooculogram.**

standing p. of the eye *See* **potential, resting of the eye.**

standing p. *See* **electrooculogram.**

visual evoked p. An electrical potential measured at the level of the occipital cortex in response to a light stimulation. Recording requires repetition of the stimulus and a computer synchronized with the onset of that stimulus, to average out the background noise produced by the spontaneous brain potentials (e.g. alpha, beta, delta, theta waves). This potential has clinical application and is used to objectively measure refraction, visual acuity, amblyopia, binocular anomalies and help in the diagnosis of some demyelinating diseases (e.g. multiple sclerosis), etc. Many abbreviations are also used. They are EP (evoked potential), VEP (visually evoked potential), VER (visual

Table P5 Power (in dioptres) of the surfaces and structures of an average adult Caucasian eye*

anterior surface of the cornea	48.21
posterior surface of the cornea	−5.97
complete corneal system	42.34
anterior surface of the lens	7.92
accommodated	13.77
posterior surface of the lens	13.54
accommodated	15.84
complete lens system	21.19
accommodated	29.42
complete eye	59.44
accommodated	67.56
refraction of the eye	+0.50
ocular accommodation	8.12

See **constants of the eye.**

evoked response), VECP (visual evoked cortical potential) and pVER (indicating that this potential is pattern-elicited).
See **accommodation, objective; alternating checkerboard stimulus; artifact; electrodiagnostic procedures.**

Potential Acuity Meter *See* **maxwellian view system, clinical.**

povidone *See* **tears, artificial.**

povidone iodine *See* **iodine-povidone.**

power General term that may refer to any power such as effective, equivalent, dioptric, focal, refractive, surface or vergence power (Table P5).

aligning p. *See* **acuity, vernier visual.**

aligning prism p. *See* **prism, aligning.**

approximate p. *See* **power, nominal.**

back vertex p. The reciprocal of the back vertex focal length. It is equal to

$$F_V' = n'/SF'$$

where n' is the refractive index of the second medium, S is the point on the back surface through which passes the optical axis and F' the second principal focus. *Symbol*: F'_v. Other formulae for the back vertex power of a lens (or an optical system) are

$$F_v' = \frac{F_1}{1-(d/n)F_1} + F_2 = \frac{F_e}{1-(d/n)F_1}$$

where d is the thickness of the lens, n the index of refraction of the lens, F_1 the power of the front surface, F_2 the power of the back surface and F_e the equivalent power. The powers are in dioptres and the length in metres. The back vertex power is the usual measurement made by a focimeter (Table P6). *Syn.* back power.
See **vergence; vertex focal length.**

dioptric p. *See* **power, refractive.**

dispersive p. *See* **dispersion.**

Table P6 Powers of the surfaces of contact lenses of thickness $d = 0.20$ mm, in which the radius of curvature of the back optic zone is constant and that of the front optic zone varies to produce various back vertex powers and equivalent powers. The index of refraction of these lenses is assumed to be 1.49.

Radius of back optic zone (mm)	Back surface power (D) f_2	Radius of front optic zone (mm)	Front surface power (D) f_1	Power of lens (D) considered thin $f_1 + f_2$	Equivalent power (D) f_e	Back vertex power (D) f'_v
7.8	−62.82	7.2	68.06	+5.24	+5.81	+5.86
7.8	−62.82	7.4	66.22	+3.40	+3.95	+3.99
7.8	−62.82	7.6	64.47	+1.65	+2.20	+2.22
7.8	−62.82	7.8	62.82	0.00	+0.53	+0.53
7.8	−62.82	8.0	61.25	−1.57	−1.05	−1.06
7.8	−62.82	8.2	59.76	−3.06	−2.56	−2.58
7.8	−62.82	8.4	58.33	−4.49	−4.00	−4.03
7.8	−62.82	8.6	56.98	−5.84	−5.36	−5.40
7.8	−62.82	8.8	55.68	−7.14	−6.67	−6.72
7.8	−62.82	9.0	54.44	−8.38	−7.92	−7.98
7.8	−62.82	9.2	53.26	−9.56	−9.11	−9.18
7.8	−62.82	9.4	52.13	−10.69	−10.25	−10.33

Table P7 Relationship between the power of the ocular refraction (or contact lens power) and the corresponding power (effective power) of a spectacle lens situated at two vertex distances

Spectacle power (D)		Ocular refraction (D)
14 mm	10 mm	
−16	−13.79	−13.07
−14	−12.28	−11.71
−12	−10.71	−10.27
−10	−9.09	−8.77
−9	−8.26	−7.99
−8	−7.41	−7.19
−7	−6.54	−6.38
−6	−5.66	−5.53
−5	−4.76	−4.67
−4	−3.85	−3.79
−3	−2.91	−2.88
+3	+3.09	+3.13
+4	+4.17	+4.24
+5	+5.26	+5.38
+6	+6.38	+6.55
+7	+7.53	+7.76
+8	+8.70	+9.01
+9	+9.89	+10.30
+10	+11.11	+11.63
+12	+13.64	+14.42

effective p. The power of a lens or surface measured in a plane other than the principal plane and usually remote from the lens or surface. If a thin lens or surface of power F is illuminated by parallel incident light, the effective power F_x of another lens placed at a distance d from the original lens and forming an image in the same position is given by the equation

$$F_x = \frac{F}{1 - dF}$$

where d is in metres and positive when measured from left to right (Table P7). *Examples*: (1) If a hyperopic eye is corrected by a lens $F = +5$ D placed at a vertex distance of 12 mm from the cornea, the ocular refraction is

$$F_x = \frac{5}{1 - (0.012 \times 5)} = +5.32 \text{ D}$$

(2) If an eye has an ocular refraction of −10 D, its spectacle refraction at a vertex distance of 10 mm is

$$F_x = \frac{-10}{1 - (-0.01 \times -10)} = -11.11 \text{D}$$

See **power, refractive; vertex distance.**
equivalent p. The refractive power of a lens or an optical system expressed with reference to the principal points. It corresponds to the refractive power of a thin lens placed in the second principal plane which would form an image of a distant object of the same size as that produced by the system that it replaces (Table P6). It is equal to

$$F_e = n'/f' = -n/f$$

where n and n' are the indices of refraction of the object and image space, respectively, f and f' the distances (in metres) between the first and second principal points and the first and second principal foci, respectively. The equivalent power (*symbol*: F_e) is in dioptres. It is also equal to

$$F_e = F_1 + F_2 - \left(\frac{d}{n}\right)F_1F_2$$

where F_1 and F_2 are the powers of the lenses or surfaces comprising the system, d is the distance between the two and n the index of refraction of the intervening medium. *Example*: If the anterior surface power of the cornea is equal to +48.21 D, the posterior surface power is equal to –5.97 D, the thickness of the cornea 0.5 mm and the index of refraction 1.376, the equivalent power will be

$$F_e = 48.21 - 5.97 - \frac{0.0005}{1.376}$$
$$\times 48.21 \times (-5.97)$$
$$= +42.34 \text{ D}$$

Syn. true power.
See length, equivalent focal; power, nominal.
equivalent viewing p. (EVP) A term used to describe the magnifying effect of a lens (or lens system). It is equal to the power resulting from the combination of a magnifier F_m assumed to be a thin lens and a near addition (or the accommodation exerted) F_a, i.e.

$$EVP = F_m + F_a - zF_mF_a$$

where z is the distance (in metres) between the magnifier and the eye (or spectacle plane). *EVP* may also be expressed as

$$EVP = M \times F_a$$

where M is the enlargement ratio (lateral magnification). If the magnifier is placed against the spectacle lens ($z = 0$),

$$EVP = F_m + F_a$$

If the magnifier is placed against the object being viewed ($z = f_a$), $EVP = F_a$. If the magnifier is held at its focal length from the eye ($z = f_m$), $EVP = F_m$. *EVP* is then equal to the power of the magnifier, irrespective of any near addition (or accommodation). *Example*: A patient uses a lens +16 D placed 12 cm from the eye and wears a near addition of +4.00 D. $EVP = 16 + 4 - 0.12 \times 16 \times 4 = +12.3$ D, the enlargement ratio ($M = EVP/F_a$) is 12.3/4 = 3.1×, and at a distance of 4 cm from the eye the enlargement is equal to 4.4×, whereas the conventional magnification remains $F_m/4 = 4\times$. The reciprocal of EVP is called the **equivalent viewing distance**. It represents the focal length of the equivalent magnifying system where the target must be placed to be seen clearly.
See magnification, lateral.
p. factor *See* magnification, spectacle.
focal p. *See* paraxial equation, fundamental; power, refractive.

front vertex p. The reciprocal of the front vertex focal length. It is equal to

$$F_V = n/SF$$

where n is the refractive index of the first medium, S is the point on the front surface through which passes the optical axis and F is the first principal focus. *Symbol*: F_V. Other formulae for the front vertex power of a lens (or an optical system) are

$$F_v = \frac{F_2}{1 - (d/n)F_2} + F_1 = \frac{F_e}{1 - (d/n)F_2}$$

where d is the thickness of the lens, n the index of refraction of the lens, F_1 the power of the front surface, F_2 the power of the back surface and F_e the equivalent power. The powers are in dioptres and the length in metres. *Syn.* front power.
See power, effective; power, equivalent; vergence; vertex focal length.
magnification p. *See* magnification, spectacle.
magnifying p. *See* magnification, apparent.
nominal p. An estimate of the power of a lens, calculated as the sum of the front and back surface powers, i.e.

$$F = F_1 + F_2$$

Syn. approximate power.
See power, equivalent; power, surface.
prism p. The amount of deviation of a ray of light transmitted through a prism or lens (outside its optical centre). It is usually expressed in prism dioptres (Δ) and given by the following approximate formula for small angle prisms (in air)

$$P = 100(n - 1)a$$

where a is the prism angle in radians and n the index of refraction of the prism. *Example*: What is the power of a prism with an apex angle of 6° (1 radian = 57.3°) and a refractive index of 1.50? $P = 100(1.50 - 1)(6/57.3) = 5.24 \Delta$ which corresponds to the deviation of a ray of light equal to 5.24 cm at 100 cm. *Syn.* prismatic power.
See dioptre, prism; law, Prentice's.
prismatic p. *See* power, prism.
refractive p. The ability of a lens or an optical system to change the direction of a pencil of rays. It is equal to

$$F = n'/f' = -n/f$$

where n and n' are the refractive indices of the object and image space, respectively, f and f' the first and second focal length, respectively, in metres, and the power F is expressed in dioptres. *Symbol*: F. *Syn.* dioptric power; focal power; vergence power.
See paraxial equation, fundamental; power, equivalent; vergence.
resolving p. *See* resolution, limit of.

surface p. The dioptric power of a single refracting or reflecting surface. It is equal to (Table P6)

$$F = n' - n/r$$

where F is the power in dioptres, n and n' are the refractive indices of the media on each side of the surface and r is the radius of curvature of the lens or mirror surface in metres. This equation forms part of the fundamental paraxial equation. For a spectacle lens in air ($n = 1$) the power of the surface becomes (Table P8)

$$F = n' - 1/r$$

Examples: Power of the corneal surfaces.
(1) Anterior surface

$$F = \frac{1.376 - 1}{0.0078} = 48.21 \text{ D}$$

where the refractive index of the cornea is 1.376 and the surface has a radius of curvature of 7.8 mm.
(2) Posterior surface

$$F = \frac{1.336 - 1.376}{0.0067} = -5.97 \text{ D}$$

where the refractive indices of the aqueous humour and the cornea are 1.336 and 1.376, respectively, and the surface has a radius of curvature of 6.7 mm.
For a thin spectacle lens in air, the sum of the powers of the two surfaces $F_1 + F_2$ represents the total power of the lens and is equal to

$$F = F_1 + F_2 = (n-1)\left(\frac{1}{r_1} - \frac{1}{r_2}\right)$$

where n is the index of refraction of the lens and r_1 and r_2 the radii of curvature of its two surfaces. *See* **paraxial equation, fundamental.**
true p. *See* **power, equivalent.**

Table P8 Surface power of the anterior surface of the cornea (in dioptres) corresponding to various radii of curvature (in mm). Calculations were made using 1.376 as the index of refraction of the cornea.

Radius	Power	Radius	Power
6.80	55.29	7.80	48.20
7.00	53.71	7.85	47.90
7.10	52.96	7.90	47.59
7.20	52.22	7.95	47.30
7.30	51.51	8.00	47.00
7.40	50.81	8.10	46.42
7.50	50.13	8.20	45.85
7.55	49.80	8.30	45.30
7.60	49.47	8.40	44.76
7.65	49.15	8.50	44.23
7.70	48.83	8.60	43.72
7.75	48.52	8.80	42.73

vergence p. *See* paraxial equation, fundamental; power, refractive; vergence.
vertex p. *See* power, back vertex; power, front vertex.

precipitates, keratic *See* keratic precipitates.

precorneal film *See* tear film.

prednisolone *See* antiinflammatory drugs.

preferential looking *See* method, preferential looking.

prelens tear film *See* tear film, prelens.

Prentice's law; rule *See* law, Prentice's.

preocular tear film *See* tear film.

preretinal haemorrhage *See* haemorrhage, preretinal.

preretinal membrane *See* membrane, epiretinal.

presbyope A person who has presbyopia.

presbyopia A refractive condition in which the accommodative ability of the eye is insufficient for near vision work due to ageing. This is due to a hardening of the lens and a reduction of the elasticity of its capsule. The main symptom is blurred vision, or difficulty in sustaining clear vision, at the working distance. It is corrected by positive lenses (called the **addition**). This condition usually occurs when the amplitude of accommodation has decreased to 4 D. It generally occurs between the age of 42 and 48 in people living in European and North American countries. People living in hot climates become presbyopic earlier. *Syn.* old sight (colloquial).
See addition, near; capsule, crystalline lens; distance, reading; lens, hyperchromatic; lens, progressive; modulus of elasticity; monovision.

presbyopia, premature *See* accommodative insufficiency.

prescription A written formula for the preparation and administration of any treatment. At a minimum, medication prescriptions should include the name of the medication to be used, instructions for its usage and the amount of medication to be dispensed. A spectacle prescription may include a spherical component (often called the **spherical error** or the **sphere**), a cylindrical component (often called the **cylindrical error**) with its axis, a prismatic component, an addition for near vision and the interpupillary distance. *Example*: +3.00 D (−1.50 D × 90°) 1.5 ΔBI, OU add: +1.75 D, 64 mm. Prescriptions for contact lenses include very specific information regarding the lenses, besides the refraction adjusted for the corneal plane. The form and terminology nowadays usually conform to the recommendations of the International Standards Organization (Table P9).
See R$_x$.

preseptal cellulites *See* cellulitis, preseptal.

preservative agents *See* antiseptic.

press-on prism *See* prism, Fresnel Press-On.

pressure The force per unit area exerted by a gas or liquid in a direction perpendicular to

Table P9 Abbreviations commonly used in prescriptions

Abbreviation	Latin	Meaning
ac	ante cibum	before meals
ad lib	ad libitum	freely, as desired
agit. ante us	agita ante usum	shake before taking
alt hor	alternis horis	every other hour
bid	bis in die	use twice a day
c	cum	with
gtt	guttae	drops
od	omni die	every day
oh	omni hora	every hour
om	omni mane	every morning
on	omni nocte	every night
pc	post cibum	after eating
po	per os	by mouth
prn	pro re nata	use as needed
qd	quaque in die	use every day
qh	quaque hora	use every hour
qid	quater in die	use four times a day
ql	quantum libet	as much as desired
qqh	quaque quarta hora	every four hours
s	sine	without
sig	signa	label
soln	solutio	solution
tab	tabella	tablet
tid	ter in die	use three times a day
ung	unguentum	ointment

that surface. The SI unit of pressure is the pascal (Pa), although blood pressure and intraocular pressure remain specified in the non-SI unit millimetres of mercury (mmHg).
See **oxygen permeability.**

blood p. *See* **sphygmomanometer.**

equivalent oxygen p. *See* **oxygen pressure, equivalent.**

intraocular p. (IOP) The pressure within the eyeball occurring as a result of the constant formation and drainage of the aqueous humour. This is measured by means of a manometer. What is actually measured in the human eye is the **ocular tension** by means of a tonometer. This is an indirect measure of the IOP as it depends on the thickness and rigidity of the tunics of the eye besides the IOP. Both terms, intraocular pressure and ocular pressure, are commonly regarded as synonymous. Normal IOP is usually considered to be between 11 mmHg and 21 mmHg (average around 16 mmHg). However, there may be cases of glaucoma with lower IOP than 21 mmHg and there are also many normal cases with IOP greater than 21 mmHg. There is a slight increase in IOP with age (about 2 mmHg), in the morning as compared to the evening (about 3 to 4 mmHg), in the supine position as compared to the sitting position (about 3 to 4 mmHg) and a decrease during accommodation (about 4 mmHg).
See **aqueous humour; diurnal variations, in intraocular pressure; glaucoma; hypertension, ocular; hypotony, ocular; indentation, scleral; law, Imbert–Fick; pathway, uveoscleral; rigidity, ocular; test, differential intraocular pressure; test, provocative; tonometer.**

osmotic p. The pressure required to stop the movement of water through a semipermeable membrane (e.g. corneal endothelium) from one solution of a given concentration to another of a different concentration. When the concentration of the solution on both sides of the membrane is equal, i.e. at equilibrium, the pressure of water on both sides of the membrane will be equal to the osmotic pressure and the movement of water will stop. The more concentrated the solution, the greater the osmotic pressure.
See **osmosis; solution, hypertonic; solution, hypotonic; solution, isotonic.**

p. phosphene *See* **phosphene.**

pulse p. *See* **sphygmomanometer.**

pretectum Either of the midbrain structures located anterior to the superior colliculus. Each pretectum contains several nuclei including the pretectal olivary nucleus, the nucleus of the optic tract and the anterior, medial and posterior pretectal nuclei. A small number of retinal fibres leave the optic tract before the lateral geniculate bodies and synapse mainly in the pretectal olivary nucleus and in the nucleus of the optic tract. Axons from the pretectal olivary nucleus project to the Edinger–Westphal nuclei. Neurons in the pretectal olivary nuclei are involved in pupillary constriction.
See **nucleus, pretectal; reflex, pupil light; tectum of the mesencephalon.**

prevalence The number of people with a disease or condition in a given population at a specific time, either at a point in time (**point prevalence**) or over a period of time (**period prevalence**). *Example*: The prevalence of keratoconus in Olmsted County, Minnesota on the third of December 1982 was 54.5 per 100 000 population.
See **incidence.**

primary action; position; visual area *See* under the nouns.

primary visual cortex *See* **area, visual.**

Prince rule *See* **rule, Prince.**

principal direction *See* **line of direction.**

principal plane; points; ray *See* under the nouns.

prism A transparent body (e.g. plastic, glass) bounded by two inclined plane surfaces, which intersect in a straight line called the apex, and form an angle called the **prism angle**. The face opposite the apex is called the **base**. A prism is an optical element used to deviate light (towards the base of the prism). The angle of deviation d of a prism in air is given by the following formula

$$d = i + i' - a$$

where i is the angle of incidence, i' is the angle of emergence and a is the prism angle (all angles in degrees) (Fig. P17 and Table P10).
See adaptation, vergence; base setting; dioptre, prism; power, prism; prism, minimum deviation of a; prism, ophthalmic; spectacles, recumbent; spectroscope.
achromatic p. Prism that deviates light without dispersion. It consists of two prisms, usually one of crown glass and the other of flint, of equal angular dispersions and mounted so that the apex of one is against the base of the other.
p. adaptation *See* adaptation, vergence; test, prism adaptation.

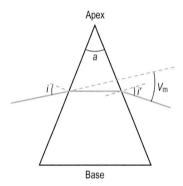

Apex

a

i i' V_m

Base

Fig. P17 Prism (a, prism angle; i, angle of incidence = i', angle of emergence; V_m, angle of minimum deviation).

aligning p. A term used to denote the prism power necessary to align the nonius markers of a fixation disparity test. It was formerly called *associated heterophoria*, but it is not strictly speaking a heterophoria because only part of the visual field of the test is dissociated while the rest of the field is fused (that fused area is often referred to as **fusion lock** or **binocular lock**). The dissociation of only part of the field is achieved by using either a method of cross-polarization (e.g. Mallet fixation disparity unit) or a septum (e.g. Turville infinity balance test). *Syn.* compensating prism.
See disparity, retinal; Disparometer; Mallett fixation disparity unit; test, Turville infinity balance.
p. ballast lens *See* ballast.
p. bar Clinical device consisting of a series of prisms of increasing strengths arranged in a convenient mount for rapid positioning in front of an eye. It can be used with the cover test or even to measure fusional responses when determining the zone of clear, single, binocular vision if rotary prisms are not available.
base-in p.; base-out p. *See* base setting.
bi-p. *See* Fresnel's bi-prism.
p. binoculars *See* binoculars.
compensating p. *See* prism, aligning; prism, relieving.
p. cover test *See* test, cover.
Crete's p. *See* prism, rotary.
p. dioptre *See* dioptre, prism.
dissociating p. A prism which, when placed in front of an eye, produces dissociation.
See dissociation.
double p. *See* Fresnel's bi-prism.
double p. test *See* test, double prism.
Dove p. An isosceles reflecting prism used to invert the image in an optical system. Light enters one side, is then refracted onto the base surface where it is internally reflected and refracted again through the other side.

Table P10 Approximate deviation of thin ophthalmic prisms of various apical angles and of two different refractive indices

Apical angle in degrees (°)	Deviation			
	Spectacle crown glass ($n = 1.523$)		Extra dense flint glass ($n = 1.70$)	
	Degrees (°)	Δ	Degrees (°)	Δ
1	0.52	0.91	0.70	1.22
2	1.05	1.84	1.40	2.45
3	1.57	2.75	2.10	3.67
4	2.09	3.66	2.80	4.90
5	2.61	4.57	3.50	6.12
6	3.14	5.49	4.20	7.35
7	3.66	6.40	4.90	8.57
8	4.18	7.31	5.60	9.80
9	4.71	8.24	6.30	11.02
10	5.23	9.15	7.00	12.25
11	5.75	10.06	7.70	13.47
12	6.28	10.99	8.40	14.70

erecting p. A prism designed to invert an image in an optical system with no change of size or shape. *Examples*: Dove prism, Porro prism. *Syn.* inverting prism.
See erector.
p. flippers *See* lens flippers.
Fresnel Press-On p. A trade name for a thin disc of transparent plastic consisting of one flat surface which can adhere to a clean lens surface when pressed in place, and another surface on which are incorporated small prismatic elements laid parallel to one another. Large optical effects can thus be provided in a much thinner and lighter form. These Press-On Fresnel prisms can be cut to any desired shape and are used commonly in orthoptics treatment.
See lens, Fresnel; orthoptics.
Herschel p. *See* prism, rotary.
induced p. Prismatic effect created when the patient's visual axis does not pass through the optical centre of an ophthalmic lens. The amount of prism power is given by Prentice's law.
See convergence, correction induced; law, Prentice's.
inverting p. *See* prism, erecting.
lacrimal p. *See* tear meniscus.
minimum deviation of a p. The deviation of light rays from their original path is minimum when light passes symmetrically through a prism so that the incident (i) and emergent (i') angles are equal (Fig. P17).
See angle of deviation; prism.
Nicol p. An optical device for producing a beam of plane polarized light. It is made from a piece of calcite crystal cut diagonally in half with the two halves cemented together. Incident light is split into ordinary and extraordinary linearly polarized rays in the prism; the ordinary ray reaches the interface and is totally reflected, while the extraordinary ray is transmitted (Fig. P18).
See analyser; birefringence; polarizer.
ophthalmic p. A prism used in the correction or in the measurement of a deviation of the eyes. The power of such a prism is usually only a few prism dioptres. The power of a thin prism in air, represented by the angle of deviation d, is given by the approximate formula

$$d = (n - 1)a$$

where n is the index of refraction of the prism and a the prism angle. *Example*: If the prism angle is equal to 10° and the index of refraction of the prism is 1.523, the deviation will be equal to 5.23° or 9.15 Δ. (Fig. P19).
See dioptre, prism; power, prism.
penta p. *See* Fig. P20.
polarizing p. A prism made from doubly refracting material. *Example*: quartz.
See analyzer; light, polarized; polarizer.
Porro p. A combination prism consisting of two 90° totally reflecting prisms arranged at right angles to each other. It is used in optical systems, such as binoculars, to invert the image and provide a shorter displacement. It is the most common erecting prism.
p. power *See* power, prism.

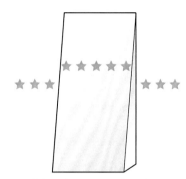

Fig. P19 A line of stars seen through a prism base down.

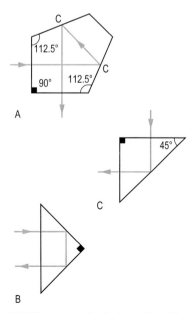

Fig. P20 Examples of reflecting prisms (A, penta prism, with surfaces C coated with silver or aluminium; B and C, in which the surfaces reflect light by total internal reflection).

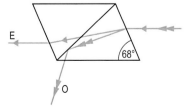

Fig. P18 Nicol prism (O, ordinary ray; E, extraordinary ray).

reflecting p. A prism in which light is internally reflected at one or more of the plane surfaces before emerging. This happens when the angle of incidence at the surface is greater than the critical angle (Fig. P20). *Syn.* total reflecting prism. *See* reflection, total.

p. reflex test *See* method, Krimsky's.

relieving p. An ophthalmic prism prescribed to relieve symptoms caused by an uncompensated heterophoria. *Syn.* compensating prism.

Risley p. *See* prism, rotary.

rotary p. A pair of identical thin prisms mounted one in front of the other, so that they can be rotated by equal amounts in opposite directions to give a resultant power in a single meridian. The power can vary from zero when the apex of one prism coincides with the base of the other to the sum of the powers of the two prisms when the apices coincide. The **Risley prism** is a very common type of rotary prism. It is used to determine the limits of the zone of clear, single, binocular vision and also in some stereoscopes (e.g. variable prism stereoscope). Other types of rotary prisms are those of Crete and Herschel. *Syn.* variable prism. *See* base setting; stereoscope, variable prism.

tear p. *See* tear meniscus.

total reflecting p. *See* prism, reflecting.

version p's. *See* prism, yoke.

Wollaston p. Two right-angle prisms of equal deviation made of a double refracting crystal such as quartz or calcite cemented together by their hypotenuse faces to form a rectangular unit. The optical axis of the crystal in one prism is perpendicular to that in the other prism and both axes are also perpendicular to the direction of the incident light. A beam of unpolarized light incident on a Wollaston prism will emerge as two diverging beams which are oppositely polarized and almost free of dispersion. This prism is used in some types of keratometers (e.g. Javal–Schiotz). *Syn.* Wollaston polarizer.

yoke p's. Two prisms, one in front of each eye, of equal deviation and direction (e.g. 2 ΔBU, OU). The apparent view moves towards the apex of the prisms. These are sometimes prescribed in the management of nystagmus, in visual training, for the bedridden (BD prisms) and, in some cases, of visual neglect and physical disability. (Fig. P21) *Note*: also spelt yoked prisms. *Syn.* version prisms. *See* base setting; neglect, visual.

prismatic effect, differential *See* effect, differential prismatic.

prismatic imbalance *See* effect, differential prismatic.

prismatic jump; power *See* under the nouns.

proband A person with a specific trait or disorder whose family is to be ascertained to evaluate the genetic transmission of that condition. *Syn.* index case; propositus. *See* neglect, visual; pedigree.

procaine hydrochloride A local anaesthetic of the amide type used in eye surgery. It is used in 1% to 10% solution and its action lasts for nearly 1 hour.

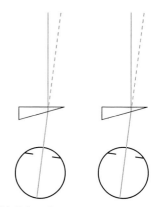

Fig. P21 Yoke prisms.

procedure A specific way of doing something. The term is commonly used for surgical operations. *See* method.

advancement p. *See* recession.

Faden p. A surgical procedure designed to weaken the action of an extraocular muscle by reattaching it to the globe posterior to its original insertion. By attaching the muscle to the eye at this point, the arc of contact of the muscle is changed, thus weakening the muscle in its field of action. The procedure can be used to treat dissociated vertical deviations, nystagmus, as well as cases of incomitant strabismus (e.g. Brown's superior oblique tendon sheath syndrome, Duane's syndrome). *Syn.* posterior fixation suture. *See* arc of contact; strabismus surgery.

frontalis sling p. A surgical intervention performed to correct ptosis, particularly severe ones, as well as the myopathic and neurogenic types. In this procedure, the upper tarsus is suspended from the frontalis muscle with a sling and adjusted accordingly. This procedure allows the patient to lift the eyelid by activating the frontalis muscle. It is also performed in the treatment of blepharophimosis syndrome. *Syn.* frontalis suspension procedure. *See* ptosis.

Harado-Ito p. *See* transposition.

Hummelsheim's p. *See* transposition.

Jensen p. *See* transposition.

Jones' p. A surgical intervention used to correct involutional entropion by folding the stretched or dehiscent lower lid retractor and reattaching it to the lower border of the tarsus, thus creating a pull on the lower eyelid, which is usually the eyelid affected. Wies' procedure is usually preferred. *See* procedure, Wies'.

Knapp p. *See* transposition.

tuck p. A strabismus surgical procedure in which a muscle or tendon is folded upon itself to effectively shorten and strengthen it. This procedure is commonly performed in cases of superior oblique paresis. It may also be used in cases of mild ptosis to shorten the levator palpebrae aponeurosis.

Wies' p. A surgical intervention to correct involutional entropion by splitting the lower lid (which is usually the affected lid) horizontally and inserting an everting suture resulting in scarring which prevents the upward movement of the preseptal portion of the orbicularis muscle.

prodrome A term indicating a precursor or an early sign or symptom of the onset of a disease. *Example*: A heightened sensitivity to light and sound may be the prodrome of a migraine attack.

prognosis The prediction of the probable course of a disease or visual anomaly based on all the relevant facts of the case.
See diagnosis; sign; test, prognostic.

progression *See* lens, progressive.

progressive myopia *See* myopia, pathological.

projection **1.** Localization of visual impressions from the eye to the apparent source of the stimulus, such as up and to the left. This is sometimes referred to as mental projection. **2.** A prominence. **3.** The imaging of an object onto a screen or a surface.
erroneous p. *See* projection, false.
false p. The false positioning in space of a visual sensation arising from a retinal image formed in an eye with paresis of an extraocular muscle. The visual sensation appears in the direction of normal action of the paretic muscle. *Example*: past-pointing. *Syn.* erroneous projection; malprojection. *See* pointing, past-.

projector An optical instrument that forms a magnified image of an object (e.g. a slide) onto a screen.

prolapse of the iris; of the lens *See* iris, prolapse of the; lens, prolapse of the.

proliferative retinopathy *See* retinopathy, proliferative.

prone test *See* test, provocative.

propamidine isethionate An antibiotic agent used topically in solution 0.1%, especially in the treatment of acanthamoeba keratitis. It is a member of the diamidine group of antibiotics. Although it may be used alone, it is most commonly used with polyhexamethylene biguanide, with neomycin or with chlorhexidine.

proparacaine hydrochloride *See* proxymetacaine hydrochloride.

prophylactic **1.** Preventing disease. **2.** An agent or a remedy that either prevents the development of a disease or prevents the worsening of a disease process.

propranolol *See* miotics.

proprioception Awareness of posture, balance or position due to the reception of stimuli, produced within the organism, which stimulate receptors (called **proprioceptors**) located within muscles, tendons, joints and the vestibular apparatus of the inner ear. The precise role of proprioception regarding the visual apparatus is uncertain.
See Table N1, p. 229; reflex, tonic neck.

proptosis Abnormal forward displacement of one eye. It is a sign of a severe orbital disorder, such as a tumour, inflammation, or thyroid eye disease. The condition may produce monocular diplopia. *See* cellulitis, orbital; disease, Graves'; exophthalmometer; exophthalmos; fistula, carotid-venous.

prosopagnosia Inability to recognize faces. It may be due to a lesion in one area of the inferotemporal (IT) cortex.
See agnosia.

prospective study *See* study, prospective

prostaglandin analogues Drugs used in the treatment of open-angle glaucoma or ocular hypertension. At specific dosages they lower the intraocular pressure (IOP), supposedly by increasing the outflow of aqueous humour via the uveoscleral pathway. Common agents include latanoprost, travoprost, bimatoprost (a synthetic prostamide structurally related to prostaglandin) and unoprostone isopropyl. Bimatoprost reduces IOP by increasing the uveoscleral outflow as well as the trabecular outflow.
See pathway, uveoscleral.

prosthesis, ocular *See* conjunctivitis, giant papillary; eye, artificial; lens, intraocular; ocularist.

protan Person who has either protanopia or protanomaly.

protanomal Person who has protanomaly.

protanomaly A type of anomalous trichromatism in which an abnormally high proportion of the red primary stimulus is needed when mixing red and green to match a given yellow. This is due to the fact that the luminosity function of a protanomal is reduced for the red radiations. The condition occurs in about 1% and 0.03% of the male and female population, respectively. *Syn.* protanomalous trichromatism; protanomalous vision; red-weakness.
See anomaloscope; colour vision, defective; plates, pseudoisochromatic; trichromatism.

protanope Person who has protanopia.

protanopia Type of dichromatism in which only two hues are seen: below 493 nm, all radiations appear bluish, whereas above it, they all appear yellowish. Around 493 nm is the neutral point. The luminosity function of protanopes is significantly decreased for red radiations (for which he or she is almost blind). The condition occurs in about 1.1% and 0.01% of the male and female population, respectively. *Syn.* red blindness.
See colour vision, defective; dichromatism; plates, pseudoisochromatic; point, neutral; sensitivity, spectral.

protective lens *See* lens, plastic.

protein Complex organic molecule composed of various combinations of any of 20 α-amino acids linked in a genetically controlled linear sequence into one or more peptide chains. Proteins are the product of gene activity occurring according to the DNA code that specifies the sequence of amino acids. Proteins are present in every living cell and

form an essential constituent of cells. They are essential in many functions, such as growth and repair of tissue, transport of molecules throughout the body (e.g. haemoglobin to carry oxygen), as enzymes to catalyse biochemical reactions, immunological responses, muscle contraction (with actin and myosin), signalling (e.g. insulin which transmits a signal from a cell where it is synthesized to other cells in other tissues) or as antibodies by binding to target receptors. Many of the 20 amino acids are produced by the body. However, nine of these have to be obtained in food.
See **DNA**.

protein removal *See* **enzyme**.

proteomics The study of proteins expressed by the genes of a particular cell, tissue or organism, especially their structures, functions and interactions, using the technologies of large-scale protein separation and identification. *Example*: the use of proteomics to study cellular protein expression in ocular tissues during eye growth in myopic and normal eyes.

prothesis *See* **eye, artificial**.

protractor **1.** Instrument used to measure or set out angles on paper. **2.** A scale containing a circle graduated in degrees and a set of axes emerging from the centre of the circle used to set the axis of an astigmatic ophthalmic lens. It also includes various other scales for positioning the optical centre of lenses.

provocative test *See* **test, provocative**.

proximal Nearest to a central point.
See **distal**.

proximal convergence *See* **convergence, proximal**.

proxymetacaine hydrochloride A topical anaesthetic, commonly used in 0.5% solution. It has a greater potency than tetracaine hydrochloride (amethocaine hydrochloride) and causes less stinging and squeezing of the eyes when instilled. *Syn.* proparacaine hydrochloride.

pseudo- Prefix meaning false or spurious (e.g. pseudochalazion, pseudoglaucoma, pseudopapilloedema, etc.).

pseudoaccommodation The attainment of functional near vision in an emmetropic or distance-corrected eye without changing the refractive power of the eye. It may occur when the pupil is very small thus increasing the depth of field, in a presbyopic eye corrected with a progressive addition lens, in a pseudophakic eye corrected with a multifocal intraocular lens implant (IOL) or occasionally as a result of spherical aberration or astigmatism induced by corneal incisions made to insert an IOL.

pseudoaphakia A congenital condition in which the crystalline lens has degenerated and been replaced by mesodermal tissue.

pseudoesotropia *See* **epicanthus**.

pseudoexfoliation Deposition of greyish-white, fibrillary, amyloid-like material on the anterior lens capsule, the iris and the ciliary processes with free-floating particles in the anterior chamber. It occurs mainly in people over the age of about 50 years. It often gives rise to secondary glaucoma (**pseudoexfoliation glaucoma**). The origin of the pseudoexfoliative material is believed to be secondary to an abnormal basement membrane, produced by ageing epithelial cells in the eye, as well as in the skin and visceral organs.
See **glaucoma, pseudoexfoliation; syndrome, pseudoexfoliation**.

pseudo-von Graefe sign *See* **aberrant regeneration**.

pseudohemianopia *See* **phenomenon, extinction**.

pseudoisochromatic plates *See* **plates, pseudoisochromatic**.

pseudomembrane A type of inflammatory response characterized by the production of mucus, which adheres to the adjacent conjunctiva. This differs from a true membrane in that the latter is firmly attached to the conjunctival surface and is composed of dead cells and debris.

pseudomyopia *See* **accommodation, spasm of**.

pseudopapilloedema A non-specific term used to describe those conditions in which the optic disc is elevated resembling papilloedema. All have normal intraocular pressure. They include optic disc drusen, small discs in hyperopia greater than 4 D, hyaloid remnant, myelinated nerve fibres, optic neuropathies and papillitis. It is usually bilateral and, unlike true papilloedema, there is no haemorrhage, the margins of the disc are relatively sharp and spontaneous venous pulsation is usually present.
See **papilloedema**.

pseudophakia A condition in which an aphakic eye has been fitted with an intraocular lens to replace the crystalline lens.
See **eye, pseudophakic**.

pseudopsia A visual defect in which objects are seen although they are not present in the field of view (e.g. visual hallucinations) or objects appear distorted (e.g. illusions).

pseudopterygium A fold of conjunctiva that has become attached to the cornea as a result of injury or ulcer near the limbus. Hard contact lens wear has occasionally given rise to pseudopterygium; refitting with soft contact lenses may then be indicated. In the case of pseudopterygium, a probe can be passed beneath it near the limbus, whereas this is impossible in true pterygium.

pseudoptosis A condition resembling ptosis, due to abnormalities other than those found in the eyelid elevator muscles. Causes include blepharophimosis, abnormal looseness of the upper lid as commonly occurs in the elderly (dermatochalasis), ipsilateral hypotropia, phthisis bulbi, microphthalmos, a decrease in orbital volume as in enophthalmos or contralateral lid retraction or after a patient has adapted to an artificial eye, and comparing both eyes. *Syn.* apparent ptosis. *See* ptosis; syndrome, blepharophimosis.

pseudosclerosis of Westphal *See* disease, Wilson's.

pseudoscope An instrument which, by means of prisms or mirrors, transposes to one eye the image seen normally by the other eye. Thus the sense of depth is reversed and peaks are seen as troughs and vice versa (Fig. P22).

pseudostrabismus *See* strabismus, apparent.

pseudotrichiasis A condition in which the eyelashes started in the normal position but have become directed towards the globe due to entropion. Management consists mainly of correcting the entropion.
See entropion; trichiasis.

pseudotumour, orbital *See* syndrome, orbital inflammatory.

pseudoxanthoma elasticum An inherited autosomal recessive disorder caused by mutation in the ABCC6 gene (in the majority of cases). It results in fragmentation and mineralization of elastic fibres in the skin and in Bruch's membrane of the choroid presenting orange looking lesions (called 'peau d'orange') in the fundus, which eventually cracks to form angioid streaks and choroidal vascularization.
See angioid streaks.

psychophysics Branch of science that deals with the relationship between the physical stimuli and the sensory response. The measurements of thresholds (e.g. visual acuity, dark adaptation) or matching of stimuli (as in the spectral luminous efficiency curve) are examples of psychophysics. *See* optometry, experimental.

pterygium A triangular fold of bulbar conjunctiva located in the interpalpebral fissure, with its apex advancing progressively towards the cornea, usually from the nasal side and which contains visible blood vessels. A pinguecula often precedes its development. It is considered to be due to a degenerative process caused by recurrent dryness or irritation from wind and dust or prolonged exposure to sunlight, especially UV and resembles pinguecula histologically in showing elastotic degeneration of vascularized collagen. It becomes more prevalent with age. Symptoms are usually absent unless the pterygium encroaches on the cornea and vision may then be affected: surgical intervention is then necessary. Some pterygia tend to recur after excision. UV absorptive lenses may help decrease the incidence (Fig. P23).
See dellen; dyskeratosis; line, Stocker's; pinguecula; pseudopterygium.

ptosis Drooping of the upper eyelid causing a narrowing of the palpebral aperture. It is often divided into two main types: congenital and acquired. The **congenital** type present at birth is usually the result of weakness of the levator palpebrae superioris or superior rectus muscle, or associated with the blepharophimosis syndrome or the Marcus Gunn jaw-winking syndrome. Management is usually carried out in the young child and consists of levator resection. The **acquired** type may result from any affection of the nerve supply of the upper eyelid musculature, i.e. from the third (or oculomotor) nerve or associated with Horner's syndrome (**neurogenic ptosis**), from a disease of the muscles themselves (e.g. myasthenia gravis, called **myasthenic ptosis**) or from mechanical interference in elevating the eyelid due to the weight of a tumour, trauma or severe oedema of the upper lid (**mechanical ptosis**). The correction is usually surgical. Sometimes a **ptosis crutch**, which is attached to the spectacles and elevates the eyelid, may be useful. There are also special contact lenses designed to support the upper eyelid (Fig. P24). *Syn.* blepharoptosis.
See ataxia, hereditary spinal; epicanthus inversus; phenomenon, jaw-winking; procedure, frontalis sling; procedure, tuck; pseudoptosis; sign, Cogan's lid twitch; spectacles, orthopaedic; syndrome, Horner's.
acquired aponeurotic p. See ptosis, involutional.
p. adiposa See dermatochalasis.
apparent p. See pseudoptosis.
involutional p. A ptosis caused by dehiscence, disinsertion or stretching of the aponeurosis of the levator palpebrae superioris muscle, which appears most commonly in the elderly. This is the most common form of acquired ptosis. It may also occur after ocular surgery or trauma. It presents usually bilaterally, with a high upper lid crease (except in severe cases when it is

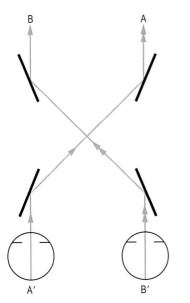

Fig. P22 Optical principle of a pseudoscope.

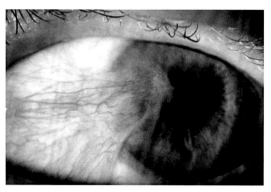

Fig. P23 Advanced case of pterygium. (From Kanski 2003, with permission of Butterworth-Heinemann)

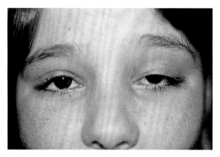

Fig. P24 Congenital ptosis. (From Kanski 2007, with permission of Butterworth-Heinemann)

absent) and a deep superior palpebral sulcus. Treatment includes levator muscle advancement. *Syn.* acquired aponeurotic ptosis.
See advancement.
neurogenic p. See ptosis.

pucker, macular *See* fibrosis, preretinal macular.

Pulfrich refractometer; stereophenomenon *See* under the nouns.

Pulsair non-contact tonometer *See* tonometer, non-contact.

pulvinar The prominence of the posterior portion of the thalamus overlapping the superior colliculus. It receives projections from the auditory, somatosensory and visual cortex regions. It is involved in visual attention, suppression of irrelevant stimuli and utilizing information to initiate eye movements.

punctal occlusion *See* occlusion, punctal.

punctal stenosis Obstruction of the lacrimal punctum, which is either idiopathic or secondary to chronic blepharitis or consequent to punctal eversion.

punctate epithelial keratitis *See* keratitis, punctate epithelial.

punctum caecum *See* spot, blind.

punctum lacrimale *See* lacrimal punctum.

punctum luteum *See* macula lutea.

punctum proximum *See* accommodation, near point of.

punctum remotum *See* accommodation, far point of.

pupil Aperture within the iris, normally circular, through which light penetrates into the eye. It is located slightly nasally to the centre of the iris. Its diameter can vary from about 2 to 8 mm. It is typically slightly smaller in old age. The function of the pupil is to regulate the amount of light admitted into the eye, to optimize the depth of focus and to mitigate ocular aberrations.
See acorea; anisocoria; corectopia; dicoria; dyscoria; hippus; iridectomy; microcoria; miosis; muscle, dilator pupillae; muscle, sphincter pupillae; mydriasis; nucleus, Edinger–Westphal; polycoria; polyopia; reflex, pupil light.
Adie's p. A pupil in which the reactions to light, direct or consensual, are almost abolished, with a reaction occurring only after prolonged exposure to light or dark. The reaction of the pupil to a near target is also delayed and slow. The condition is usually unilateral, with the affected pupil being the larger of the two (anisocoria). It is due to an abnormal parasympathetic supply from the ciliary ganglion or the short ciliary nerves to the sphincter pupillae muscle of the iris and to the ciliary muscle, possibly as a result of a viral illness which has caused a denervation. The pupil is larger than in the unaffected eye. If the condition is bilateral, the cause may be syphilis. The condition is typically associated with the Holmes-Adie syndrome. Reading spectacles help as well as dark lenses or low-dose concentration of a parasympathomimetic drug (e.g. pilocarpine) may be used to mitigate photophobia incurred with a large pupil (Table P11). *Syn.* myotonic pupil; pupillotonia; tonic pupil (some authors use this last term when the cause is known and Adie's pupil when the cause is unidentified).
See **pupillary defect, efferent; syndrome, Holmes-Adie; reflex, pupil light.**
amaurotic p. Miotic pupil that does not react to direct and consensual ipsilateral light stimulation, but does react consensually to contralateral

Table P11   Examples of pupil abnormality

Defect	Appearance	Light response*	Consensual light response*	Near response
Adie's pupil	large	impaired	impaired	slow
Argyll Robertson	both pupils small, unequal + irregular	almost abolished	almost abolished	normal
blindness in one eye	normal	abolished	abolished	normal
Horner's syndrome	small + ptosis	normal	normal	normal
Hutchinson's pupil	large	abolished	abolished	abolished
optic neuritis	normal/large	impaired	impaired	normal
3rd nerve paralysis†	large + ptosis	abolished	abolished	abolished

*To stimulation of the affected eye
†When caused by an aneurysm of the posterior communicating artery

stimulation. It results from a complete optic nerve lesion. The diseased eye is blind, both pupils are equal in size and the near reflex is normal. *Syn.* absolute afferent pupillary defect.
See **pupil, Marcus Gunn.**
apparent p. See **pupil entrance p. of the eye.**
Argyll Robertson p. Pupil that reacts when the eye accommodates and converges but fails to react directly and consensually to light. The condition is bilateral, and the pupils are small and usually unequal. It is usually a sign of neurosyphilis (Table P11).
See **iridoplegia; tabes dorsalis.**
artificial p. 1. Pupil made by iridectomy. 2. A circular aperture made in a diaphragm which can be mounted in front of the eye to provide a constant and smaller pupil size. It is used in research but also as a clinical test.
See **disc, pinhole.**
p. block See **pupillary block.**
p. constriction See **miosis; reflex, pupil light.**
p. dilatation See **mydriatic; reflex, pupil light.**
ectopic p. See **corectopia.**
entrance p. of the eye This is the image of the iris aperture formed by the cornea. It is what one sees when one looks at an eye. It is some 13% larger than the real pupil and located slightly in front of it. *Syn.* apparent pupil (Fig. P25).
exit p. of the eye This is the image of the iris aperture formed by the crystalline lens. It is slightly larger (about 3%) than the real pupil and situated slightly behind it (Fig. P25).
Horner's p. See **syndrome, Horner's.**
Hutchinson's p. A pupil that is dilated and completely inactive to all stimuli. It is associated with lesions of the central nervous system, as may occur in head injury (Table P11).
keyhole p. A pupil shaped like a keyhole due to iridectomy in which a section of the iris extending from the pupillary margin to the periphery has been excised, or due to coloboma or trauma to the iris.
p. light reflex See **reflex, pupil light.**
Marcus Gunn p. A defect of the pupillary reflex characterized by a smaller constriction of both pupils when the affected eye is stimulated by

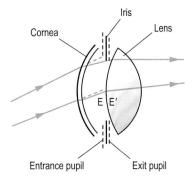

Fig. P25 The entrance and exit pupils of the eye. E and E′ are the centres of the entrance and exit pupils, respectively (diagram not to scale). (After Atchison et al 2000, with permission of Butterworth-Heinemann)

light as compared to that occurring when the normal eye is stimulated. It is easier, however, to observe this phenomenon when swinging a light from one eye to the other in a darkened room while the subject is fixating a distant object (this is called the **swinging flashlight test**) (Fig. P26). Stimulation of the normal eye will cause constriction of both pupils whereas rapid stimulation of the affected eye will lead to a small dilatation (a paradoxical reaction, sometimes referred to as **pupillary escape**). This condition is due to a lesion in one retina or in one of the optic nerves, optic chiasma, optic tract or the pretectal olivary nucleus that affects the afferent pupillary pathway. It is often the result of central or branch retinal or vein occlusion, extensive retinal detachment, retrobulbar optic neuritis, compressive optic neuropathy or optic tract lesion, etc. *Syn.* relative afferent pupillary defect.
See **pupil, amaurotic.**
myotonic p. See **pupil, Adie's.**
p. reflex See **reflex, pupil.**
tonic p. See **pupil, Adie's.**
white p. See **leukocoria.**

pupillae ectopia *See* **corectopia.**

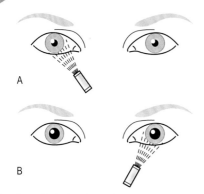

A

B

Fig. P26 Swinging flashlight test performed in a darkened room. A, stimulation of the normal eye results in bilateral pupil constriction. B, stimulation of the affected eye results in a small bilateral dilatation.

pupillae muscle, dilator *See* muscle, dilator pupillae.

pupillary axis *See* axis, pupillary.

pupillary block A blockage of the normal flow of aqueous humour from the posterior to the anterior chamber of the eye. It may be caused by a posterior annular synechia occurring during anterior uveitis, by luxation of the lens anteriorly occluding the pupil or by adhesion of the iris to the vitreous or to the posterior capsule following extracapsular cataract extraction (called **aphakic pupillary block**). It may produce an attack of acute angle-closure glaucoma as the iris may be pushed forward blocking the drainage angle. *Syn.* pupil block.
See iris bombé; seclusion pupillae.

pupillary defect, afferent *See* pupil, Marcus Gunn.

pupillary defect, efferent A defect of the pupillary reflex caused by a lesion along the pathway of either the parasympathetic supply from the Edinger–Westphal nucleus to the sphincter pupillae muscle of the iris (Adie's pupil) or the ocular sympathetic supply from the ciliospinal centre to the dilator pupillae muscle of the iris (Horner's syndrome). The main sign of efferent pupillary defect is non-physiological anisocoria.
See pupil. Marcus Gunn; reflex, pupil light; syndrome, Horner's.

pupillary defect, relative afferent; escape *See* pupil, Marcus Gunn.

pupillary membrane *See* membrane, pupillary.

pupillary reflex *See* reflex, pupil light.

pupillometer 1. Instrument for measuring the diameter of the pupil. There exist several types, but the most common is a series of graduated filled circles whose sizes are compared with the pupil (**Haab's pupillometer**). It is also common to measure pupil size by photography or video after appropriate calibration of the method

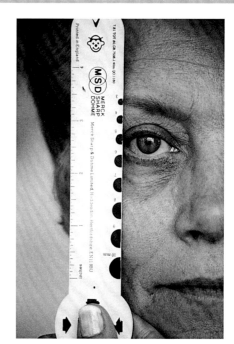

Fig. P27 Typical pupillometer.

(Fig. P27). *Syn.* coreometer. **2.** Although incorrectly used, it refers to an instrument for measuring the interpupillary distance (PD). These instruments are based either on using the pupil centres or the corneal reflections, but the latter can be used on the basis of the pupil centres as well. In the instruments using corneal reflections the subject views the image of a small illuminated target surrounding the observation aperture used by the examiner or made to appear as if it came from the observer's eye. That image is formed at infinity by a lens placed in front of the subject's eyes. The examiner moves a hair line to coincide with the centre of the corneal reflections and reads the monocular and total interpupillary distances. *Syn.* interpupillometer (this is the most appropriate term for this instrument); PD gauge; PD meter.
See rule, PD.

pupillometer, Broca's A subjective instrument for measuring the diameter of the pupil. It consists of a pair of very small light sources placed at the anterior focal plane of the eye. The two sources are separated until the circular out-of-focus images on the retina are seen in juxtaposition. The distance between the two sources represents the diameter of the pupil.

pupilloscope Instrument for observing the pupil.

pupillotonia *See* pupil, Adie's.

purity *See* colorimetric purity; saturation.

Purkinje after-image *See* after-image; Bidwell's ghost.

Purkinje cell *See* cell, Purkinje.

Purkinje figures; shadows *See* angioscotoma.

Purkinje shift Reduction in the luminosity of a red light relative to that of a blue light when the luminances are reduced from photopic to scotopic levels of illumination. This is due to the shift of the spectral sensitivity curve from a maximum at 555 nm to 507 nm when passing from light to dark adaptation. *Syn.* Purkinje's phenomenon. *See* interval, photochromatic; theory, duplicity.

Purkinje tree *See* angioscotoma.

Purkinje–Sanson images *See* image, Purkinje–Sanson.

purple A mixture, in suitable proportions, of short-wave radiations (less than 400 nm) and long-wave radiations (greater than 700 nm). It is a complementary colour to yellow-green. Purples are colour stimuli represented on the chromaticity diagram by the straight line joining the ends of the spectrum locus. *Syn.* non-spectral colour; non-spectral purple. *See* chromaticity diagram.

pursuit movement *See* movement, pursuit.

push-up *See* method, push-up; test, push-up.

p value *See* significance.

Q

quadrantanopia A loss of vision in a quarter of the visual field. The defect is usually bilateral as it is typically caused by a lesion past the optic chiasma. It may be homonymous (binasal, bitemporal, upper or lower), crossed (one upper and the other lower), congruous (equal size of the defects) or incongruous (unequal size of the defects). *Syn.* quadrantanopsia; quadrantic anopsia; quadrantic hemianopia. *See* gland, pituitary; hemianopia.

quadrantanopia, inferior An inferior homonymous loss of vision in two quarters due to a lesion of the superior fibres of the optic radiations in the parietal lobe on the contralateral side of the visual pathway. *Syn.* 'pie on the floor' defect.

quadrantanopia, superior A superior homonymous loss of vision in two quarters due to a lesion of the most anterior and inferior fibres of the optic radiations in the temporal lobe involving Meyer's loop, on the contralateral side of the visual pathway (Fig. Q1). *Syn.* 'pie in the sky' defect. *See* loop, Meyer's; radiations, optic.

quadrigemina, corpora *See* colliculi.

quantity of light *See* light, quantity of.

quantum *See* photon.

quantum theory *See* theory, quantum.

Fig. Q1 Complete, right, superior homonymous quadrantanopia due to a lesion of the optic radiations in the left temporal lobe.

quartz A silicon dioxide (SiO_2) material which is transparent to visible and ultraviolet light and can produce polarized light. *See* light, polarized; prism, Wollaston.

quinine amblyopia *See* amblyopia.

quinolones A class of broad-spectrum antibacterial drugs of which the main ophthalmic agents are **ciprofloxacin** and **ofloxacin**. They are used topically in 0.3% solution. They are effective against the majority of gram-negative pathogens, including *Haemophilus, Neisseria gonorrhoeae, Chlamydia trachomatis, Pseudomonas aeruginosa* (especially ciprofloxacin), staphylococci and streptococci. They are used in the treatment of conjunctivitis, blepharitis, keratoconjunctivitis and corneal ulcers.

See antibiotic.

R

radiant energy Effect of electromagnetic waves considered with regard to their physical properties and not as to their effects on the eye. The SI unit of measurement is the joule. *See* photon; radiometry; SI unit.

radiant flux Power emitted in the form of radiation. The SI unit of measurement is the watt. The corresponding photometric quantity is luminous flux. *See* luminous flux; radiant energy; SI unit.

radiation 1. Emission or transfer of energy expressed in the form of electromagnetic waves or particles. 2. A group of nerve fibres that diverge in all directions from a point of origin. *Example*: the optic radiations.
See spectrum, electromagnetic.

radiation, black body The radiation emitted by a heated black body.
See body, black; colour temperature.

radiations, optic The part of the visual pathway which consists of axons arising in the lateral geniculate body and terminating in a fan-shaped manner in the visual area of the occipital lobe. As they emerge from the lateral geniculate body, the inferior fibres loop forward in the temporal lobe before swinging back towards the occipital cortex. These fibres form what is called **Meyer's loop** (**Archambault's loop**). They receive impulses from the inferior retinal quadrants (corresponding to the superior aspect of the contralateral visual field) and terminate on the inferior lip of the calcarine fissure. *Syn.* optic radiations of Gratiolet; geniculocalcarine pathway; geniculostriate pathway.
See test, optokinetic nystagmus.

radiology A science dealing with techniques that use radiant energy (e.g. X-rays) for diagnosis and therapy.
See angiography, fluorescein; magnetic resonance imaging; tomography, computed.

radiometry The measurement of radiant energy irrespective of its effect on vision.
See radiant energy; photometry.

radiotherapy, plaque A form of therapy used to treat intraocular tumours such as uveal melanoma and particularly choroidal melanoma, retinoblastoma and choroidal haemangioma. It consists of radioactive seeds (most often using iodine-125) or a ruthenium-106 isotope film attached within a gold or steel carrier shaped like a bowl called a plaque, which is sewn in place to the outer surface of the eye near the tumour. This procedure provides localized concentrated radiotherapy. It has been shown to be very effective. The dose of radiation depends upon various factors including the length of time exposure (no more than 7 days), *Syn.* brachytherapy; plaque brachytherapy.
See melanoma, choroidal.

radiuscope Instrument used for measuring the radius of curvature of the surfaces of a contact lens. It is based on the Drysdale method. *Syn.* optical microspherometer.
See method, Drysdale's; Toposcope.

Raman effect *See* effect, Raman.

rami oculares Small bundle of parasympathetic fibres emerging from the ciliary ganglion. They continue along, but separate from, the short ciliary nerves and terminate in the choroid.

Ramsden eyepiece *See* eyepiece, Ramsden.

ramus communicans *See* ganglion, ciliary; nerve, ophthalmic.

random-dot stereogram; random-dot E test *See* stereogram, random-dot.

randomized controlled trial *See* trial, randomized controlled.

range of accommodation *See* accommodation, range of.

range of visible luminances The human visual system can operate over a large range of luminances from bright sunlight with a luminance of about 10^4 cd/mm^2 to the absolute threshold of around 10^{-6} cd/mm^2, a range of about 10 log units (10,000,000,000 : 1).
See luminance; vision, photopic; vision, scotopic.

ranibizumab *See* anti-VEGF drugs; macular degeneration, age-related; retinopathy, diabetic.

raphe, retinal *See* retinal raphe.

ratio, Arden *See* electrooculogram.

ratio, AV The ratio of the diameter of the retinal arteries to that of the retinal veins. It is usually around two-thirds. Deviations from this value may indicate a vascular disease (e.g. hypertension).
See arteriosclerosis; AV crossing; retinopathy, hypertensive.

ratio, cup-disc *See* cup-disc ratio.

Raubitschek chart *See* chart, Raubitschek.

ray In geometrical optics, a straight line representing the direction of propagation of light.
axial r. A ray that is coincident with the axis of an optical system.
chief r. Ray joining an object point to the centre of the entrance pupil of an optical system (Fig. R1). *See* light, pencil of.
emergent r. A ray of light in image space either after reflection (**reflected ray**) or after refraction (**refracted ray**).
extraordinary r. A ray which does not obey Snell's law of refraction in passing through a birefringent medium.
See birefringence.
incident r. Ray of light in object space that strikes a reflecting or refracting surface.
marginal r. Ray joining the axial point of an object to the edge or margin of an aperture or pupil (Fig. R1).
ordinary r. A ray which obeys Snell's law of refraction in passing through a birefringent medium.
See birefringence.

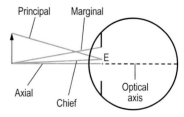

Fig. R1 Rays of light incident to the eye (E, centre of the entrance pupil of the eye).

Table R1 Differences between the sine and the tangent values of various angles (in degrees and radians). The error is calculated between the sine value and the value in radians and between the value in radians and the tangent value.

Angle (deg)	Angle (rad)	Sine value	Tangent value	Error (%) sine error	Error (%) tangent error
0.5	0.008 727	0.008 727	0.008 727	0.00	0.00
1	0.017 453	0.017 452	0.017 455	0.01	0.01
2	0.034 907	0.034 899	0.034 921	0.02	0.04
3	0.052 360	0.052 336	0.052 408	0.05	0.09
4	0.069 813	0.069 756	0.069 927	0.08	0.16
5	0.087 266	0.087 156	0.087 489	0.13	0.25
6	0.104 720	0.104 528	0.105 104	0.18	0.37
7	0.122 173	0.121 869	0.122 785	0.25	0.50
8	0.139 626	0.139 173	0.140 541	0.33	0.65
10	0.174 533	0.173 648	0.176 327	0.51	1.03
15	0.261 799	0.258 819	0.267 949	1.15	2.35
20	0.349 066	0.342 020	0.363 970	2.06	4.27
30	0.523 599	0.500 000	0.577 350	4.72	10.27

paraxial r. Light ray that forms an angle of incidence so small that its value in radians is almost equal to its sine or its tangent. (i.e. sin θ = θ or tan θ = θ). These are approximate expressions referred to as the **paraxial approximation** (or the **gaussian approximation**) (Table R1). *See* **optics, paraxial; paraxial region; theory, gaussian.**

principal r. Ray joining the extreme off-axis object point to the centre of the entrance pupil or aperture (Fig. R1).

r. tracing Technique used in optical computation consisting of tracing the paths of light rays through an optical system by graphical methods or by using formulae. Nowadays, computer methods are used. *See* **sign convention.**

Rayleigh criterion *See* **criterion, Rayleigh.**

Rayleigh equation A colour equation representing a match of yellow (usually 589 nm) with a mixture of red (usually 670 nm) and green (usually 535 nm). It is used to differentiate certain types of colour deficiencies. The anomaloscope is built on this principle. *See* **anomaloscope; colour vision, defective.**

Rayleigh scattering *See* **scattering, Rayleigh.**

reaction time The time interval between the onset of a stimulus and the response of a subject. Visual stimulations with a flash of light give rise to reaction times varying between 130 and 180 ms. This figure increases significantly with age.

reactive oxygen species *See* **oxidative stress.**

reading The act of viewing and interpreting letters, words, sentences, etc. It consists of a pattern of eye movements. The eyes proceed along a line in a series of step-like **saccades**, separated by **fixation pauses** during which information from the text is acquired. The amount of reading matter correctly identified during the fixation pause is called the **span of recognition** or the **perceptual span**. Most saccades are made from left to right, but some occur in the opposite direction (called **regression**) to return to text recently read but not yet fully perceived. At the end of the line, the eyes make a return sweep to the next line of text (Fig. R2). *See* **movement, saccadic eye; test, developmental eye movement.**

reading addition *See* **addition, near;** Table R3, p. 305.

reading distance; lens *See* under the nouns.

reading portion *See* **segment of a bifocal lens.**

reading slit *See* **typoscope.**

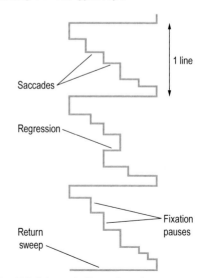

Fig. R2 Schematic illustration of eye movements during reading. Horizontal lines represent eye movements and vertical lines fixation pauses.

receptive field *See* field, receptive.

receptor *See* photoreceptor.

recession A surgical procedure used in strabismus in which an extraocular muscle is removed from its insertion and repositioned elsewhere on the globe posteriorly to weaken and slacken it. *See* advancement; resection; strabismus surgery.

recessive inheritance *See* inheritance.

reciprocal innervation *See* law of reciprocal innervation, Sherrington's.

reciprocal metre *See* curvature of a surface.

reciprocity, law of *See* law, Bunsen–Roscoe.

von Recklinghausen's disease *See* neurofibromatosis type 1.

recovery point *See* point, recovery.

rectus muscles *See* Table M6, p. 220.

recumbent spectacles *See* spectacles, recumbent.

recurrent corneal erosion *See* corneal erosion, recurrent.

red One of the hues of the visible spectrum evoked by stimulation of the retina by wavelengths beyond 630 nm. The complementary colours to red are blue-green (between 490.4 and 492.4 nm).

red blindness *See* protanopia.

red-free ophthalmoscopy *See* ophthalmoscopy, red-free.

red glass test *See* test, red glass.

red reflex *See* reflex, fundus.

red-green colour deficiency A general term indicating a colour vision deficiency, which is either of the deutan (green colour vision defect) or of the protan (red colour vision defect) type. These defects are mostly hereditary and affect both eyes equally. Most cases are inherited in X-linked recessive manner. *See* colour vision, defective; rule, Kollner's.

reduced eye *See* eye, reduced.

refixation reflex *See* reflex, refixation.

reflectance A measure of reflection equal to the ratio of reflected luminous flux Φ' to the incident luminous flux Φ, i.e. $\rho = \Phi'/\Phi$. *Syn.* reflection factor. *See* Fresnel's formula.

reflecting prism; telescope *See* under the nouns.

reflection Return or bending of light by a surface such that it continues to travel in the same medium.
　angle of r. *See* angle of reflection.
　diffuse r. Reflection from a surface that is not polished and light is reflected in many or all directions (Fig. R3). *Syn.* irregular reflection. *See* diffusion; glossmeter; matt surface.
　direct r. *See* reflection, specular.
　r. factor *See* reflectance.
　irregular r. *See* reflection, diffuse.
　law of r. *See* law of reflection.
　mixed r. The simultaneous occurrence of diffuse and specular reflection.

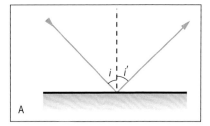
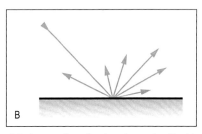

Fig. R3 A, specular reflection; the angle of incidence *i* is equal to the angle of reflection *i'*. B, diffuse reflection.

　regular r. *See* reflection, specular.
　specular r. Reflection from a polished surface in which there is no scattering and light travels back in a definite direction (Fig. R3). *Syn.* direct reflection; regular reflection. *See* microscope, specular.
　surface r. Light reflected at a surface according to Fresnel's formula.
　total r. Reflection occurring when light is incident at an angle greater than the critical angle. *Syn.* total internal reflection. *See* angle, critical; prism, reflecting.
　total internal r. *See* reflection, total.

reflector Any device that reflects light (e.g. glass-plate, prism, mirror).

reflex 1. Involuntary response to a stimulus. 2. Reflection or an image formed by reflection (e.g. corneal reflex).
　accommodative r. *See* accommodation, reflex; reflex, near.
　r. arc *See* reflex, pupil light.
　blinking r. Blinking in response to various stimulations such as a light source, a mechanical threat or an auditory stimulus. It serves as a protection of the cornea and conjunctiva. *See* blink; pathway, retinotectal.
　cat's eye r. A whitish bright reflection observed in the normally black pupil in several conditions, such as leukocoria, retinoblastoma, Coats' disease or persistent hyperplastic primary vitreous. It resembles the reflection from the tapetum lucidum of a cat when a light is shined at night.
　consensual light r. *See* reflex, pupil light.
　corneal r. 1. Blinking in response to a threat or to tactile stimulation of the cornea. Associated responses include lacrimation and miosis. *Example*: blinking which occurs when approaching the cornea with a pointed instrument. 2. Image

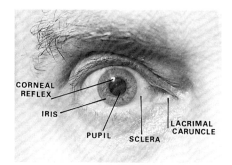

CORNEAL REFLEX

IRIS

PUPIL

SCLERA

LACRIMAL CARUNCLE

Fig. R4 Frontal view of the right eye.

formed by reflection of light from the cornea (Fig. R4).
See **aesthesiometer; blink; method, Hirschberg's; method, Krimsky's; pupillometer; strabismus, apparent.**

direct light r. See **reflex, pupil light.**

eyeball compression r. See **reflex, oculocardiac.**

fixation r. Psycho-optical reflex consisting of an involuntary movement of the eye (or eyes) aimed at placing on the foveola the retinal image of an object that was formed in the retinal periphery.
See **reflex, psycho-optical; reflex, re-fixation.**

foveal r. Tiny reflection from the concave surface of the foveal depression of the retina seen in ophthalmoscopy. It is not usually visible in old eyes, because the index of refraction of the vitreous is believed to become very nearly equal to that of the retina in the elderly.

fundus r. Light reflected by the fundus of the eye, as seen in retinoscopy and ophthalmoscopy. It appears as a red glow in the plane of the pupil in retinoscopy because it is reflected from the blood in the choroid and the retina, and media in front are transparent. It is absent in the elderly or when the eye has a dense cataract or a vitreous haemorrhage. *Syn.* red reflex.
See **fundus, ocular; fusion, motor.**

fusion r. See **fundus, ocular; fusion, motor.**

hemianopic pupillary r. In hemianopia, a loss of pupillary constriction when light falls on the blind side of the retina while pupillary constriction is maintained when light stimulates the unaffected side of the retina. It is caused by an optic tract lesion. *Syn.* Wernicke's hemianopic pupil; Wernicke's pupillary reaction; Wernicke's pupillary reflex; Wernicke's sign.
See **hemianopia, incongruous; tract. optic.**

indirect light r. See **reflex, pupil light.**

lacrimal r. Secretion of tears in response to irritation of the cornea or conjunctiva as, for example, when first wearing contact lenses (hard in particular), but it may also be induced by eyestrain, glare, laughing, etc. *Syn.* lacrimation reflex; tearing reflex; weeping reflex.
See **lacrimal apparatus; tear secretion; test, Schirmer's.**

lacrimation r. See **reflex, lacrimal.**

light r. **1.** That light which appears in the pupil in retinoscopy. It is light reflected by the retina. *Syn.* retinoscopic light. **2.** Any reflected light.
See **reflex, pupil light.**

near r. Reflex evoked by a blurred retinal image, as when fixating from far to near. It consists of three responses: (1) increased convexity of the crystalline lens; (2) constriction of the pupils; and (3) convergence of the eyes. This reflex is not a pure reflex as each of the three components can act independently of the other two; convergence by means of prisms, accommodation by means of lenses and miosis by light stimulation. Moreover, accommodation and convergence are linked to form the AC/A ratio. Innervation is parasympathetic. The response is produced in the pathway from neurons in the Edinger-Westphal nucleus passing to the ciliary ganglion and short ciliary nerves to the sphincter pupillae muscle for miosis and ciliary muscles for accommodation and other separate oculomotor fibres to the medial recti for convergence. *Syn.* accommodative reflex; near triad reflex; synkinetic near reflex.
See **accommodation, mechanism of; accommodation, reflex; accommodative response.**

near triad r. See **reflex, near.**

oculocardiac r. Decrease in pulse rate following compression of the eyeball or traction on the extraocular muscles during ocular surgery. It may produce a systolic cardiac arrest. *Syn.* Ascher's phenomenon; Ascher's reflex; eyeball compression reflex.

optokinetic r. See **reflex, vestibulo-ocular.**

postural r. A reflex which helps to maintain static or dynamic posture of the body, for example, the **righting reflex**, in which visual stimuli help to maintain a correct position of the head in space by activating the muscles of the neck and limbs.
See **reflex, static eye.**

psycho-optical r. Reflex involving the eye which is mediated by the occipital cortex such as the accommodative, fixation, fusion, version and vergence reflexes.

pupil r. Any alteration of the pupil size in response to stimuli other than light (e.g. a sudden noise).
See **reflex, pupil light.**

pupil light r. **1.** Constriction of the pupil in response to light stimulation of the photoreceptors of the retina. The response of an eye to light stimulation can occur either with a light shining on it directly (the **direct light reflex**) or when the other eye is stimulated (the **consensual** or **indirect light reflex**). The reflex arc consists of four neurons beyond the ganglion cells. The **first** afferent neuron transmits nervous impulses from the retina to the two pretectal olivary nuclei located on the lateral and anterior side of the superior colliculi. Impulses from the nasal retina terminate in the contralateral pretectal nucleus, while those originating on the temporal retina terminate in the ipsilateral nucleus. The **second** neurons, called the internuncial neurons, connect each pretectal olivary nucleus to both Edinger–Westphal nuclei which form part of the oculomotor nuclei. The

third efferent neurons connect the latter nuclei via the third nerve (oculomotor nerve) to the ciliary ganglion where there is a synapse. The **fourth** efferent neurons connect the latter via the short ciliary nerves, to the sphincter pupillae muscle of each iris and constrict the pupils. Light stimulation of the central region of the retina produces a greater pupillary response than peripheral stimulation. The efferent path for pupil constriction represents the **parasympathetic** innervation (Fig. R5). *Note*: Some research points to a different pathway for the second afferent neuron; almost all of the fibres from each pretectal olivary nucleus project to the contralateral Edinger–Westphal nucleus. **2.** Dilatation of the pupil in response to a reduction of the light stimulation of the retina. It is effected by **sympathetic** innervation through three neurons. The **first** neuron fibres originate in the hypothalamus and descend down the brainstem to the ciliospinal centre (of Bulge), located between the cervical C8 and the thoracic T2 of the spinal column. The **second** neuron fibres pass from the ciliospinal centre to the superior cervical ganglion in the neck. The **third** neuron efferent fibres ascend along the internal carotid artery until they join the ophthalmic division of the trigeminal nerve. The fibres reach the dilator pupillae muscle of the iris via the nasociliary and long ciliary nerves, which enter the eyeball behind the equator. *Syn.* light reflex.
See **brachium; fibre, pupillary; pathway, retinotectal; pretectum; pupillary defect, efferent.**
red r. *See* **reflex, fundus.**
re-fixation r. This reflex occurs while fixating one object and another in the visual field attracts the attention. The eye then turns to fixate on the new object. This is a special case of the fixation reflex.
retinoscopic r. *See* **reflex, light; retinoscope.**
righting r. *See* **reflex, postural.**

static eye r. Higher order postural reflex which helps to maintain the eye static with respect to the visual environment by action on the extraocular muscles (possibly via the utricular receptors of the vestibular system) during head or body movements. *Syn.* compensatory eye movements.
r. tearing *See* **reflex, lacrimal.**
tonic neck r. Orientation of the head, eyes and body in response to proprioceptive information provided by the activity of the muscles of the neck. *See* **proprioception.**
vergence r. Disjunctive eye movements in response to an object that moves closer or farther than the original position of the fixation point. *See* **movement, disjunctive eye; vergence.**
version r. Conjugate fixation reflex in response to an object moving in the same frontal plane. *See* **version.**
vestibulo-ocular r. Conjugate movement of the eyes in the direction opposite to a head movement. This reflex is triggered by stimulation of the semicircular canals. It is aimed at maintaining a stable image on the retina during head movement. This reflex responds best at high velocities and frequencies of the visual stimulus. At low velocities and frequencies, the stabilization of the retinal image is attempted by the **optokinetic reflex**, which is triggered only by retinal stimulation; this latter reflex complements the vestibulo-ocular reflex.
See **nystagmus; optokinetic; phenomenon, doll's head.**
weeping r. *See* **reflex, lacrimal.**
Wernicke's pupillary r. *See* **reflex, hemianopic pupillary.**
white pupillary r. *See* **leukocoria.**

refract 1. To bend a ray of light as it passes through a surface separating two media of different refractive indices. **2.** To measure the refractive state of the eye.

refracting angle *See* **angle, prism.**

refracting unit *See* **phoropter.**

refraction 1. The change in direction of the path of light as it passes obliquely from one medium to another having a different index of refraction (Fig. R6). **2.** The process of measuring and correcting the refractive error of the eyes. *Syn.* refraction of the eye; sight testing (obsolete term). **3.** *See* **refractive error.**
See **law of refraction.**
angle of r. *See* **angle of refraction.**
binocular r. Clinical procedure in which the subjective measurement of refraction of each eye is performed while both eyes are viewing a test. The visual examination is thus carried out under more natural conditions than when one eye is closed; the sizes of the pupils are similar and the accommodation-convergence relationship is maintained. There are various such methods: using polarized targets (e.g. Vectograph slides; using a septum (e.g. Turville Infinity Balance test), or fogging (e.g. Humphriss Immediate Contrast test). These methods give better results than refracting

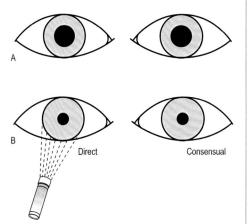

Fig. R5 A, pupils under low illumination. B, direct pupil light reflex of the right eye in response to light stimulation, accompanied by a consensual light reflex of the left eye.

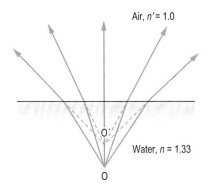

Air, $n' = 1.0$

Water, $n = 1.33$

O

Fig. R6 Refraction of light from water into air. Object O forms an image at O′ which appears closer to the surface than it actually is. Thus the apparent thickness t′ of a pool of water (or block of glass), in air, is smaller than its true thickness t and the greater the index of refraction n, the smaller it appears, i.e. $t' = t/n$

monocularly, especially in latent hyperopia, hyperopic anisometropia, pseudomyopia, cyclophoria, etc., and no additional step for binocular balancing is necessary.
See method, Humphriss; test, balancing; test, Turville, infinity balance.
cycloplegic r. Assessment of the refractive state of the eye when accommodation has been totally or partially paralysed by a cycloplegic (e.g. cyclopentolate 1% eyedrops, or atropine 0.5 or 1% ointment). This may be carried out in children to reveal the full extent of a hyperopia or in the initial assessment of accommodative esotropia, but only occasionally in adults as fogging methods usually suffice for them.
See cycloplegia; esotropia, accommodative.
double r. Splitting of an incident ray into two (ordinary and extraordinary) by a birefringent medium.
See anisotropic; birefringence; prism, Nicol; prism, Wollaston.
dynamic r. Determination of the refractive state of the eye when accommodation is stimulated, as distinct from **static refraction** which is the determination of the refractive state of the eye when accommodation is at rest or paralysed.
See refractive error; retinoscopy, dynamic.
error of r. See ametropia; refractive error.
r. of the eye 1. *See* refraction. 2. Refraction of light by the optical media of the eye. 3. *Syn.* for ametropia.
See ametropia; refractive error.
index of r. See index of refraction.
laser r. Method of subjective refraction in which the patient observes a slowly rotating drum, on the surface of which is perceived a speckle pattern resulting from illumination by a laser. The speckle pattern appears to move only when the eye is not focused for the fixation distance. If the perceived movement of the pattern is opposite to that of the drum, the eye is myopic, and if the perceived movement of the pattern is in the same direction

as the drum, the eye is hyperopic. Correction can be determined by placing a lens in front of the eye, which will neutralize the movement; at that point, the eye is focused for the fixation distance. Astigmatism can be measured by rotating the drum in various meridians. The drum can be placed at infinity or at near (an allowance for the radius of curvature of the drum and the distance must then be made). This method can be useful for mass screening, especially children, as accommodation is not stimulated as much as with Snellen letters. It has been very useful as a research tool for accommodation studies where it is arranged as part of a Badal optometer.
manifest r. Refractive error or the process of determining it when accommodation is at rest (but not paralysed).
See refraction, cycloplegic.
objective r. Measurement of the refraction of the eye that is not based on the patient's judgments, as when using an objective optometer or a retinoscope.
See photorefraction.
ocular r. See refractive error.
spectacle r. See refractive error.
static r. See refraction, dynamic; refractive error.
subjective r. Measurement of the refraction of the eye based on the patient's judgments.
See method, fogging; optometer; test, duochrome; test, fan and block; test, plus 1.00 D blur.

refractionist One who measures and corrects the refractive state of the eye.
See optometrist.

refractive amblyopia; correction *See* under the nouns.

refractive error The dioptric power (K) of the ametropia of the eye. It is equal to 1/k in dioptres, where k is the distance between the far point and either the spectacle plane (**spectacle refraction**), the principal point of the eye or the refracting surface of the reduced eye (**ocular refraction**) in metres. Thus

$$K = 1/k$$

when the milieu facing the eye is air. *Syn.* ametropia (although this is not strictly so as ametropia is the anomaly); refraction of the eye; refractive status; static refraction.
See accommodation, far point of; correction; experiment, Scheiner's; power, effective.

refractive index *See* index of refraction.

refractive surgery Surgical procedure aimed at correcting ametropia. Most procedures are performed on the cornea, but some involve either an intraocular lens implant, or more rarely crystalline lens extraction.
See epikeratoplasty; Intacs; keratomileusis; keratophakia; keratectomy, photorefractive; LASIK; LASEK.

refractive power *See* power, refractive.

refractivity *See* dispersion.

refractometer **1.** An instrument for measuring the refractive index of transparent objects. There exist several types: **Abbé's refractometer,** which is based on the measurement of the critical angle at the interface between a sample and a prism of known index of refraction and uses white light whereas that of **Pulfrich,** which is based on the same principle as Abbé's, uses monochromatic light. As the refractive index of some materials is related to their water content, the hand-held **Atago CL-1 Soft Lens Refractometer** has been calibrated to provide a reading of the percentage of water content of soft contact lenses. **2.** *See* optometer; water content.

refractometry **1.** Measurement of the refractive error of the eye with a refractometer or optometer. *See* optometer. **2.** Measurement of the index of refraction of a medium with a refractometer (e.g. Abbé's refractometer).

refractor *See* phoropter.

refractory period *See* potential, action.

Refsum's disease *See* disease, Refsum's.

regeneration Reproduction of tissue. *Examples*: nerve regeneration; restoration of rhodopsin following bleaching. *See* bleaching.

regeneration, aberrant An abnormal regeneration process following paralysis or paresis of the fibres of the third cranial nerve (oculomotor) in which the upper lid fails to follow the eye on downward gaze or even retracts on downward gaze or adduction with occasional contraction of the pupil. *Syn.* pseudo-von Graefe sign.

regression **1.** *See* reading. **2.** In statistics, it represents a method of analysing the association between one or more independent variables and a dependent variable. When there is more than one independent (also called predictor) variable, it is called **multiple regression**, otherwise it is referred to as **linear regression**. *See* correlation; statistics.

Reis–Buckler dystrophy *See* dystrophy, Reis–Buckler.

Reiter's syndrome *See* syndrome, Reiter's.

Rieger's syndrome *See* syndrome, Rieger's.

relapse Recurrence of a disease after recovery had apparently occurred or a worsening of a disease from which a patient was apparently recovering. *Example*: the recurrence of an iris melanoma after it had been excised.

relative afferent pupillary defect *See* pupil, Marcus Gunn.

relative amplitude of accommodation; convergence; scotoma *See* under the nouns.

reliability The extent to which multiple measurements of the same thing, made on separate occasions, yield approximately the same results. The reliability between two sets of scores can be assessed by determining the correlation coefficient (**test-retest reliability** coefficient). *See* validity.

relief **1.** The quality of an object or of different parts of a surface to stand out from the background or general plane in which it is situated. The perception of relief is a special case of depth perception. **2.** A feeling of gladness that something unpleasant or painful has not occurred or has ceased. *See* perception, depth; stereopsis.

relieving prism *See* prism, relieving.

remission Period of time during which signs and symptoms are absent or greatly diminished. A disease may present alternate remissions and recurrences (relapses) over a period of time.

remotum, punctum *See* accommodation, far point of.

Remy separator A simple hand-held instrument for separating the vision of both eyes and commonly used for antisuppression or divergence training. It consists of a vertical septum in the median plane, which is attached to and divides a target holder at one end. The other end of the septum rests against the patient's nose so that a target on either side of the septum is seen by only one eye (Fig. R7). *See* suppression.

resection Surgical procedure used in strabismus or in congenital ptosis in which a portion of an extraocular muscle is excised (usually at its insertion) and the muscle is reattached at or near the original site of insertion. This is carried out to shorten and strengthen the muscle. *See* enophthalmos; recession; strabismus surgery.

residual astigmatism *See* astigmatism, residual.

residual error of refraction *See* over-refraction.

reserve of accommodation *See* addition, near.

reserve, convergence fusional *See* convergence, relative.

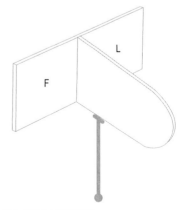

Fig. R7 Remy separator.

resolution, limit of Minimum separation of two images so that they are seen as separate when viewed through an optical instrument. This is usually evaluated in terms of the separation between the maximum of the intensity distribution curve of the diffraction pattern (or Airy's disc) of the images; it is commonly assumed that two points will be resolved if the centre of one pattern falls on the first dark ring of the other. The limit of resolution is greater as the aperture of the system becomes larger. *Syn.* resolving power; resolution threshold.
See **criterion, Rayleigh; minimum separable.**

resolution, spurious If the contrast sensitivity function (CSF) is measured when the eye is not in focus for the grating (e.g. due to a lack of correction or an erroneous correction), the CSF will suffer appreciably and fall much more rapidly with increasing spatial frequency towards zero contrast sensitivity. At this point, the grating can no longer be resolved and appears a uniform grey. At spatial frequencies greater than this threshold value, there may occur a phenomenon known as spurious resolution in which the CSF rises above zero. Thus, the grating may become visible again at higher spatial frequencies than that at which it first disappeared. *Example*: Spurious resolution can be observed when looking at a radial grating (or star sector target) in which the spatial frequencies increase towards its centre. If the grating is held close to the eye with the accommodation relaxed, one can see a grey annulus (and sometimes two) separating a zone (or two) of spurious resolution.
See **function, contrast sensitivity.**

resolution visual acuity See **acuity, visual.**

response, SILO An acronym for *small in large out*. It refers to the presumed change of the perceived size of a test object that a patient experiences, while maintaining fusion when convergence or divergence is varied. When convergence is increased with BO prisms, the object may appear to become smaller and nearer. When divergence is increased with BI prisms, the object may appear larger and further away. The SILO is not universal; children tend to respond that way, but adults commonly respond in the opposite way, that is, if the test object becomes smaller, they report it as moving away from them. The acronym is then given as SOLI. The response is used in visual therapy as a feedback mechanism to patients about their performance.
See **base setting; biofeedback; fusion, sensory.**

restriction An interference in normal eye movement. This is most often due to the development of abnormal tissue that acts to limit free movement of the eye.
See **disease, Graves'.**

ret See **retinoscopy.**

reticular formation See **brainstem.**

reticule See **graticule.**

reticulosis See **syndrome, Mikulicz's.**

retina The light-receptive innermost nervous tunic of the eye. It is a thin transparent membrane (about 125 μm near the ora serrata, 350 μm near the macula and 560 μm near the optic disc). The retina proper has an area of about 266 mm^2. It lies between the vitreous body and the choroid, and extends from the optic disc to the ora serrata. Near the posterior pole and temporal to the optic disc is the macula, at the centre of which is the foveola which provides the best visual acuity. The retina contains at least 10 distinct layers, of which there are two synaptic layers. They are from the outermost layer to the innermost: (1) the pigment epithelium; (2) the photoreceptor layer of rods and cones; (3) the external limiting membrane; (4) the outer nuclear layer; (5) the outer molecular (outer plexiform) layer; (6) the inner nuclear layer (which contains the bipolar, amacrine and horizontal cells and nuclei of the fibres of Mueller); (7) the inner molecular (inner plexiform) layer; (8) the ganglion cell layer; (9) the nerve fibre (layer stratum opticum) and (10) the internal limiting membrane. The two synaptic layers where visual signals must synapse as they emerge from the rods and cones on their way to the optic nerve are the two molecular layers (5 and 7) (Fig. R8). The blood supply to the retina is composed of the capillaries from the central retinal artery, which supply the inner two-thirds of the retina up to the outer plexiform layer, and the choriocapillaris, which supplies the outer one-third. There is no retinal circulation in the foveola (**avascular zone**). A **blood-retina barrier** is created by the walls of the retinal capillaries which restrict the movement of molecules, which could be damaging to neural tissue or interfere with function, from the inside to the outside of the capillaries. The blood-retina barrier in the outer third of the retina is formed by the tight junctions of the retinal pigment epithelium cells (Table R2).
Plural: retinae.
See **astrocytes; cone pedicle; cup, optic; disc, optic; ectoderm; fundus, ocular; layer of Henle, fibre; macula; neurotransmitter; retina, neurosensory; retinitis; retinopathy; rhodopsin; rod spherule; space, subretinal; transduction.**
converse r. See **retina, inverted.**
fleck r. Term referring to a retina with multiple, small or yellow spots, which are seen in various conditions: actinic keratopathy, drusen, fundus albipunctatus, fundus flavimaculatus, Alport's syndrome.
inverted r. Term referring to the fact that the retina of vertebrates is orientated so that the light has to pass through all the neuronal layers before reaching the photoreceptors. However, the retina of invertebrates is normally orientated so that light passes first through the photoreceptors as it traverses the retina; such a retina is called a **verted** or **converse retina**.
lattice degeneration of the r. Vitreoretinal degeneration usually found between the equator and the ora serrata leading to a thinning of the retina and characterized by a lesion made up of fine white lines and some pigmentation. It may

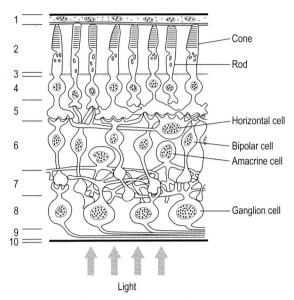

Light

Fig. R8 Schematic representation of the cells and layers of the central primate retina (1: retinal pigment epithelium; 2: photoreceptor layer of rods and cones; 3: external limiting membrane; 4: outer nuclear layer; 5: outer plexiform (or molecular) layer; 6: inner nuclear layer; 7: inner plexiform (or molecular) layer; 8: ganglion cell layer; 9: nerve fibre layer; 10: internal limiting membrane).

Table R2   Some approximate retinal dimensions

Structure	Diameter		Distance from centre of foveola
	mm	Degrees	
foveola	0.4	1.3	
fovea centralis	1.5	5.0	
macula lutea	4.0	14	
optic disc*			
horizontal	1.8	6.0	
vertical	2.1	7.5	
nasal disc margin			5.5 mm or 18.5°
temporal disc margin			3.5 mm or 12.5°
centre of disc			4.6 mm or 15.5°

*The figures given for the size of the disc are those corresponding to the blind spot. Anatomically the optic disc is slightly smaller.

result in holes or tears and in rhegmatogenous retinal detachment by which time the patient usually complains of floaters. The condition is most common in myopes and often found in patients with connective tissue syndromes such as Marfan's or Stickler's.
See **retinal break; retinal detachment; retinoschisis; syndrome, Marfan's; syndrome, Stickler's.**
leopard r. See **fundus, leopard.**
neurosensory r. This is composed of all the layers of the retina, except the outer pigmented layer (called retinal pigment epithelium). It comprises three main groups of neurons: (1) the photoreceptors, (2) the bipolar cells and (3) the ganglion cells. In addition, there are other connecting neurons: the horizontal and amacrine cells. The neurosensory layer is derived embryologically from the inner layer of the optic cup, whereas the pigmented layer is derived from the outer layer of the optic cup and they are separated by a potential space which facilitates their separation, as occurs in detached retina. *Syn.* neuroretina; sensory retina.
tessellated r. See **fundus, tessellated.**
tigroid r. See **fundus, tessellated.**
verted r. See **retina, inverted.**

retinal 1. Pertaining to the retina. **2.** *See* **rhodopsin.**

retinal artery occlusion Occlusion of the central retinal artery is characterized by a sudden loss of vision and a defective direct pupil light reflex. The retinal arterioles are constricted while the veins are full but a venous pulse is absent. The retina appears white and swollen, especially near the posterior pole, and the choroid is seen through it as a cherry-red spot (Fig. S11, p. 323). If the occlusion persists, the cherry-red spot disappears after several weeks, the retinal arterioles remain attenuated, eventually becoming white threads, and the optic disc becomes atrophic.

Occlusion is more frequently limited to one branch of the central retinal artery. In this case, the clinical picture is limited to the area supplied by the branch and this is associated with a visual field defect in that region. Causes include retinal emboli due to a cardiovascular disease, systemic hypertension, temporal arteritis, oral contraceptives, syphilis, intravenous drug abuse or trauma. Treatment is urgent as there is an extremely serious risk of blindness.

See **amaurosis fugax; angiography, fluorescein; atheroma; plaques, Hollenhorst's; spot, cherry-red.**

retinal break A full-thickness opening in the neurosensory retina. It may be a hole, usually due to atrophy of the retina and often overlaid by an operculum; a tear, horseshoe-shaped (U-shaped), round or slit-like, usually caused by posterior vitreous detachment in which the vitreous adheres to the retina and pulls it from the point of adherence during or just after an abrupt eye movement; or a giant retinal tear which involves 90° or more of the circumference of the globe and is commonly associated with Marfan's syndrome or Stickler's syndrome; or retinal dialysis which is usually the result of trauma. The patient may complain of photopsia, seeing floaters or flashes and some visual field defects, and they may present with a vitreous haemorrhage. Management of retinal breaks includes localized laser photocoagulation (laser retinopexy) or cryopexy, and without delay as the defect may lead to rhegmatogenous or tractional retinal detachment.

See **cryopexy; horseshoe tear; macular hole; retinal dialysis; retinopexy; retinoschisis; scleral buckling; sign, Shafer's.**

retinal correspondence, abnormal (ARC) A type of retinal correspondence in which the fovea of one eye is associated with an extrafoveal area of the other eye to give rise to a perception of a single object. This phenomenon is common in strabismus, but may also occur as a result of a macular lesion. ARC is often classified in three types: (1) **Harmonious**, in which the angle of anomaly is equal to the objective angle of deviation. This indicates that the ARC fully corresponds to the strabismus. (2) **Unharmonious**, in which the angle of anomaly is less than the objective angle of deviation. (3) **Paradoxical**, when the angle of anomaly is greater than the objective angle of deviation. ARC can be detected by examination with a major amblyoscope, with the after-image test, or by comparison between the objective and the subjective angles of deviation measured with the alternate cover test and either a Maddox rod or the von Graefe's test, respectively (a difference between the objective and the subjective angles indicates ARC) (Fig. R9). *Syn.* anomalous retinal correspondence; retinal incongruity.

See **diplopia, incongruous; diplopia, physiological; phenomenon, phi; test, after-image; test, Bagolini's.**

retinal corresponding points Two points (or small areas), one in each retina, which when simultaneously stimulated give rise to the perception of a single object. These points share a common line of direction and this explains why stimulating them is perceived as arising from the same point in space. *Syn.* normal retinal correspondence.

See **area, Panum's; disparity, retinal; horopter; law of identical visual directions; test, after-image transfer.**

retinal detachment Separation of the neurosensory retina from the pigment epithelium layer. There are three main types: **rhegmatogenous retinal detachment**, which is the most common type, **exudative (serous or secondary) retinal detachment** and **traction retinal detachment**.

See **cryotherapy; horseshoe tear; macular hole; metamorphopsia; photocoagulation; retina, lattice degeneration of the; retinal break; retinal dialysis; retinopathy, central serous; retinopathy of prematurity; space, subretinal; striae retinae; syndrome, Ehlers–Danlos; syndrome, Marfan's; syndrome, Stickler's; ultrasonography; vitreoretinopathy, familial exudative; vitreous detachment.**

exudative r. d. Separation of the neurosensory retina from the retinal pigment epithelium due to fluid accumulating in the subretinal space in the absence of a retinal break or preretinal traction following damage to the blood-retina barrier of the choriocapillaris. Common causes are choroidal tumour, posterior uveitis, exudative age-related

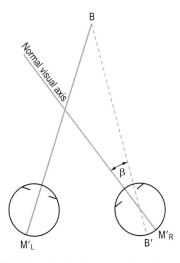

Fig. R9 Abnormal retinal correspondence between M′L and B′ in right esotropia (M′R, fovea of the right eye).

macular degeneration, uveal effusion syndrome, Coats' disease, central serous chorioretinopathy or idiopathic. The patient notices a loss of vision in the area of the visual field corresponding to the detached area, reduced visual acuity if the macula is involved and floaters if there is an associated inflammation. The elevation is smooth and convex, and the subretinal fluid shifts the area which is detached when the head moves (referred to as 'shifting fluid'). Treatment is aimed at the primary cause. *Syn.* serous retinal detachment; secondary retinal detachment.

rhegmatogenous r. d. A separation of the neurosensory retina from the retinal pigment epithelium due to fluid from the vitreous entering the subretinal space through a tear or break in the retina. The retinal breaks are most commonly the result of posterior vitreous detachment, which is found in a large percentage of patients older than 70 years, in aphakic eyes, and in degenerative myopic eyes. Retinal breaks may also occur as a result of trauma and occasionally ocular surgery. The patient notices floaters, flashes, photopsia and a loss of vision in one area of the visual field corresponding to the detached area and pigment granules 'tobacco dust' floating in the anterior vitreous. It is imperative that management be commenced as soon as possible. It may involve **scleral buckling** (indenting the sclera over the retinal break) or **vitrectomy**, and usually draining the subretinal fluid, or **pneumatic retinopexy** (the retinal break is sealed and the retina reattached using an intravitreal gas bubble) (Fig. R10). *See* **retinopexy; scleral buckling; vitrectomy.**

tractional r. d. Separation of the neurosensory retina from the retinal pigment epithelium due to contraction of vitreoretinal fibroproliferative membranes, which pull the retina away from the pigment epithelium. The main causes are proliferative diabetic retinopathy, retinopathy of prematurity, sickle-cell retinopathy and perforating ocular injury. Ophthalmoscopically, the detachment typically appears concave. The condition is often asymptomatic. Treatment is aimed at releasing the vitreoretinal traction. *See* **incontinentia pigmenti; vitrectomy.**

retinal dialysis A full-thickness retinal tear at the ora serrata. It usually results from trauma, although some tears occur spontaneously. If the trauma is intense, there may also be a retinal break at the optic disc, but the most frequent location is in the lower temporal quadrant. The condition is most typically asymptomatic. However, as it often gives rise to retinal detachment, the patient may report some of the symptoms associated with the latter. Perimetry and binocular indirect ophthalmoscopy are essential in the examination of this condition. In some cases, the tear does not progress, but because of the risk of retinal detachment, patients must be referred to a retinal specialist. *Syn.* retinal dehiscence; retinal disinsertion. *See* **retinal break.**

retinal disinsertion *See* retinal dialysis.

retinal disparity *See* disparity, retinal.

retinal embolism Obstruction of a retinal artery or arteriole by a clot (embolus), which may result in atrophy or blindness in the area of the retina affected. *See* **retinal artery occlusion.**

retinal glioma *See* retinoblastoma.

retinal hypoxia *See* hypoxia.

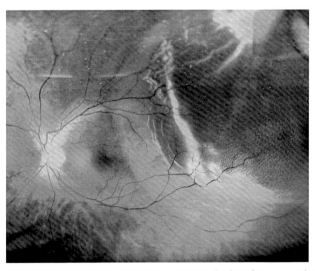

Fig. R10 Retinal detachment as observed with fundus angiography (autofluorescence) showing a circular area surrounding the detached retina which indicates the extent of fluid spread. (From Bowling 2016, with permission of Elsevier)

retinal illuminance Luminous flux incident on the retina. The simplified formula is

$$T = LS$$

where L is the luminance of the stimulus in cd/m^2 and S is the area of the pupil in mm^2. The retinal illuminance T is then given in trolands. Retinal illuminance decreases with age due to absorption of the lens and to a reduction in pupil size. It may represent a reduction of at least tenfold in an 80-year-old eye as compared to a 20-year-old eye. *Syn.* retinal illumination.
See troland; vignetting.

retinal image, stabilized *See* stabilized retinal image.

retinal incongruity *See* retinal correspondence, abnormal.

retinal line *See* line, retinal.

retinal mosaic Pattern formed by the distribution of the retinal visual cells and their interspaces.

retinal necrosis, acute A necrotizing retinitis caused by the varicella-zoster virus or herpes simplex virus types 1 and 2, which may infect healthy individuals of any age. The patient usually presents with ocular discomfort or pain, reduced visual acuity and floaters. The signs are those of anterior granulomatous uveitis. There are typically many areas of retinitis, which eventually coalesce ending in full-thickness retinal necrosis. Treatment is with antiviral agents, followed by systemic steroids.

retinal necrosis, progressive outer A very rare and devastating necrotizing retinitis typically caused by the varicella-zoster virus, usually occurring in patients with AIDS. There is less inflammation than in the acute form, many lesions on the retina eventually end in full-thickness retinal necrosis and rapid progressive visual loss due to rapidly coalescing white areas of retinal necrosis. The prognosis used to be poor, but the use of Highly Active Antiretroviral Therapy (HAAT) combined with other antiviral agents has greatly improved the prognosis.
See syndrome, acquired immunodeficiency.

retinal nerve fibre layer *See* glaucoma detection.

retinal pigment epithelium (RPE) A brown monolayer of hexagonal cells of the retina, in contact with Bruch's membrane, composed of cells joined by tight junctions and filled with pigment, mainly melanin and lipofuscin (Fig. R8). Depending upon the amount of pigment, the fundus will appear dark or light. The main functions of the RPE are control of the flow of fluid and nutrients entering the retina (blood-retina barrier), transport of metabolic waste material from the photoreceptors across Bruch's membrane to the choroid, absorption of scattered light, visual pigment metabolism, vitamin A metabolism which contributes to visual pigment regeneration, ingestion and digestion of photoreceptor discs (phagocytosis), retinal adhesion and synthesis of growth factors of adjacent tissues. A dysfunction of this tissue can be detected with the electrooculogram. With age, there is an accumulation of lipids within the tissue hindering the flow of fluids, which may contribute to age-related macular degeneration.
See membrane, Bruch's; syndrome, Usher's.

retinal pigment epithelium, congenital hypertrophy of the A benign congenital proliferation of the retinal pigment epithelium which may appear unilaterally as a small dark-grey or black round or oval lesion in the fundus (**typical** form) or, in other cases, as multiple smaller lesions grouped together and resembling '**bear tracks**'. The photoreceptor layer overlying the RPE usually shows marked degeneration. In the **atypical** form the lesions are bilateral. The latter is associated with familial adenomatous polyposis (an autosomal dominant condition characterized by neoplasms derived from epithelial tissue which appear as polyps throughout the rectum and colon and may become malignant) and its variants, Turcot's syndrome or Gardner's syndrome.

retinal pigment epithelium and retina, hamartoma of the An abnormal proliferation of retinal pigment epithelium (RPE), retinal astrocytes, usually congenital. This condition is thought to be due to persistent abnormal traction on the RPE, causing it to proliferate. It may be associated with neurofibromatosis type 2. It presents with decreased visual acuity and an elevated pigmented lesion and a whitish epiretinal membrane, tortuosity of vessels. Treatment for amblyopia may be sufficient.

retinal raphe A horizontal line of demarcation, on the temporal side of the macula, separating the arcuate nerve fibres from the upper and lower retina.
See fibre, papillomacular; scotoma, arcuate; scotoma, Bjerrum's.

retinal rivalry When the two eyes are simultaneously or successively stimulated on corresponding retinal areas by dissimilar images (e.g. a green source to one eye and a red to the other or lines orientated in one direction to one eye and in the other direction to the other), there results either an alternation of perception (complete or partial) or even a constant dominance of one eye. (Fig. R11) *Syn.* binocular rivalry.
See effect, Cheshire cat; suppression.

retinal slip *See* disparity, retinal.

retinal tear *See* retinal break.

retinal telangiectasia *See* disease, Coats'; telangiectasia.

retinal vasculitis *See* disease, Eales'; uveitis, intermediate; uveitis, posterior.

retinal vein occlusion Occlusion of the central retinal vein (CRVO) can be either **non-ischaemic CRVO** (sometimes referred to as **venous-stasis retinopathy**), which is the most common type, or **ischaemic** CRVO. Predisposing causes are

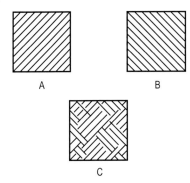

Fig. R11 Retinal rivalry. Target A is seen by one eye. Target B is seen by the other eye. Target C is seen by both eyes simultaneously.

cardiovascular disease, systemic hypertension, diabetes or raised intraocular pressure. Non-ischaemic CRVO is characterized by some loss of vision, metamorphopsia, slight impairment of the pupil responses to light and partial or complete central scotoma due to macular oedema. The ophthalmoscopic picture shows retinal haemorrhages, blot and flame-shaped in appearance and distributed throughout the whole fundus, dilated and tortuous veins, a swollen optic disc and an oedematous macular area. In some cases, cotton-wool exudates are also noted. When the condition affects young adults, it is commonly referred to as **papillophlebitis (optic disc vasculitis)** in which the clinical picture is similar except that the pupillary responses to light are normal and the patient is often asymptomatic. Ischaemic CRVO, which usually affects older people, is a more severe type and the signs and symptoms are much more marked than in the non-ischaemic type.

Occlusion is more frequently limited to one branch of the central retinal vein (**BRVO**). In this case, the clinical picture is limited to the retinal area drained by the occluded branch, but most patients will have some loss of vision depending on the extent of the macular oedema, as well as metamorphopsia and visual field defect. Many eyes with BVRO have been found to be hyperopic, and hypertension is commonly associated with BRVO. Treatment depends on the primary cause. Photocoagulation is used in some cases (Fig. R12). A rare form is called **hemiretinal vein occlusion** in which the central retinal vein is occluded. It may lead to retinal and iris neovascularization and possibly neovascular glaucoma.

See **angiography, fluorescein; rubeosis iridis; vein, central retinal.**

retinex A theory proposed to explain colour and brightness perception and constancies. It postulates that the colour of an object is not determined by the spectral composition of the light stimulus coming from the object but is determined by information obtained from a comparison of three lightnesses generated by the light absorption of the three types of cone cell. The name of the theory 'retinex' reflects the fact that the perception of the image results from the retina and the cortex. *See* **pigment, visual.**

retinitis Inflammation of the retina. This usually follows inflammations of the vitreous body, retinal vessels and especially of the choroid. Retinitis leads to an exudation of cells into the vitreous body and, if serious, vision will be affected. If the inflammation affects the macular area there will be a loss of central vision. Haemorrhages and oedema (producing a blurring of the margins of the optic disc) are also usually present. *See* **retinal necrosis.**

retinitis, cytomegalovirus (CMV retinitis) Rare, chronic, diffuse infection of the retina caused by the cytomegalovirus (CMV), a member of the herpesvirus group. It affects people with an impaired immune system as a result of either AIDS, organ transplantation or chemotherapy for some malignancies such as leukaemia. The signs are whitish retinal lesions, which look granular (not fluffy cotton-wool spots). These lesions progress into retinal necrosis with absolute visual field loss in that area. The lesions are usually accompanied by haemorrhages. Eventually the lesions coalesce and involve the entire fundus, resulting in complete visual loss. In the initial phase of the disease, most patients are usually asymptomatic while those with symptoms will complain of floaters, blurred vision, photopsia, scotomas, metamorphopsia, etc. In some cases, retinal detachment follows the disease. Treatment with dihydroxy propoxymethyl guanine and ganciclovir produces some regression of the disease. *See* **syndrome, acquired immunodeficiency.**

retinitis pigmentosa A primary pigmentary dystrophy of the retina followed by migration of pigment. It is, in most cases, an inherited disease caused by abnormalities of many genes and characterized by night blindness (nyctalopia) and constricted visual fields. The inheritance can be autosomal dominant, autosomal recessive or X-linked. Many cases are caused by mutations in the rhodopsin gene (RHO). The condition is usually bilaterally symmetrical. The rod system is damaged, but cones are also involved to some degree and the electroretinogram amplitude is subnormal. The disease usually begins in adolescence with night blindness, followed by a ring scotoma in the periphery that spreads until only a small contracted central field remains and vision is greatly reduced or completely lost. Ophthalmoscopic examination reveals a yellowish atrophy of the optic disc, severe arterial attenuation and conspicuous pigment proliferation, which begins in the equatorial region. The areas of pigment have dense centres and irregular processes shaped like 'bone spicules'. There are several variants (atypical RP) of pigment distributions and patterns throughout the fundus (e.g. in mainly one quadrant) or as **retinitis punctata albescens** (scattered white dots most numerous at the equator, arteriolar attenuation

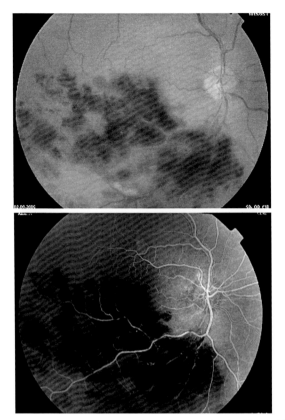

Fig. R12 Major inferior branch retinal vein occlusion. Note the extensive dot-blot and flame-shaped haemor-rhages affecting the sector of the retina drained by the obstructed vein. The bottom photo is a fluorescein angiogram showing hypofluorescence due to the blockage by blood. (From Kanski 2007, with permission of Butterworth-Heinemann)

and cone abnormalities unlike fundus albipunc-tatus). Associated systemic syndromes include Bassen–Kornzweig, Kearns–Sayre, Bardet–Biedl, Refsum's and Usher's. *Syn.* primary pigmentary retinal dystrophy.
   See **bone spicule; field; visual field; fundus, leopard; tritanopia; vision, tunnel.**

retinitis proliferans *See* retinopathy, proliferative.

retinitis punctata albescens *See* retinitis pigmentosa.

retinitis, solar *See* retinopathy, solar.

retinoblastoma A congenital malignant tumour of the retina usually noted in the first 2 years of life, although in some cases it may not be until after age 5 years. It is the most common intraocular tumour of childhood occurring in about 1 of every 15000 to 18000 births. The tumour is composed of small immature cells of the developing retina (retinoblasts) with large nuclei and thin cytoplasms. The condition is inherited in about 40% of all cases. The predisposing gene (RB1) is located on chromosome 13q14. Most individuals who inherit a mutant copy of the retinoblastoma gene

sustain a second hit to the remaining normal copy of the gene and develop the disease. The most common ocular manifestations are leukokoria and strabismus and sometimes, red eye, glaucoma, reduced vision and orbital cellulitis. Diagnosis is usually made by the appearance of a greyish reflex of light observed at the pupil, although often by that time the pupil is fixed and the eye is blind. Computerized tomography is useful in imaging the tumour. Treatment includes chemotherapy, external beam radiotherapy, photocoagulation, cryotherapy and plaque radiotherapy while advanced tumours are managed by enucleation. *Syn.* retinal glioma.
   See **chromosome; cryopexy; penetrance; reflex, cat's eye.**

retinochoroiditis Inflammation of both the retina and the choroid.
   See **toxoplasmosis.**

retinochoroidopathy, birdshot A bilateral chronic condition which appears in middle-aged individu-als, over 90% of whom are HLA-A29 positive, suggesting a genetic predisposition. The clinical picture is varied: multiple cream-yellow circular or oval spots spread throughout the posterior fundus, vitritis, cystoid macular oedema and eventually optic atrophy. Choroidal neovascularization is a common complication. Symptoms are reduction of visual acuity, floaters, colour vision defects and nyctalopia. Treatment includes corticosteroids and/or immunosuppressants. *Note*: HLA (human leukocyte antigen) is a product of a gene complex located on chromosome 6p21.3.

retinopathy A disease of the retina.
See **retinitis; tritanopia.**

arteriosclerotic r. See **arteriosclerosis.**

background diabetic r. Progressive microangiopathy of the retinal vessels occurring in the early stage of diabetic retinopathy. It is characterized by microaneurysms, dot-blot haemorrhages, flame-shaped haemorrhages, hard exudates and retinal oedema. Retinal veins may also become dilated and tortuous. If the microvascular occlusion progresses, there will be signs of ischaemia and occasionally cotton-wool spots will appear, as well as more venous changes and maculopathy, producing the clinical picture of **pre-proliferative diabetic retinopathy**. If the macular oedema is not clinically significant, the patient remains asymptomatic. *Syn.* non-proliferative diabetic retinopathy.

diabetic r. Retinal changes occurring in long-standing cases of diabetes mellitus. It is the most common retinal vascular disease. In general, the severity of the retinopathy parallels the duration of the diabetes. The retinopathy is characterized by the presence of new blood vessels (neovascularization), which proliferate on or near the optic disc and on the surface of the retina, microaneurysms (small round red spots), cotton-wool spots and sharply defined white or yellowish waxy exudates. Vitreous detachment is a likely outcome. If the vessels bleed, there can be a preretinal haemorrhage with visual loss. Both eyes are usually involved although to different degrees. Visual acuity may be unaffected unless the fovea is involved with the appearance of scattered microaneurysms and small haemorrhages (**diabetic maculopathy**). After the condition has reached the stage of proliferative retinopathy, the principal treatment is with laser photocoagulation, which reduces the risk of further visual loss. Other treatments include intravitreal injections of a corticosteroid or of an anti-VEGF drug such as aflibercept, bevacizumab or ranibizumab. Low vision aids may be needed afterward. *Syn.* diabetic retinitis; proliferative diabetic retinopathy.
See **angiography, fluorescein; diabetes; maculopathy, diabetic; microaneurysm; retinopathy, pre-proliferative diabetic; retinopathy, proliferative diabetic.**

haemorrhagic r. A retinopathy marked by profuse haemorrhage in the retina. It may be due to diabetes, hypertension or retinal vein occlusion.
See **retinal vein occlusion.**

hypertensive r. Retinal changes occurring as a result of systemic hypertension (**essential hypertension**). Most cases are chronic but in a very small percentage of patients it is acute (malignant hypertension). The condition is characterized by local and/or generalized narrowing of the arterioles, changes at arteriovenous crossings (Salus' sign) and 'copper-wire' arteriolar light reflex (grades 1 and 2). As the condition progresses, flame-shaped haemorrhages, cotton-wool exudates, oedema and changes at arteriovenous crossings (Gunn's crossing sign) and 'silver-wire' arteriolar reflex appear (grade 3). At the most advanced stage (grade 4), there is optic disc swelling; this is **malignant hypertension** (**accelerated hypertension**). Patients are usually asymptomatic. A rare more damaging feature is involvement of the choroidal arteries (**hypertensive choroidopathy**), along with Elschnig's spots and Siegrist's streaks, optic neuropathy and exudative retinal detachment. *Note:* The grading of hypertensive retinopathy is the Keith–Wagener–Barker classification.
See **arteriosclerosis; exudate; hypertension; macular star; sphygmomanometer.**

non-proliferative r. See **retinopathy, background diabetic.**

pigmentary r. A term commonly used as a synonym of retinitis pigmentosa.

r. of prematurity A bilateral retinal disease which commonly affects premature infants exposed to high ambient oxygen concentrations. It ranges from mild to a severe condition and classified in five stages. The moderate to advanced stages are characterized by proliferation and tortuosity of blood vessels, usually with haemorrhages and retinal detachment accompanied by an accumulation of fibrous tissue on the surface of the retina. Some infants may develop cicatricial complications, which may be innocuous or may progress to cover the central region of the retina and cause blindness. Other complications may be myopia or glaucoma. This condition is less common nowadays thanks to tight control of the amount of oxygen provided to preterm infants. *Syn.* retrolental fibroplasias (RLF).
See **leukocoria.**

pre-proliferative diabetic r. Early stage in the development of diabetic retinopathy. It is characterized by microaneurysms, intraretinal microvascular abnormalities, venous changes (beading/loops), cotton-wool spots, exudates and retinal haemorrhages (dot and blot, flame-shaped). *Syn.* non-proliferative diabetic retinopathy.
See **retinopathy, diabetic; retinopathy, pre-proliferative diabetic.**

proliferative diabetic r. Neovascularization of the retina extending into the vitreous with connective tissue proliferation surrounding the vessels. Vitreous haemorrhage is also present. The vessels usually arise from a retinal vein near an arteriovenous crossing at the posterior pole and from the surface of the optic disc. It occurs as a result of certain inflammatory conditions and in diabetes. Visual acuity may be affected. Management is with laser photocoagulation. *Syn.* retinitis proliferans.
See **membrane, epiretinal; retinopathy, diabetic; vitrectomy; retinopathy, pre-proliferative diabetic.**

radiation r. A retinopathy which may develop following plaque therapy (brachytherapy) to treat an intraocular tumour, particularly choroidal melanoma, or irradiation of the globe, orbit or nasopharyngeal malignancies. The condition only appears after half a year and is characterized by capillary occlusion with microaneurysms, macular oedema, retinal haemorrhages and cotton-wool spots. Treatment is by photocoagulation for macular oedema and also if proliferative retinopathy has developed.

solar r. Macular damage caused by fixating the sun without adequate protection, usually viewing a solar eclipse, but also in people staring at the sun as part of sun worship or psychosis. The retina presents at first with retinal oedema, which may develop into an atrophy of the tissue and produce a circumscribed hole or cyst in the fovea. This latter event results in a permanent central scotoma. There is no specific treatment, but the condition can be prevented by wearing very dense light filters or viewing through photographic films. *Syn.* eclipse retinopathy; foveomacular retinitis; solar retinitis.
See actinic; macular hole.

toxaemic r. of pregnancy Sudden angiospasm of retinal arterioles, later followed by the typical picture of advanced hypertensive retinopathy. Restitution follows rapidly after the pregnancy has reached full term.

venous-stasis r. *See* retinal vein occlusion.

retinopexy A surgical procedure performed to produce an adhesion of the retina to the pigment epithelium and choroid. It is used to repair retinal detachment or breaks and posterior vitreous detachment. There are several forms of retinopexy: **laser retinopexy** in which the lesion is sealed by absorption of the light generating heat and coagulation in several confluent burns with the practitioner looking into the eye with a binocular indirect ophthalmoscope; **pneumatic retinopexy** in which a gas (sulfur hexafluoride SF6, perfluoropropane C3 F8 or hexafluoroethane C2F6, which serve as a tamponade agent) is injected into the vitreous and a bubble presses against the torn retina. It is usually combined with cryopexy or laser photocoagulation and it is used when the retinal break is located in the upper half of the retina; and **diathermy** in which heat is applied locally to the retina. It is usually performed with a scleral incision.
See cryopexy; retinal break; scleral buckling; tamponade; vitrectomy.

retinoschisis A vitreoretinal degeneration characterized by splitting of the retina into two layers. It occurs either as a hereditary disease or as an acquired condition (70% of these patients are hyperopic). The X-linked hereditary condition (called **juvenile X-linked retinoschisis**) affects only males and usually involves the macula with loss of central vision. The congenital condition is characterized by a splitting of the nerve fibre layer from the sensory retina and the prognosis is poor, whereas the acquired form (called **degenerative retinoschisis**), which is the most common, results in a splitting at the level of the outer plexiform layer/inner nuclear layer. The latter usually begins in the temporal periphery appearing as a coalescence of microcystoid degenerations with a smooth transparent elevation and associated with an absolute localized scotoma, although the condition is usually asymptomatic. The condition may spread to involve the entire peripheral fundus. Holes in the two layers are common and are a sign of progression. The inner layer contains blood vessels and sometimes has small whitish flakes on it, which are called 'snowflakes'. A possible but rare complication is retinal detachment.

retinoschisis, degenerative; juvenile *See* retinoschisis.

retinoscope An instrument for determining objectively the refractive state of the eye. It consists of a light source, a condensing lens and a mirror. The mirror is either semitransparent or has a hole through which the retinoscopist can view the patient's eye along the retinoscope's beam of light. A patch of light is formed on the patient's retina and, by moving that patch in a given direction and observing the direction in which it appears to move after refraction by the patient's eye, the retinoscopist can determine whether the patient's retina is focused in front of, at or behind the retinoscope's sight hole. If the light reflected from the patient's fundus (called the **retinoscopic reflex** or **light reflex**) and observed in the patient's pupil through the retinoscope moves in the same direction as the movement of the mirror (this is referred to as a **with movement**), the eye is hyperopic. If the reflex moves in the opposite direction to that of the mirror (**against movement**), the eye is myopic. Sometimes it is impossible to see a clear movement one way or the other but only a bipartite reflex, showing opposite movements in the two sectors of the pupils (this is called a **split reflex** or a **scissors movement**). The refractive error is determined by placing lenses of various powers in front of the patient's eye until no movement is seen, i.e. the whole pupil is either illuminated or dark and the image of the patient's retina is then conjugate with the plane of the retinoscope's sight hole. When this phenomenon occurs, the **neutral point** has been reached. The neutral point is measured for each principal meridian of the eye if it is astigmatic. To arrive at the patient's error of refraction, the dioptric power corresponding to the distance between patient and retinoscope (called the **working distance**) is subtracted from the total lens power used to obtain neutralization. The amount of dioptric power subtracted is called the **allowance**. (Fig. R13) *Syn.* skiascope.
See band, retinoscopic; chromoretinoscopy; reflex, fundus; velonoskiascopy.

spot r. Retinoscope that projects a circular beam of light upon the patient's retina.

streak r. Retinoscope that projects into the patient's eye an oblong streak, which can be

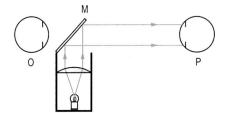

Fig. R13 Optical principle of a retinoscope (O, observer's eye; P, patient's eye; M, semi-silvered mirror).

adjusted in width and rotated in various meridians. It is more efficient than the spot retinoscope in determining astigmatism.

retinoscopic artefact An error encountered in determining the refractive error by retinoscopy. This error is due to the fact that the retinal layer which reflects the retinoscopic light is not situated within the photoreceptors (where an image must be formed to appear in focus) but in front of them. Retinoscopic light is reflected by the vitreous-retina interface due to the difference in their refractive indices (that difference may not exist in some species and in old eyes). Consequently, retinoscopic results tend to be more hyperopic or less myopic than is actually the case. The smaller the eye is, the greater the error because the thickness of the retina is nearly constant across species. This error is equal to about 0.25 D in young human adults, about 1 D in infant eyes and can reach some 8 D in very small animals. *Syn.* retinoscopic error; small eye artifact (so called because the effect is much greater for small eyes than for large eyes).

retinoscopy (ret) The determination of the refractive state of the eye by means of a retinoscope. *Syn.* skiascopy; shadow test.
See **chromoretinoscopy.**
Cross-Nott r. Technique of dynamic retinoscopy in which the patient wears the distance correction and fixates a near target (e.g. a card with letters). The practitioner performs retinoscopy close behind the near target moving closer or farther away until neutrality is achieved. The reciprocal of the distance at which neutrality is observed indicates the accommodative response.
dynamic r. Retinoscopy performed with the patient fixating binocularly a near object such as a letter, a word or a picture mounted on, or held close to, the retinoscope and wearing the distance correction. The method can be used to assess a patient's accommodative system. If the patient accommodates accurately, the retinoscopic reflex will indicate a neutral point and the accommodative response will be equal to the accommodative demand. If the patient overaccommodates (**lead of accommodation**), the retinoscopic reflex will show an 'against movement'. The amount of lead of accommodation

is given by the dioptric difference between the position of the neutral point and that of the target, the retinoscope having been moved towards the patient. If the patient underaccommodates (**lag of accommodation**), the retinoscopic reflex will show a 'with movement'. The amount of lag of accommodation is given by the dioptric difference between the position of the neutral point and that of the target, the retinoscope having been moved away from the subject. A lag of accommodation of up to about 0.75 D is a common response in nonpresbyopic patients. If it exceeds 1.00 D, it may be due to insufficiently corrected hyperopia or reduced amplitude of accommodation. If there is no lag, it may indicate latent hyperopia, pseudomyopia or spasm of accommodation. The method can also be used to determine the reading addition by placing the retinoscope at the usual reading distance and obtaining the neutral point. No working distance lens power is subtracted or added to the finding because the plane of regard is at the same distance as the retinoscope. *Syn.* book retinoscopy (this term is restricted to the case when the patient is reading a text); cognitive retinoscopy (when the patient fixates a single letter or reads some words); near point retinoscopy.
See **accommodation, lag of; accommodation, objective; retinoscopy, MEM; retinoscopy, Mohindra's technique of; retinoscopy, static.**
MEM r. A type of dynamic retinoscopy in which the retinoscope is held in the same plane as the near fixation target and lenses are interposed very briefly in front of one eye while the other eye fixates the target. The aim of the method is to estimate the fundus reflex motion without disturbing the accommodative stance, that is, by leaving each lens in front of one eye for less than 1 second until the neutral point is achieved. The results in non-presbyopic subjects generally showing a lag of accommodation of 0 to +0.75 D. *Note:* MEM is an acronym of 'monocular estimation method'.
Mohindra's technique of r. Retinoscopy performed in a darkened room at 50 cm (20 inches) with the patient fixating the retinoscope light monocularly (the other eye being occluded). Distance retinoscopic refraction is derived by adding −1.00 D (to take into account the working distance and the state of accommodation in the dark) to the value found by near retinoscopy. The technique is used in paediatric optometry. *Syn.* monocular near retinoscopy.
See **accommodation, resting state of; retinoscopy, dynamic; retinoscopy, MEM.**
near point r. *See* **retinoscopy, dynamic; Mohindra's technique of.**
static r. Retinoscopy performed with the patient fixating a target at distance or with accommodation paralysed.

retinotectal pathway *See* **pathway, retinotectal.**

retinotopic map Term referring to the fact that the precise spatial arrangement of the retina is maintained throughout the visual pathway. *Syn.* retinotopic organization.
See **geniculate body, lateral; pathway, visual.**

retraction syndrome, Duane's *See* syndrome, Duane's.

retractor muscles, eyelid *See* muscle, levator palpebrae superioris; muscles, Müller's palpebral.

retrobulbar Behind the eyeball as, for example, retrobulbar optic neuritis.
See neuritis, optic.

retrobulbar block *See* injection, retrobulbar.

retrobulbar optic neuritis *See* neuritis, optic.

retrography *See* mirror writing.

retro-illumination *See* illumination, retro-.

retrolental fibroplasia *See* retinopathy of prematurity.

retrolental space of Berger *See* postlenticular space, Berger's.

retroscopic angle *See* angle, retroscopic.

retrospective study *See* study, retrospective.

reverse-geometry contact lens *See* lens, reverse-geometry contact; lens, ortho-k.

reversed image *See* image, inverted.

reversible spectacles *See* spectacles, reversible.

rhegmatogenous retinal detachment *See* retinal detachment, rhegmatogenous.

rheumatoid arthritis *See* arthritis, rheumatoid.

rhinoconjunctivitis, allergic *See* conjunctivitis, allergic.

rhodopsin Visual pigment contained in the disc membranes of the outer segments of the rod cells of the retina and involved in scotopic vision. It is estimated that each disc membrane contains approximately 150,000 rhodopsin molecules. Each rhodopsin molecule contains a large protein called *opsin* and a small attached molecule called *retinal*, which is vitamin A aldehyde. *Retinal* is the portion of the photopigment first affected by light absorption. When light stimulates the retina, a chain bleaching reaction is initiated which results in the breaking off of opsin and the photoisomerization of the chromophore of the pigment molecule *retinal* from '11-*cis*' isomer into the 'all-*trans*' isomer of *retinal*. Rhodopsin is regenerated during darkness by converting all-*trans* back to 11-*cis* *retinal* and recombining *retinal* and *opsin* with some enzymes. The isomerization from '11-*cis*' to 'all-*trans*' gives rise to the process of **transduction** in which the membrane potential covering the pigment molecules in the outer segment changes towards a hyperpolarization of the cell. This is the first step in the nervous response to a light stimulation of the retina. The absorption spectrum of rhodopsin has a maximum around 498 nm. *Syn.* visual purple (not used any more); erythropsin.
See adaptation, dark; bleaching; isomerization; optogram; pigment, visual; potential, receptor; spectrum, absorption; transduction.

rhythm, circadian The characteristic of some processes to repeat at approximately 24-hour intervals. *Examples*: Intraocular pressure is at its lowest every evening and highest every morning; corneal sensitivity is at its lowest every morning and highest every evening. *Syn.* diurnal cycle (provided the variation in activity or behaviour is more or less divided equally between night and day).
See melanopsin; nucleus, suprachiasmatic.

Ricco's law *See* law, Ricco's.

Riddoch phenomenon *See* phenomenon, Riddoch.

Rieger's anomaly; syndrome *See* syndrome, Rieger's.

rigid lens *See* lens, contact.

rigidity, ocular The resistance of the coats of the eye to indentation. This factor is taken into account in the tables used when determining the intraocular pressure by means of an indentation tonometer such as that of Schiötz. The tables are based on an eye of average ocular rigidity, but if the eye has high or low rigidity, an error is introduced into the readings. Means of minimizing this effect have been devised.
See law, Imbert-Fick; tonometer, impression.

Riley–Day syndrome *See* syndrome, Riley–Day.

rim That part of a spectacle frame which partly or completely surrounds the lens.

rim, neuroretinal *See* neuroretinal rim.

rimexolone *See* antiinflammatory drug.

rimless fitting Fitting an edged lens to a rimless mount. The process may include drilling, slotting, strap adjustment, etc. (British Standard).
See lens groove.

rimless spectacles *See* spectacles, rimless.

ring Any line, object or structure that is circular in shape.
anterior limiting r. of Schwalbe *See* line of Schwalbe.
capsular tension r. A plastic device placed within the lens capsule during cataract surgery to stabilize the remaining capsular bag with its implant. It may be used if the zonule of Zinn is partially missing.
Coat's white r. A small, oval or circular, whitish-grey ring opacity in the cornea found at the level of Bowman's layer, usually near the periphery. It is composed of a deposition of iron, possibly located at the site of a previous foreign body injury. No treatment is necessary.
See line, iron.
Fleischer's r. A narrow ring of brownish or greenish pigment containing iron, deposited in the epithelium of the cornea and surrounding (completely or partially) the base of the cone in keratoconus. It is not always present in that disease. *Syn.* Fleischer's line.
See line, iron.
Kayser–Fleischer r. A ring of pigment granules containing copper located in Descemet's membrane around the periphery of the cornea. It has a brown or greyish-green colour to the unaided eye or golden brown to reddish colour when viewed

through the slit-lamp and appears in nearly all cases of Wilson's disease.

Landolt r. *See* Landolt ring.

Newton's r's. Circular concentric interference fringes surrounding a point of contact when two glass surfaces are pressed together. The thicker the air film separating the two surfaces, the greater the number of concentric rings.

scleral r. Appearance of a white patch of sclera adjacent to the optic disc when the retinal pigment epithelium and the choroid do not extend to the optic disc.

See crescent, congenital scleral.

r. scotoma *See* scotoma, ring.

Soemmering's r. Lens remnants found within the periphery of the capsular bag. It may occur as a result of trauma, but more commonly following extracapsular cataract extraction. The pupillary area is usually left relatively free.

See after-cataract; Elschnig's pearls.

Vossius' r. An annulus-shaped opacity which is imprinted on the anterior lens capsule and which contains pigments from the posterior epithelium of the iris. It occurs as a result of a blunt trauma to the eye in which the aqueous pressure throws the iris forcefully against the lens. The ring is usually located sufficiently off-axis not to impair vision.

Wessley's r. A disc-shaped greyish opacity made up of inflammatory cells consisting of antigen-antibody complexes located in the corneal stroma. It is seen in stromal disciform keratitis. The ring may attract neovascularization. *Syn.* immune ring of Wessley.

Weiss' r. A greyish circular floater found in the vitreous when it detaches from the optic nerve head. It occurs in posterior vitreous detachment.

Riolan muscle *See* muscle of Riolan.

Risley prism *See* prism, rotary.

rivalry, binocular *See* retinal rivalry.

river blindness *See* onchocerciasis.

Rizzuti's sign *See* sign, Rizzuti's.

rock, accommodative *See* accommodative facility.

rod cell *See* cell, rod.

rod-free area *See* foveola.

rod monochromat *See* monochromat.

rod spherule The onion-shaped synaptic terminal of a rod photoreceptor located in the outer molecular (plexiform) layer of the retina. There is a deep pit (invagination) in the base of the terminal, which contains the dendrites of bipolar and horizontal cells, often two of each. The neurotransmitter is glutamate, which is stored in vesicles contained in the terminal, and when the photoreceptors are stimulated by light, the release of glutamate is decreased.

See cell, rod; hyperpolarization; neurotransmitter.

Roenne's nasal step When scotomata occur above and below the fixation point, they meet in the nasal field and form a horizontal step-like defect. It is one of the signs of glaucoma.

See scotoma, Bjerrum's.

room, Ames A specially constructed room in which all the visible features have been distorted to make the room appear cubic from one specific point of observation. In particular, the back wall of the room appears perpendicular to the line of sight, with left and right corners appearing equidistant to the observer, although in reality one corner is much farther away. The true shape of the room is trapezoidal with the ceiling and the floor at an incline. To an observer looking into the room through a peephole, people of identical heights standing one in each corner of the room appear of clearly different height. The person standing in the far away left corner where the floor is much lower than the right near corner does indeed produce a smaller retinal image, but because the observer believes that they are at the same distance and because the illusion of a cubic environment is so strong, it overrides size constancy, the person standing closer 'must be larger'. The Ames room demonstrates how perceived distance influences perceived size. *Syn.* Ames distorted room.

See illusion, moon; perception, depth.

room, leaf A cubical box, about 2 metres square, with its walls vertical and one open side. The interior surfaces are covered with artificial leaves of various sizes, which stick out in a random manner. An observer who is looking binocularly into the room from the centre of the open side will see its cubical shape due to stereopsis. However, monocularly the room appears almost flat as the monocular cues to depth perception are almost completely eliminated in this room. The leaf room is used to detect and measure spatial distortions resulting from aniseikonia. It can also be used to demonstrate spatial distortion using meridional size lenses.

See lens, aniseikonic; perception, depth.

rosacea, acne *See* acne rosacea.

rosacea keratitis *See* keratitis, rosacea.

rose bengal An iodine derivative of fluorescein having vital staining properties, but unlike fluorescein it is a true histological stain, which binds strongly and selectively to cellular components. The colour of this stain is red. It has the disadvantage of causing some pain in a good percentage of eyes. It stains dead or degenerated epithelial cells but not normal cells and is used to help in the diagnosis of corneal abrasion, keratitis, keratoconjunctivitis sicca, lagophthalmos, etc.

See fluorescein; lissamine green.

Rosenmuller, valve of *See* valve of Rosenmuller.

rostral Relating to either the anterior or superior part of the brain.

See caudal; dorsal; ventral.

rotary prism *See* prism, rotary.

Roth's spots *See* spots, Roth's.

rouge A powder consisting of iron oxide used to polish lenses, metals, etc.

See polishing; surfacing.

roughing Grinding of the surface of a lens to the approximate curvature and thickness with a coarse abrasive. It is the first step in the grinding process performed in the preparation of an ophthalmic lens or optical surface (e g. mirror). The surface is made to the desired curvature by having a grinding tool slide back and forth over the lens surface with a mixture of water and abrasive powder (e.g. carborundum), which has been brushed over the surfaces. *See* blocking; grinding; smoothing; surfacing.

rubella syndrome *See* syndrome, rubella.

rubeosis iridis Neovascularization of the iris characterized by numerous coarse and irregular vessels scattered on the surface and stroma of the iris. The new blood vessels may cover the trabecular meshwork, cause peripheral anterior synechia and give rise to secondary glaucoma. The most frequent causes are diabetes mellitus and central retinal vein occlusion. *See* glaucoma, neovascular; iritis; retinal vein occlusion.

Rubin's vase An ambiguous drawing, which may be perceived either as a vase or as two human profiles facing each other (Fig. R14). *See* figure, Blivet; Necker cube; Schroeder's staircase.

rule 1. A guiding principle governing an action or a procedure. **2.** A rigid graduated rod for measuring length.

Javal's **r.** Relationship that relates corneal astigmatism to the total astigmatism of the eye. It states that

$$A_t = 1.25A_c - 0.50 \text{ axis } 90°$$

where A_t and A_c are the total and corneal astigmatism, respectively. This relationship is relatively accurate in predicting the total astigmatism of the eye when corneal astigmatism is greater than 2 D. For smaller amounts of corneal astigmatism, a more appropriate version of Javal's rule is

$$A_t = 1.0A_c - 0.50 \text{ axis } 90°$$

Kestenbaum's **r.** A procedure designed to estimate the power of the addition needed to read ordinary newsprint (about Jaeger 5 or N7–8) in low-vision patients. It consists of dividing the denominator of the Snellen visual acuity fraction by its numerator (i.e. 1/Snellen visual acuity). *Example*: If the Snellen visual acuity is 6/60 (20/200), the power of the add will be +10 D, which corresponds to a magnification of 10/4 = 2.5× (Table R3). *Syn.* Kestenbaum's formula.

Knapp's **r.** *See* law, Knapp's.

Kollner's **r.** Lesions of the outer retinal layers and changes in the ocular media cause a blue-yellow colour vision defect, whereas lesions of the inner retinal layers, the optic nerve and the visual

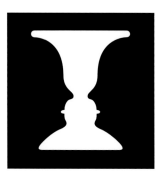

Fig. R14 Rubin's vase.

Table R3 Power of the addition required (and corresponding focal length) to read ordinary newsprint (about J5 or N8) in low vision patients for various acuities. The add is calculated according to Kestenbaum's rule and is an estimate.

Acuity at 40 cm	Snellen equivalent at 40 cm		Power of add (D)	Focal distance of add (cm)
	(m)	(ft)		
40/80	6/12	20/40	+2	50
40/100	6/15	20/50	+2.5	40
40/120	6/18	20/60	+3	33
40/140	6/21	20/70	+3.5	29
40/160	6/24	20/80	+4	25
40/200	6/30	20/100	+5	20
40/250	6/38	20/125	+6.25	16
40/320	6/48	20/160	+8	12.5
40/400	6/60	20/200	+10	10
40/500	6/75	20/250	+12.5	8
40/600	6/90	20/300	+15	6.7
40/800	6/120	20/400	+20	5
40/1200	6/180	20/600	+30	3.3
40/1600	6/240	20/800	+40	2.5

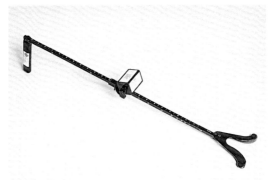

Fig. R15 The RAF near point rule.

pathway produce a red-green defect. *Examples:* Age-related maculopathy causes a blue-yellow defect; optic neuritis causes a red-green defect. There are exceptions to this rule, particularly during the evolution of a disease. *Syn.* Kollner's law.

near point r. Device for measuring the near points of accommodation and convergence. The RAF rule consists of a graduated four-sided bar on which is mounted a movable target holder which can be moved in the median plane of the head. The bar is calibrated in centimetres and dioptres (Fig. R15).
See **method, push-up.**

PD r. A ruler calibrated in millimetres used for measuring the interpupillary distance. Some have the zero point in the middle and the gradations on each side to measure two half-distances thus taking into account facial asymmetry. Many PD rules also have facilities for measuring frames (Fig. R16). *Syn.* pupillometer (although it is an incorrect use of this term, it is frequently used as a synonym).
See **pupillometer.**

Prentice's r. *See* **law, Prentice's.**

Prince's r. A device used for determining the location of the monocular near point of accommodation and the amplitude of accommodation. It consists of a ruler scaled in dioptres on one side and in millimetres on the other. One end of the ruler is held against the face and a test card is moved along the ruler towards the eye until a

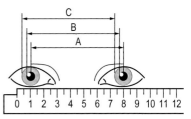

Fig. R16 PD rule. Measurement of the interpupillary distance is made by measuring the distance A between the two corneal images, B between the edges of the pupils (if both pupils are of the same size) or C between the edges of the limbus. In normal use, the PD rule is typically placed along the horizontal diameter of the cornea.

blur is noticed. The amplitude of accommodation in dioptres represents either the ocular accommodation (if the reference point is the cornea) or the spectacle accommodation (if the reference point is the spectacle plane).
See **accommodation, amplitude of; method, push-up.**

Rₓ Traditionally this symbol, which is an abbreviated form of the Latin word 'recipe', meaning 'take', appears before the main part of a prescription. It is nowadays commonly used as a synonym for prescription.
See **prescription.**

S

sac, lacrimal *See* lacrimal apparatus.

saccade *See* movement, fixation.

saccadic eye movement *See* movement, saccadic eye.

saccadic oscillation *See* flutter, ocular; myoclonus, ocular; opsoclonus.

saddle bridge *See* bridge, saddle.

safety glass *See* glass, safety.

sag Abbreviation for sagitta or sagittal depth; the height of a segment of a circle or sphere.
See lens measure; vertex depth.

sagittal depth *See* sag; vertex depth.

sagittal focus *See* astigmatism, oblique.

sagittal plane *See* plane, sagittal.

saline, physiological A 0.9% sterile solution of sodium chloride in water. This concentration of sodium chloride is considered approximately isotonic with the tears. It is used to store and rinse soft contact lenses, to irrigate the eye, etc. *Syn.* normal saline; NaCl 0.9%.
See eyewash; irrigation; solution, isotonic.

salt and pepper fundus *See* fundus, salt and pepper.

Salus' sign *See* sign, Salus'.

Salzmann's nodular degeneration *See* degeneration, Salzmann's nodular.

sample *See* sampling.

sampling The selection of a group of subjects from a population. This is usually done for the purpose of experimentation. The part of the population selected is called the **sample**; it is usually considered to be representative of a given population. A good sample must be **random**, i.e. every possible member of that population has an equal chance of being selected. Otherwise, it is said to be **biased**. Sampling can extend either across geographical areas (**spatial sampling**) or over a period of time (**temporal sampling**).

Sampaolesi's line *See* line, Sampaolesi's.

Sandhoff's disease *See* disease, Sandhoff's.

sarcoidosis An idiopathic multisystem granulomatous disorder in which the eye is affected in about 20% to 25% of patients in their third (acute form) and fourth or fifth (insidious form) decade of life. Ocular manifestations are (according to the International Workshop on Ocular Sarcoidosis): (1) 'mutton-fat' keratic precipitates (KP) and/or granulomatous KPs and/or iris nodules (Koeppe's and/or Busacca's), (2) trabecular meshwork nodules and/or tent-shaped peripheral anterior synechia, (3) vitreous opacities: snowballs and/or 'string of pearls', (4) multifocal chorioretinal peripheral lesions, (5) nodular and/or segmental periphlebitis and/or retinal microaneurysms in an inflamed eye, (6) optic disc nodule(s)/granuloma(s) and/or solitary choroidal nodule and (7) bilaterality. In addition, there may be dry eye, lacrimal gland infiltration and orbital and scleral lesions.
See dacryoadenitis; iridocyclitis; keratopathy, band; keratopathy, exposure; syndrome, Mikulicz's; uveitis.

sarcoma Malignant tumour formed by proliferation of mesodermal cells.

Sattler's layer *See* layer, Sattler's.

Sattler's veil Clouding of vision accompanied by seeing coloured haloes around lights caused by corneal oedema resulting from contact lens wear, more frequently the hard lens type without gas permeability such as PMMA lenses. The cause has been shown to be due to a circular diffraction pattern formed by the basal epithelial cells and the extracellular spaces. *Syn.* Fick's phenomenon.
See corneal clouding, central.

saturation Attribute of a visual sensation, which permits a judgment to be made of the proportion of pure chromatic colour in the total sensation. *Note:* This attribute is the psychosensorial correlate, or nearly so, of the colorimetric quantity purity (CIE). Note that all wavelengths do not elicit the same saturation. A monochromatic stimulus of wavelength 570 nm appears less saturated (i.e. with more white) than any other wavelengths.
See colorimetric purity.

scale, Snell–Sterling visual efficiency *See* visual efficiency scale, Snell–Sterling.

scanning laser polarimetry *See* polarimetry, scanning laser.

scatter Dispersion of a beam of light in various directions as it passes through a medium in which there are spatial variations in the refractive index due to inhomogeneities. Scatter is due to a combination of diffraction, refraction and reflection. **Forward scatter** occurs when the angle of deviation is less than 90° from the direction of the incident light and **backward scatter** when the angle is larger than 90°. The amount of light scattered is proportional to the intensity of the incident light, and the angular distribution depends on the size, shape and refractive index of the scattering particles. In the eye, light is scattered in the cornea and lens due to the presence of inhomogeneities and fundus due to its pigmentation. In the healthy eye, forward scatter does not exceed 1% to 2% of the incident light, but it increases significantly with age mainly caused by new lens proteins and affects visual performance in the presence of a bright light source. If a cataract is present, forward scatter produces a veiling glare and backward scatter reduces the amount of light reaching the retina.
See scattering, Rayleigh.

scatter illumination, sclerotic *See* illumination, sclerotic scatter.

scatter, Tyndall *See* effect, Tyndall.

scattering, Rayleigh Diffusion of radiation in the course of its passage through a medium containing particles the size of which is small compared with the wavelength of the radiation (CIE). The amount of forward and backward scatter is approximately equal, and it is proportional to the inverse of the fourth power of the wavelength, i.e. $1/\lambda^4$; thus blue light of wavelength 400 nm is scattered 9.4 times more than red light of 700 nm.

Scheimpflug photography An imaging technique that provides an assessment of the anterior segment of the eye in a sagittal plane. The principle of the technique is that the film plane, lens plane and subject plane (plane of focus) are tilted in such a way that all three planes intersect along a straight line. In this condition, a subject will be completely in focus. The technique can be used to detect and monitor opacities in the media of the anterior segment (e.g. in the lens), to document these changes and to carry out biometric evaluation (e.g. depth of the anterior chamber, corneal and lens thickness measurements, anterior and posterior corneal curvatures) by having a Scheimpflug camera and a monochromatic slit-light source rotating together around the optical axis of the eye and supplying three-dimensional images (Fig. S1).

Scheiner's disc; experiment; test *See* under the nouns.

schematic eye *See* eye, schematic.

Schiötz tonometer *See* tonometer, impression.

Schirmer's test *See* test, Schirmer's.

Schlemm's canal *See* canal, Schlemm's.

Schroeder's staircase This is an ambiguous figure that gives rise to two different perceptions. It consists of a drawing of parallel step-like lines extending from the upper corner of a parallelogram to the lower opposite corner. One either sees a staircase from underneath or a staircase from above and, upon continuous viewing, the impression alternates (Fig. S2). *Syn.* Schroeder's staircase visual illusion.
See figure, Blivet; Necker cube; Rubin's vase.

Schwalbe, anterior limiting ring of; line *See* line of Schwalbe.

Schwann cell *See* cell, Schwann.

science of vision *See* vision science.

scimitar scotoma *See* scotoma, arcuate.

scintillans, synchisis *See* synchisis scintillans.

scintillating scotoma *See* scotoma, scintillating.

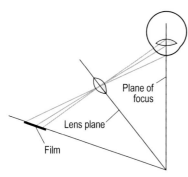

Plane of focus

Lens plane

Film

Fig. S1 Principle of Scheimpflug's photography. The whole optical section of the anterior segment of the eye is in sharp focus.

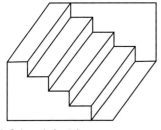

Fig. S2 Schroeder's staircase.

scissors movement *See* movement, scissors.

sclera The tough, white, opaque, fibrous outer tunic of the eyeball covering most of its surface (the cornea contributes 7% of, and completes, the outer tunic). It is avascular and made up of densely woven collagen fibres (thicker than those of the cornea), elastin, proteoglycans and fibroblasts. Its anterior portion is visible and constitutes the 'white' of the eye. In childhood (or in pathological conditions) when the sclera is thin, it appears bluish, while in old age, it may become yellowish due to a deposition of fat. The sclera varies in thickness and stiffness. It is thickest posteriorly around the optic nerve (about 1 mm), thin at the equator (0.4 mm) and posterior to the recti insertions (0.3 mm) and thickens to about 0.8 mm near the limbus, although there are wide individual variations. It is a sieve-like membrane at the lamina cribrosa. The sclera is pierced by three sets of apertures: (1) the posterior apertures around the optic nerve and through which pass the long and short posterior ciliary vessels and nerves; (2) the middle apertures, 4 mm behind the equator which give exit to the vortex veins and (3) the anterior apertures through which pass the anterior ciliary vessels. The tendons of insertion of the extraocular muscles run into the sclera as parallel fibres and then spread out in a fan-shaped manner. The sclera is commonly considered to be divided into three layers from without inward: (1) the episclera, (2) the lamina fusca (scleral stroma), which blends with (3) the suprachoroid (also called epichoroid), which is interposed between choroid and sclera. *Syn.* sclerotic. *Note*: Some authors consider the suprachoroid as belonging to the choroid. However, when choroid and sclera are separated, part of the suprachoroid adheres to the choroid and part to the sclera.
See cribriform plate; episclera; plexus, scleral; evisceration.

blue s. A hereditary defect in which the sclera has a bluish appearance. The sclera is thinner than normal and is susceptible to rupture if the person engages in contact sports. It is often associated with fragility of the bones and deafness as part of a condition called **osteogenesis imperfecta** (**fragilitas ossium, van der Hoeve's syndrome**) with keratoconus or with acquired scleral thinning (e.g. necrotizing scleritis). *Syn.* blue sclerotic.
See episclera; syndrome, Ehlers–Danlos; syndrome, Marfan's; syndrome, Turner's.

scleral buckling A surgical procedure aimed at repairing retinal breaks or detachment. It usually consists of one or more soft or hard silicone bands (called an explant) inserted through a small opening in Tenon's capsule overlying the retina and sutured onto the sclera. It presses the retinal pigment epithelium against the neurosensory retina. In case of extensive retinal breaks, a circumferential buckle is used.
See retinal detachment, rhegmatogenous.

scleral crescent *See* crescent, myopic.

scleral contact lens; ectasia; rigidity; ring *See* under the nouns.

scleral discolouration *See* alkaptonuria.

scleral foramen *See* lamina cribrosa.

scleral indentation A clinical procedure used in conjunction with indirect ophthalmoscopy in which some slight pressure is applied to the sclera to bring the peripheral retina into view. Observation of a lesion and retinal detachments and tears, for example, are more easily seen with this procedure. Pressure is usually applied with an instrument called an **indentor**. The technique is contraindicated in patients with elevated intraocular pressure. *See* **ophthalmoscope, indirect.**

scleral size, back Maximum internal diameter of the back surface of a scleral contact lens before the outer sharp edge has been rounded. *Syn.* back haptic size.

scleral spur A ridge of the sclera at the level of the limbus interposed between the posterior portion of Schlemm's canal and the anterior part of the ciliary body. The scleral spur is the structure to which some of the ciliary muscle fibres are attached. *See* **gonioscopy; sulcus, internal scleral.**

scleral sulcus *See* **sulcus, external scleral; sulcus, internal scleral.**

scleral zone The portion of a scleral contact lens designed to lie in front of the sclera. *Syn.* haptic.

sclerectasia *See* **ectasia, scleral.**

sclerectomy Surgical removal of a portion of the sclera performed in glaucoma surgery. A common procedure is to make a conjunctival flap at the limbus, followed by a full thickness scleral opening and iridectomy.

deep s. A type of non-penetrating filtration surgery aimed at lowering intraocular pressure by dissecting a superficial scleral flap and excising a deeper partial-thickness scleral flap below leaving a thin membrane consisting of trabeculum and Descemet's membrane through which the aqueous humour diffuses. It then passes from the anterior chamber to the subconjunctival space or though Schlemm's canal. *See* **trabeculectomy.**

scleritis Inflammation of the sclera, which in its severe necrotizing or in the posterior type may cause sight-threatening complications such as keratitis, uveitis, angle-closure glaucoma or optic neuropathy. Most scleritis are non-infectious. Infectious scleritis are rare and usually associated with surgical complications or linked with an inflammation of the cornea or conjunctiva, which has been caused by a systemic condition such as herpes zoster, syphilis, tuberculosis, etc. It is characterized by pain, redness, oedema and tearing, and some patients may develop nodules (**nodular scleritis**). It is often associated with a systemic disease (e.g. rheumatoid arthritis, Wegener's granulomatosis, polyarteritis nodosa).

anterior s. Scleritis involving the anterior sclera. It is classified as **diffuse non-necrotizing scleritis,** which affects females more commonly than males in the fourth to sixth decades of life. It presents with a red eye, pain, eyelid oedema and tearing, and it may recur; or **nodular non-necrotizing scleritis,** which presents suddenly with moderate to severe pain, redness, tearing and multiple bluish-red nodules.

The other anterior types are necrotizing and are the more aggressive form of scleritis. They are **anterior necrotizing scleritis with inflammation,** which presents in older patients than the other forms, with severe pain, redness, tearing, oedematous sclera and may result in scleral necrosis with complications such as keratitis, uveitis, glaucoma, or more rarely perforation; or **anterior necrotizing scleritis without inflammation,** which presents with small yellow areas of necrotic sclera which coalesce into a large area, and scleral thinning revealing the underlying uvea. It is a form of **scleromalacia perforans** and occurs most typically in women with rheumatoid arthritis. Treatment includes topical and systemic steroids, immunosuppressive drugs and surgery if perforation is present or at risk, although this very rare. *See* **keratitis, acute stromal; keratolysis; scleromalacia; syndrome, Brown's superior oblique tendon sheath.**

necrotizing s. *See* **scleritis, anterior.**

s. necroticans See scleritis, anterior; scleromalacia.

posterior s. Inflammation of the sclera involving the posterior segment of the eye. The condition is often associated with a systemic disease (e.g. rheumatoid arthritis). It is more difficult to diagnose because the eye remains white, unless the anterior sclera is involved, but it is characterized by pain and reduced visual acuity. The severity of the visual impairment depends on the involved tissue and its location, but the condition is potentially sight-threatening. Signs include eyelid oedema, proptosis, limitation of ocular movements and, if anterior scleritis is present, redness. The ocular fundus may present disc swelling, choroidal folds, macular oedema and exudative retinal detachment. Treatment consists mainly of systemic steroids and immunosuppressive agents. *See* **choroidal folds.**

sclerochoroiditis Inflammation of the sclera and the choroid. It can occur as a result of pathological myopia and it presents with a posterior staphyloma in the region of the optic disc.

scleroconjunctival Pertains to the sclera and the conjunctiva.

scleroconjunctivitis Inflammation of the sclera and of the conjunctiva.

sclerocornea Rare congenital condition in which the sclera and cornea are considered as a single layer. The limbus is ill-defined, and portions of opaque scleral tissue with conjunctival vessels cover the cornea. The condition is usually bilateral and frequently associated with cornea plana. Visual acuity is reduced and often it is merely

light perception if the entire cornea is involved. The eye is usually hyperopic. Systemic associations include mental retardation, deafness and craniofacial abnormalities. Treatment includes correction of the refractive error but in cases of central corneal opacification, keratoplasty may be indicated.
See **cornea plana.**

scleroderma An autoimmune condition characterized by thickening and hardening of the skin due to new collagen formation. It occurs in middle age, either in localized or in systemic disease as systemic sclerosis which affects blood circulation and internal organs as well as the skin. It may very occasionally produce keratoconjunctivitis sicca. *Syn.* dermatosclerosis.

scleroiritis Inflammation of the sclera and of the iris.

sclerokeratitis Inflammation of the sclera and of the cornea.

scleromalacia A bilateral and painless degenerative thinning of the sclera occurring in people with rheumatoid arthritis. In this condition, rheumatoid nodules may develop in the sclera and cause perforation (**scleromalacia perforans**). *Syn.* necrotizing scleritis without inflammation; scleritis necroticans.
See **scleritis, anterior.**

sclerosis, central areolar choroidal *See* dystrophy, central areolar choroidal.

sclerosis, multiple An autoimmune disease in which there are disseminated patches of demyelination and sclerosis (or hardening) of the brain, spinal cord and peripheral and optic nerves causing paralysis, tremor, disturbance of speech, nystagmus, diplopia due to involvement of the extraocular muscles and frequently retrobulbar optic neuritis.
See **myokymia; neuritis, demyelinating optic; ophthalmoplegia, internuclear; oscillopsia; potential, visual evoked cortical; pupil, Marcus Gunn; Uhthoff's symptom.**

sclerosis, tuberous A rare phakomatosis characterized, in severe cases, by epilepsy, mental impairment and adenoma sebaceum. Many cases are sporadic and others are autosomal dominant. There are visceral tumours, most commonly renal and of the heart, as well as cerebral with consequent mental defects and epilepsy and also a host of skin lesions such as red papules with butterfly distribution around the nose and cheeks; ash leaf spots of hypopigmentation on the trunk and limbs; and shagreen patches (collagenous plaques) over the lumbar region. Ocular signs are retinal tumours of astrocyte cells (cells with a large number of branching processes) around the optic disc, which may produce visual field defects and patchy iris hypopigmentation. *Syn.* Bourneville's disease.
See **phakomatoses.**

sclerotic *See* **sclera.**

sclerotic scatter illumination *See* **illumination, sclerotic scatter.**

sclerotomy Surgical incision of the sclera. It may be performed to extract an intraocular cyst or to drain a choroidal haemorrhage.

scopolamine hydrobromide *See* hyoscine hydrobromide.

scotoma An area of partial or complete blindness surrounded by normal or relatively normal visual field. *Plural*: scotomata.
See **angioscotoma; hemianopia; quadrantanopia.**
absolute s. Scotoma in which vision is entirely absent in the affected area.
See retinoschisis; scotoma, relative.
annular s. *See* scotoma, arcuate; scotoma, ring.
arcuate s. Scotoma running from the blind spot into the nasal visual field and following the course of the retinal nerve fibres. A double arcuate scotoma extending both in the upper and lower part of the field may join to make an **annular scotoma** or **ring scotoma**. A common cause is glaucoma. *Syn.* comet scotoma; scimitar scotoma.
See **fibre, arcuate; retinal raphe; scotoma, Bjerrum's; scotoma, ring.**
Bjerrum's s. Arcuate scotoma extending around the fixation point (usually located between the 10° and 20° circles) which occurs in open-angle glaucoma. It often extends from the horizontal midline to the optic disc (Fig. S3). *Syn.* Bjerrum's sign.
See **Roenne nasal step; scotoma, Seidel's.**
central s. Scotoma involving the fixation area.
centrocaecal s. Scotoma involving the macular area and continuous with the area surrounding the blind spot. It appears as a horizontal oval defect. It may result from optic nerve compression (e.g. from pituitary gland adenoma, nutritional optic neuropathy).
comet s. *See* scotoma, arcuate.
congruous s'. Identical scotomas noted in the two visual fields. They form a single defect in the binocular visual field. Such scotomas are often the result of lesions in the visual cortex.

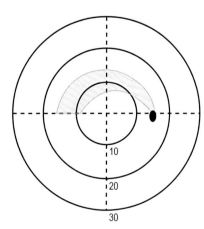

Fig. S3 Bjerrum's scotoma.

flittering s. *See* scotoma, scintillating.

incongruous s'. Scotomas seen in the two visual fields but differing in one or more ways. Such scotomas are often the result of lesions in the optic tract.

junction s. A visual defect due to a lesion (e.g. a pituitary tumour) at the junction of one optic nerve with the chiasma where it is believed that the inferior nasal fibres of the contralateral optic nerve loop before passing backward to the optic tract. The visual defects typically consist of an upper temporal quadrantanopia in the field of the contralateral eye with, usually, a temporal hemicentral scotoma in the ipsilateral eye. Some authors attribute these visual defects to prechiasmal compression of one optic nerve plus compression of the whole chiasma. *See* gland, pituitary; Wilbrand's knee.

negative s. Scotoma of which the person is unaware. The physiological blind spot is an example of a negative scotoma, but it is usually referred to as a **physiological scotoma.**

paracentral s. Scotoma involving the area adjacent to the fixation area.

physiological s. *See* scotoma, negative.

positive s. Scotoma of which the person is aware.

relative s. A scotoma in which there is some vision left or in which there is blindness to some stimuli, but not to others. *See* scotoma, absolute.

ring s. **1.** An annular scotoma surrounding the fixation point. It may be formed by the development of two arcuate scotomas. *Syn.* annular scotoma. *See* scotoma, arcuate. **2.** A circular area in the peripheral field of view at the edge of a strong convex spectacle lens which is not seen (Fig. S4). This scotoma is due to the prismatic effect at the edge of the lens and, unlike other scotomas, not from a pathological or physiological condition. When the head turns, the ring scotoma also turns, and it is then called a **roving ring scotoma.**

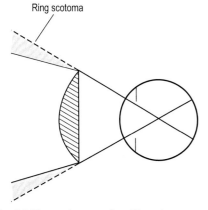

Ring scotoma

Fig. S4 Ring scotoma produced by a strong convex spectacle lens (shaded area).

See phenomenon, jack-in-the-box.

roving ring s. *See* phenomenon, jack-in-the-box; scotoma, ring.

scimitar s. *See* scotoma, arcuate.

scintillating s. The sudden appearance of a transient shimmering scotoma with a zigzag outline of brightly coloured lights (also called a **fortification spectrum** or **fortification figures**). It usually occurs as one of the first symptoms of a migraine attack. *Syn.* flittering scotoma. *See* migraine; teichopsia.

Seidel's s. An arcuate scotoma extending above and below the blind spot found in glaucoma. *Syn.* Seidel's sign. *See* scotoma, Bjerrum's.

scotometer An instrument such as a campimeter or a perimeter for detecting and plotting the position and magnitude of a scotoma. *See* campimeter; perimeter.

scotopia *See* vision, scotopic.

scotopic eye *See* eye, dark-adapted.

scotopic sensitivity syndrome *See* syndrome, Meares–Irlen.

scotopic vision *See* vision, scotopic.

screen, Bjerrum's *See* screen, tangent.

screen, Hess A black tangent screen for measuring and classifying strabismus. It consists of a chart divided by red lines into small sections of 5° separations. As the screen is flat, the lines are curved in a pincushion pattern (i.e. the middle of the lines is closer to the centre of the screen than the ends of the lines). At the respective positions on the lines in the eight major meridians are small red dots indicating positions 15° and 30° from the fixation point. Two green threads extend from the upper corners of the screen and meet a third green thread, which originates on the end of a pointer. The three threads form a figure Y. The patient, wearing a red lens in front of one eye and a green lens in front of the other, moves the pointer until the common origin of the green threads is superimposed on each of the red dots. The discrepancy between the two on the screen indicates the extent of the deviation in various directions of gaze. It is a particularly useful test to indicate an incomitant strabismus as the field plots obtained with each eye are compared and an estimate of which muscle(s) is affected can be made. Moreover, if the inner (15°) and outer (30°) plots are affected differently, the incomitancy is of mechanical origin. *Note*: There exists a computerized version of the Hess screen.

screen, Lees An instrument similar to the Hess screen. It consists of two internally illuminated screens placed at right angles. One eye views one screen directly, and the other views the second screen via a mirror; hence, the eyes are dissociated. When one eye fixates a point on one illuminated screen, its position as seen by the second eye is indicated with a wand on the second, non-illuminated screen. When this is illuminated, the position of the wand relative to the screen markings indicates whether a muscle or set of muscles is paretic or not.

screen, tangent A large plane surface for detecting and plotting the central visual field (about 50° in diameter) by moving the position of a stimulus (e.g. a white 1-mm pinhead). It consists of dull black cloth or other material perpendicular to the line of sight and placed usually 1 m away from the subject (2 m gives more accuracy). In the centre of the screen is a white spot that provides a fixation point and a series of radial and circumferential lines are sewn or drawn to facilitate the localization of the stimulus. *Syn.* Bjerrum's screen.
See campimeter; perimeter.

screen test *See* test, cover.

screener, vision *See* vision screener.

SEAL *See* staining, fluorescein.

sebaceous gland carcinoma; cyst *See* under the nouns.

sebum *See* gland, meibomian.

seclusio pupillae A complete blocking of the anterior chamber from the posterior chamber by a posterior annular synechia. It usually occurs as a result of an inflammation of the iris membrane. The pupil is immobile, so the aqueous flow is prevented from leaving the posterior chamber and the intraocular pressure becomes very high causing angle-closure glaucoma.
See aqueous humour; glaucoma, inflammatory; pupillary block.

secondary Refers to a disease that results from or follows a primary event, although it may differ in character from the primary event.

secondary deviation; glaucoma; position *See* under the nouns.

secretion 1. The substance produced by a cell or organ (e.g. a lacrimal gland). **2.** Production by a cell or organ of a physiologically active substance. The flow released out of a cell is driven by an osmotic pressure gradient across the membrane, which is created by active transport of one or more ion species from one side to the other.
See tear secretion; transport, active; ultrafiltration.

see 1. To perceive by the eye. **2.** To discern. **3.** To note; to understand.

see-saw nystagmus *See* nystagmus.

segment height The vertically measured distance from the lowest point on the lens to the top of the segment of a bifocal (or trifocal) ophthalmic lens. *Syn.* seg height.

segment of a bifocal lens (seg) An area of a bifocal lens of a power different to that of the main portion. *Syn.* portion. There is the **distance portion**, which has the correction for distance vision, and the **near** or **reading portion**, which has the correction for near vision.
See portion, intermediate.

segment of the eye, anterior *See* eye, anterior segment.

segment of the eye, posterior *See* eye, posterior segment.

Seidel aberration *See* aberration, monochromatic.

Seidel's scotoma; test *See* under the nouns.

semidecussation *See* hemidecussation.

semi-finished lens *See* lens, semi-finished.

semilunar fold *See* plica semilunaris.

senile macular degeneration *See* macular degeneration, age-related.

senilis, arcus *See* corneal arcus.

sensation The conscious response to the effect of a stimulus exciting any sense organ.
See perception.

sensation, visual A sensation produced by the sense of sight.

sense Any faculty (or ability) by which some aspect of the environment is perceived. The five main senses are those of sight, hearing, smell, taste and touch. The sense of sight may be further divided into the colour sense, the form sense, the light sense, the space sense, etc.

sense organ A structure especially adapted for the reception of stimuli and the transmission of the relevant information to the brain. The organ of sight is the eye, in which light is transduced into nerve signals in the photoreceptors of the retina.

sensitive period *See* period, critical.

sensitivity 1. The capability of responding to or transmitting a stimulus. **2.** The reciprocal of the threshold. **3.** The extent to which a test gives results that are free from **false negatives** (i.e. people found not to have the defect when they actually have it). The fewer the number of false negatives, the greater is the sensitivity of the test. It is usually presented as a percentage of the number of people truly identified as defectives, referred to as **true positives**, A (or hit), divided by the total number of defective people tested. The total number includes all the true positives, A, plus the false negatives, C (or **miss**). Hence

$$\text{sensitivity (in \%)} = \frac{A}{A+C} \times 100$$

See specificity.
contrast s. The ability to detect luminance contrast. In psychophysical terms, it is the reciprocal of the minimum perceptible contrast. The measurement of the contrast sensitivity of the eye is a more complete assessment of vision than standard visual acuity. It provides an evaluation of the detection of objects of varying spatial frequencies and of variable contrast, and a contrast sensitivity function (CSF). *Example:* Following amblyopia treatment, some cases still have the same visual acuity while the CSF is improved (Table S1).
See chart, contrast sensitivity; function, contrast sensitivity; resolution, spurious; test, Arden grating; test, Melbourne Edge; Vistech.

corneal s. The capability of the cornea to respond to stimulation. Corneal sensitivity to touch is assessed with an aesthesiometer that measures the **corneal touch threshold**, which is the reciprocal of corneal sensitivity. Sensitivity varies across the cornea, with the centre being the most sensitive. Diseases (e.g. neurotrophic keratopathy), ageing and rigid contact lens wear of low transmissibility greatly reduce the sensitivity of the cornea.
See aesthesiometer; corneal touch threshold; hyperaesthesia, corneal.

spectral s. The reciprocal of the radiant energy of a light source observed at a given wavelength. It is usually represented as a function of wavelength for a given individual or a given visual pigment. An average compounded value (usually referred to as spectral luminous efficiency) has been proposed by the CIE. The average spectral sensitivity (1/threshold energy) of the human eye has a peak at 555 nm in photopic vision and 507 nm in scotopic vision. If the observer is colour deficient, the photopic spectral sensitivity curve is displaced toward shorter wavelengths than 555 nm in protanopes and only slightly toward longer wavelength in deuteranopes.
See efficiency, spectral luminous; colour vision, defective; theory, duplicity; vision, photopic; vision, scotopic.

sensitization 1. State or condition in which the response to a second or later stimulus (e.g. a drug) is greater than the response to the original stimulus (e.g. first administration of the drug). **2.** The process in which exposure to an antigen results in the development of hypersensitivity.

sensory fusion; neuron *See* under the nouns.

Table S1 Relationship between contrast sensitivity and contrast threshold (contrast sensitivity = 1/contrast threshold). Neither values have units.

Contrast sensitivity	Log$_{10}$ contrast sensitivity	Contrast threshold	
		Decimal	%
1000	3.00	0.001	0.1
100	2.00	0.01	1
20	1.30	0.05	5
10.00	1.00	0.1	10
5.00	0.70	0.2	20
3.33	0.52	0.3	30
2.50	0.40	0.4	40
2.00	0.30	0.5	50
1.67	0.22	0.6	60
1.43	0.15	0.7	70
1.25	0.10	0.8	80
1.11	0.05	0.9	90
1.00	0.00	1	100

septo-optic dysplasia *See* syndrome, de Morsier.

septum orbitale *See* orbital septum.

serous chorioretinopathy *See* chorioretinopathy, central serous.

sessile drop test *See* test, sessile drop.

sex chromosome *See* chromosome.

sex-linked recessive inheritance *See* inheritance.

Shack-Hartmann aberrometry *See* aberration, wavefront.

shadow A darkened area from which rays from a source of light are excluded. The shadow pattern cast by an object placed in a light beam (e.g. sunlight, ceiling fixtures) is a common sight so that if light shines from the opposite direction (e.g. from the ground upward) the normal shadow pattern will be reversed and so will perception; depressions will appear as mounds or vice versa. Shadows offer a cue to depth perception, as when trying to judge the shape of objects.
See penumbra; perception, depth; umbra.

shadow test *See* test, shadow.

Shaffer classification *See* gonioscopy; method, van Herick, Shaffer and Schwartz.

Shafer's sign *See* sign, Shafer's.

shagreen, crocodile Polygonal greyish-white corneal opacities separated by relatively clear spaces and located in the stroma, either near Bowman's layer (**anterior crocodile shagreen**) or occasionally near Descemet's membrane (**posterior crocodile shagreen**). They are the result of an irregularity of the stromal collagen lamellae. The condition occurs in old people who are asymptomatic, with little or no effect on vision.
Syn. crocodile shagreen of Vogt.

shagreen of the crystalline lens The slightly irregular or granular appearance of the surfaces of the crystalline lens when viewed with the slit-lamp with specular reflection illumination. The posterior lens shagreen has a slightly yellower tint and is less coarse than the anterior. It is believed to represent variations in the refraction of light within the lens capsule.
See sign, Vogt's.

shaken baby syndrome *See* syndrome, shaken baby.

shape constancy *See* constancy, shape.

shape factor; magnification *See* magnification, shape; magnification, spectacle.

Sheard criterion *See* criterion, Sheard.

sheath syndrome *See* syndrome, Brown's superior oblique tendon sheath.

shedding Process by which some discs situated at the tip of the outer segment of the photoreceptors are discarded at regular intervals.
See cell, cone; cell, rod; phagocytosis.

shell *See* eye impression.

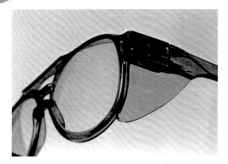

Fig. S5 Spectacles with protective shield.

Sheridan–Gardner test *See* test, Sheridan–Gardner.

Sherrington's law of reciprocal innervation *See* law of reciprocal innervation, Sherrington's.

shield, eye 1. *See* occluder. **2.** A protecting screen against injury or light (Fig. S5).
See goggles; spectacles, industrial.

shield ulcer *See* ulcer, shield.

shingles *See* herpes zoster.

short-pointing *See* pointing, short-.

short sight *See* myopia.

shutter A device that provides a means (mechanical or electro-optical) for letting a beam of light pass during a given length of time.

SI unit Abbreviation of **Système International d'unités** (or International System of Units). It is derived from the metric system of physical units. There are seven base units, two supplementary units and many derived units (Table S2).
See candela per square metre; lumen; lux; micrometre (micron); nanometre.

sickle-cell disease *See* disease, sickle-cell.

side An attachment to the front of a spectacle frame passing towards or over the ear for the purpose of holding the frame in position. *Syn.* temple.
See spectacle frame markings; spectacles; temple, library.
curl s. End of the side of a spectacle frame that lies along the greater part of the groove behind the ear. It contributes to the stability of the frame and it is particularly useful to children and to people engaged in sports. *Syn.* earpiece.

siderosis bulbi Deposit of iron produced by a foreign body in the ocular tissues, especially in the lens epithelium and retinal pigment epithelium. It is characterized by a reddish-brown discoloration of the surrounding tissue and its toxicity causes reduced visual acuity, constricted visual field, relative afferent pupillary defect, anterior capsular cataract and secondary glaucoma. The b-wave of the electroretinogram is attenuated.
See heterochromia; line, iron; pupil, Marcus Gunn.

Siegrist's streaks Line of pigment spots seen along choroidal arteries in the ocular fundus in advanced

Physical quantity	Name	Symbol
Base Units		
length	metre	m
mass	kilogram	kg
time	second	s
electric current	ampere	A
thermodynamic temperature	kelvin	K
luminous intensity	candela	cd
amount of substance	mole	mol
Supplementary Units		
plane angle	radian	rad
solid angle	steradian	sr
Some Derived Units		
area	square metre	m^2
electric potential difference	volt	V
electric resistance	ohm	Ω
energy	joule	J
force	newton	N
frequency	hertz	Hz
illuminance	lux	lx
luminance	candela per square metre	cd/m^2
luminous flux	lumen	lm
power	watt	W
velocity	metre per second	m/s
volume	cubic metre	m^3

Table S2 Base and supplementary SI units, and some derived units

hypertensive retinopathy. They are indicative of fibrinoid necrosis.

sight The special sense by which the colour, form, position, shape, etc. of objects is perceived when light from these objects impinges upon the retina of the eye.

sight, line of *See* line of sight.

sight, night *See* hemeralopia.

sight, old *See* presbyopia.

sight, partial *See* vision, low.

sight, second Improvement of near vision in the elderly resulting from increased refraction of the nucleus of the crystalline lens. It often occurs in people with incipient cataract. *Syn.* gerontopia; senile lenticular myopia.

sight, sense of *See* sense.

sight-testing *See* refraction.

sign Objective evidence of a disease as distinct from **symptom**, which is a subjective complaint of a patient.
See diagnosis; prognosis; symptom.
Argyll Robertson s. See pupil, Argyll Robertson.
Bard's s. An increase of the oscillations in organic nystagmus when a patient is directed to follow a

moving target across the field of view from one side to the other alternatively and a decrease in congenital nystagmus under the same conditions.

Bell's s. Bell's phenomenon occurring on the affected side of the face in Bell's palsy. *See* palsy, Bell's; phenomenon, Bell's.

Bjerrum's s. *See* scotoma, Bjerrum's.

Cogan's lid twitch s. A twitch of the upper eyelid in an eye with ptosis when the patient is asked to look in the primary position following a downward look. The eyelid then returns to its ptosis position. This condition occurs in myasthenia gravis.

Collier's s. Unilateral, or more commonly bilateral, eyelid retraction that exposes an unusual amount of the sclera of the eye above and below the iris; it gives the person a frightened or startled expression. It is due to a midbrain lesion. *See* syndrome, Parinaud's.

s. convention A set of conventions regulating the direction of distances, lengths and angles measured in geometrical optics. The most common is the **New Cartesian Sign Convention**. It stipulates: (1) All distances are measured from the lens, refracting surface or mirror. Those in the same direction as the incident light, which is drawn travelling from left to right, are positive. Those in the opposite direction are negative. (2) All vertical distances are measured from the axis. Those above are positive. Those below are negative. (3) Angles are measured from the incident ray to the axis, with anticlockwise angles positive and clockwise angles negative. (4) The power of a converging lens is positive and that of a diverging lens is negative (Fig. S6). *See* length, focal; law, Lagrange's; law of refraction; Newton's formula; paraxial equation, fundamental.

Dalrymple's s. Retraction of the eyelids causing an abnormally widened palpebral fissure, in primary gaze. This is a sign of Graves' disease. The patient appears to stare and to be frightened as some white sclera may be seen above the upper limbus. *See* disease, Graves'.

doll's eye s. *See* phenomenon, doll's head.

double-ring s. *See* hypoplasia, optic nerve.

von Graefe's s. Immobility or lagging of the upper eyelid when looking downward. This is a sign of Graves' disease.

Gunn's crossing s. Tapering of veins on either side of the arteriovenous crossings seen in hypertensive retinopathy.

Hutchinson's s. A triad of signs present in congenital syphilis. They are interstitial keratitis, notched teeth and deafness.

Kocher's s. Spasmodic retraction of the upper eyelid on attentive fixation. This is a sign of Graves' disease.

local s. *See* direction, oculocentric.

Moebius' s. Convergence weakness occurring in Graves' disease.

Mizuo's s. *See* phenomenon, Mizuo's.

Munson's s. A sign observed in keratoconus in which the lower lid is bulging as a cone when the patient looks downward. *See* keratoconus.

pseudo-von Graefe s. *See* aberrant regeneration.

Rizzuti's s. An arrowhead pattern near the nasal part of the corneoscleral limbus, sometimes seen in advanced keratoconus.

Salus' s. Retinal vein deflection from its normal course at arteriovenous crossings seen in hypertensive retinopathy.

Seidel's s. *See* scotoma, Seidel's.

Shafer's s. The presence of pigment granules of various sizes floating in the anterior vitreous. They usually result from a retinal break(s), which may progress into rhegmatogenous retinal detachment. Then the pigment cells appear as small, black, dust-like particles ('**tobacco dust**') seen on clinical examination. *See* retinal detachment, rhegmatogenous.

Vogt's s. Loss of the normal shagreen of the front surface of the crystalline lens indicating anterior capsular cataract. *See* shagreen, crocodile.

Uhthoff's s. *See* Uhthoff's symptom.

significance In statistics, an indication that the results of an investigation on a population (e.g. patients) differ from those of another population

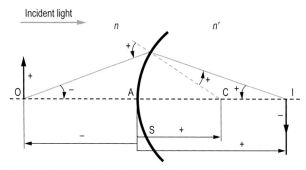

Fig. S6 Sign convention at a spherical refracting surface S (O, object; A, vertex; C, centre of curvature; I, image; n, n', refractive indices).

(e.g. general) by an amount that could not happen by chance alone. This is evaluated by establishing a **significance level**, that is the probability, called **p value**, which leads us to reject or accept the **null hypothesis** H$_o$, that there is no significant difference between two populations, and accept or reject the **alternative hypothesis** H$_1$, that there is a statistically significant difference between two populations. A p value of $p < 0.05$ is often considered significant, but the lower this figure, the stronger the evidence.
See hypothesis; regression; Student's t-test; trial, randomized controlled.

silicone hydrogel lens *See* lens, silicone hydrogel.

silicone rubber A polymeric elastomeric, transparent material that is used in the manufacture of silicone rubber contact lenses. It has very high oxygen permeability but it is also very hydrophobic (wetting angle greater than 90°). The surfaces must be specially treated to render them wettable. A silicone component is used in silicone hydrogel and gas permeable contact lenses. *Syn.* poly(dimethyl siloxane).
See angle, contact; index of refraction; lens, silicone hydrogel; modulus of elasticity.

simultanagnosia An inability to perceive more than one element of a picture or sustain visual attention across simultaneous elements, although its constituent elements may be recognized. Objects may look fragmented or even sometimes disappear, hence the patient may have difficulty reading or recognizing a face as only one part is seen. Visual acuity and visual fields are normal. This is often a symptom of Balint's syndrome or the result of a lesion, usually, in both parietal visual cortices, although temporal lobes may also be involved. *Syn.* simultagnosia; visual disorientation.
See syndrome, Balint's.

SILO response *See* response, SILO.

silver wire artery *See* arteriosclerosis.

simple astigmatism; cell *See* under the nouns.

simultaneous binocular vision *See* vision, Worth's classification of binocular.

simultaneous vision *See* lens, bifocal contact.

Simultantest Trade name for an accessory to be inserted in the lens aperture of a phoropter or trial frame used to refine both the sphere and cylindrical components of a refraction. It provides simultaneous viewing of a distant test object through either a plus and minus sphere lens (+0.25 D and −0.25 D) or through two +0.25 D sphere, −0.50 D cylinder lens systems with their cylindrical axes perpendicular to each other. Either mode of viewing is obtained by turning a knob, which actually rotates one of the lenses in the system.
See phoropter; trial frame.

sine condition The elimination of distortion and coma in an image formed in an optical system is met when

$$M = n \sin u/n' \sin u' \text{ or } nh \sin u = n'h' \sin u'$$

where M is the lateral magnification, n and n' the refractive indices of the media in the object and image space, u and u' are the angular apertures on the object and image sides, and h and h' the sizes of the object and image, respectively. *Syn.* Abbé's condition.
See aperture, angular; coma; correction; distortion.

single binocular vision *See* vision, binocular single.

single-vision lens *See* lens, single-vision.

sinus A hollow space in bone or other tissue.
cavernous s. One of the two venous sinuses located in the dura mater of the brain extending on each side of the pituitary body, behind the orbit. It receives blood from the superior and the inferior ophthalmic veins and the central retinal veins. The third, fourth, fifth and sixth nerves pass through as well as the internal carotid artery. The cavernous plexus is located within this sinus.
See fistula, carotid-cavernous; plexus, cavernous.
s. circularis iridis *See* canal, Schlemm's.
ethmoidal s. Mucus-lined air cavities within the ethmoid bone, between the nose and the orbit. They drain into the nasal cavity. They contain the anterior and posterior ethmoidal nerves and blood vessels and are filled with air. They are separated from adjacent areas by very thin plates through which infection can pass easily and in particular ethmoiditis, which is the most common cause of orbital cellulitis.
s. of Maier *See* lacrimal apparatus.
scleral s. *See* canal, Schlemm's.
s. venosus sclerae *See* canal, Schlemm's.

situs inversus of the disc *See* disc, situs inversus of the.

sixth cranial nerve *See* nerve, abducens.

sixth nerve paralysis *See* palsy, sixth nerve.

size, angular The size of an object measured in terms of the angle it subtends. The point of reference for the eye can be either the nodal point or the centre of the entrance pupil.
See object, extended; size, apparent.
apparent s. 1. The size of an object represented by its angular size. 2. The perceived size of an object as distinct from the actual size (Fig. S7).
s. constancy *See* constancy, size.
s. lens *See* lens, aniseikonic.

Sjögren's syndrome *See* syndrome, Sjögren's.

skiascope *See* retinoscope.

skiascopy *See* retinoscopy.

skull The skeleton of the head. It consists of the cranium enclosing the brain, the facial skeleton and the mandible. The cranium comprises a set of bones, the ethmoid, frontal, parietal (2), occipital, sphenoid and temporal (2) bones, which are immobile and separated by sutures. An injury to the occipital bone involving the occipital cortex can cause visual field defects, scotomas or even

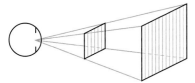

Fig. S7 Objects of different size seen in the same direction and with the same angular size stimulate the same retinal points and thus have the same apparent size.

blindness (cortical blindness). A fracture involving the orbital plate of the frontal bone results in a haemorrhage underneath the conjunctiva and into the orbital cavity causing proptosis.
See **blindness, cortical; orbit.**

slab-off lens *See* **lens, slab-off.**

slit-lamp Instrument producing a bright focal source of light with a slit of variable width and height used in the examination of ocular structures. It consists of a binocular microscope of variable magnification and an illumination system linked on a common pivot so that both are focused in the same plane. It may be used to examine the tissues of the anterior segment of the eye with and without fluorescein. To examine the internal structures of the eye including the retina, an auxiliary lens is required. Many such lenses exist, some which do not make contact with the eye (e.g. Hruby lens, Volk lens) and others which come in contact with the eye, usually like a scleral type of lens (e.g. Goldmann lens, Thorpe four mirror fundus lens, Wilson three mirror fundus lens). A slit-lamp is essential in contact lens practice. This instrument is also commonly called a **biomicroscope** (although strictly speaking this only forms part of the instrument) (Fig. S8).
See **biomicroscopy, fundus; fluorescein; gonioscope; illumination; method, van Herick, Shaffer and Schwartz; method, Smith's; microscope, slit-lamp; polymegethism, endothelial.**

small angle strabismus *See* **microtropia.**

small eye artifact *See* **retinoscopic artifact.**

smooth pursuit *See* **movement, pursuit.**

Smith's method *See* **method, Smith's.**

smoothing Grinding of the surface of a lens to the exact curvature and thickness with a very fine abrasive. This procedure comes after the roughing process and prior to polishing. *Syn.* fining.
See **abrasive; grinding; polishing; roughing; surfacing.**

Snell's law *See* **law of refraction.**

Snellen acuity *See* **acuity, Snellen.**

Snellen chart *See* **chart, Snellen.**

Snellen equivalent *See* **acuity, near visual.**

Snellen fraction A representation of visual acuity in the form of a fraction (e.g. 6/6 [20/20], 6/24

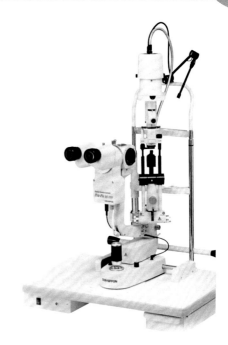

Fig. S8 Slit-lamp. (Shin Nippon SL500D, courtesy of Grafton Optical Co.)

[20/80], etc.) in which the numerator is the testing distance, usually expressed in metres (or in feet), and the denominator is the distance at which the smallest Snellen letter read by the eye has an angular size of 5 minutes (Table S3).
See **acuity, decimal visual; acuity, near visual; acuity, visual.**

Snellen test type *See* **chart, Snellen.**

Snell–Sterling visual efficiency scale A representation of visual efficiency as a function of visual acuity, in which other factors are taken into account such as perception, experience, etc. in estimating how much vision a person has for a given visual acuity (Table S4).

snow blindness *See* **keratoconjunctivitis, actinic.**

sodium chloride *See* **saline, physiological; tears, artificial.**

sodium cromoglicate *See* **conjunctivitis, giant papillary; conjunctivitis, vernal; keratoconjunctivitis, superior limbic; mast cell stabilizers.**

sodium fluorescein *See* **fluorescein.**

sodium pump *See* **potential, action.**

sodium/potassium pump *See* **potential, action; transport, active.**

Soemmering's ring *See* **ring, Soemmering's.**

soft drusen; exudate *See* **under the nouns.**

solar retinopathy; spectrum *See* **under the nouns.**

Table S3 Relationship between Snellen fractions in metres and feet (20 feet), and for two testing distances (4 and 6 metres)

(6 m)	(20 ft)	(4 m)
6/3	20/10	4/2
6/4.8	20/16	4/3.2
6/6	20/20	4/4
6/7.5	20/25	4/5
6/9.5	20/32	4/6.3
6/12	20/40	4/8
6/15	20/50	4/10
6/18	20/60	4/12
6/21	20/70	4/14
6/24	20/80	4/16
6/30	20/100	4/20
6/38	20/125	4/25
6/48	20/160	4/32
6/60	20/200	4/40
6/90	20/300	4/60
6/120	20/400	4/80
6/150	20/500	4/100
6/180	20/600	4/120
6/240	20/800	4/160
6/300	20/1000	4/200

Table S4 Relationship between visual acuity and the Snell–Sterling visual efficiency scale (in percentage round figures)

Visual acuity		Efficiency	Loss of vision
(M)	(ft)	(in %)	(in %)
6/6	20/20	100	0
6/7.5	20/25	96	4
6/9	20/30	91	9
6/12	20/40	84	16
6/15	20/50	77	23
6/18	20/60	70	30
6/24	20/80	59	41
6/30	20/100	49	51
6/48	20/160	29	71
6/60	20/200	20	80
6/90	20/300	8	92
6/120	20/400	3	97
6/150	20/500	1.5	98.5

solution A liquid, usually aqueous, in which a substance is dissolved. Most eyedrops are presented as a solution.

hypertonic s. A solution with an osmotic pressure greater than that of an isotonic solution. Hypertonic ophthalmic solutions cause some stinging when instilled. *Examples*: sodium chloride 5%: when applied to an oedematous cornea, this solution reduces oedema by drawing water from it; sulfacetamide sodium 30%; glycerol (or glycerin), at a dose of 1 to 1.5 g/kg body weight given as a solution with water or other liquid, which draws water from the eye into the blood and thereby reduces the intraocular pressure.

See **hydrops, corneal; hyperosmotic agent; pressure, osmotic; saline, physiological.**

hypotonic s. A solution with an osmotic pressure lower than that of an isotonic solution. Hypotonic ophthalmic solutions generally cause less irritation than hypertonic ones.

See **pressure, osmotic.**

isotonic s. A solution with an osmotic pressure equal to that on the other side of a semipermeable membrane. *Example*: Sodium chloride 0.9% is considered to be approximately isotonic with the tears and is commonly used as an eyewash.

See **pressure, osmotic; saline, physiological.**

soma 1. The body of an organism (e.g. head, nerve trunk) as distinct from the mind or the internal organs (viscera). **2.** The body of a nerve cell, which contains the nucleus, mitochondria, Golgi complex, lysosomes, etc. and from which the axon and dendrites project.

somatic Pertaining to the body.

source A point of origin.

coherent s. See **coherent sources.**

extended s. A source consisting of many point sources separated laterally and such that it has a very low degree of coherence. Thus, an extended source has a given size and subtends a given angle.

See **coherent sources; light, beam of; light, diffuse.**

glare s. See **glare.**

light s. See **illuminants, CIE; light source.**

point s. A source whose dimensions are sufficiently small to produce radiations with a high degree of coherence. If the point source is situated on the axis of an optical system it gives rise to an axial ray and it is referred to as an **axial point source.**

See **coherent sources; ray, axial.**

space 1. An area or a cavity within the body. **2.** A limited area, usually three-dimensional.

Berger's postlenticular s. A space situated between the posterior surface of the crystalline lens and the hyaloid fossa of the vitreous. The space is believed to be filled with aqueous humour. *Syn.* retrolental space of Berger.

colour s. A two- or three-dimensional representation of colour stimuli. *Example*: CIE chromaticity diagram.

See **chromaticity diagram.**

free s. Refers to a visual environment which is observed in natural viewing conditions, that is viewing an object that is neither housed inside an instrument (e.g. in a synoptophore) nor viewed through an optical system. *Syn.* open environment; true space.

gaussian s. See **paraxial region.**

horopter s. Horopter consisting of all object points in space which stimulate corresponding retinal points, as distinct from the two-dimensional cases such as the apparent frontoparallel plane, longitudinal or nonius horopters.

image s. Region on one side of an optical system in which the image is formed.
See **space, object.**
intertrabecular s. See **trabecular meshwork.**
object s. Region on one side of an optical system or a lens in which the object is situated.
See **space, image.**
Panum's fusional s. An area in space corresponding to Panum's area within which there is fusion and stereopsis of a non-fixated target.
See **area, Panum's; horopter.**
perichoroidal s. See **space, suprachoroidal.**
subarachnoid s. The space between the arachnoid mater and the pia mater that surrounds the brain and spinal cord which is filled with cerebrospinal fluid and through which pass arteries, veins and nerves. It extends around the optic nerve to the back of the lamina cribrosa. If there is increased intracranial pressure, the space may be compressed as well as the optic nerve and central retinal vein.
See **haemorrhage, subarachnoid; meninges; papilloedema; syndrome, Terson's.**
subretinal s. Small extracellular space between the photoreceptor outer segments and the retinal pigment epithelium. It is filled with a viscous matrix composed of proteins and glycosaminoglycans that provide adhesive properties for the apposition of the adjacent cell layers. It is a space into which oedema penetrating either from the choriocapillaris or the vitreous may lead to retinal breaks and detachment.
See **retinal detachment.**
suprachoroidal s. A potential space located between the choroid and the sclera. Anteriorly it is continuous with the supraciliary space. It contains thin pigmented strands of collagen fibres and it is traversed by the long and short posterior ciliary arteries and nerves. *Syn.* perichoroidal space.
See **haemorrhage, suprachoroidal.**
supraciliary s. A potential space located between the ciliary body and the sclera. In this space are thin strands of collagen fibres derived partly from the suprachoroid and partly from layers of the ciliary muscle. This space together with the suprachoroidal space form part of the unconventional route of aqueous humour outflow, the uveoscleral pathway.
See **pathway, uveoscleral.**
true s. See **space, free.**

span of recognition The amount of reading matter that can be correctly identified or perceived during a brief exposure. It is often evaluated in testing and training reading ability.
See **reading.**

sparing of the macula See **macula, sparing of the.**

spasm of accommodation; of the near reflex See **accommodation, spasm of.**

spasm of the lid See **blepharospasm.**

spasmus nutans A pendular rapid nystagmus of small amplitude which presents in infancy. It is generally bilateral, although asymmetrical and horizontal in most cases. Rotary and vertical types have been reported. The condition is associated with head nodding and less frequently with torticollis. The cause is unknown and the condition subsides spontaneously in early childhood. It must be differentiated from other disorders, such as congenital nystagmus and intracranial tumours, which also result in head nodding, and nystagmus.

spatial frequency; induction; summation See under the nouns.

spatial vision See **perception, depth.**

specificity The extent to which a test gives results that are free from **false positives** (i.e. people found to have the defect when they are actually free of it). The fewer the number of false positives, the greater is the specificity of the test. It is usually presented as the percentage of people truly identified as not defectives, or normal, referred to as **true negatives**, D (or correct reject), divided by the total number of not defectives or normal people tested. The total number includes all the true negatives, D, plus the false positives, B (or false alarm). Hence

$$\text{Specificity (in \%)} = \frac{D}{B+D} \times 100$$

See **sensitivity.**

spectacle blur See **blur, spectacle.**

spectacle crown See **glass, crown.**

spectacle frame See **spectacles.**

spectacle frame markings Numbers shown on a spectacle frame. They are usually the eyesize, the distance between lenses and the side length. Metal frames may also indicate the amount of gold (if any) found in the frame (e.g. 12 k meaning that the material is one-half gold and one-half of another metal). *Example*: 52/22 on the front of the frame means that the eyesize is 52 mm and the DBL is 22 mm, and 140 on the side means that the total length of the side is 140 mm.
See **distance between lenses; eyesize; side.**

spectacle frame, metal A structure in metal for enclosing or supporting ophthalmic lenses. Common materials include nickel/silver, Hi-nickel alloy, bronze, stainless steel, gold, gold plated, gold coating (commonly referred to as gold filled in which the base metal is most often nickel silver and for better quality frames, monel), copper, beryllium, titanium and sometimes aluminium. Metal spectacle frames are usually more rigid and maintain their shape better than plastic spectacle frames. However, the contacts with the skin of the nose and ears are done with plastic (or silicone) nose pads and temple covers.

spectacle frame, plastic A structure in plastic for enclosing or supporting ophthalmic lenses. Common materials include carbon fibre composite materials, which are a mixture of principally carbon and nylon in different percentages, cellulose

acetate, cellulose propionate, nylon, epoxy resin (trade name Optyl) and Perspex and Plexiglas (which are both trade names for acrylic plastics containing mainly polymethyl methacrylate). Most of the plastics used are thermoplastic, i.e. a material which softens with heat and can thus be manipulated to fit the patient's head and to insert and remove the lenses.
See **frame heater; polymethyl methacrylate.**

spectacle lens See **lens, spectacle.**

spectacle magnification See **magnification, spectacle.**

spectacle refraction See **refractive error.**

spectacles An optical appliance consisting of a pair of ophthalmic lenses mounted in a frame or rimless mount, resting on the nose and held in place by sides extending towards or over the ears. Syn. eyeglass frame; eyeglasses; eyewear (colloquial); glasses; spectacle frame.
See **acetone; angle, pantoscopic; angle, retroscopic; angling; bridge; clipover; eczema; endpiece; eyesize; front; hinge; lens washer; lorgnette; mount; pad; plastic; rim; side; spectacle frame markings; sunglasses; temple; tortoiseshell.**

aphakic s. Spectacles mounted with aphakic lenses used to compensate the loss of optical power resulting from a cataract extraction when no intraocular lens implant has been inserted. Syn. cataract glasses.
See **lens, aphakic.**

billiards s. Spectacles incorporating joints that enable the wearer to adjust the angle of the sides (British Standard).

folding s. Spectacles that are hinged at the bridge and in the sides, so as to fold with the two lenses in apposition.

half-eye s. A pair of spectacles for near vision, designed so that the lenses cover only half of the field of view, usually the lower half. The wearer looks in the distance over the spectacles. (Fig. S9). Syn. half-eyes.

hemianopic s. Spectacles incorporating a device that provides a lateral displacement of one or both fields of view. The device is usually a prism such as a Fresnel Press-On prism, which is placed over the blind (hemianopic) side of the visual field. A mirror system may also be used. The view within that side of the field is imaged on the seeing side of the visual field of the eye.

industrial s. Spectacles made with plastic or safety glass and solid frame, sometimes with side shields. They are used in industrial occupations where there are possible hazards to the eye.
See **Fig. S5, p. 314; glass, safety; goggles; lens, safety.**

library s. Plastic spectacle frame with heavyweight front and sides. Syn. library frame.

magnifying s. Spectacles containing lenses of high convex power (+10 D or higher) used for near vision.

orthopaedic s. Spectacles with attachments designed to relieve certain anatomical deformities such as entropion, ptosis, etc.
See **ptosis; syndrome, Horner's.**

pinhole s. Spectacles fitted with opaque discs having one or more small apertures. They are used as an aid in certain types of low vision (e.g. corneal scar).
See **spectacles, stenopaeic; vision, low.**

recumbent s. Spectacles intended to be used while recumbent. They usually incorporate a prism that deflects a beam of light through approximately 90° while keeping the image erect.
See **prism, yoke.**

reversible s. Spectacles that are designed to be worn with either lens before either eye.

rimless s. Spectacles without rims, the lenses being fastened to the frame by screws, clamps or similar devices.
See **lens groove; rim.**

stenopaeic s. Spectacles fitted with opaque discs having a slit. They are used as an aid in certain types of low vision.
See **disc, stenopaeic; spectacles, pinhole; vision, low.**

supra s. Spectacles in which the lenses are held in position by thin nylon threads attached to the rims.
See **lens groove; rim.**

telescopic s. See **lens, telescopic.**

spectral 1. Relating or belonging to a spectrum. **2.** Relating to wavelength.

spectral luminous efficiency See **efficiency, spectral luminous.**

spectral transmission factor See **spectrophotometer.**

spectral sensitivity See **sensitivity, spectral.**

spectrometer An instrument for making measurements of the angle of a prism and of the index of refraction. It consists of a collimator, an astronomical telescope, a table for carrying a prism and a graduated circle.

spectrophotometer An instrument for measuring the relative intensities of the spectrum, wavelength by wavelength. Specifically, it measures the spectral **transmission factor** (i.e. the ratio of radiant flux transmitted through a medium to that incident

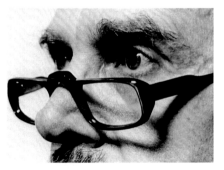

Fig. S9 Half-eye spectacles.

Table S5 Approximate values of the velocity, frequency and wavelength of electromagnetic radiations in a vacuum (the values represent a point within a range of radiations)

Radiation	Velocity (m/s)	Frequency (Hz)	Wavelength (m)	Wavelength (nm)
AM radio	3×10^8	1×10^6	3×10^2	3×10^{11}
television	3×10^8	1×10^8	3	3×10^9
radar	3×10^8	1×10^9	3×10^{-1}	3×10^8
microwave	3×10^8	1×10^{10}	3×10^{-2}	3×10^7
thermal infrared	3×10^8	1×10^{13}	3×10^{-5}	3×10^4
near infrared	3×10^8	1×10^{14}	3×10^{-6}	3000
Light				
red	3×10^8	3.94×10^{14}	7.6×10^{-7}	760
yellow	3×10^8	5.45×10^{14}	5.5×10^{-7}	550
violet	3×10^8	7.50×10^{14}	4.0×10^{-7}	400
ultraviolet	3×10^8	1×10^{16}	3×10^{-8}	30
X-rays	3×10^8	1×10^{18}	3×10^{-10}	0.3
gamma rays	3×10^8	1×10^{21}	3×10^{-13}	0.0003

on it) of a medium for a given wavelength. This factor is usually plotted as a graph against many wavelengths providing a spectral transmission curve. Ophthalmic lenses, contact lenses and any other substances (e.g. tear lipids) through which light may be passed can thus be analysed. *See* density.

spectroscope An instrument for producing and observing spectra. It consists of a slit, a diffraction grating or a prism to disperse the radiations, achromatic lenses and an eyepiece to observe them. *See* monochromator; spectrum.

spectrum 1. Spatial display of a complex radiation produced by separation of its monochromatic components. **2.** Composition of a complex radiation, e.g. continuous spectrum, line spectrum (CIE). *Plural*: spectra.
See light.
absorption s. Curve representing the relative absorption of a pigment or chemical substance as a function of the wavelength of light. *Example*: the absorption spectrum of rhodopsin. *Syn.* absorbance spectrum.
action s. Graphical representation of the relative energy necessary to produce a constant biological effect. *Example*: frequency of action potentials in a ganglion cell as a function of wavelength.
continuous s. A spectrum in which, over a considerable range, all wavelengths exist without any abrupt variation in intensity. *Example*: the spectrum of hot solids.
See lamp, filament.
electromagnetic s. The total range of all electromagnetic waves. It extends from the longest radio waves of some thousands of metres in wavelength through radar, microwave, infrared rays, visible rays (between wavelengths 780 nm and 380 nm) to ultraviolet rays, X-rays, gamma rays and cosmic rays with wavelengths as short as 8×10^{-13} m. All these electromagnetic waves differ only in frequency (and wavelength)

but have the same speed as light in a vacuum (Table S5).
equal energy s. Spectrum in which all wavelengths have about the same amount of energy. *See* achromatic; light, white.
fortification s. See scotoma, scintillating.
invisible s. Portions of the entire electromagnetic spectrum that are made up of radiations other than those of the visible spectrum.
line s. Spectrum consisting of a series of discrete monochromatic lines (or narrow bands of monochromatic light) with large intensity differences and separated by intervals without radiations. *Example*: the spectrum emitted by an electric discharge through a gas or vapour under low pressure. *See* line, Fraunhofer's.
s. locus The representation of the spectral colour stimuli on a chromaticity diagram.
solar s. The spectrum formed by sunlight. It is crossed at intervals by Fraunhofer's lines.
visible s. Portion of the electromagnetic spectrum that can be perceived by the visual system. It is composed of radiations of wavelengths in the range between 380 nm and 780 nm in younger eyes. This range decreases with age especially due to lens absorption of short wavelengths becoming closer to 420 nm than 380 nm.
See light; Table L3, p. 195.

specular microscope; reflection *See* under the nouns.

speculum, eye *See* eye speculum.

speed of light *See* light, speed of.

sphenoid bone *See* orbit.

sphere A term commonly used to denote the spherical component of a prescription or of the power of a lens or even a spherical lens.
See lens, spherical; prescription.
far point s. The imaginary spherical surface on which lie the far points of accommodation for all directions of gaze.

See **accommodation, far point of.**

near point s. The imaginary spherical surface on which lie the near points of accommodation for all directions of gaze.

See **accommodation, near point of.**

spherical aberration *See* **aberration, spherical.**

spherical equivalent A spherical power whose focal point coincides with the circle of least confusion of a spherocylindrical lens. Hence, the spherical equivalent of a prescription is equal to the algebraic sum of the value of the sphere and half the cylindrical value, i.e. sphere + cylinder/2. *Example*: the spherical equivalent of the prescription −3 D sphere −2 D cylinder, axis 180° is equal to −4 D.

spherical error *See* **prescription.**

spherical lens *See* **lens, spherical.**

spherometer *See* **lens measure.**

sphero-cylindrical lens *See* **lens, spherocylindrical.**

spherophakia A congenital bilateral defect in which the crystalline lens is smaller and more spherical than normal. The zonule of Zinn may also be defective or absent and the lens may be subluxated or luxated into the vitreous. The lens may need to be excised as it could cause secondary glaucoma.

See **luxation of the lens; syndrome, Weill–Marchesani.**

spherule, rod *See* **rod spherule.**

sphincter oculi muscle *See* **muscle, orbicularis.**

sphincter pupillae muscle *See* **muscle, sphincter pupillae.**

sphingomyelin lipidosis *See* **disease, Niemann–Pick.**

sphygmomanometer An instrument for measuring the arterial blood pressure. There are various types, the most common consisting of an inflatable cuff that is placed around the upper arm (usually the left) and air pressure within the cuff is balanced against the pressure of the blood in the brachial artery. The pressure is estimated by means of a mercury or an aneroid manometer. A stethoscope is normally used in conjunction with the instrument to listen to the blood pressure sounds (a stethoscope is not needed with an electronic sphygmomanometer). Normal systolic and diastolic blood pressures in a young adult are about 120/80, respectively. The difference between the two pressures is called the **pulse pressure**. Blood pressure varies with age, gender, altitude, disease, stress, fear, excitement, exercise, etc. A normal range for systolic pressure is usually considered to be 100–140 mmHg, and for diastolic pressure below 90 mmHg.

See **arteriosclerosis; hypertension; retinopathy, hypertensive.**

Spielmeyer–Stock disease *See* **disease, Batten–Mayou.**

spin-cast contact lens *See* **lens, spin-cast contact.**

spindle, Krukenberg's *See* **Krukenberg's spindle.**

spindle, muscle *See* **muscle, extraocular.**

spiral, Plateau's *See* **Plateau's spiral.**

spiral of Tillaux A line forming a spiral which connects the insertions of the four recti muscles starting with the medial rectus, which has its insertion closest to the limbus (5.5 mm) and going around to the insertion of the inferior rectus (6.5 mm), then to the lateral rectus (6.9 mm) and ending at the superior rectus with its insertion farthest from the limbus (7.7 mm).

sporadic Adjective describing a disease that occurs occasionally or haphazardly in an individual.

See **epidemic.**

spot A small circumscribed area visibly different in colour or texture from the surrounding tissue.

baring of the blind s. A visual field defect in which there is such a marked contraction of the peripheral temporal visual field that it lies on, or nasal to, the blind spot. Although it may occur in open-angle glaucoma, it is not indicative of the disease as it also occurs in other conditions (e.g. miosis).

See **scotoma, Bjerrum's.**

Bitot's s. A foamy patch found on the bulbar conjunctiva near the limbus in xerophthalmia and due to vitamin A deficiency. *Syn.* Bitot's patch.

blind s. Physiological negative scotoma in the visual field corresponding to the head of the optic nerve. It is not seen in binocular vision, as the two blind spots do not correspond in the field. In monocular vision, it is usually not noticed. It has the shape of an ellipse with its long axis vertical and measuring approximately 7.5°, whereas its shorter axis along the horizontal measures approximately 5.5°. Its centre is located 15.5° to the temporal side of the centre of the visual field and 1.5° below the horizontal meridian. *Syn.* blind spot of Mariotte; physiological blind spot; punctum caecum (Fig. S10).

See **fibre, myelinated nerve; image, retinal.**

blind s. enlargement A visual field defect in which the blind spot appears larger than normal. One of the common causes is papilloedema.

blind s. esotropia; syndrome *See* **syndrome, Swann's.**

Brushfield's s's. Small, white or yellow spots in the periphery of the iris associated with Down's syndrome. They may be present in normal children.

cherry-red s. Bright red appearance of the macular area in an eye with occlusion of the central retinal artery, Tay–Sachs disease or Niemann–Pick disease. In the case of central retinal artery occlusion, the surrounding area is white due to ischaemia but the reddish reflex from the intact

+

Fig. S10 Demonstration of the blind spot. Looking at the cross with the right eye at a distance of about 15 to 20 cm, one sees the black circle disappear.

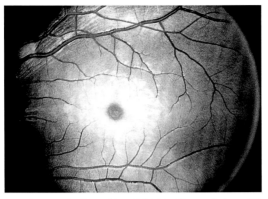

Fig. S11 Cherry-red spot at the macula. (From Kanski 2007, with permission of Butterworth-Heinemann)

choroidal vessels beneath the fovea shows at that spot since the retina is thinnest there. There is a very marked, if not complete, loss of vision which appears suddenly. In cases of storage disease (i.e. Niemann–Pick or Tay–Sachs), the area surrounding the fovea is artificially whitened and opaque, offsetting the normal pinkish colour of the fovea (Fig. S11).
See commotio retinae; disease, Niemann–Pick; disease, Sandhoff's; disease, Tay–Sachs; retinal artery occlusion.

cotton-wool s's. *See* bodies, cytoid; exudate.

Elschnig's s's. Small yellowish spots found in the fundus in advanced hypertensive retinopathy. They are choroidal infarcts caused by insufficient blood supply.

Forster-Fuchs s. *See* spot, Fuchs'.

Fuchs' s. A round or elliptical pigmented spot, usually located in the macular or paramacular area. It occurs in patients who have pathological myopia. It is due to breaks in Bruch's membrane (called **lacquer cracks**) and to the development of a choroidal neovascular membrane followed by subretinal haemorrhage which has changed colour and has become pigmented. The patient may notice photopsia when the membrane breaks but eventually it causes a loss of vision with a central scotoma. *Syn.* Forster–Fuchs spot.

Maxwell's s. An entopic phenomenon in which the subject can observe a dark or greyish spot in the visual field corresponding to the fovea. This is accomplished by viewing a diffusely illuminated field through a purple-blue or dark blue filter. (These are the best colours for this observation.) This phenomenon is used clinically to detect eccentric fixation by placing a fixation point in the diffusely illuminated field. The degree of eccentric fixation can thus be estimated by asking the subject to describe the position of the grey spot with respect to the fixation point. *See* image, entoptic.

s. retinoscope *See* retinoscope, spot.

Roth's s. A small white spot consisting of coagulated fibrin seen in the middle of a retinal haemorrhage. It is associated with leukaemia, but it can be seen in subacute bacterial endocarditis, diabetic retinopathy, hypertensive retinopathy and vascular conditions with capillary fragility.

spring catarrh *See* conjunctivitis, vernal.

scleral spur *See* scleral spur.

spurious resolution *See* resolution, spurious.

squamous cell *See* corneal epithelium.

squamous cell carcinoma *See* carcinoma, squamous cell.

squint *See* esotropia; strabismus.

squinting eye *See* eye, deviating.

SRK formula An approximate formula established by Sanders, Retzlaff and Kraft to determine the power of an intraocular lens implant *P*, in aqueous, to render the eye emmetropic (and ignoring the lens thickness)

$$P = A - 2.5X - 0.9K$$

where *A* is a numerical term specific to the implant and to the manufacturer. It is equal, on average, to 115 for anterior chamber implants and 116.8 for posterior chamber implants. *X* is the axial length of the eye (in mm) and *K* is the average keratometer reading (in dioptres). The formula gives satisfactory results for eyes of average length. *Example*: *A* = 116.8, *X* = 23 mm and *K* = 43 D, *P* = 116.8 – 57.5 – 38.7 = 20.6 D.
The power of the intraocular lens implant differs in air and is given by the following formula

$$P \text{ air} = \frac{nl - n \text{ air}}{nl - n \text{ aqueous}} \times P$$

where *nl* is the index of refraction of the implant and *P* its power in aqueous. *Example*: Assuming *nl* is equal to 1.523 and the power is 20.6 D, P_{air} = (1.523 – 1.0)/(1.523 –1.333) × 20.6 = 56.70 D.
There are several other formulae used to predict the power of an intraocular lens implant (e.g. Holladay, Hoffer Q).
See biometry of the eye; lens, intraocular.

stabilized retinal image Image formed on the retina when neutralizing the fixation movements of the eye. The effect of these movements is thus eliminated and the image usually disappears after a few seconds. The methods used for stabilizing a retinal image are: (1) The target is placed at the end of a tube mounted on a tightly fitted contact lens. The whole device moves with every movement of the eyeball and the retinal image remains on the same retinal spot. (2) The subject is also fitted with a tight contact lens on the side of which is attached a small mirror. A test projected on the mirror is reflected onto a screen. The subject views the test through a compensating system of four mirrors and therefore as the eye moves, the retinal image moves along with it and stimulates the same retinal spot. (3) Presentation of a target for a length of time smaller than the time necessary for the eye to perform a small eye movement. Presentations of less than 0.01 s usually fulfill this requirement.
See **movement, fixation; phenomenon, Troxler's.**

stage The platform, at right angles to the optical axis of a microscope, on which the object to be examined is mounted.

staining, fluorescein The artificial coloration of tissue by fluorescein. Under ultraviolet illumination, it stains dead or degenerated corneal epithelial cells due to abrasions, old age or following inadequate contact lens fit, a yellowish-green colour. It also stains the tears, thus facilitating the evaluation of tear drainage or the blood flow through the retina and choroid when injected intravenously. Corneal staining resulting from contact lens wear may present in various shapes, locations, depths or severity. A very common form is punctate staining as appears in punctate epithelial keratitis. There may be arcuate stains located in different parts of the cornea, some inferiorly (called **inferior epithelial arcuate lesions**) or superiorly (called **superior epithelial arcuate lesions** [*acronym*: **SEAL**] or **epithelial splitting**), which usually do not give rise to symptoms and appear mainly with soft or silicone hydrogel lenses. A very severe form of staining is called epithelial plug. It is typically round in shape and represents a loss of the full thickness of the epithelium. Corneal staining resulting from contact lens wear typically disappears after cessation of contact lens wear. *See* **angiography, fluorescein; test, dye dilution; test, fluorescein.**

staining, 3 and 9 o'clock Punctate corneal staining located just inside the limbus usually on the horizontal meridian on both sides, hence called 3 and 9 o'clock staining (or 4 and 8 o'clock). It may appear only on one side. It is observed with the biomicroscope after instillation of fluorescein. It is very useful to have the patient look nasally to inspect the temporal cornea and then temporally for the nasal portion. This staining is associated with hard corneal contact lens wear, although in some rare cases mild staining is observed without contact lens wear. It is due to inadequate spreading of the tear film over these areas of the cornea as a result of incomplete and/or infrequent blinking. Another cause for this type of staining is a small contact lens that is too thick. This condition is a mild form of exposure keratitis.
See **keratopathy, exposure; lamp, Burton; test, fluorescein.**

standard axis notation *See* **axis notation, standard.**

standard deviation A descriptive statistics test designed to estimate the degree of dispersion or variability of a set of data from the mean value of the set. It is expressed in the same unit as the data themselves and expressed as the square root of the variance. *Symbol*: σ (sigma). The **variance** is equal to the mean of the squared deviations of the data from their mean, hence

$$s^2 = \sum (x_1 - m)^2 / n - 1$$

where x_1 is a data point, m the mean and n the sample size The standard deviation is σ = s.
See **statistics.**

standard illuminants *See* **illuminants.**

staphyloma A bulging of the sclera, or very rarely the cornea, due to injury, inflammation, glaucoma or pathological myopia, and containing adherent uveal tissue. Staphylomas can occur anywhere within the eye, and they are then referred to as anterior or ciliary scleral staphyloma, which is partly overlaid by prolapsed tissue of the ciliary body, or more frequently posterior staphyloma, which is typically associated with degenerative myopia. If only the cornea or sclera stretches without uveal tissue, the condition is called **ectasia**.
See **ectasia, corneal.**

staphyloma, anterior A congenital disease characterized by an opacity of one or both corneas, which become protuberant, often with adherent iris tissue. It is possibly due to a faulty embryonic development or intrauterine inflammation. *Syn.* keractectasia (if there is no uveal lining).

stare To look at something fixedly for a long time.

Stargardt's disease *See* **disease, Stargardt's.**

static eye reflex; perimetry; visual acuity *See* under the nouns.

statistics The science that deals with collection, classification, analysis and interpretation of information expressed in numbers and in accordance with the theory of probability and the application of various test assessments. There are two major branches: **descriptive statistics**, which present data using various tests, including mean, median, mode, standard deviation, range, correlation, etc. and **inferential statistics** which deals with hypothesis testing and significance level.
See **correlation; hypothesis; mean; median; mode; regression; significance; standard deviation; Student's t-test; study.**

stem cells *See* **cell, stem.**

stem cell deficiency, limbal A rare condition in which the stem cells located at the limbus are diminished as a result of topical medication, previous ocular surgery or ultraviolet exposure. Conjunctival cells are then able to ingress into the cornea leading to surface irregularity and vascularization with consequent visual impairment. It is often associated with pterygium.
See cell, stem; limbus.

stenopaeic disc; slit *See* disc, stenopaeic.

stenopaeic spectacles *See* spectacles, stenopaeic.

stenosis, punctal *See* punctal stenosis.

stereo-acuity *See* acuity, stereoscopic visual.

stereo-blindness Complete lack of perception of stereopsis. It may result from blindness in one eye or strabismus, but also from some unknown cause in people with otherwise normal vision in both eyes. Stereo-blindness in some parts of the visual field also occurs in people who have had their corpus callosum or optic chiasma cut or destroyed. However, some depth perception may still exist thanks to monocular cues (e.g. aerial perspective, light and shadow, overlap, relative size).
See perception, depth.

stereo-threshold *See* acuity, stereoscopic visual.

stereogram Paired similar photographs or drawings which when viewed in a stereoscope give the sensation of stereopsis. Some stereograms are used only to explore fusion. Stereograms can also be used in free space that is in natural viewing conditions (called **free space** stereograms), which require over- or underconvergence to obtain fusion.
Syn. stereoslide.
See space, free.

stereogram, random-dot A stereogram in which the eyes see an array of little characters or dots of a roughly uniform texture and containing no recognizable shape or contours. The only difference is that a certain region in one target has been laterally displaced with respect to the other, to produce some retinal disparity. When they are viewed in a stereoscope, that region is seen in stereoscopic relief. The shape in that region can be any pattern. The effect is remarkable, as the shape usually appears to float out from the surround.
Syn. Julesz random-dot stereogram.
The **random-dot E test** uses a polarized random test pattern and requires the use of Polaroid spectacles to detect whether a subject has stereopsis. The subject will see a raised letter E in the random-dot pattern of one of the test plates. At 50 cm, the retinal disparity induced by the E is 500 seconds of arc.
The **TNO test** for stereoscopic vision also uses random-dot stereograms in which the half-images have been superimposed and printed in complementary colours, like anaglyphs. The test plates, when viewed with red and green spectacles, elicit stereopsis. There is a series of plates inducing retinal disparities ranging from 15 to 480 seconds of arc.

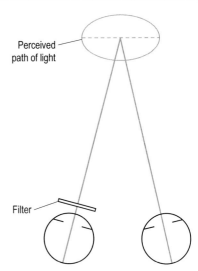

Fig. S12 Pulfrich stereophenomenon. Observer looks at an oscillating object moving along the dotted line. When one eye is covered by a light-absorbing filter, the object appears to move in depth along the path represented by the ellipse.

See acuity, stereoscopic visual; anaglyph; disparity, retinal; stereotest, Frisby; stereotest, Lang; test, two-dimensional; vectogram.

stereophenomenon, Pulfrich If an object swings in the frontal plane and the observer places in front of one eye a light-absorbing filter (any value between 5% and 40%), that object will appear to move along an ellipse. This elliptical movement is virtually horizontal, with one part in front and the other behind the frontal plane. If the filter is placed in front of the other eye, the object will appear to swing along an ellipse but in the opposite direction. One explanation for the perception of depth of the moving object is a hypothesized difference in the latent periods of the two eyes caused by the filter, which induces a reduced level of illumination in one eye. The covered eye presents a position of the moving target, which lags behind that of the uncovered eye. Therefore at any given moment, this unilateral delay gives rise to binocular disparity and depth perception (Fig. S12). *Syn.* Pulfrich effect; Pulfrich phenomenon.

stereophotography Photography performed to produce pictures that give rise to the perception of stereopsis when viewed in a stereoscope. It has been used for determining corneal and optic disc topography.
See photokeratoscopy.

stereopsis Awareness of the relative distances of objects from the observer, by means of binocular vision only and based on retinal disparity. *Syn.* stereoscopic vision; third-degree fusion.
See acuity, stereoscopic visual; anaglyph; angle of stereopsis; column, cortical; disparity, retinal;

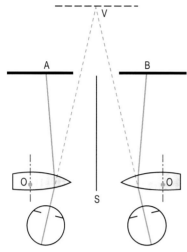

Fig. S13 Principle of the Brewster–Holmes stereoscope (S, septum; A and B, stereograms; O, optical centre of the convex lenses decentred to produce BO prisms; V, fused images formed by the lenses).

> perception, depth; room, leaf; stereo-blindness; stereogram, random-dot; stereoscopy; test, Howard-Dolman; test, three needle; test, two-dimensional.

stereopsis, chromatic *See* chromostereopsis.

stereoscope An instrument that allows targets to be presented independently to the two eyes. The separation of the targets is produced either by tubes, a septum or an arrangement of mirrors. Stereograms are the targets used with a stereoscope. Stereoscopes are used to test and train binocular fusion and stereopsis, evaluate suppression and view images in three dimensions.
Brewster's s. A stereoscope consisting of two tubes separating the two fields of view and convex lenses. The distance between the tubes can be adjusted to suit the viewer's PD. *Syn.* lenticular stereoscope; Brewster–Holmes stereoscope (although this instrument uses a septum to separate the two visual fields, a sliding stereogram holder and decentred convex lenses, usually +5.25 D, to produce BO prisms) (Fig. S13).
See Telebinocular.
Brewster–Holmes s. See stereoscope, Brewster's.
lenticular s. See stereoscope, Brewster's.
Pigeon–Cantonnet s. A stereoscope consisting of three black cardboard leaves attached together as in a book, with a plane mirror placed on one face of the middle leaf and targets on the other two leaves. The subject places the central leaf as a septum and one eye sees one target directly while the other eye sees the other by reflection in the mirror. The angle of convergence may be controlled by the angle between the leaves. This instrument is often used in visual training as well as in orthoptics.

variable prism s. A stereoscope incorporating two Risley prisms and a septum positioned so that each eye sees one half of a stereogram card which can be moved to and fro from the eyes in the median plane of the head. To maintain the normal relationship between accommodation and convergence at a given fixation distance, BO prisms are adjusted before each eye. This instrument is particularly well suited to measure and train fusional reserves of convergence and divergence.
See prism, rotary.
Wheatstone s. See amblyoscope, Wheatstone.

stereoscopic vision *See* stereopsis.

stereoscopic visual acuity *See* acuity, stereoscopic visual.

stereoscopy The science dealing with the perception of three-dimensional effects and of producing them.
See stereopsis.

stereoscopy, colour *See* chromostereopsis.

stereotest, Frisby A stereoacuity test consisting of a transparent square plate on which four similar patterns (resembling a random-dot stereogram) are printed on one side. In the central part of one of the four patterns is a circular area, which is printed on the other side of the plate and can appear in depth. The plate (made of plastic or glass) comes in three thicknesses: 6 mm, 3 mm and 1 mm. By using the three plates and presenting them at different distances, the test can produce a retinal disparity of the circular area between 7 and 600 seconds of arc. In this test, the patient's head must be kept still to avoid monocular cues. The plate can be turned upside down or rotated to alter the position of the pattern with relief. *Syn.* Frisby test.
See stereogram, random-test.

stereotest-housefly *See* vectogram.

stereotest, Lang A random-dot stereogram upon which is imprinted a series of parallel strips of cylindrical lenses, which act to separate the views seen by each eye. There are three stereoscopic shapes that the patient has to identify: a cat (inducing 1200 seconds of arc of retinal disparity), a star (600 seconds of arc) and a car (550 seconds of arc). The test is administered at 40 cm and exactly in the frontoparallel plane. As there is no need to use special spectacles, it is a very useful test for young children. *Syn.* Lang test.
See stereogram, random-dot.

stereotest, Titmus *See* vectogram.

stereothreshold *See* acuity, stereoscopic visual.

sterile infiltrates A condition characterized by the presence of infiltrates, which are often noted in the cornea of contact lens wearers. These lesions differ from infectious infiltrates in so much that the overlying epithelium is usually intact, there is typically little or no pain, and the lesions tend to be small (less than 1.5 mm). The lesions consist of subepithelial infiltrates of leukocytes.

It is postulated that these lesions are an immune response to a specific antigen (likely contact lens or solution-related), and not related to a bacterial infection. Treatment is often supportive with cessation of contact lens wear.
See corneal infiltrates.

sterilization The process or act of killing all microorganisms from a surface, equipment, medication, contact lenses, etc. It is achieved through the application of heat (dry or moist), chemicals, irradiation, supersonic waves, etc.
See antiseptic; disinfection.

steroid One of a group of hormonal substances produced mainly by the adrenal cortex. They fall into three main groups: glucocorticoids (or glucocorticosteroids), mineralocorticoids and sex hormones. The **glucocorticoids** have anti-inflammatory properties reducing vasodilatation, stabilizing mast cells thus decreasing the release of histamine and maintaining the normal permeability of blood thus preventing oedema. They also inhibit the production of prostaglandins, which mediate some of the effects of inflammation. They are widely used in the treatment of a variety of inflammatory diseases of various organs including the eye (e.g. allergic and vernal conjunctivitis, corneal diseases, iritis, uveitis and sympathetic ophthalmia). The natural glucocorticoids, such as cortisone and hydrocortisone, are effective only at high doses. Synthetic and more potent steroids are used in ophthalmic treatment (when used as ophthalmic preparations they are called **corticosteroids**). They include, betamethasone, dexamethasone, fluorometholone, prednisolone and triamcinolone.
See antiinflammatory drug; gland, adrenal.

Stevens–Johnson syndrome *See* syndrome, Stevens–Johnson.

Stevens' law *See* law, Fechner's.

stigmatic lens *See* lens, anastigmatic.

stigmatism The condition of an optical system in which light from a point source forms an image which is also a point, as distinct from astigmatism.
See astigmatism.

stigmatoscope An instrument for observing or measuring the refractive state of the eye based on the position of best focus of a very small point source.

stigmatoscopy A method of determining the refractive state of the eye based on the criterion of sharpness of an image. The observer determines the position at which a point source appears in the best focus, while the eye is unaccommodated: this indicates the far point of the eye. If the eye is astigmatic, the point source will appear as a line or streak when at the far point of each principal meridian. The distance between the two foci corresponds to the cylinder correction and the slant of the streaks from the horizontal or vertical indicates the axis of the astigmatism.
See refractive error; stigmatoscope.

Stiles–Crawford effect *See* effect, Stiles-Crawford.

Stilling canal *See* canal, hyaloid.

Still's disease *See* disease, Still's.

Stilling–Turk–Duane syndrome *See* syndrome, Duane's.

stimuli, heterochromatic *See* heterochromatic stimuli.

stimulus Any agent or environmental change that provokes a response. *Plural*: stimuli.
See potential, action.
   adequate s. Stimulus of sufficient intensity and of appropriate nature to provoke a response in a given receptor. Visible light is the adequate stimulus for the eye, but pressure on the eye that may nevertheless produce a response (called a phosphene) is an **inadequate stimulus**.
   inadequate s. *See* stimulus, adequate.
   liminal s. A stimulus of intensity such that it just provokes a response that is at threshold. *Syn.* threshold stimulus.
   threshold s. *See* stimulus, liminal.

Stocker's line *See* line, Stocker's.

Stokes lens *See* lens, Stokes.

stop *See* diaphragm.

strabismometer An instrument for measuring the angle of strabismus.

strabismus The condition in which the lines of sight of the two eyes are not directed towards the same fixation point when the subject is actively fixating an object. Thus the image of the fixation point is not formed on the fovea of the deviated eye and there may be diplopia, although in most cases, the diplopic image is suppressed and vision is essentially monocular. The prevalence of concomitant strabismus in children is 2% to 5% and is far more common than paretic strabismus. Management depends on the type of strabismus. However, in all cases, the refractive errors must be accurately corrected. If the deviation still prevails, orthoptics and, sometimes, pharmacological (e.g. miotics in accommodative esotropia) treatment is attempted, but in many cases surgery is necessary (except where accommodation is faulty or when the deviation is small), usually followed by some orthoptics treatment aimed at developing fusion and stereopsis. *Syn.* heterotropia; squint (this term is commonly used by the general public); tropia.
See angle of anomaly; angle of strabismus; botulinum toxin; chemodenervation; deviation, dissociated vertical; deviation, skew; esotropia; eye, deviating; eye, fixating; hypertropia; method, Javal's; microtropia; phenomenon, phi; point, zero; pointing, past-; retinal correspondence, abnormal; suppression; syndrome, Apert's; syndrome, Brown's superior oblique tendon sheath; syndrome, Crouzon's; syndrome, Duane's; syndrome, Marfan's; test, Bruckner's; test Hirschberg's; test, Krimsky's; test, cover; test, three-step.
   accommodative s. *See* esotropia, accommodative.

acquired s. Abnormal alignment of the visual axes that occurs after the age of 6 months.

alternating s. Strabismus in which either eye may deviate.
See **strabismus, unilateral.**

angle of s. *See* **angle of deviation.**

apparent s. Condition simulating the appearance of strabismus. It may be due to epicanthus, to an abnormally large angle lambda (or kappa) or to the breadth of the nose, etc. It can be distinguished from a real strabismus by noting that the corneal light reflexes are centrally located in relation to the pupils or by means of the cover test. *Syn.* pseudostrabismus.

comitant s. *See* **strabismus, concomitant.**

concomitant s. Strabismus in which the angle of deviation remains the same whichever eye is fixating and in whichever direction the eyes are looking. *Syn.* comitant strabismus.
See **concomitance; strabismus, incomitant.**

congenital s. *See* **esotropia, infantile.**

consecutive s. A deviation of the eye in the opposite direction to what it was previously. This condition may follow surgery although it may occur spontaneously. There are two types: **consecutive exotropia** in a patient who previously had esotropia or esophoria and **consecutive esotropia** in a patient who previously had exotropia or exophoria. *Syn.* postoperative overcorrection.
See **esotropia; exotropia.**

convergent s. *See* **esotropia; Fig. S14.**

cyclic s. *See* **esotropia, cyclic.**

deorsumvergens s. *See* **hypertropia.**

divergent s. *See* **exotropia; Fig. S14.**

s. fixus A rare, congenital condition in which one or both eyes are firmly fixed in a position of extreme adduction or abduction, although the most common position is adduction (esotropia). It is due to an anatomical anomaly (e.g. anomalous

insertion of the medial or lateral rectus muscle) or muscle fibrosis (e.g. of the two medial recti muscle in esotropia). Voluntary movements of duction and version, as well as passive movements as in the forced duction test, are either absent or negligible.
See **test, forced duction.**

incomitant s. Strabismus in which the angle of deviation varies with the direction of gaze and with the eye used for fixation. It may be congenital or acquired. The *congenital* type is due to some developmental anomaly of one or more of the extraocular muscles or of the neural component that serves them. The *acquired* type may be due to head injury, disease of the oculomotor system or systemic disease (e.g. multiple sclerosis, myasthenia gravis, thyroid eye disease, aneurysms). The main symptom of incomitant strabismus is diplopia, and it suddenly appears in the acquired type. Abnormal head posture and past-pointing may be present. The affected muscle(s) may be detected by the motility test. Treatment is aimed first at the primary cause but, in general, this type of strabismus does not respond well to orthoptic procedures. In large deviation, surgery is usually the only remedy. *Syn.* non-concomitant strabismus.
See **head posture, abnormal; incomitance; pointing past-; screen, Hess; strabismus, paralytic; test, motility.**

infantile s. *See* **esotropia, infantile.**

intermittent s. Strabismus that is not present at all times.
See **esotropia, cyclic.**

monocular s. *See* **strabismus, unilateral.**

non-accommodative s. *See* **esotropia, non-accommodative.**

non-concomitant s. *See* **strabismus, incomitant.**

paralytic s. Strabismus due to a paralysis of the extraocular muscles. It usually gives rise to incomitance. The paralysis is usually due to a disorder of the third, fourth or sixth cranial nerve. Diplopia is noticed if the paralysis is recent and it is usually accompanied by an abnormal head posture. In most cases, there is not a complete loss of action of a muscle but a partial loss and the condition is referred to as **paretic strabismus**, whether it is congenital or acquired. Orthoptic treatment is very limited in these cases and is not normally appropriate if the deviation was caused by injury or a recent disease. Cosmetic surgery is often necessary.
See **head posture, abnormal; incomitance; palsy, fourth nerve; palsy, sixth nerve; palsy, third nerve; test, motility.**

paretic s. *See* **strabismus, paralytic.**

periodic s. Strabismus in which the deviation occurs only at certain distances or in certain directions of fixation. *Syn.* relative strabismus.

relative s. *See* **strabismus, periodic.**

secondary s. Strabismus resulting from a sensory deficit, surgical intervention, tumour, trauma or stroke.
See **strabismus, consecutive; strabismus, sensory.**

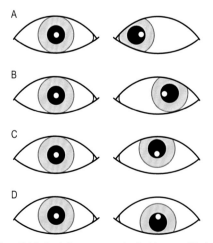

Fig. S14 A, left convergent strabismus; **B,** left divergent strabismus; **C,** left hypertropia; **D,** left hypotropia.

sensory s. Strabismus caused by a unilateral reduction in visual acuity which disrupts binocular vision, such as unilateral cataract, optic atrophy, uncorrected anisometropia or other unilateral visual impairments.

small angle s. *See* microtropia.

s. surgery *See* advancement; botulinum toxin; myectomy; myotomy; procedure, Faden; procedure, tuck; recession; resection; transposition.

sursumvergens s. *See* hypertropia.

unilateral s. Strabismus in which the deviating eye is always the same, as distinct from alternating strabismus. *Syn.* monocular strabismus.

strain 1. The change in dimension of a tissue, cell or body caused by mechanical force. It is equal to elongation divided by the original length and expressed in per cent, i.e.

$$s = (l - L/L) \times 100$$

where *l* is the final length and *L* the original length. **2.** Internal tension in a lens due to poor annealing, to glass of a non-uniform coefficient of expansion or from external pressure on the edge of a glass spectacle lens. It results in birefringence, which is observed with a polariscope. **3.** To overwork a faculty (e.g. eyestrain caused by sustained vision of near point objects), a part of the body (e.g. muscles) or a system (e.g. the effect on corneal metabolism of a closed eye wearing a PMMA lens. This is often referred to as **hypoxic stress**). *Note*: The strain can be either the cause or the effect. Strain is often regarded erroneously as a synonym of stress, but a lot of strain leads to stress.

See annealing; asthenopia; hypoxia; polariscope; stress.

stratum opticum Nerve fibre layer of the retina.

strawberry naevus *See* haemangioma, capillary orbital.

stray light *See* light, stray.

streak retinoscope *See* retinoscope, streak.

streaks, angioid *See* angioid streaks.

streaks, Siegrist's *See* Siegrist's streaks.

stress 1. Any potentially damaging factor which is capable of inducing a disease, injury or behavioural anomaly. **2.** In physics, the force per unit area and usually applied to a body and usually expressed in newtons/m^2 (or pascals, Pa).

See oxidative stress; strain.

stress, hypoxic *See* strain.

stress, near point *See* asthenopia; syndrome, Meares–Irlen.

stria 1. A narrow stripe or channel, usually one of several that are close together or parallel and distinct from the surrounding tissue by colour, texture or elevation. *Plural*: striae. **2.** Slight dark ridges in the pars plana of the ciliary body, which run parallel with each other from the teeth of the ora serrata to the valleys between the ciliary processes. *Syn.* striae ciliares. **3.** A line in the posterior corneal stroma associated with corneal oedema and sometimes keratoconus. **4.** A vein or streak seen in optical glass which has been contaminated during manufacture or in which the ingredients have been imperfectly mixed.

See ciliary body; glass; oedema.

striae ciliares *See* stria.

striae, Haab's Horizontal or concentric striae caused by tears in Descemet's membrane found in congenital glaucoma (Fig. S15).

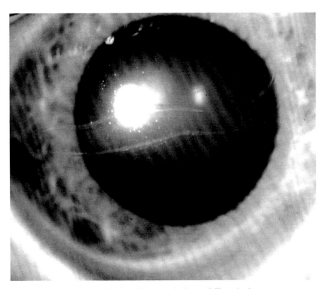

Fig. S15 Haab's striae. (From Bowling 2016, with permission of Elsevier.)

striae retinae Concentric lines on the surface of the retina, which appear after spontaneous or surgical retinal reattachment.
See retinal detachment.

striae, Vogt's Thin vertical streaks located in the posterior corneal stroma. These folds disappear with external pressure on the globe. They are often present in patients with keratoconus. *Syn.* Vogt's line.

striate area; cortex *See* area, visual.

stroboscope An instrument that produces brief flashes of illumination at a variable frequency. The frequency can be synchronized or asynchronized with the frequency of a moving object, which can be made to appear stationary, to rotate slowly or to rotate in the opposite direction to its real rotation. This apparent change of motion or immobilization of an object, when the object is illuminated by a periodically varying light of appropriate frequency, is called a **stroboscopic effect**. Stroboscopes have various uses in medicine, industry (e.g. to study the stresses of machine parts in motion), scientific research, etc.
See aliasing; movement, stroboscopic.

stroke *See* blindness, cortical; hemianopia, homonymous; ophthalmodynamometer.

stroma, ciliary *See* ciliary body.

stroma, corneal *See* corneal stroma.

Student's t-test An inferential statistical test designed to establish the significance of the difference between the means of two samples of data. It is calculated by the formula

$$t = x_1 - x_2 / s\sqrt{(1/n_1 + 1/n_2)}$$

where x_1 and x_2 are the means of the two samples, respectively, s is the standard deviation and n_1 and n_2 the size of each sample. The denominator in this equation is called the 'standard error of the difference between two means'. If the comparison is made with more than two groups of data, the test used is the analysis of variance (ANOVA).
See significance.

study A research project, a detailed examination or a procedure.
case s. A method designed to give a detailed description of a single case (**case report**) or of more than one case (**case series**). It may be used to describe a rare condition, a new procedure and how cases with the same condition vary.
case-control s. A longitudinal retrospective study in which two groups of individuals, the **cases-** people who have the disease and the **controls** who do not have the disease, are compared for specific characteristics that may be more commonly found in the diseased group (risk factors) than in the control group. This type of study may be affected by confounding factors (e.g. imprecise records, mismatch of the two groups). A variation of this type of study is the **nested case-control study** in which a subset of controls is compared to the cases. This is especially useful when conducting a survey for a rare condition in which a very large number of people are tested and few cases detected. It is then essential to reduce the number of controls by matching according to various risk factors (e.g. age, gender, geographical location).
cohort s. A longitudinal study in which a group of subjects, called a **cohort**, is followed over a period of time. It can be either followed into the future (prospective study) or analysing past records (retrospective study). It is usually compared to another cohort, the controls, who do not possess the attribute being investigated.
cross-over s. An experimental design in which the effect of two or more treatments on a particular feature (e.g. a drug therapy) are given to each individual, one treatment after the other in random order.
cross-sectional s. Study in which the prevalence of a condition in a group of individuals is determined at a given point in time.
See study, longitudinal.
double-blind s. An experimental design in which neither the person receiving the treatment (or recording the results of a test) nor the person administering it knows the identity of the treatment or test.
See trial, randomized controlled.
longitudinal s. A design in which subjects are followed over a period of time with data collected at various intervals. *Examples*: prospective study, retrospective study.
See study, cross-sectional.
nested case-control s. *See* study, case-control.
observational s. A research method designed to draw inferences about the possible effect of exposure on an established outcome (e.g. a disease, a therapy) without the investigator's intervention. *Examples*: case-control study, cohort study, cross-sectional study.
prospective s. A longitudinal study aimed at establishing an association between a specific risk factor (or therapy) and the development of a disease (or cure). Two groups of individuals (cohorts), one group exposed to a specific risk factor and the other not exposed, are examined over a period of time and the incidence rates of the outcome are compared between the two groups. It is a more powerful design than a retrospective study to determine an association because the experimenter can control the variables.
See trial, randomized controlled.
retrospective s. A longitudinal study aimed at establishing the presence of specific factors that are associated with a given outcome (e.g. disease, a cure) by analysing the past records of patients with the outcome as compared to patients without the outcome. *Example*: case-control study.
single-blind s. A method of testing in which the treatment assignment or procedure is unknown to the patient or subject.

See **placebo.**

triple-blind s. An experimental design in which the subject, practitioner and the person administering the test do not know the identity of the treatment or test.
See **trial, randomized controlled.**

Sturge–Weber syndrome *See* **syndrome, Sturge–Weber.**

Sturm, conoid of The bundle of rays formed by an astigmatic optical system consisting of a primary focal line (called **Sturm's line**), a circle of least confusion and a secondary focal line (Sturm's line) perpendicular to the first.
See **astigmatism; circle of least confusion.**

Sturm, interval of The linear distance between the two focal lines of an astigmatic optical system.
Syn. astigmatic interval; focal interval.
See **astigmatism, oblique.**

Sturm's line *See* **line, focal; Sturm, conoid of.**

stye *See* **hordeolum.**

subarachnoid haemorrhage; space *See* under the nouns.

subclinical Pertains to the early stage of a disease when it is insufficiently developed to produce clear signs and symptoms, as in the early development of cataract.

subconjunctival haemorrhage; injection *See* under the nouns.

subhyaloid haemorrhage *See* **haemorrhage, preretinal.**

subjective refraction *See* **refraction, subjective.**

subliminal perception *See* **perception, subliminal.**

subluxation of the lens An incomplete dislocation of the crystalline lens. It is a cause of monocular diplopia and is associated with spherophakia.
See **luxation; spherophakia.**

subnormal vision *See* **vision, low.**

subretinal space *See* **space, subretinal.**

substantia propria *See* **cornea; corneal stroma.**

subtarsal sulcus *See* **sulcus, subtarsal.**

successive contrast *See* **contrast, successive.**

sulcus A depression or a groove found on the surface of an organ or tissue, as on the surface of the brain separating adjacent convolutions. Large sulci that divide the brain into lobes as well as the two hemispheres are more often called fissures. *Plural*: sulci.
See **fissure.**
calcarine s. *See* **fissure, calcarine.**
ciliary s. A groove situated between the posterior root of the iris and the ciliary body. It may be used, sometimes, as a site of fixation of an intraocular lens implant.
See **lens, intraocular.**
external scleral s. A shallow circular narrow furrow found on the outer surface of the limbus. It appears where the radius of curvature of the cornea changes to that of the sclera. It corresponds approximately to the periphery of the visible iris.
See **sulcus, internal scleral.**
inferior palpebral s. A furrow found in the skin of the lower eyelid. It separates the tarsal from the orbital portion of the lid. It is often not very distinct although it becomes more so with age.
internal scleral s. A circular large groove situated at the margin between the posterior surface of the cornea and the sclera on the inner surface of the limbus. It contains the trabecular meshwork and the canal of Schlemm. The posterior lip of the sulcus forms a projecting ridge called the scleral spur.
See **scleral spur; sulcus, external scleral.**
optic s. *See* **pit, optic.**
subtarsal s. A groove on the inner surface of the eyelid, near the eyelid margin and parallel to it, which forms the border separating the marginal from the tarsal conjunctiva. Foreign bodies are commonly lodged in this groove.
See **eversion, lid; irrigation.**
superior palpebral s. A furrow found in the skin of the upper eyelid. It separates the tarsal portion, which is closest to the lid margin from the orbital portion, which extends from the tarsus to the eyebrow. This furrow becomes more prominent with age.
See **aperture, palpebral; Fig. A16, p. 27.**

sulfacetamide sodium An anti-infective bacteriostatic drug of the sulfonamide family, used topically against infections and injuries as well as minor abrasions of the conjunctiva and cornea. It should not be used immediately following a local anaesthetic. However, **antibiotics** (e.g. bacitracin, chloramphenicol, erythromycin, gentamicin, neomycin, norfloxacin, polymyxin B, tetracycline, tobramycin), which inhibit or destroy a wide range of microorganisms, are used more commonly than local sulfonamides.
See **antibiotic; antifungal agent; antiinflammatory drug; bacteriostatic; sulfonamide.**

sulfonamide Denotes a group of organic derivatives containing $SO_2 NH_2$. *Example*: sulfacetamide sodium.

summation Increased effect produced by a series of stimuli applied either simultaneously or successively (provided the intervals are greater than the latent period of perception). **Binocular summation** usually occurs when the two eyes are stimulated; thus binocular brightness is greater than monocular, except in the unusual Fechner's paradox. Two or more stimuli falling within the excitatory region of a receptive field will increase the excitatory response and similarly two or more stimuli falling within the inhibitory region of a receptive field will increase the inhibition; this is called **spatial summation**. The summation may also occur if successive stimulations are received by the same retinal region; this is called **temporal summation**.

See cell, complex; cell, simple; Fechner's paradox; field, receptive; inhibition, lateral.

sun gazing *See* retinopathy, solar.

sunflower cataract *See* chalcosis lentis.

sunglasses Spectacles that have tinted lenses. They are used to protect the eyes from bright sunlight, for special cases (e.g. fear of light) or for cosmetic reasons.
See cataract; lens, tinted; photophobia; pterygium; ultraviolet.

sunlight *See* light, solar.

supercilium *See* eyebrow.

superimposition The ability to see two similar images superimposed but not mentally fused. *Examples*: seeing a bird in a cage with both eyes in a synoptophore when one eye is presented with a bird and the other with a cage; seeing the letter E in a synoptophore when one eye is presented with the letter F and the other with the letter L.
See vision, Worth's classification of binocular.

superior cervical ganglion; colliculus; limbic keratoconjunctivitis; oblique muscle; oblique sheath syndrome; ophthalmic vein; orbital fissure; quadrantanopia; rectus muscle *See* under the nouns.

superior transverse ligament *See* muscle, levator palpebrae superioris.

suppression The process by which the brain inhibits the retinal image (or part of it) of one eye, when both eyes are simultaneously stimulated. This occurs to avoid diplopia as in strabismus, in uncorrected anisometropia, in retinal rivalry, etc. *Syn.* suspenopsia (this term actually refers to voluntary suppression as occurs, for example, when using a monocular microscope with one eye); suspension (sometimes used when referring to partial suppression, although the term **foveal suppression** is preferred when central viewing is involved).
See cheiroscope; diplopia, physiological; grid, Javal's; Mallett fixation disparity unit; Remy separator; retinal rivalry; test, Bagolini lens; test, bar reading; test, four prism dioptre base out; test, FRIEND; test, Turville infinity balance; test, Worth's four dot; vectogram.

suppression, foveal *See* suppression.

supra *See* spectacles, supra.

suprachoroid *See* choroid; sclera.

suprachiasmatic nucleus *See* nucleus, suprachiasmatic.

suprachoroidal space *See* space, suprachoroidal.

supraciliaris *See* ciliary body.

supraciliary space *See* space, supraciliary.

supraduction *See* elevation of the eye.

supranuclear In general, referring to nerve fibres situated above a nucleus.

supranuclear gaze palsy *See* palsy, supranuclear gaze.

supraorbital artery *See* artery, supraorbital.

supraorbital nerve *See* nerve, ophthalmic.

supraorbital notch An indentation in the orbital margin of the frontal bone, one-third of the way from the nose. The supraorbital nerve and vessels pass through that indentation. Occasionally it is converted into a foramen by ossification.

supravergence Movement of one eye upward relative to the other. *Syn.* sursumvergence.
See infravergence; vergence.

supraversion *See* version.

surface colour; power *See* under the nouns.

surface, diffusing; matt *See* matt surface.

surface, optical Surface at which light is either refracted or reflected, or both simultaneously.

surface, toroidal *See* lens, toric.

surfacing The combined grinding processes of roughing, smoothing and polishing of a glass lens surface to a given curvature.
See cerium oxide; blocking; grinding; lens blank; lens, finished; moulding; rouge.

surfactant An agent that reduces the surface tension of oil or solid-water interfaces and therefore has cleaning properties. *Note*: The term is an acronym made from the following italic letters; *surf*ace *act*ive *a*ge*nt*. *Example*: poloxamine, which is used in multipurpose solutions for soft contact lenses.
See deposits, contact lens; disinfection; enzyme; wetting solution.

surrounding field *See* field, surrounding.

sursumduction *See* elevation.

sursumvergence *See* supravergence.

sursumversion *See* version.

suspenopsia *See* suppression.

suspension 1. *See* suppression. 2. A pharmaceutical preparation of an undissolved substance presented in a liquid. A few eyedrop agents are presented as a suspension and the container needs to be shaken before use.

suspensory apparatus of the lens; ligament *See* Zinn, zonule of.

suture 1. The lines of fusion of the separate bones which unite to form the cranium. *See* **skull**. 2. The technique of closing a wound. *Example*: the suture made to secure a corneal graft with the host in penetrating keratoplasty. 3. The material with which the two surfaces of a wound are kept together.

sutures, lens *See* lens sutures.

swab A small piece of absorbent material (e.g. cotton) usually attached to the end of a stick or rod used to apply medication, to take specimens for analysis (e.g. from the bulbar conjunctiva or eyelids) or, in surgery, for cleaning a wound.

Swann's syndrome *See* syndrome, Swann's.

Swedish Interactive Thresholding Algorithm (SITA) *See* algorithm.

sweep VEP *See* potential, visual evoked.

swinging flashlight test *See* pupil, Marcus Gunn.

symblepharon Adhesion, partial or complete, of the palpebral conjunctiva of the eyelid to the bulbar conjunctiva of the eyeball. It results from disease (e.g. erythema multiforme) or trauma, but is rarely congenital. *See* syndrome, Stevens–Johnson.

sympathetic eye; nervous system; ophthalmia *See* under the nouns.

sympatholytic drugs Drugs that inhibit nerve impulses in the sympathetic nervous system. They may block the effect of alpha-adrenergic receptors (e.g. thymoxamine, which is used to reverse pupillary blockage caused by a mydriatic) or the effect of beta-adrenergic receptors. The latter are called **beta-blockers** (e.g. betaxolol which block beta 1 receptors; timolol maleate, levobunolol, metipranolol and carteolol which block beta 1 and beta 2 receptors). Beta-blockers are used in the treatment of glaucoma. *Syn.* adrenergic blocking agents. *See* alpha-adrenergic antagonist; beta-blocker.

sympathomimetic drugs Drugs that produce an effect similar to that obtained by stimulation of the sympathetic nervous system. Some of these predominantly act on the adrenergic alpha-receptors (e.g. noradrenaline [norepinephrine]), while others act on the adrenergic beta-receptors (e.g. isoproterenol). Others have little direct effect on the adrenergic receptors but enhance the release of natural catecholamine from the sympathetic nerve terminals (e.g. amphetamine, phenylpropanolamine). Sympathomimetic drugs are used (1) in the treatment of open-angle glaucoma by decreasing aqueous humour secretion and increasing the outflow through the trabecular meshwork thus reducing the intraocular pressure (e.g. apraclonidine and brimonidine tartrate, which are both alpha-2 adrenergic agonists and dipivefrine hydrochloride. Adrenaline [epinephrine] was used initially but not anymore), (2) dilate the pupil without affecting accommodation (e.g. phenylephrine) and (3) constrict conjunctival blood vessels (e.g. naphazoline, tetrahydrozoline, xylometazoline). *Syn.* adrenergic agonist; adrenergic stimulating agent. *See* alpha-adrenergic agonist; mydriatic.

symptom Subjective complaint of a patient indicating the presence of a disease or of an unusual condition (e.g. blurred vision). *See* sign.

synapse The place where a nerve impulse is transmitted from one neuron to another. This transmission is usually mediated by neurotransmitters (e.g. acetylcholine, noradrenaline [norepinephrine], glutamate, etc.) that are released by the presynaptic neuron, then diffuse across the **synaptic cleft** (about 20 to 50 nm wide) to bind to receptor sites on the postsynaptic membrane and generate an electrical change in the postsynaptic neuron, which results in either depolarization (excitation) or hyperpolarization (inhibition). This is often referred to as a **chemical synapse**. There is another type of synapse called an **electrotonic synapse** (or **electrical synapse**) in which electrical impulses are transmitted via ionic currents from one neuron to another by direct propagation across a **gap junction** (2 to 3 nm wide). Electrotonic synapses are rare in vertebrates and have been found at only a few central nervous sites. It is estimated that a cortical neuron, for example, makes some 5000–10 000 synapses with surrounding neurons. *See* neuron; neurotransmitter; potential, receptor.

synaesthesia A sensory experience in which stimulation of one sensory modality (e.g. hearing) elicits an involuntary response in another sensory modality (e.g. colour), as well as its own.

synchisis scintillans Degenerative condition noticed in old eyes, in myopia or after injuries, vitreous detachment and inflammation of the eye (e.g. posterior uveitis) and characterized by the presence of bright shiny particles floating in a liquified vitreous body. The particles are believed to be composed of cholesterol. Vision may be impaired if the particles float across the visual axis but is restored when the eye is immobile, as they settle at the bottom of the vitreous. *See* asteroid hyalosis; floaters; vitreous humour; uveitis.

syndrome The aggregate of signs and symptoms associated with a disease, lesion, anomaly, etc. *A s. See* pattern, alphabet.
Aarskog's s. A rare hereditary disorder characterized by short stature and facial and genital anomalies and syndactyly. One type is X-linked, and others are either dominant or recessive. Ocular signs are megalocornea, hypertelorism and strabismus.
acquired immunodeficiency s. (AIDS) A viral disease characterized by a relentless transition from asymptomatic lymphadenopathy to a wasting condition with infections (e.g. pneumonia, toxoplasmosis) and malignancies (e.g. Kaposi's sarcoma). It has a long incubation period and a poor prognosis. It is caused by the human immunodeficiency virus (**HIV**, a retrovirus composed of RNA), which breaks down the immune response and is transmitted by exchange of body fluids (e.g. blood, semen) or transfused blood products. The main ocular features are reduced vision, floaters, retinitis (caused by the herpesvirus, cytomegalovirus) with haemorrhage and necrosis (with the appearance of a 'pizza pie') sometimes granular and there may be complications such as areas of retinal necrosis where inflammation has subsided, optic nerve disease, keratoconjunctivitis sicca, reddish-purple nodular tumours in the eyelids and conjunctiva and blepharitis as part of Kaposi's sarcoma. Progression and severity of the condition has now been greatly reduced with Highly Active AntiRetroviral Therapy (HAART) combined with other antiviral agents. *See* retinal necrosis, progressive outer; retinitis, cytomegalovirus; uveitis, viral.

adherence s. Uncommon complication of strabismus surgery where the posterior Tenon's capsule is severed, allowing retrobulbar fat to scar and adhere to the ocular surface. The scarring produces a restriction in ocular movements and thus a form of restrictive strabismus. It can be diagnosed by a positive forced duction test and/or a restriction in ocular motility. The condition can be prevented by careful strabismus surgical technique and care not to disturb the posterior Tenon's capsule. *Syn.* adhesive syndrome; cicatricial syndrome.
See **test, forced duction; Tenon's capsule.**

Adie's s. *See* **syndrome, Holmes–Adie.**

Aicardi's s. Inherited disorder seen in females, consisting of retinal, optic nerve as well as central nervous system anomalies with seizures and retardation. Inheritance is X-linked. Retinal findings consist of multiple, round, chorioretinal depigmented lesions. Additional abnormalities include optic nerve head colobomas, microphthalmos, partial or complete absence of the corpus callosum (agenesis).

Alagille's s. An autosomal dominant inherited disorder of the liver accompanied with abnormalities of the heart, spine and face. Ocular findings include posterior embryotoxon, hypertelorism, iris abnormalities, optic disc drusen and fundus hypopigmentation.

Albright's s. A disorder characterized by a host of findings, including cutaneous pigmentation, precocious puberty in females and fibrous dysplasia of the orbital bone(s), which may lead to proptosis and optic atrophy.

Alport's s. Hereditary disorder characterized by three major phenotypes: progressive nephritis, sensorineural deafness and ocular lesions including anterior lenticonus, anterior polar or cortical cataract, fleck retina and recurrent corneal erosions. There are several modes of inheritance: 85% of the case are X-linked due to mutation in the gene encoding the alpha-5 chain of basement membrane collagen type IV (COL4A5); autosomal recessive caused by mutation in the COL4A3 or COL4A4 gene and autosomal dominant with mutation in the COL4 A3 gene.

Alstrom–Olsen s. A very rare autosomal recessive disorder characterized by obesity, diabetes mellitus, sensorineural deafness and heart failure. The principal ocular manifestation is a cone-rod dystrophy.

anterior chamber cleavage s. *See* **Peter's anomaly.**

Andersen–Warburg s. *See* **disease, Norrie's.**

Anton's s. Bilateral blindness characterized by a lack of awareness of being blind and near normal pupil reflexes. It is due to a destruction of the cortical visual area (e.g. head injury, stroke). *Syn.* Anton–Babinski syndrome.
See **blindness, cortical.**

Apert's s. Congenital craniofacial malformation due to premature fusion of the cranial sutures. Some cases are inherited as autosomal dominant and caused by mutation in the gene encoding fibroblast growth factor receptor-2 (FGFR2). It is characterized by an abnormally high, peaked or conically shaped head and complete or partial webbing of the fingers and toes. There is also intellectual retardation in many cases. The ocular signs include shallow orbits with prominent globes, hypertelorism, strabismus, reduced visual acuity and, as a result of hydrocephalus, the patient may have optic atrophy. It may be associated with keratoconus. *Syn.* acrocephalosyndactyly.
See **syndrome, Crouzon's.**

Axenfeld–Rieger s. A group of inherited ocular developmental anomalies occurring in the fetus caused by defective neural crest cells and composed of Axenfeld' anomaly, Rieger's anomaly and Rieger's syndrome.
See **Axenfeld's anomaly; ectoderm; syndrome, Rieger's.**

Balint's s. An entity characterized by an inability to fixate voluntarily in different parts of the visual field, to see two objects simultaneously (simultanagnosia) and to mislocate when reaching for, or pointing to, an object (ocular apraxia). Patient has normal visual acuity. This is usually due to a bilateral lesion of an area within the parieto-occipital region of the brain. *Syn.* Balint–Holmes syndrome.
See **apraxia, ocular motor; simultanagnosia.**

Bardet–Biedl s. An heterogeneous hereditary disorder characterized by mental handicap, polydactylism, hypogenitalism and obesity. The associated ocular abnormalities are retinitis pigmentosa, optic nerve atrophy with reduced visual acuity, night blindness and myopia. There is evidence of an overlapping phenotype with the Laurence–Moon syndrome, although without obesity or polydactyly, and some authors have proposed unifying the two and referring to it as a *Syn.* Laurence–Moon–Bardet–Biedl syndrome.

Bassen–Kornzweig s. An autosomal recessive hereditary disorder characterized by a congenital inability to absorb fats. By the end of the first decade of life, the patient develops pigmentary retinopathy, which resembles retinitis pigmentosa, although the pigment clumps are scattered throughout the fundus and not confined to the periphery, and night blindness. Treatment with large doses of vitamin A, E and D may retard the progression of the condition. *Syn.* abetalipoproteinaemia; acanthocytosis.

Behçet's s. *See* **disease, Behçet's.**

Behr's s. An autosomal recessive inherited disorder caused by mutation in the OPA1 gene on chromosome 3q28. It presents in childhood with optic atrophy, visual loss and nystagmus, as well as ataxia and mental handicap.

Benedikt's s. A syndrome caused by a lesion (usually vascular) within the midbrain in the fibres of the fasciculus joining the third nerve nucleus (oculomotor) that pass through the red nucleus to the cerebral peduncle. It is characterized by an ipsilateral third nerve palsy and ataxia and tremor of the limbs on the other side of the body.
See **palsy, third nerve; syndrome, Weber's.**

Bernard–Horner s. *See* **syndrome, Horner's.**
blepharophimosis s. A rare, autosomal, dominant, inherited disorder characterized by ptosis, poor levator function, shorter than normal width of the palpebral aperture, telecanthus, commonly epicanthus inversus, partial ectropion of the lower lid and flattening of the supraorbital ridges. Amblyopia and strabismus are present in about half of the cases. The syndrome is caused by mutations in the FOXL2 gene on chromosome 3. Treatment usually begins with surgical correction of the epicanthus and telecanthus before ptosis surgery. A combination of the following three features is called **blepharophimosis, ptosis and epicanthus inversus syndrome.**
See **blepharophimosis; ectropion, congenital; epicanthus inversus; procedure, frontalis sling.**
blind spot s. *See* **syndrome, Swann's.**
Bloch-Sulzberger s. *See* **incontinentia pigmenti.**
Brown's superior oblique tendon sheath s. This syndrome is characterized by limitation of elevation of the eye in adduction but normal or near normal elevation when the eye is in abduction. There is limitation of movement of the affected eye in the forced duction test when attempting to elevate the eye from the adducted position. The eyes are usually straight in the primary position. The condition seems to be due to a short tendon sheath of the superior oblique muscle and an apparent anomaly of the inferior oblique muscle. It may be congenital and idiopathic or acquired due to inflammation of the tendon as a result of scleritis or rheumatoid arthritis or trauma. *Syn.* Brown's syndrome; sheath syndrome; superior oblique sheath syndrome.
See **pattern, alphabet; procedure, Faden.**
cat's eye s. A condition caused by an extra fragment of a copy of chromosome 22. It is characterized by partial iris coloboma (usually a vertical portion) which makes the patient's eye look like a cat's eye. There are also optic disc coloboma, optic nerve degeneration and microphthalmos. The systemic manifestations include mental and growth retardation and low-set or malformed ears.
Chandler's s. A syndrome characterized by a severe corneal endothelial degeneration resulting in corneal oedema and blurred vision. There is also mild iris atrophy and secondary glaucoma. It tends to affect mainly women between 20 and 40 years of age. The therapy is aimed at treating the glaucoma. *Syn.* iridocorneal syndrome.
See **syndrome, ICE.**
Charles Bonnet s. A rare condition characterized by visual hallucinations in an individual who is aware of the unreal nature of the hallucinations. Almost all subjects have reduced vision bilaterally. The condition is often associated with age-related macular degeneration, diabetic retinopathy, other retinal diseases or cataracts.
Cogan's s. *See* **keratitis, interstitial.**
Cogan–Reese s. *See* **syndrome, ICE.**
computer vision s. A condition resulting from extensive viewing of computer screens, video display terminals or visual display units. The patient may complain of eyestrain, dry red eyes, headaches, transient blurred vision or diplopia, as well as neckache or backache. The ocular symptoms are caused by continuous accommodative demands produced by the pixels or tiny dots of the computer screen that are difficult to keep in focus, unlike print on a page. Other causes are frequent saccadic eye movements, convergence demands and position of the screen. Management includes exact correction for the distance at which the display unit appears, viewing it about 10° to 20° below the straight-ahead position and special optical dispensing.
corneal exhaustion s. An intolerance to continue wearing contact lenses after many years of wear, probably due to endothelial dysfunction as a result of chronic hypoxia and acidosis. It occurs primarily with PMMA lenses but also with other lenses with low oxygen transmissibility. Some of the signs associated with this syndrome are endothelial polymegethism, corneal oedema, loss of corneal sensitivity, variations in corneal curvature and refractive error, blurred vision, lacrimation, hyperaemia and discomfort. Management usually consists in discontinuing contact lens wear. Refitting with lenses with high oxygen transmissibility is often successful. *Syn.* corneal fatigue syndrome; corneal exhaustion phenomenon.
See **hypoxia; syndrome, overwear.**
corneal fatigue s. *See* **syndrome, corneal exhaustion.**
Cornelia de Lange s. A congenital anomaly characterized by growth and mental retardation, limb malformation, syndactyly, bushy eyebrows meeting in the midline, hairline down on the forehead, depressed bridge of the nose and low-set ears. Ocular manifestations may include ptosis, nystagmus, microcornea and most commonly high myopia. The pathogenesis of the condition is unknown.
Crouzon's s. An autosomal dominant inherited craniofacial malformation due to premature fusion of the cranial sutures. It is caused by a mutation in the gene encoding the fibroblast growth factor receptor-2 (FGFR2). It is characterized by an abnormally wide cranium, high forehead and short anteroposterior head distance. The ocular signs include exophthalmos, hypertelorism, ectopia lentis, iris coloboma and strabismus. The incidence of this syndrome is much higher than that of Apert's syndrome, another craniofacial anomaly. *Syn.* craniofacial dysostosis.
dorsal midbrain s. *See* **syndrome, Parinaud's.**
Down's s. A disorder caused by a chromosomal anomaly, a trisomy 21, and in which many genes are involved resulting in intellectual and physical handicaps with small stature, obesity and developmental heart defects, etc. Ocular signs include epicanthus, blepharoconjunctivitis, cataract, keratoconus, nystagmus and iris spots (Brushfield's). Cases of high myopia are noted, but most subjects tend to have hyperopia and there is a high prevalence of strabismus. Visual

acuity is also reduced, even after correction of the ametropia. *Syn.* trisomy 21 syndrome.

Duane's s. A complex disorder found in about 1% of patients with strabismus; it occurs in three different types. All three types are characterized by retraction of the globe into the orbit and by narrowing of the palpebral fissure on attempted adduction. The left eye is affected more often than the right eye and the condition is bilateral in about 20% of patients. In addition, each type presents an abnormal pattern of ocular motility. **Type 1**, the most common affecting more than three-quarters of all cases, presents limited or absent abduction and slight esotropia in the primary position, and typically a head turn towards the involved side. **Type 2** presents limited adduction, slight exotropia and relatively normal or slightly limited abduction, and usually a head turn away from the involved side. **Type 3**, the rarest (about 1% of all cases), presents limited abduction and adduction. The aetiology is believed to be a congenital absence of the sixth cranial nerve and its nucleus (partial absence in type 2) associated with aberrant co-innervation of the lateral and medial recti muscles. The degree of this paradoxical innervation determines the severity of the disorder. Management is frequently surgical especially in types 2 and 3, but prismatic corrections have been found to be beneficial in selected cases. *Syn.* Duane retraction syndrome; Duane's phenomenon; retraction syndrome; Stilling–Turk–Duane syndrome; Turk's disease. *See* **procedure, Faden.**

Edwards' s. A congenital condition in which an extra chromosome 18 is present. The major systemic findings are congenital heart defects and intellectual and physical retardation, and the major ocular manifestations are epicanthal folds, corneal opacities, congenital cataract, ptosis and microphthalmos. The life expectancy of patients with this syndrome is less than 1 year. *Syn.* syndrome, trisomy 18.

Ehlers–Danlos s. Syndrome characterized by hyperelasticity of the skin, hyperextensibility of the joints and fragile blood vessels. It is inherited as an autosomal dominant disorder of connective tissue with an increase in dermal elastic tissue and a decrease in collagen. The ocular signs include blue sclera, eye elongation and myopia, angioid streaks, ectopia lentis, keratoconus and retinal detachment.

exfoliation s. *See* **syndrome, pseudoexfoliation.**

fallen eye s. A condition occurring after a prolonged paresis of the superior oblique muscle of one eye, in which the other eye may not elevate completely, if the paretic eye was always the fixating eye.

Fisher's s. A rare developmental anomaly due to a fusion of the fascial sheaths of some of the extraocular muscles giving rise to a variety of paralyses depending on the muscles or tendons which have adhered to each other. It can be acquired or congenital. Therapy is mainly surgical.

floppy eyelid s. A condition often occurring in very obese middle-aged males, characterized by a very loose upper eyelid allowing it to be very easily everted and sometimes injured during sleep resulting in papillary conjunctivitis. If severe, treatment is by lid shortening.

Foster Kennedy s. A syndrome in which there is optic atrophy in one eye and papilloedema in the other. This is due to direct pressure by a tumour on one optic nerve giving rise to optic atrophy, and as a result of raised intracranial pressure papilloedema develops in the other eye. It is often caused by a tumour at the base of the frontal lobe or an olfactory meningioma. In some cases, the patient also reports a loss of smell. *Syn.* Kennedy's syndrome.

Foville's s. A disorder of the inferior cerebellar artery that causes a pontine lesion involving the abducens (sixth) and the facial (seventh) nucleus or its fasciculus as it leaves the brainstem at the pontine paramedian reticular formation. It is characterized by a paralysis of the conjugate eye movements (versions) towards the affected side (horizontal gaze palsy), ipsilateral facial paralysis, hemianaesthesia of the face, contralateral paralysis of the limbs, Horner's syndrome and deafness. *Syn.* inferior medial pontine syndrome.

fragile X s. An inherited syndrome caused by a constriction and nearly broken long arm of an X chromosome at q27.3. Although males are mainly affected, females are also affected to a lesser extent and carry the genetic defect. Systemic manifestations are intellectual retardation (the second most common cause after Down's syndrome), enlarged testes, high forehead, large jaws and long ears. The ocular manifestations are strabismus (typically esotropia), large refractive errors (most commonly hyperopic) and poor eye contact.

Fuchs' uveitis s. *See* **heterochromia; iridocyclitis, Fuchs' heterochromic.**

Gardner's s. An autosomal dominant variant of familial adenomatous polyposis associated with congenital hypertrophy of the retinal pigment epithelium. It is caused by mutation in the APC gene on chromosome 5q22. It is characterized by osteomas of the skull, mandible and orbit, and multiple soft tissue tumours. *See* **retinal pigment epithelium, congenital hypertrophy of the.**

Gerstmann s. A disorder believed to result from a lesion at the occipitoparietal border, the angular gyrus and the interparietal sulcus. It is characterized by finger agnosia, agraphia, acalculia and right-left disorientation. Ocular findings may include homonymous hemianopia and visual agnosia for colours.

Goldenhar's s. A syndrome characterized by preauricular appendages and vertebral and facial bones anomalies with epibulbar dermoids, upper eyelid coloboma as well as a microphthalmos and optic disc coloboma. *Syn.* oculoauriculovertebral dysplasia. *See* **coloboma; cyst, dermoid.**

Gradenigo's s. An inflammation of the middle ear (**otitis media**) and mastoid bone (**mastoiditis**) extending to the apex of the petrous temporal bone. It results in ipsilateral deafness, pain in or near the eye on the side of the face (fifth nerve involvement), paralysis of the lateral rectus muscle (sixth nerve involvement), facial paralysis, reduced corneal sensitivity (fifth nerve involvement) and some increase in body temperature. The condition responds well to antibiotics.

Gregg s. See **syndrome, rubella.**

Hallermann-Streiff-Francois s. A rare congenital disorder that causes a lack of body growth with cranial deformities and reduced hair growth. Main ocular signs are microphthalmos and cataract. *Syn.* oculomandibulofacial syndrome.

Hermansky–Pudlak s. See **albinism.**

von Hippel–Lindau s. An autosomal, dominant, inherited disorder caused by mutation in the VHL gene on chromosome 3p25. It is characterized by retinal haemangioblastoma involving one or both eyes associated with similar tumours in the cerebellum and spinal cord and sometimes cysts of the kidney and pancreas. Ophthalmoscopic examination shows a reddish, slightly elevated tumour of the retina. *Syn.* von Hippel–Lindau disease.

See **haemangioma, capillary; phakomatoses; syndrome, Sturge–Weber; syndrome, Wyburn–Mason.**

histoplasmosis presumed ocular s. See **syndrome, presumed ocular histoplasmosis.**

van der Hoeve's s. See **sclera, blue.**

Holmes–Adie s. A dilated pupil in which all reactions to light are barely existent, with slowed and impaired focusing at near, together with the absence of tendon reflexes. It typically affects adult women. Reading spectacles help as well as dark lenses or low-dose concentration of a parasympathomimetic drug (e.g. pilocarpine) may be used to mitigate photophobia. *Syn.* Adie's syndrome.

See **anisocoria; pupil, Adie's; reflex, pupil light.**

Horner's s. Interruption of the sympathetic nerve supply to the dilatator pupillae muscle resulting in miosis, slight ptosis (1 or 2 mm), slight elevation of the lower lid, enophthalmos, anisocoria (greater in dim illumination), heterochromia (mainly in the congenital type) and reduced or absence of ipsilateral sweating if the lesion is preganglionic to the superior cervical ganglion. Possible causes are central (e.g. tumour, vascular, demyelination, cervical spinal cord lesion), preganglionic (tumour, common carotid and aortic aneurysms and dissection) or postganglionic (e.g. otitis media, internal carotid dissection, tumour). *Syn.* Bernard–Horner syndrome.

See **pupillary defect, efferent; Table P11, p. 283.**

Hurler's s. An autosomal recessive inherited disorder caused by mutation in the gene encoding the enzyme alpha-L-iduronidase (IDUA). It is characterized by dwarfism, skeletal and facial dysmorphism (gargoyle-like) and intellectual retardation. Ocular features include pigmentary retinopathy, optic atrophy and corneal clouding. Patients excrete excessive amounts of heparan sulfate and dermatan sulfate in the urine. A subtype of this condition is called **Hurler–Scheie syndrome** (**Scheie syndrome**) in which the enzyme deficiency is less severe and the systemic features are less pronounced. *Syn.* mucopolysaccharidosis type 1; gargoylism.

ICE s. A syndrome involving the proliferation of corneal endothelium cells, which migrate onto the anterior surface of the iris, the iridocorneal angle and the trabecular meshwork resulting in secondary glaucoma. ICE is an abbreviation of iridocorneal endothelial. The syndrome consists of three clinical entities: Chandler's syndrome, essential iris atrophy (progressive iris changes) and iris naevus (Cogan–Reese syndrome which is an appearance of pigmented iris nodules). *Syn.* iridocorneal endothelial syndrome; iris naevus syndrome.

See **naevus, iris; syndrome, Chandler's.**

immobile lens s. See **contact lens acute red eye.**

infantile esotropia s. See **esotropia, infantile.**

iridocorneal endothelial s. See **syndrome, ICE.**

iris naevus s. See **syndrome, ICE.**

Irlen's s. See **syndrome, Meares–Irlen.**

Irvine–Gass s. See **oedema, cystoid macular.**

ischaemic ocular s. A syndrome occurring in individuals over the age of 50 with a history of cardiovascular disorders. It is characterized by, usually, unilateral loss of vision which may be acute or may develop over days or months, rubeosis iridis and there may be fadeouts of vision and pain. The fundus may have dilated congested veins with some haemorrhages and macular oedema. Management is directed at the cardiovascular disorder.

Joubert's s. A rare disorder of the brain which causes physical impairment and sometimes, abnormal eye movements, poor vision and/or difficulty fixating. Although some cases are sporadic, most are inherited as an autosomal recessive disorder caused by a mutation in the INPP5E gene on chromosome 9q34.3.

Kearns–Sayre s. See **ophthalmoplegia, chronic progressive external.**

Kennedy's s. See **syndrome, Foster Kennedy.**

Kjer's s. See **atrophy, Kjer-type optic.**

Laurence–Moon-Bardet-Biedl s. See **syndrome, Bardet-Beidl.**

Lowe's s. A rare X-linked, inherited disorder of amino acid metabolism. Systemic features include muscular hypotonia, mental handicap, craniofacial deformities and renal tubules disturbances. Ocular manifestations are congenital cataract, and in half of the cases, a coexisting congenital glaucoma, as well as microphakia. *Syn.* oculocerebrorenal syndrome.

Marcus Gunn jaw-winking s. See **phenomenon, jaw-winking.**

Marfan's s. A widespread autosomal dominant inherited disorder of connective tissue that affects many organs, including the skeleton, lungs, heart and blood vessels. The syndrome appears to be due to a mutation in the fibrillin-1 gene (FBN1), which is located on chromosome 15. The patient exhibits musculoskeletal (long-limbed, arachnodactyly, kyphoscoliosis) and cardiovascular (aortic dilatation, aortic dissection, mitral valve prolapse) abnormalities. The ocular signs are subluxation or dislocation of the lens which results from a defective suspensory ligament, myopia due to increased axial length, retinal detachment as well as heterochromia, keratoconus, blue sclera, strabismus and glaucoma due to developmental anomalies of the angle of the anterior chamber. *See* **luxation of the lens.**

Meares–Irlen s. A visual disorder characterized by difficulties with reading (**visual stress**). The patient often complains of headaches and eyestrain and observes illusions of motion, colour and shape distortion of a stationary striped pattern (e.g. grating or text). The patient may also have low amplitude of accommodation and reduced stereoscopic visual acuity. Coloured filters (called **Irlens lens**) individually selected have been found to help in the management of this condition. *Syn.* Irlen's syndrome; scotopic sensitivity syndrome. *See* **dyslexia.**

Mikulicz's A bilateral, painless, symmetrical enlargement of the lacrimal and salivary glands, causing hyposecretion of tears and saliva. It is usually associated with reticulosis, sarcoidosis, tuberculosis or syphilis. *See* **dacryoadenitis; keratoconjunctivitis sicca; syndrome, Sjögren's.**

Millard–Gubler s. A disorder caused by a lesion in the ventral part of the pons involving the fasciculus (bundle of nerve fibres) of the sixth and seventh nerve, caused by vascular disease, tumour or demyelination. It results in ipsilateral sixth (abducens) and seventh (facial) nerve palsies and contralateral hemiplegia. *See* **pons; syndrome, one and a half.**

Möbius' s. (or Moebius') A congenital condition due to a deletion on the long arm of chromosome 13. It is characterized by varying dysfunctions of the sixth (abducens) and seventh (facial) in particular, but other cranial nerves may be involved (third and fourth). The patient may exhibit an expressionless facial appearance, webbed fingers or toes, limb defects, deafness, feeding difficulties and mild mental handicap. The ocular signs include unilateral or bilateral esotropia with inability to abduct the eyes, horizontal gaze palsy and sagging of the lower lids.

monofixation s. A condition in which there is an inability in binocular fixation to fuse images formed on the fovea of each eye while peripheral fusion remains normal. There is limited stereopsis in most cases. One eye is usually amblyopic with a small central scotoma, which accounts for the absence of diplopia. There are cases in which there is no strabismus, although anisometropia is present. When there is strabismus (most commonly esotropia), the angle of deviation is small (less

than 8 Δ) and the condition is frequently regarded as a type of microtropia. Management usually consists in correcting the refractive error and often occlusion treatment. *See* **fusion, sensory; microtropia; occlusion treatment.**

Moon–Bardet–Biedl s. *See* **syndrome, Bardet–Biedl.**

de Morsier s. A disorder caused by midline brain abnormalities, including hypoplasia of the pituitary gland, absence of septum pellucidum, and corpus callosum and optic nerve hypoplasia. *Syn.* septo-optic dysplasia. *See* **hypoplasia; gland, pituitary.**

nystagmus blockage s. A condition in which convergence or adduction of one eye reduces nystagmus.

'one and a half' s. An eye movement disorder resulting from a brainstem lesion of the medial longitudinal fasciculus and the paramedian pontine reticular formation on the same side of the body. It is characterized by a horizontal palsy when the eye looks towards the same side as the lesion and an internuclear ophthalmoplegia when the eyes look to the side of the body opposite to that of the lesion. It is thus named because there is a complete ipsilateral gaze palsy and a contralateral half gaze palsy. *Syn.* paralytic pontine exotropia. *See* **brainstem; ophthalmoplegia, internuclear; syndrome, Millard–Gubler.**

orbital apex s. *See* **syndrome, orbital fissure.**

orbital fissure s. A disorder caused by trauma or tumour involving the superior orbital fissure through which pass the third, fourth and sixth cranial nerves, which supply the extraocular muscles, and also the ophthalmic division of the trigeminal nerve. It is characterized by diplopia, corneal and facial anaesthesia (about half the forehead), proptosis and pain behind the eyeball. If the trauma, tumour or orbital inflammation expands to the orbital apex (**orbital apex syndrome**) it involves the optic nerve and the results are more severe than the orbital fissure syndrome, with optic nerve compression, loss of vision, diplopia, proptosis, limitation of eye movements and corneal and facial anaesthesia. *Syn.* orbital apex-sphenoidal syndrome.

orbital inflammatory s. An idiopathic inflammation of orbital tissues causing sudden pain, restricted ocular motility (including diplopia), proptosis, lid oedema and decreased vision. It may occur in children or adults. The abnormality is thought to be due to an inflammation of the orbital structures including the extraocular muscles (myositis) and tendons, vascular system, sclera, and optic nerve sheath. Lesions may be noted bilaterally, in which case, in the adult population, the possibility of systemic vasculitis or lymphoproliferative disease is raised. *Syn.* orbital pseudotumour.

overwear s. Ocular pain, which may be very intense, accompanied by corneal epithelium damage, conjunctival injection, lacrimation,

blepharospasm, photophobia, and hazy vision following corneal hypoxia caused by overwear of contact lenses, principally the PMMA type, but also lenses with very low oxygen transmissibility. The symptoms usually begin to appear 2 to 3 hours after the lenses are removed and recovery usually occurs within 24 hours, although an antibiotic may be needed.
See **corneal abrasion; hypoxia; oedema; syndrome, corneal exhaustion.**

Parinaud's s. A disorder caused by a lesion at the level of the superior colliculi or in the subthalamic region resulting in a supranuclear upgaze palsy and sometimes downgaze palsy with paralysis of convergence, fixed pupils and lid retraction. Causes include pinealoma, demyelination, cerebrovascular accidents or tumour in the elderly. *Syn.* dorsal midbrain syndrome; tectal midbrain syndrome.
See **nystagmus, convergence-retraction; palsy, supranuclear gaze; sign, Collier's.**

Parinaud's oculoglandular s. A rare disorder characterized by unilateral conjunctivitis with granulomatous nodules surrounded with follicles, and systemic manifestations (malaise, fever). Causes include cat-scratch disease, tularaemia, tuberculosis and syphilis.

Patau's s. A disorder caused by a chromosomal abnormality, trisomy 13. Major systemic features are cleft lip and palate, microcephaly and heart defects. Ocular signs are anophthalmia, microphthalmia, optic disc coloboma, retinal dysplasia and cataract. Life expectancy is less than one year. *Syn.* trisomy 13 syndrome.

pigment dispersion s. A degenerative process in the iris and ciliary body epithelium in which pigment granules are disseminated and deposited on the back surface of the cornea, the lens, the zonules and within the trabecular meshwork. On the corneal endothelium, it may form a vertical spindle shape (called Krukenberg's spindle). Deposition of pigment in the trabecular meshwork may give rise to secondary glaucoma (called **pigmentary glaucoma**).
See **glaucoma, pigmentary; Krukenberg's spindle; line, Sampaolesi's.**

plateau iris s. See **iris plateau.**

Posner–Schlossman s. A condition characterized by recurrent episodes of high intraocular pressure (40 to 80 mmHg) associated with intraocular inflammation. Keratic precipitates commonly appear with each attack, especially on the trabecular meshwork. Patients are typically young adult males. Main complaint is blurred vision, due to corneal oedema. The cause is unknown, although herpes simplex virus has been implicated. With repeated attacks, which last a few hours to a few weeks, chronic uveitis and open-angle glaucoma may develop. Treatment usually consists of topical steroids to control the inflammation and carbonic anhydrase inhibitors or beta-blockers to reduce the secretion of aqueous humour and decrease the intraocular pressure. *Syn.* glaucomatocyclitic crisis.

presumed ocular histoplasmosis s. An infection which can be caused by inhalation of the fungus *Histoplasma capsulatum* found in soil dust, most likely in individuals with an abnormal immune response. It manifests by a self-limited pneumonitis, which occasionally progresses and may affect the eye. It is then characterized by a disseminated choroiditis with small, yellowish scattered lesions called **'histo spots'** which represent atrophic choroidal scars appearing as 'punched-out' spots. At a later stage, the patient may present subretinal neovascularization with blurred vision. Many cases have been reported in parts of the world where the fungus is non-existent. Thus the condition has been termed **'presumed ocular histoplasmosis syndrome'**. The main treatment for neovascularization consists of laser photocoagulation and intravitreal anti-VEGF injection.
See **anti-VEGF drugs.**

pseudoexfoliation s. A systemic disorder in which a greyish-white fibrillogranular basement membrane material is deposited on the anterior lens capsule, zonules, ciliary body, iris, trabeculum and conjunctiva, as well as other organs such as the skin, heart, lungs, kidneys and meninges. With gonioscopy, Sampaolesi's line of pigment can be seen on the surface of the trabecular meshwork anterior to Schwalbe's line. Secondary glaucoma may occur as a result. *Syn.* exfoliation syndrome.
See **glaucoma, capsular; pseudoexfoliation.**

Refsum's s. See **disease, Refsum's.**

Reiter's s. A systemic syndrome characterized by a triad of three diseases: urethritis, arthritis and conjunctivitis. Keratitis and iridocyclitis may follow as complications. It occurs mainly in young men typically following urethritis and less commonly after an attack of dysentery (infection of the intestines) or acute arthritis, which usually affects the knees, ankles and Achilles tendon. *Syn.* Reiter's disease.

retraction s. See **syndrome, Duane's.**

Rieger's s. A rare hereditary (usually autosomal dominant) developmental anomaly of the cornea, iris and the angle of the anterior chamber. It is characterized by posterior embryotoxon, stromal hypoplasia of the iris, ectropion uveae, pupillary anomalies (corectopia) and adhesion of strands of iris tissue to the cornea at the angle of the anterior chamber which comprise **Rieger's anomaly**. **Rieger's syndrome** includes, in addition to the features of the anomaly, glaucoma in about half of the cases, as well as dental and facial abnormalities. It is a more severe disorder than Axenfeld's syndrome with which it forms part of the **Axenfeld–Rieger syndrome**. *Syn.* mesodermal dysgenesis of the cornea and iris.
See **Axenfeld's anomaly; Peter's anomaly; syndrome, Axenfeld–Rieger.**

Riley–Day s. A hereditary disorder of the nervous system largely confined to Ashkenazic Jews. It is characterized by alacrima, corneal hypoaesthesia, exotropia, myopia and excessive sweating, vomiting, attacks of high fever, incoordination and lack of pain sensitivity. Few patients survive to adulthood as most die from pneumonia and cardiovascular collapse. *Syn.* familial autonomic dysfunction; familial dysautonomia.

See **keratopathy, neurotrophic.**

rubella s. Congenital defects in infants whose mothers contracted rubella in the first few months of pregnancy. The infant may have cardiac malformation, cataract, pigment epithelium disorders, deafness, microcephaly and mental handicap. *Syn.* Gregg syndrome.

See **deaf-blind.**

Scheie s. *See* **syndrome, Hurler's.**

scotopic sensitivity s. *See* **syndrome, Meares–Irlen.**

shaken baby s. Malicious injury to an infant which causes cerebral (especially intracranial haemorrhage) and ocular damage particularly retinal haemorrhage, but in whom external signs of ocular or head injury are typically absent. It is due to ruptures of retinal vasculature as a result of violent shaking of the baby.

Sjögren's s. An autoimmune chronic connective tissue disease characterized by a failure of lacrimal secretion and diminished salivary flow due to impaired function or destruction of lacrimal and salivary glands. It leads to keratoconjunctivitis sicca, with dryness of the mouth, of the upper respiratory tract and other mucous membranes and is often associated with rheumatoid arthritis. The condition occurs predominantly in women after menopause. Main features are dry eye, grittiness, burning, redness and blepharitis. Management involves artificial tears, corticosteroids, punctal occlusion and in very severe cases tarsorrhaphy may be required.

See **alacrima; keratoconjunctivitis sicca; syndrome, Mikulicz's; tears, artificial.**

Steele–Richardson–Olszewski s. *See* **palsy, progressive supranuclear.**

Stevens–Johnson s. An acute form of erythema exudativum multiforme involving the mucous membranes and large areas of the body. Some form of conjunctivitis occurs in most cases, but symblepharon and keratoconjunctivitis sicca with corneal opacification and loss of vision may also occur. Common causes include reaction to some drugs (e.g. sulfonamides, penicillin, NSAIDs), secondary to an infection (e.g. herpes simplex virus, *Mycoplasma pneumoniae*). Management consists of systemic and ocular medication (ocular lubricants, steroids) and sealed scleral contact lenses with high permeability which can retain physiological saline bathing the cornea have been found to alleviate symptoms.

See **conjunctivitis, pseudomembranous; entropion; erythema multiforme; test, ocular ferning.**

Stickler's s. Autosomal dominant hereditary, progressive connective tissue disorder. One form of the syndrome is caused by mutation in the collagen, type 2, alpha-1 gene (COL2A1), another by mutation in COL11A1 gene and another by mutation in COL11A2 gene. It is characterized by a flattened face, maxillary hypoplasia, progressive arthritis, cleft palate and deafness. The ocular

manifestations include progressive vitreoretinal degeneration, which results in an empty vitreous cavity, vitreous bands, retinal vascular sheathing, chorioretinal atrophy, high myopia, cataract and retinal detachment.

See **retina, lattice degeneration of the; syndrome, Wagner's.**

Stilling–Turk–Duane s. *See* **syndrome, Duane's.**

Sturge–Weber s. A rare congenital disorder characterized by vascular abnormalities such as a reddish pigmentation or 'port-wine' stains (**naevus flammeus**), usually on one side of the face in the area supplied by the trigeminal nerve. It is associated with a haemangioma of the choroid (diffuse), iris and ciliary body and high intraocular pressure, which give rise to megalocornea or glaucoma, as well as haemangioma of the brain and meninges and sometimes heterochromia. *Syn.* Sturge–Weber disease, encephalotrigeminal angiomatosis.

See **haemangioma, choroidal; phakomatoses; syndrome, von Hippel–Lindau; syndrome, Wyburn–Mason; telangiectasia.**

superior oblique sheath s. *See* **syndrome, Brown's superior oblique tendon sheath.**

Swann's s. Esotropia in which the angle of deviation is such that the retinal image of the fixation object in the deviated eye falls on the optic disc. *Syn.* blind spot esotropia; syndrome, blind spot.

Terson's s. Subarachnoid haemorrhage followed by retinal haemorrhage (in about 30% of patients) which breaks through the inner limiting membrane of the retina into the vitreous. It is likely due to an acute rise in intracranial pressure. The condition commonly subsides spontaneously; otherwise treatment usually consists of vitrectomy.

See **haemorrhage, preretinal; space, subarachnoid.**

tight lens s. *See* **contact lens acute red eye.**

tilted disc s. *See* **crescent, congenital scleral.**

Treacher Collins s. An autosomal dominant inherited disorder characterized by deformities of the skull and face with hypoplasia of the zygomatic and mandible bones, ear defects, antimongoloid slants of the palpebral fissures, colobomas of the lower lids and absence of eyelashes medially. It is caused by mutation in the 'treacle' gene (TCOF1). *Syn.* mandibulofacial dysostosis.

trisomy 13 s. *See* **syndrome, Patau's.**

trisomy 18 s. *See* **syndrome, Edwards'.**

trisomy 21 s. *See* **syndrome, Down's.**

Turcot s. A variant of familial adenomatous polyposis associated with congenital hypertrophy of the retinal pigment epithelium. It is characterized by tumours of the central nervous system, medalloblastoma and glioma. The main ocular sign is atypical congenital hypertrophy of the retinal pigment epithelium and there can also be diplopia, ptosis, nystagmus or papilloedema.

See **retinal pigment epithelium, congenital hypertrophy of the.**

Turner's s. A disorder caused by the absence of, or sometimes defective, X chromosomes

in females. It is characterized by shortness of stature, webbing of the skin and neck, congenital heart disease and genitourinary anomalies. The ocular manifestations include epicanthus, ptosis, strabismus, blue sclera, myopia, cataract, and colour vision deficiencies. *Note*: As female patients are born with only a single X chromosome, this is designated as monosomy 45XO.
See **chromosome; inheritance.**

UGH syndrome A disorder characterized by uveitis, glaucoma and hyphaema. The main cause is as a complication of intraocular lens implantation.

Usher's s. An autosomal recessive inherited condition characterized by retinitis pigmentosa associated with deafness. One form of the syndrome is caused by mutation in the MYO7A gene (myosin, unconventional, family 7, member A) and CDH23 gene. Other types are caused by mutations in the USH2A and CLRN1 genes.
See **deaf-blind.**

uveal effusion s. A condition characterized by choroidal detachments associated with exudative retinal detachment and frequent localized areas of retinal pigment epithelium hypertrophy. The cause may be idiopathic, trauma, intraocular surgery or chronic uveitis. Treatment is aimed at the primary cause.
See **choroidal detachment.**

V s. *See* **pattern, alphabet.**

Vogt–Koyanagi–Harada s. A severe multisystem disorder of unknown origin. It is characterized by inflammation of various tissues such as the ears (deafness, vertigo) brain (meningitis), skin (vitiligo) and hair (alopecia, poliosis). The ocular manifestations, bilateral in nature, are granulomatous anterior uveitis with posterior synechia, iris nodules and posterior uveitis with exudative retinal detachment, choroidal depigmentation and Dalen–Fuchs nodules. Loss of vision, headaches, pain in the eye and vertigo are the principal symptoms. Complications include choroidal neovascularization, cataract and glaucoma. The condition affects predominantly pigmented individuals. Management includes high-dose steroids with mydriatics (if there uveitis) and if persistent, immunosuppressive agents. *Syn.* Vogt–Koyanagi–Harada disease.
See **disease, Harada's.**

Waardenburg's s. An autosomal dominant inherited disorder characterized by pigmentary anomalies of the skin, hair (a white forelock) and eye (choroidal depigmentation), such as heterochromia, as well as hypertelorism, telecanthus and deafness.

Wagner's s. An autosomal dominant inherited disease caused by mutation in the VCAN gene. The condition is characterized by an empty vitreous cavity or dense membranes within the vitreous, myopia, retinal perivascular pigmentation, retinal degeneration, cataract and, less frequently, retinal detachment. Vision is usually normal until adulthood. The condition is not associated with systemic diseases. *Syn.* vitreoretinal degeneration.
See **syndrome, Stickler's.**

Weber's s. A syndrome caused by a lesion (usually vascular) in the region of the cerebral peduncles of the brain. It is characterized by an ipsilateral third nerve paralysis associated with facial paralysis and contralateral hemiplegia.
See **palsy, third nerve; syndrome, Benedikt's.**

Weill–Marchesani s. A connective tissue disorder inherited as autosomal dominant caused by mutations in the fibrillin 1 gene (FBN1) or recessive dominant, which can be caused by mutations in the ADAMTS10 gene. The syndrome is characterized by spherophakia, lenticular myopia and glaucoma, which result from lens subluxation and pupil block, associated with brachydactyly and short stature.
See **syndrome, Marfan's.**

Wernicke's s. *See* **disease, Wernicke's.**

white dot s's. A group of idiopathic inflammatory conditions involving the retina and choroid (chorioretinopathy). They are so-called because they are characterized by the appearance of white dots in the fundus. They all present with reduced visual acuity, mild vitritis, some with photopsia. They include multiple evanescent white dot syndrome, acute posterior multifocal placoid pigment epitheliopathy, birdshot chorioretinopathy, punctate inner choroidopathy, serpiginous choroidopathy, multifocal choroiditis and panuveitis, and subretinal fibrosis and uveitis. Some recover spontaneously (the first two), the others with steroids and immunosuppressants.
See **retinochoroidopathy, birdshot.**

Wyburn–Mason s. A disorder caused by arteriovenous malformation of the retina, orbit and brainstem with facial nevi and mental handicap.
See **phakomatoses; syndrome, von Hippel-Lindau; syndrome, Sturge–Weber.**

Zellweger's s. A severe autosomal recessive inherited disorder caused by a dysfunction of the cell structures (called peroxisomes) that break down toxic substances and synthesize lipids that are essential for normal cell function. The condition is characterized by generalized hypotonia, enlarged liver, renal cysts, prominent forehead and cognitive impairment. Ocular signs include corneal clouding, cataract, optic nerve hypoplasia and retinal abnormalities. Life expectancy is less than 1 year. A mild form of the syndrome is infantile Refsum's disease. *Syn.* cerebrohepatorenal syndrome.
See **disease, Refsum's.**

synechia Adhesion of parts of the body. In the eye, it refers to the iris. *Note*: also spelt synechiae.

annular s. A posterior synechia in which there is an adhesion of the entire pupillary margin of the iris to the capsule of the crystalline lens. *Syn.* ring synechia.
See **iris bombé; pupillary block; synechia, posterior.**

anterior s. Adhesion of the iris to the cornea. It may give rise to angle-closure glaucoma. *Syn.* goniosynechia (if at the AC angle).
See **glaucoma, inflammatory; gonioscopy, indentation; iris, prolapse of the; Peter's anomaly; syndrome, Rieger's.**

posterior s. Adhesion of the iris to the capsule of the crystalline lens. It often forms at the site of Koeppe's nodules.
See **capsule, crystalline lens; iris bombé; iritis; nodule, Koeppe's; uveitis.**
ring s. *See* **synechia, annular.**

syneresis A degenerative shrinkage of the vitreous humour in which the gel separates and breaks into liquid-filled particles, which coalesce and render it partially or completely fluid. It occurs in elderly individuals and may precede vitreous detachment.
See **synchisis scintillans; vitreous detachment.**

synergist muscle *See* **muscle, synergistic.**

synaesthesia Phenomenon in which the stimulation of one of the senses produces a response from another sensory modality. *Example*: seeing the colour red when a particular sound is heard.
See **modality.**

synkinetic reflex, near *See* **reflex, near.**

Synoptiscope *See* **amblyoscope, Worth.**

Synoptophore A type of major amblyoscope (Fig. S16).
See **amblyoscope, Worth.**

syphilis An infection caused by the microorganism *Treponema pallidum*, which affects the skin, mucous membranes and various ocular tissues.
See **anisocoria; conjunctivitis; dacryoadenitis; fundus, salt and pepper; keratitis, interstitial; luxation of the lens; madarosis; neuritis, optic; pupil, Adie's; pupil, Argyll Robertson; sign, Hutchinson's; tabes dorsalis; uveitis, acute anterior; uveitis, bacterial; syndrome, Parinaud's oculoglandular.**

system 1. A group of body organs serving a common function (e.g. the nervous system). **2.** A combination of parts or things forming a unitary whole (e.g. optical system). **3.** A method of arrangement or classification.
autonomic nervous s. (ANS) A part of the nervous system involved in the regulation of the internal environment (homeostasis) which is achieved mostly by controlling cardiovascular, digestive, respiratory and reproductive functions of the body, as well as salivation, perspiration, pupil size, urinary and genital systems. Most of these activities are involuntary, although, for example, breathing can be partly voluntary. Sensory information from the **visceral sensory neurons (afferent)** located in the peripheral nervous system (PNS), such as monitoring the composition of the blood and stomach, is conveyed to the central nervous system (CNS), especially the hypothalamus and medulla oblongata, where it is integrated. *Motor neurons* (efferent) of the ANS consist of a set of two neurons: the first with its cell body in the CNS project to an autonomic ganglion (preganglionic neuron) and a second motor neuron (postganglionic neuron) outside the CNS, innervates visceral effectors (target organs). The efferent part of the ANS has two principal divisions: sympathetic and parasympathetic. Many organs receive autonomic fibres from both divisions. The **preganglionic sympathetic** neurons have their cell bodies in the lateral horn and the first two or three lumbar segments of the spinal cord, while the **parasympathetic preganglionic** neurons are found in the brainstem and their axons leave the brain via the third, seventh, ninth and tenth cranial nerves. **Sympathetic postganglionic** neurons project to sympathetic ganglia from which axons project to the eyes, lacrimal glands, salivary glands, respiratory, cardiovascular, digestive, urinary and reproductive systems. **Parasympathetic postganglionic** neurons are located in or near the target organs. They also innervate the eyes, lacrimal glands, salivary glands, respiratory, cardiovascular, digestive, urinary and reproductive systems. *Examples*: Sympathetic stimulation causes pupil dilatation and relaxation of the ciliary muscle, while parasympathetic stimulation causes pupil constriction, accommodation and lacrimal secretion.
The *sympathetic nervous system* dominates in stressful situations causing a 'fight or flight' response, while the **parasympathetic nervous system** primarily regulates those activities that conserve and restore energy. Acetylcholine is the neurotransmitter for sympathetic and parasympathetic preganglionic neurons and for postganglionic parasympathetic neurons, which act on muscarinic receptors, while noradrenaline (norepinephrine) is the neurotransmitter for all postganglionic sympathetic neurons (except for the sweat glands) which act on adrenergic receptors.
See **acetylcholine; adrenergic receptors; neurotransmitter.**
boxing s. A method of measurement of the eyesize of spectacle frames. It is based on a rectangle with its horizontal and vertical length tangential to the edges of the lens. The horizontal lens size is equal to the horizontal length of the rectangle. *Syn.* box system of lens measurement; boxing method.
See **centre, boxing; centre, standard optical position.**
catadioptric s. Optical system employing both reflecting and refracting components as used, for example, in a lighthouse. This design makes long focal length more compact, and mirrors, unlike lenses or prisms, are free of chromatic aberration.

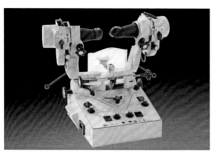

Fig. S16 Clement Clarke synoptophore. (Courtesy of Haag-Streit UK)

See **image, catadioptric.**

central nervous s. The largest part of the nervous system, comprising the brain and the spinal cord. The brain is encased and protected by the skull and the spinal cord by the vertebrae, as well as the meninges and the blood-brain barrier that protects against blood-borne toxins. The central nervous system processes and integrates sensory information received from the peripheral nervous system and issues appropriate motor responses. *See* **system, autonomic nervous; system, peripheral nervous.**

centred optical s. *See* **system, optical.**

compound optical s. An optical system consisting of more than one lens (e.g. the eyepiece of a telescope).

immune s. Complex system that protects the body against infection, disease and malignant cells by producing the immune response. The system includes skin and mucous secretions, white blood cells (leukocytes), lymphocytes (B cells and T cells), killer T cells, complement system (proteins in the blood) and antibodies. Disorders of the immune system can cause disease; they include immunodeficiencies due to aging, alcoholism, malnutrition, etc., immune responses against its own cells (autoimmunity), or damaging effects caused by the immune system (hypersensitivity). *See* **disease, autoimmune; hypersensitivity.**

koniocellular s. That part of the visual pathway from the ganglion cells to layers 3 (in the cytochrome oxidase blobs) and 4A, and to a lesser extent layer 1, of the primary visual cortex. It is mainly responsible for processing colour vision, especially the blue end of the spectrum. *See* **blobs.**

Lens Opacity Classification S. *See* **grading scale.**

magnocellular visual s. That part of the visual pathway from the photoreceptors in the retina to layer $4C\alpha$ (and to a lesser extent in layer 6) of the visual cortex and then projected to area V5. It is mainly responsible for transmitting information about movement, depth perception and high-contrast targets. Action potentials are transmitted faster in this pathway because of the large-diameter axons of these neurons than in the parvocellular pathway. *Syn.* dorsal stream; parietal pathway; transient visual system; 'where' system. *See* **cell, M; dyslexia; geniculate body, lateral; theory, two visual systems.**

optical s. A collection of lenses, prisms, mirrors, etc. which act together to produce an image of an external object. If the axes of all the components coincide, the system is called a **centred optical system**.

parvocellular visual s. That part of the visual pathway from the photoreceptors in the retina to layer $4C\beta$ (and to a lesser extent in layers 4A and 6) of the primary visual cortex and then projected to area V4. It is mainly responsible for transmitting information about visual acuity, form vision, colour vision and low-contrast targets. *Syn.* sustained visual system; ventral stream; 'what' system. *See* **area, visual association; cell, ganglion; cell, P; geniculate body, lateral; theory, two visual systems.**

peripheral nervous s. The part of the nervous system which consists of the nerves and neurons that are outside the brain and spinal cord. It comprises the cranial nerves, spinal nerves and the autonomic nervous system. The primary role of the peripheral nervous system is to transmit sensory information about the external and internal milieus to the central nervous system and to transmit motor commands to the effectors such as muscles and glands. *Note*: Some authors do not consider the autonomic nervous system as part of the peripheral nervous system. It is, however, a separate entity, which is part central and part peripheral. *See* **system, central nervous.**

'what' s. *See* **system, parvocellular visual.**

'where' s. *See* **system, magnocellular visual.**

systemic Adjective usually referring to medication affecting the whole body. Some systemic drugs have ocular side effects (e.g. steroids may cause cataract, antimalarials may cause keratopathy or retinal toxicity, etc.).

See **topical.**

T

tabes dorsalis A degenerative disease of the posterior columns of the spinal cord, the posterior spinal roots and the peripheral nerves accompanied by a number of ocular signs and symptoms such as atrophy of the optic nerve, visual field defects, ptosis, Argyll Robertson pupil and paralysis of one or more of the extraocular muscles. The disease is a result of neurosyphilis.

TABO notation *See* **axis notation, standard.**

tachistoscope An instrument that presents visual stimuli for a brief and variable period of time (usually less than 0.1 s).

tacrolimus *See* **immunosuppressants.**

Talbot-Plateau law *See* **law, Talbot-Plateau.**

tamponade agent A gas, pad, silicone oil, perfluorocarbon liquid or semifluorinated alkanes used to plug a cavity, stop a haemorrhage or compress a part. In the eye, it may be employed in vitreous surgery to fill the vitreous space with either gas or silicone, and in retinal detachment therapy.
See **retinopexy; scleral buckling.**

tangent scale *See* **Maddox cross.**

tangent screen *See* **screen, tangent.**

tangential focus *See* **astigmatism, oblique.**

tapetoretinal degeneration *See* **degeneration, tapetoretinal.**

tapetoretinal dystrophy, progressive *See* **choroideremia.**

tapetum lucidum A reflecting pigment layer lying behind the visual receptors of the retina of certain mammals (e.g. cats, dogs), birds and fish, which gives a shining appearance to the eyes when illuminated in the dark. The tapetum is located either in the pigment epithelium or in the choroid and covers either the whole fundus or, more often, only the upper and central portion. The role of the tapetum lucidum is to increase the probability of visual stimulation of the photoreceptors by reflecting light back after having already traversed them once, thus aiding vision in dim illumination. In some species, the tapetum consists of guanine crystals.

target A pattern or an object of fixation such as a red dot or an optotype.
See **optotype.**

tarsal Pertaining to the tarsus.

tarsal gland *See* **gland, meibomian.**

tarsal muscles *See* **muscle, Müller's palpebral.**

tarsal plate *See* **tarsus.**

tarsorrhaphy A surgical procedure consisting of suturing the upper and lower eyelids together either partially or completely. It provides a temporary or permanent protection to the eye (e.g. in exposure or neurotrophic keratopathy) or forms part of the treatment of dry eyes.
See **alacrima; blepharorrhaphy; keratoconjunctivitis sicca; keratopathy.**

tarsus Thin flat plate of dense connective tissue, situated one in each eyelid, which gives it shape and firmness. Each tarsus extends from the orbital septum to the eyelid margin. The upper tarsal plate, shaped like the letter D placed on its side, is much larger than the lower. Its width is 11 mm in the centre whereas the corresponding measurement in the lower tarsus, which is somewhat oblong in form, is 5 mm. Each tarsus is about 29 mm long and 1 mm thick. Within each tarsus are the meibomian glands, approximately 25 in the upper and 20 in the lower. *Syn.* tarsal plate.
See **ligament, palpebral; orbital septum.**

Tay's choroiditis *See* **drusen, familial dominant.**

Tay–Sachs disease *See* **disease, Tay–Sachs.**

tear drainage The process of excreting tears via the lacrimal puncta and into the lacrimal apparatus. Some 70% is drained through the inferior canaliculus and 30% through the superior. Following a blink, it is believed that contraction of the orbicularis muscle compresses the canaliculi and lacrimal sac. This is followed by a decrease in the orbicularis contraction, which results in an expansion of the lacrimal sac and canaliculi thus reducing the pressure within and allowing an influx of tears, which then flows into the nasolacrimal duct. Blockage of the tear drainage (e.g. at the puncta) causes dry eye.
See **keratoconjunctivitis sicca; lacrimal apparatus; tears.**

tear duct One of about a dozen ducts of the lacrimal gland. It originates in the orbital part of the gland, traverses the palpebral part of the gland and opens into the lateral superior fornix of the conjunctival sac. *Syn.* lacrimal duct.
See **lacrimal apparatus.**

tear exchange *See* **lens, fenestrated.**

tear film The film covering the anterior surface of the cornea which consists of lacrimal fluid and of the secretion of the meibomian and conjunctival glands. Its total thickness is thought to be about 9 μm. It is composed of three layers: (1) The deepest and densest is the **mucin layer (mucous layer)** which derives from the conjunctival goblet cells, as well as some secretion from the lacrimal gland. It lubricates and renders the corneal epithelium hydrophilic. (2) The watery lacrimal fluid is the middle layer, called the **lacrimal (aqueous layer)**. It is secreted by the lacrimal gland and the accessory glands of Krause and Wolfring. It forms the bulk of the film and contains most of the bactericidal lysozyme, IgA and other proteins, inorganic salts, sugars, amino acids, urea, etc. and provide oxygen to the corneal epithelium (3) The **oily layer (lipid layer)** is the most superficial and is derived principally from the meibomian glands in the lids as well as some secretion from the glands of Zeis. It greatly slows the evaporation of the watery layer and may provide a lubrication effect between lid and cornea (Fig. T1). *Note:* Some authors have suggested that the tear film is made up of only two layers: an innermost aqueous and mucin gel layer, and an outer lipid layer. *Syn.* lacrimal layer; precorneal film; preocular tear film; tear layer.
See **hyperlacrimation; mucin; tear secretion; Tearscope; test, break-up time.**

tear film break-up test *See* **test, break-up time.**

tear film, prelens Tear film found on the front surface of a contact lens on the eye. The oily layer of the film is slightly thinner with soft lenses than in the precorneal film and almost absent with rigid lenses. The aqueous layer is thinner with rigid lenses than in the precorneal film. The exact composition of the prelens tear film varies with the characteristics of the contact lens on the eye.
See **tear film.**

tear layer *See* **tear film.**

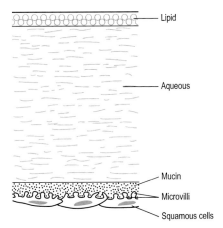

Fig. T1 Diagram of the three layers of the tear film attached to the squamous epithelial cells of the cornea.

tear meniscus A thin strip of tear fluid with concave outer surfaces at the upper and lower lid margins. It contains most of the exposed tear volume. In normal eyes, the meniscus is about 1 mm in height. The absence of a tear meniscus is an indication of a dry eye. *Syn.* marginal tear strip; lacrimal prism; tear prism.
See **tear film; lacrimal lake.**

tear prism *See* **tear meniscus.**

tear pumping The mechanism involving blinking, which acts to bring fresh tears with oxygen and nutrients to the cornea behind a contact lens and pumping stale tears containing carbon dioxide, lactic acid and other waste products from beneath the lens. It occurs most readily with hard contact lenses (between 14% and 20% of the tear volume is exchanged with each blink) and to a much smaller extent with soft lenses (between 1% and 5% of the tear volume is exchanged with each blink).
See **hypoxia; oxygen transmissibility.**

tear, retinal *See* **retinal break.**

tear secretion There are two types of tear secretion: (1) **Basal (basic) tear secretion**, which occurs normally without any stimulation. It ensures the cornea and conjunctiva are continuously moist but is reduced in dry eyes (e.g. keratoconjunctivitis sicca) and in elderly individuals. (2) **Reflex tear secretion**, which is produced in response to a corneal or conjunctival irritant and also depends on psychological factors. It is reduced by topical anaesthesia. Basal and reflex secretion are produced principally by the lacrimal gland, about 95%, and the rest by the accessory glands of Krause and Wolfring. The amount of tears secreted amounts to 14 to 33 g per 24 hours or 0.5 to 2.2 μl/minute, being about 2 μl/minute at 15 years of age and less than 1 μl/minute at 65 years of age. *Note*: It was formally thought that basal secretion was produced solely by the accessory glands and reflex secretion by the lacrimal gland, but it is now thought that they all contribute to both forms of tear secretion.
See **occlusion, punctal; reflex, lacrimal; test, basic secretion; test, Norn's; test, Schirmer's.**

tear stasis The slowing down or stoppage of tear flow behind a contact lens. It can lead to **lens adherence (lens binding)** to the cornea with the possible consequences of acute red eye, arcuate corneal staining, and, if severe, corneal ulceration. Fitting or refitting in such a way that some lens movement is maintained usually prevents this condition.
See **lens adherence; staining, fluorescein.**

tear strip, marginal *See* **tear meniscus.**

tearing reflex *See* **reflex, lacrimal.**

tears The clear watery fluid secreted by the lacrimal gland which, together with the secretions from the meibomian glands, the goblet cells, the gland of Zeis, as well as the accessory lacrimal glands of Krause and Wolfring, helps to maintain the conjunctiva and cornea moist and healthy. Periodic involuntary blinking spreads the tears over the cornea and conjunctiva and causes a pumping action of the lacrimal drainage system, through the lacrimal puncta into the nasolacrimal duct. Approximately 25% of the tears is lost by evaporation, the remaining 75% is pumped into the nasal cavity and more than 60% of the tear volume is drained through the lower canaliculus. Tears contain water (98.2%), salts, lipids (e.g. wax esters, sterol esters, hydrocarbons, polar lipids, triglycerides and free fatty acids), proteins (e.g. lysozyme, lactoferrin, lipocalin, albumin, IgA, IgE, IgG, complement proteins C3, C4, C5 and C9 and beta-lysin), magnesium, potassium, sodium, calcium, chloride, bicarbonate, urea, ammonia, nitrogen, citric acid, ascorbic acid and mucin. Tears have a pH varying between 7.3 and 7.7 (shifting to a slightly less alkaline value when the eye is closed), and the quantity secreted per hour is between 30 and 120 ml. Tears provide atmospheric oxygen to the corneal epithelium and have antibacterial properties due to proteins (e.g. IgA, lysozyme and lactoferrin). *Syn.* lacrimal fluid.
See **alacrima; blink; epiphora; hyperlacrimation; keratoconjunctivitis sicca; lacrimal apparatus; lacrimal lake; lysozyme; mucin; staining, fluorescein; tear drainage; tear film; test, break-up time; test, non-invasive break-up time; test, phenol red cotton thread; test, Schirmer's.**
artificial t. An eyedrop solution that can replace tears by approximating its consistency in terms of viscosity and tonicity and may contain many of the substances found in tears. The most common agents found in artificial tears are cellulose derivatives, such as methylcellulose, hydroxymethylcellulose, hydroxypropylcellulose, hydroxypropyl guar. hypromellose (hydroxypropylmethylcellulose), hydroxyethylcellulose, and polyvinyl alcohol, povidone (polyvinyl pyrrolidine), sodium hyaluronate and sodium chloride, all of which have low viscosity. Carbomer (polyacrylic acid), carmellose (carbomethylcellulose), liquid

paraffin and yellow soft paraffin have medium to high viscosity. Acetylcysteine, a **mucolytic agent** prepared with hypromellose, is used when the tear deficiency is associated with threads and filaments of mucus to soften and make the mucus more fluid, as well as shrinking the mucous membranes (**astringent**). *Syn.* ocular lubricant.
See **alacrima; corneal erosion, recurrent; ectropion; eye, dry; hypromellose; keratoconjunctivitis sicca; methylcellulose; palsy, Bell's; xerophthalmia.**
crocodile t. Copious secretion of tears occurring during eating in cases of abnormal regeneration of the seventh cranial nerve after recovery from Bell's palsy. *Syn.* paradoxic lacrimation.

Tearscope plus Trade name of a hand-held instrument designed to view the tear film non-invasively. It uses a cold light source to minimize any drying of the tear film during the examination. It can be used directly in front of the eye or in conjunction with a slit-lamp biomicroscope to gain more magnification. Evaluation of the interference patterns of the anterior surface of the tear film lipid layer facilitates the diagnosis of the cause of dry eye symptoms, as well as screening patients for contact lens wear. The instrument also allows the measurement of the non-invasive break-up time.
See **tear film; test, non-invasive break-up time.**

technique *See* **method; test.**

tectal midbrain syndrome *See* **syndrome, Parinaud's.**

tectum of the mesencephalon Structure comprising the plate of grey and white matter (called the **tectal lamina**) that forms the roof of the midbrain and from which project the inferior and superior colliculi. The area anterior to it is called the pretectal region. *Syn.* tectum of the midbrain; optic tectum. *Note*: The word tectum comes from the Latin and means roof. The word mesencephalon is made up of two parts that come from the Greek and means middle brain.
See **colliculi, inferior; colliculi, superior; fibre f., pupillary; nystagmus, convergence-retraction; pathway, retinotectal; pretectum.**

tectum of the midbrain *See* **tectum of the mesencephalon.**

teichopsia A transient shimmering visual sensation. *Example*: the fortification spectrum of a scintillating scotoma seen in the initial stage of a migraine.

telangiectasia A dilatation of small blood vessels (arterioles, capillaries, venules), often multiple in character. Telangiectasias create small red lesions, sometimes spidery in appearance, usually in the skin or mucous membranes, which blanch on pressure. They can develop into naevus flammeus ('port-wine stain'), a birthmark found usually on the head or neck. It can occur in the retina and macula, either secondary to a retinal disorder (e.g. central retinal vein occlusion, diabetic retinopathy), idiopathic (**idiopathic macular telangiectasia**) or in Coat's disease.
See **syndrome, Sturge–Weber.**
retinal t. See **disease, Coat's.**

Telebinocular A trade name for a stereoscope based on that of Brewster–Holmes and used to investigate distance and near visual functions such as acuity, stereopsis, etc.
See **stereoscope, Brewster's.**

telecanthus Excessive separation between the medial canthi of the eyelids. It may occur in isolation or form part of the blepharophimosis syndrome. Treatment consists in shortening and re-fixating the medial canthal tendons to the lacrimal crest. This condition is distinct from hypertelorism in which the whole orbits are widely separated.
See **hypertelorism; syndrome, Aarskog's; syndrome, blepharophimosis; syndrome, Waardenburg's.**

telecentric Pertains to an optical system in which its aperture stop is positioned so that the entrance pupil falls in the first focal plane, the exit pupil is at infinity, and the rays through the centre of the entrance pupil from all points on the object are parallel to the axis in the image space. Similarly, if the exit pupil lies in the second focal plane, the entrance pupil will be at infinity, and the rays through the centre of the exit pupil will be parallel to the axis in the object space.

telemedicine The provision of consultation and education services by practitioners to others situated anywhere in the world, via the internet, closed-circuit television or the telephone. *Example*: Digitized imaging of the eye or its fundus makes it possible to facilitate the diagnosis and treatment of an eye disease by consulting an expert in another part of the country or the world.

teleopsia Anomaly of visual perception in which objects appear to be much farther away than they actually are. It may be due to vision in a hazy atmosphere, intoxication, neurosis, etc.
See **metamorphopsia.**

telescope An optical instrument for magnifying the apparent size of distant objects. It consists, in principle, of two lenses: (1) the objective, being a positive lens which forms a real inverted image of the distant object and (2) the eyepiece through which the observer views a magnified image of that formed by the objective. The eyepiece may be either positive (**astronomical** or **Kepler telescope**) or negative (**galilean telescope**). The magnification M of a telescope is given by the following formula

$$M = f'_o/f_e = D_o/D_e$$

where f'_o is the second focal length of the objective, f_e the first focal length of the eyepiece, and D_o and D_e are the diameters of the entrance and exit pupils of the telescope (approximately equal to the diameters of the objective lens and the eyepiece). There are also some telescopes that do not use a lens (or lens system) as objective, as these are difficult to produce if large apertures and minimum aberrations are required. These telescopes use a concave mirror (usually parabolic) as the objective.

They are called **reflecting telescopes**. Light from a distant object is collected by the large concave mirror and reflected onto a small mirror (positive in the **Cassegrain telescope** and negative in the **gregorian telescope**). This mirror is located on the optical axis, and light is then transmitted through a central hole in the concave mirror onto the eyepiece. In the **newtonian telescope**, the light collected by the large concave mirror is reflected onto a small plane mirror at a 45° angle to the optical axis and transmitted to the eyepiece, which is at right angles to the optical axis (Fig. T2).
See binoculars; eyepiece; magnification, telescopic; objective.

astronomical t. See telescope.

bioptic t. A system of lenses forming a galilean or Kepler telescope which is mounted high on a plastic spectacle or carrier lens with the distance correction, so as to allow the patient to look through either the telescope, or below, by moving his or her head. It is used to magnify distant objects for patients with low vision. *Syn.* bioptic position telescope.

Cassegrain t. See telescope.

Dutch t. See telescope, galilean.

galilean t. Simple optical system that allows observation of far objects with a low magnification and without image inversion. It consists of a convex lens, which acts as the objective, and a concave lens as the eyepiece. Magnification of such a telescope rarely exceeds 5×. This optical system is used in opera glasses and as a low vision aid (Fig. T2). *Syn.* Dutch telescope.
See binoculars; minification.

gregorian t.; Kepler t.; newtonian t. See telescope.

reflecting t. Telescope that uses a concave mirror as the objective.

refracting t. Telescope that uses a positive lens system as the objective.

reverse t. See field, visual expander.

terrestrial t. Telescope that provides an erect image of a distant object. The image is usually erected by means of a lens system placed between the objective and the eyepiece. It does, however, make the terrestrial telescope relatively longer than an astronomical telescope.
See binoculars; erector.

telescopic spectacles *See* lens, telescopic.

telestereoscope, Helmholtz Instrument designed to produce an exaggerated perception of depth by optically increasing the length of the base line of the viewer, using a system of mirrors or prisms (Fig. T3).

Teller acuity cards *See* acuity cards, Teller.

temple 1. *See* side of a spectacle frame. **2.** The lateral area of the human head between the outer canthi and the ears and above the zygomatic arch.

temple, library A straight side of a spectacle frame.
See spectacles, library.

temporal arteritis; induction; summation *See* under the nouns.

temporal cortex *See* areas, visual association.

tendon A dense band of connective tissue, mainly composed of collagen fibres, which attaches the end of a muscle to a bone or other structure.
See muscle, extraocular.

tendon of Zinn *See* annulus of Zinn.

Tenon's capsule The fibrous membrane that envelops the globe from the margin of the cornea to the optic nerve. Its outer surface is loosely attached to the stroma of the conjunctiva. Its inner surface is in close contact with the episclera to which it is connected by fine trabeculae. These trabeculae also attach it to the extraocular muscles. The posterior surface of the capsule is in contact with the orbital fat. Anteriorly, it becomes thinner and merges gradually into the subconjunctival

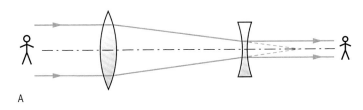

A

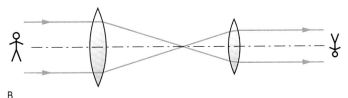

B

Fig. T2 Telescopes: A, galilean; B, Kepler.

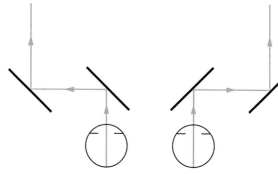

Fig. T3 Optical principle of a telestereoscope.

connective tissue. *Syn.* Bonnet's capsule; capsule of the eyeball; fascia bulbi.
See injection, sub-Tenon's; ligament of Lockwood.

tension, ocular *See* pressure, intraocular.

Terrien's disease; marginal degeneration *See* degeneration, Terrien's marginal; ectasia, corneal.

Terson's syndrome *See* syndrome, Terson's.

tertiary action; position *See* under the nouns.

test 1. A method of examination used to determine a disease or a performance. **2.** To try; to prove. **3.** The equipment used to carry out the test.
after-image t. A subjective test used to determine the presence or absence of abnormal retinal correspondence (ARC). The subject is instructed to fixate the centre of a vertical light filament for some 15 s with one eye and then the centre of a horizontal light filament for some 15 s with the other eye. Looking at the after-images of the two filaments on a uniform surface (e.g. a wall) the subject sees either a cross, which indicates normal retinal correspondence or two separated filaments, indicating ARC. *Syn.* Hering's after-image test.
See after-image; retinal correspondence, abnormal.
after-image transfer t. Test aimed at detecting and measuring the angle of eccentric fixation in an amblyopic eye in a patient with normal retinal correspondence. The normal eye fixates an illuminated vertical line (often produced by a photographic flash gun) and is then occluded, while the amblyopic eye fixates a dot (or a Snellen letter). If the after-image and the fixation point coincide, the amblyopic eye has no eccentric fixation, otherwise the relative position of one to the other indicates the angle of eccentric fixation. *Syn.* Brock's after-image test.
See fixation, eccentric; retinal corresponding points.
alternate cover t. See test, cover.
Ammann's t. See test, neutral density filter.
Arden grating t. Clinical test designed to evaluate contrast sensitivity. It consists of photographic plates, each with a sinusoidal grating of constant spatial frequency but of increasing contrast from top to bottom. There are seven plates, one being for demonstration. The other six, each with a different spatial frequency, are used for testing. The spatial frequencies are: 0.2, 0.4, 0.8, 1.6, 3.2 and 6.4 cycles per degree when viewed at a distance of 50 cm. Contrast levels are numbered from 1 to 20 on a vertical scale on the side of the plate. The testing procedure consists of slowly removing each plate from its folder until the grating becomes visible to the patient, at which point the contrast level is noted. The testing is carried out monocularly with optical correction, if any. The procedure is repeated for each plate and all the contrast levels are added to arrive at a score, which is compared with normal values provided in the instructions. *Syn.* Arden gratings; Arden plates.
See chart, contrast sensitivity; function, contrast sensitivity; Vistech.
Bagolini's lens t. Test to detect binocular sensory and motor anomalies such as abnormal retinal correspondence and suppression. Two Bagolini lenses, one in front of each eye with their striations oriented 90° apart (typically 135° for one eye, 45° for the other) are used. The patient fixates a punctate light source at distance and near. Each eye sees a diagonal line perpendicular to that seen by the fellow eye. For example, if one line or part of one line is missing, there is suppression. If the two diagonal lines cross at the source, the patient is orthophoric or, if strabismic as indicated by the cover test, the patient has harmonious abnormal retinal correspondence (Fig. T4). *Syn.* Bagolini's striated lens test.
See glass, Bagolini's.
balancing t. A test designed to obtain equal focusing or equal accommodative states in the two eyes. This is accomplished either objectively (by retinoscopy) or, more commonly, subjectively using either the duochrome test, or comparing the visual acuity in the two eyes simultaneously or successively, or using prisms (for example, a 3Δ base-down in front of one eye and a 3Δ base-up in front of the other) to present two images of a chart and ask the patient to compare these images, or using a binocular refraction technique (e.g. Turville infinity balance test). *Syn.* equalization test.

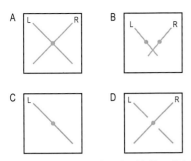

Fig. T4 Possible results found with Bagolini test. A, either orthophoria, or harmonious ARC if strabismic; B, esotropia (homonymous diplopia); C, suppression of the right eye; D, central suppression in the left eye. R, view of the left eye. L, view of the left eye. ARC, abnormal retinal correspondence.

See **balance, binocular; method, Humphriss; test, Turville infinity balance; vectogram.**

bar reading t. A test used for determining the presence of binocular vision or central suppression. It can also be used in the management of amblyopia and when there is central suppression in heterophoria. It consists of a narrow bar (or a pencil) held vertically and interposed between the reader's eyes and a page of print. The bar occludes a vertical strip of print from each eye. If binocular vision is present, the subject will experience no difficulty reading the text. *Syn.* Welland's test. *See* **grid, Javal's.**

Barany's caloric t. See, **test, caloric.**

basic secretion t. Measurement of the basal tear secretion independently of reflex tear secretion. A filter paper strip (e.g. Whatman No. 41) is placed in the anaesthetized lower fornix and, after 5 minutes, the strip is removed and the amount of wetting measured from the folded end. *See* **tear secretion; test, Schirmer's.**

Bielschowsky's head tilt t. A test designed to determine which of the inferior or superior extraocular muscles, and of which eye, is paretic. The test is based on the following fact: if the head is tilted to the right, the right intorters of the right eye (superior oblique and superior rectus muscles) contract as well as the extorters of the left eye (inferior oblique and inferior rectus muscles). If the head is tilted to the left, the inferior oblique and inferior rectus muscles of the right eye contract to cause extorsion while the superior oblique and superior rectus of the eye contract to cause intorsion. Thus, tilting the head towards one side will indicate the palsied muscle. For example, in the right superior rectus muscle palsy, when the head is tilted to the left, there will be no change in the vertical deviation, because contraction of the right superior rectus muscle is not involved. However, when the head is tilted to the right, there will be an increase in downward movement. This test is not reliable in an adult with congenital ocular palsy. *See* **test, forced duction; test, Parks' three-step.**

Bielchowsky's phenomenon t. A test used to differentiate between dissociated vertical deviation (DVD) and alternating hypertropia. After the occlusion of one eye (which elevates behind the cover), an optical wedge of increasing density is placed in front of the fixating eye; if the patient has DVD, the eye behind the cover will perform a gradual downward movement with increasing filter density and a gradual upward movement if the wedge is moved in the opposite direction. *Syn* dark wedge test. *See* **deviation, dissociated vertical; phenomenon, Bielchowsky's.**

binocular Esterman t. See **test, Esterman.**

blind t. See **study, single-blind; study, double-blind.**

blue field entoptoscope t. See **entoptoscope, blue field.**

blur back t. See **test, plus 1.00 D blur.**

break-up time t. (BUT) A test for assessing the precorneal tear film. Fluorescein is applied to the bulbar conjunctiva and the patient is asked to blink once or twice and then to refrain from blinking. The tear film is scanned through the slit-lamp using a cobalt blue filter with a wide beam, while the examiner counts or records the time between the last blink and the appearance of the first dry black spot which indicates that the tear film is breaking up. In normal subjects, break-up times vary between 15 and 35 s (in Caucasians). A BUT of 10 s or less is abnormal and may be due to mucin deficiency, and is often considered to be a negative factor for success in contact lens wear, especially soft lenses. However, this test has been shown to be flawed, because fluorescein can disrupt the tear film. *See* **eye, dry; lens, cobalt; mucin; tear film; test, non-invasive break-up time.**

broad H t. A test designed to evaluate the integrity of the extraocular muscles and their innervation. The patient is asked to fixate a penlight while keeping the head still. The penlight is moved slowly horizontally to one side of the straight-ahead position, then moved vertically, back down to the horizontal line, then below it and back up again to the horizontal line. The penlight is now moved along the horizontal line to the other side of the straight-ahead position and the same procedure is repeated thus completing the shape of the letter with a wide horizontal dimension. Overaction or underaction of one eye and the patient's report of diplopia in any position of gaze are recorded to identify the paretic muscle/s. *See* **test, motility.**

Brock's after-image t. See **test, after-image transfer.**

Brock's string t. See **Brock's string.**

Bruckner's t. An objective method performed to detect the presence of strabismus. The examiner illuminates both eyes of the patient simultaneously with an ophthalmoscope from a distance of about 1 metre. Looking through the ophthalmoscope, the examiner focuses on the fundus reflexes seen in the two pupils. If one pupil appears brighter, it is considered that this eye may be strabismic and perhaps amblyopic. The reason may be due to the fact that this eye will be deviated and optical aberrations will make the pupil area appear brighter and whiter. The examiner may also note the position of the corneal reflexes when carrying out this test. This test is more reliable when patients are wearing their correction. *Syn.* Bruckner's method. *See* **test, Hirschberg's; test, Krimsky's.**

caloric t. A method used to detect disorders of the vestibular system in which irrigating the ear with either warm or cold water elicits a nystagmus. If warm water is introduced into the right ear, a right jerk nystagmus appears (fast phase to the right). If cold water is introduced into the right ear, a left jerk nystagmus appears (fast phase to the left). In vestibular disease (e.g. Meniere's disease), the nystagmus may be either reduced or absent. The mnemonic COWS (cold–opposite, warm–same) is used to describe this effect. By placing the subject at a 30-degree upright position, heated or cooled water stimulates the vertical horizontal semicircular canals. *Syn.* Barany's caloric test. *See* **caloric testing; nystagmus, vestibular.**

Cardiff acuity t. A test designed to measure the visual acuity of young children. It consists of a series of cards, each with a different picture (either a car, a dog, a duck, a fish, a house or a train) drawn with a white band, which is surrounded by a black line half the width of the white, on a neutral grey background. Thus the average luminance of the target is equal to that of the grey background. The picture is situated either in the top or bottom half of the card. The pictures remain of the same overall size on each card; only the width of the black and white bands decreases in size. There are 11 acuity levels ranging from 6/60 (20/200 or 1.00 logMAR) to 6/6 (20/20 or 0.00 logMAR) at a viewing distance of 1 metre, in 0.1 log steps. The acuity is given by the narrowest white band for which the picture is still recognizable, but the child's eye movements are also noted to confirm or establish recognition. This test is best used with toddlers and children with intellectual impairment (Fig. T5).

See **Glasgow acuity cards; method, preferential looking; test, Lea-Hyvarinen acuity.**

City University colour vision t. A set of 10 pseudoisochromatic plates, each consisting of a central coloured spot surrounded by four differently coloured spots. The subject is asked to choose the spot that most closely matches the colour of the central spot in each plate viewed at a normal reading distance. For each plate, there is a normal response and a response corresponding to each of the colour defects, deutan, protan and tritan. *See* **test, Farnsworth-Munsell 100 Hue.**

t. chart *See* **chart, test.**

colour vision t. *See* **Edridge–Green lantern; plates, pseudoisochromatic; test, City University colour vision; test, Farnsworth-Munsell 100 Hue; test, lantern; test, wool.**

confrontation t. A rough method performed to determine the approximate extent of the visual field. The patient, with one eye occluded, faces the examiner at a distance of about 60 cm and fixates the opposite eye of the examiner. The test object is moved in a plane midway between the examiner and the patient, starting far in the periphery and moving it towards the patient and in various meridians until it is seen.

contrast sensitivity t. *See* **chart, contrast sensitivity; function, contrast sensitivity; sensitivity, contrast; test, Arden grating; Vistech.**

corneal reflex t. *See* **method, Hirschberg's; method, Javal's; method, Krimsky's.**

cortical vision screening t. A test designed to detect visuoperceptual impairments caused by a cerebral disease (e.g. Alzheimer, stroke) or injury in individuals who have normal or near-normal vision (with or without correction). It consists of an A4-size bound book containing a sequence of 10 cards, each one assessing a different aspect of visual processing by cortical centres and prefaced by a description of its aim, instructions and significance. The test includes symbol acuity, shape discrimination, size discrimination, shape detection, hue discrimination, scattered dot

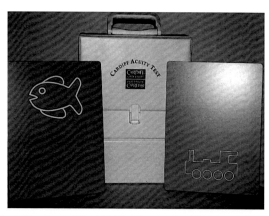

Fig. T5 Cardiff acuity test. (Courtesy of Dr. J M Woodhouse, Cardiff University)

counting, fragmented numbers, word reading, crowding and face perception.

cotton thread t. *See* **test, phenol red cotton thread.**

cover t. A test performed to determine the presence and the type of heterophoria or strabismus. The subject fixates a small letter or any fine detail at a given distance. Strabismus is usually tested first. The opaque cover or occluder is placed over one eye and then removed, while the examiner observes the other eye and then the same operation is repeated on the other eye (this is called the **unilateral cover test**). If neither uncovered eye moves, the subject does not have strabismus. If the unoccluded eye moves when a cover is placed in front of the other, **strabismus** is present. In esotropia, the unoccluded eye will move temporally to take up fixation, while in exotropia, the unoccluded eye will move nasally, and an upward or downward movement indicates hypotropia or hypertropia, respectively. In alternating squint, in which either eye can take up fixation, the eye behind the cover will appear deviated when uncovered and will move as the cover is shifted to the other eye.

The type of **heterophoria** can be detected by observing the eye behind the cover. If there is no movement of the eye behind the cover, the subject is orthophoric. If the eye behind the cover moves inward and outward when the cover is removed, the subject has esophoria. If the eye behind the cover moves outward and inward when the cover is removed, the subject has exophoria. A similar procedure is used for hyperphoria and hypophoria. As it is difficult to view the eye behind the cover without allowing sufficient peripheral fusion to stop the eyes going to the phoria position, the observer usually watches for the recovery movement as the occluder is removed. By placing prisms of increasing power in front of one of the eyes until no movement is evoked, one can evaluate the approximate amount of the phoria. The cover test is the only objective method of measuring heterophoria. The determination of the magnitude of the deviation of the strabismus or heterophoria can also be done with the **alternate (alternating) cover test**. The subject fixates a target and the cover is successively placed in front of one eye and then the other while watching the eye that has just been uncovered to see the direction of the deviation. The amount of deviation can be estimated by using prisms of appropriate strength and base direction until the movement of the eye is neutralized when the cover is alternated from one eye to the other (**prism cover test**). Although these tests are objective, they are sometimes used subjectively, i.e. the patient indicates the apparent movement of the fixation object. The alternate cover test is the most appropriate test for subjective testing. An apparent movement of the fixation object in the same direction as the cover indicates exophoria, while an apparent movement of the fixation object in the opposite direction to the cover indicates esophoria. An apparent downward movement of the fixation indicates hyperphoria of the eye from which the occluder is moved. Again, prisms can be placed in front of the eyes until the apparent movement disappears, thus giving a measure of the heterophoria. This subjective perception of a movement of a stationary fixation object in people with heterophoria or strabismus is a particular example of the phi phenomenon. *Syn.* occlusion test; screen test. *See* **phenomenon, phi.**

cross-cylinder t. for astigmatism A subjective test for measuring the axis and the amount of astigmatism using a cross-cylinder lens. Having obtained the best visual acuity with a spherical lens, the cross-cylinder lens is placed before the eye being tested with its axes at 45° to the cylinder axis determined by retinoscopy. The patient looks at a single circular target, often a letter (O or C or Verhoeff's circles), the cross-cylinder lens is then flipped and, if one position provides a clearer image of the target, the axis of the correcting (minus) cylinder should be turned towards the minus axis of the cross-cylinder lens until vision is equally blurred in both positions of the cross-cylinder lens. That point indicates the correct axis of the correcting cylinder. The determination of the power of the correcting cylinder is carried out by placing the cross-cylinder lens with one of its axes parallel to the axis of the correcting cylinder. The cross-cylinder lens is flipped and the position that provides the clearer vision indicates whether to increase the cylinder power (when the minus axis of the cross-cylinder is parallel) or decrease cylinder power (when the plus axis is parallel). The proper amount of cylinder correction is obtained when the vision is equally blurred in both positions of the cross-cylinder lens. *Syn.* cross-cylinder method; cross-cylinder test; Jackson crossed cylinder test. *See* **lens, cross-cylinder.**

cross-cylinder t. at near A subjective test to determine the addition for near vision. It is performed (monocularly or binocularly) at a distance of usually 40 cm with the patient wearing his or her subjectively determined lenses and cross-cylinder lenses with axes horizontal and vertical and viewing a test chart composed of parallel, horizontal and vertical black lines. Beginning with sufficient fogging lens power, the plus lens power is reduced until the patient reports that the vertical and horizontal lines are equally distinct. *See* **addition; method, fogging.**

dark filter t. *See* **test, neutral density filter.**

dark room t. *See* **test, provocative.**

dark wedge t. *See* **test, Bielchowsky's phenomenon.**

Denver Developmental Screening t. *See* **test, developmental and perceptual screening.**

development and perceptual screening t. A test used to assess children's perceptual and processing skills, such as gross motor coordination, directionality, laterality, visual form perception, visual memory and visualization, visual-motor integration and auditory and language development.

There are many such tests, each evaluating one or several of the above skills. The most common ones are: (1) The **Denver Developmental Screening Test**, which is used for children up to about 6 years of age. It is easy to administer and covers a wide range of skills, which fall into four sectors: personal-social, fine motor-adaptive, language and gross motor. Treatment and/or referral will depend on the type of skills found to be abnormal. (2) The **Test of Visual Analysis Skills** assesses the child's visual perceptual skills. It consists of 18 squares containing dots and lines, each forming a different pattern. The child is given a pencil and a special test form on which to reproduce the visual stimuli. The test comes with an expected score for each grade up to grade 3 and failure to reach that score may indicate that the child has a perceptual skills disorder. (3) The **Gardner Reversal-Frequency Test** in which the child is asked to mark those letters and numbers which are printed backward. This test assesses the directionality skill.

developmental eye movement t. An indirect test for saccadic eye movements in which the subject reads numbers placed in 4 vertical columns (total of 80 numbers) and 16 horizontal rows (total of 80 numbers). The lengths of time taken to perform the horizontal and the vertical subtests are measured independently and assessed as a ratio, as well as the number of errors (omissions, additions, transpositions, or substitutions). All results are compared to test norms for the age of the subject. The vertical array mainly gives an indication of visual-verbal number skills (automaticity), whereas the horizontal array provides additional information on oculomotor function.

differential intraocular pressure t. A test performed to differentiate between a muscle paresis and a mechanical restriction of the eye. The intraocular pressure is measured in the primary position and then again with the patient turning his or her eyes in the direction of action of the suspected paretic muscle. An increase in intraocular pressure of 6 mmHg or more indicates a mechanical restriction (e.g. a fracture of the orbital floor), whereas no change in pressure suggests a muscle paresis. This test produces less discomfort to the patient than the forced duction test.
See **test, forced duction.**

diplopia t. **1.** A test for measuring heterophoria in which the fusion reflex is prevented by displacing the retinal image of one eye with a prism as in the **von Graefe's test** in which the magnitude of the phoria is estimated by the amount of prism necessary to align the two images. To measure lateral phorias the images are displaced vertically and aligned one above the other, whereas to measure vertical phorias the images are displaced horizontally and realigned horizontally (if a phoria is present). *Syn.* displacement test; prism dissociation test. **2.** A test to investigate the integrity of the extraocular muscles in strabismus, in which the patient is required to view a light source in

the dark with a red filter in front of one eye and a green filter in front of the other, to produce diplopia (prisms are sometimes necessary). The direction and extent of diplopia are evaluated relative to the size and direction of the angle measured with the cover test at the same distance.
See **dissociation; test, red glass.**

displacement t. *See* **test, diplopia.**

dissociating t. Any test for measuring heterophoria in which fusion is dissociated.
See **dissociation; Maddox rod; test, diplopia.**

distortion t. A test for measuring heterophoria, in which the images presented to the two eyes are so unlike that they cannot be fused. The most common such test is the Maddox rod test.

doll's head t. *See* **phenomenon, doll's head.**

Dolman's t. *See* **test, hole in the card.**

double-blind t. *See* **study, double-blind.**

double prism t. A test for determining the presence of cyclophoria, in which a double prism (a pair of prisms set base to base) with the base line horizontal is placed before one eye. The patient is requested to fixate a horizontal line (or row of letters), which through the double prism appears as two lines (or two rows) vertically separated. On uncovering the other eye, the patient sees three lines (or rows). If there is no cyclophoria, all three lines (or rows) will appear parallel, but lack of parallelism indicates cyclophoria. The double prism used in this test consists of two weak prisms (about 4 or 5 Δ); this clinical type of double prism is commonly called a **Maddox double prism** (Fig. T6).
See **Fresnel's bi-prism; test, Maddox rod.**

double Maddox rod t. *See* **test, Maddox rod.**

Dunlop t. A test used for determining motor ocular dominance. It consists in having the eyes fusing two slightly different targets in, for example, a synoptophore, and diverging the targets until diplopia appears. Just beforehand, fixation disparity occurs in one eye. That eye is called the non-dominant or non-reference eye. The other eye is the dominant or reference eye.

duochrome t. A subjective refraction test in which a subject compares the sharpness of black targets (e.g. Landolt rings) of similar sizes on a red background on one side and on a green background on the other side (blue is sometimes used) of a chart. In undercorrected myopia or overcorrected hyperopia, the letters on the red background will appear more distinct, while in overcorrected myopia or undercorrected hyperopia, the letters on the green background will appear more distinct, and in emmetropia or corrected ametropia, the letters should appear equally distinct on both sides. The test makes use of the chromatic aberration of the eye and assumes that when the eye is looking at distant objects, it is focused on the yellow part of the visible spectrum. *Syn.* bichrome test; duochrome method.
See **lens, cobalt; Verhoeff's circles.**

dye dilution t. A test used for detecting a blockage in the lacrimal (or drainage) system. It

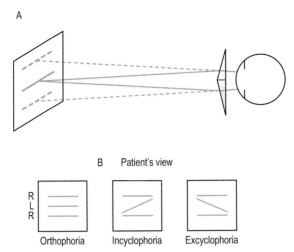

A

B Patient's view

R
L
R

Orthophoria   Incyclophoria   Excyclophoria

Fig. T6 A, Maddox double prism used to measure cyclophoria. If, for example, the double prism is placed in front of the right eye (ensuring that the common base exactly bisects the the pupil horizontally) the patient sees two parallel horizontal lines (discontinuous lines); B, with both eyes the patient sees three lines: if the central line L seen by the left eye appears parallel to both the upper and lower lines R produced by the double prism, the subject is free of cyclophoria, otherwise cyclophoria is present.

consists of instilling a few drops of fluorescein (or a mixture of rose bengal and fluorescein) into the conjunctival sac and observing how long it takes before it dilutes, which is shown by the change in colour. No change in colour indicates a blockage or a lack of tear production.
See **dilation and irrigation; lacrimal apparatus; staining, fluorescein; test, Jones 1.**
'E' t. *See* **'E' game; chart, E.**
equalization t. *See* **test, balancing.**
Esterman t. A method used for quantifying visual field disability. It consists of a grid made up of rectangles of different sizes placed across the field, being smaller centrally, inferiorly and along the horizontal meridian than at other locations, as these areas are considered to be most important functionally. Each rectangle contains a dot in the centre. There is a grid for the monocular field with 100 rectangles and a grid for the binocular field with 120 rectangles. The grid is placed on top of the results of the field chart. A percentage score is calculated on the basis of the number of spots seen by the patient. The grids are incorporated into most automated perimeters.
fan and block t. A test designed to determine the axis and the amount of astigmatism of the eye. It consists of an astigmatic fan chart with an inner rotating central disc on which are printed an arrowhead forming an acute angle of typically 60° and two sets of mutually perpendicular lines or 'blocks'. The test follows the subjective determination of the best vision sphere that places the circle of least confusion on the retina. A positive spherical lens, of a power equal to half the estimated amount of astigmatism, is placed in front of the eye to create simple myopic astigmatism.

The patient is asked to indicate the clearest line(s) on the chart, and the arrowhead is rotated until its two sides appear equally blurred. The axis of the correcting negative cylindrical lens is then read on the fan chart. The amount of astigmatism is found when that cylindrical lens is of a power such that the two blocks appear equally clear. *Syn.* fan and block method.
See **chart, astigmatic fan; method, fogging.**
Farnsworth t. *See* **test, Farnsworth–Munsell 100 Hue.**
Farnsworth-Munsell 100 Hue t. A colour vision test consisting of 85 small discs made up of Munsell colours of approximately equal chroma and value, but of different hue for normal observers. The examinee must place the discs so that they appear in a continuous and smooth series. Errors are scored and a diagnosis of the type and severity of the colour defect can be made. A smaller version of the Farnsworth test called the **Farnsworth D-15** exists (Figs. T7 and T8). It consists of only 15 small discs and the procedure is the same, but it is a more rapid test, which does not give as much information as the large version. However, it has been found to be very valuable for detecting severe colour vision defects, including tritanopia. There exist also some versions of this test in which the colour samples are less saturated than the standard ones: (1) The **Lanthony desaturated D-15 test** in which the colour samples are less saturated by 2 units of Munsell chroma but also lighter by 3 units of Munsell value than the standard D-15 test, and (2) the **Adams desaturated D-15 test** in which only the saturation (or chroma) has been reduced by 2 units. These desaturated D-15 tests are more

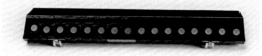

Fig. T7 Farnsworth D-15 test.

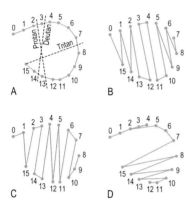

Fig. T8 Score sheet of the Farnsworth D-15 colour test as arranged by a subject. A, with normal colour vision; B, with a protan defect; C, with a deutan defect and D, with a tritan defect (0 is the fixed reference cap and 1 to 15 are the moveable caps which the subject must arrange in a logical sequence of colours).

effective in detecting mild colour vision deficiencies than the standard D-15 test. *Syn.* Farnsworth test; FM 100 Hue test.

See **colour vision, defective; lamp, Macbeth; Munsell colour system; test, City University colour vision.**

fluorescein t. **1.** A test performed to assess the fit of hard contact lenses. Fluorescein is instilled between the cornea and the contact lens, and under ultraviolet illumination, areas where the lens touches the cornea appear purple or blue, whereas areas where there is a space between the lens and the cornea appear yellowish green. This appearance is often referred to as **fluorescein pattern. 2.** Test using fluorescein and ultraviolet illumination to detect abrasions or other corneal epithelial defects, which stain yellowish green.

See **bearing, apical; fluorescein; lamp, Burton; rose bengal; staining; test, Jones 1; test, Jones 1.**

fogging t. See **method, fogging.**

forced duction t. A test designed to differentiate between a muscle paresis and a mechanical restriction of the eye. The eye in which the conjunctiva is anaesthetized is grasped with toothless forceps and passively rotated in the direction of action of the suspected paretic muscle. If the eye cannot be rotated further than the point where the patient can voluntarily rotate it, a mechanical restriction exists (e.g. a fracture of the orbital floor); if the examiner can passively rotate the eye to its full extent, the muscle is paretic. *Syn.* traction test.

See **palsy, third nerve; strabismus fixus; syndrome, adherence; syndrome, Brown's superior oblique tendon sheath; test, Bielschowsky's head tilt; test, Parks' three-step.**

four dot t. See **test, Worth's four dot.**

four prism dioptre base-out t. A test used for the detection of microtropia and for the assessment of the suppression area. A 4Δ BO is placed momentarily in front of the fixating eye (or the eye with the best acuity) and if the other eye moves outward but does not refixate inward, it indicates suppression in that eye and a small angle strabismus. Microtropia is also indicated if, when the prism is placed BO in front of the eye that showed suppression, there is no movement of either eye. The extent of the suppression area can be assessed by momentarily placing prisms, of various powers and in various directions, in front of the affected eye until diplopia is noticed. The observation of the patient's eye movements is difficult because of the small angle of deviation and because of the variation in size of the suppression area. *Syn.* Irvine's prism displacement test.

See **microtropia.**

FRIEND t. A subjective test for simultaneous binocular vision in which the word FRIEND printed with the letters FIN in green and RED in red is viewed through red and green filters, one before each eye. People with simultaneous binocular vision see all the letters, whereas those with suppression see only some of the letters.

See **test, Worth's four dot.**

Frisby stereo t. See **stereotest, Frisby.**

Gardner Reversal-Frequency t. See **test, developmental and perceptual screening.**

gradient t. See **AC/A ratio.**

von Graefe's t. See **test, diplopia.**

Hering after-image t. See **test, after-image.**

Hess–Lancaster t. A test used for measuring and classifying strabismus using the Hess screen.

Hirschberg's t. Method performed to estimate the objective angle of strabismus. The examiner's eye is placed directly above a small penlight source fixated by the subject and observes the position of the corneal reflex of the deviating eye. The angle of strabismus can be estimated on the basis that each mm of deviation, relative to the corneal reflex in the fixating eye, represents approximately 7° (12 Δ) of strabismus (Fig. T9). *Syn.* Hirschberg's method.

See **test, Bruckner's; test, Krimsky's.**

hole in the card t. A test for determining which eye is dominant. It consists of a card with a hole in it through which the patient views a spotlight (or a letter) on a distant test chart while holding

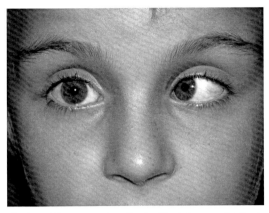

Fig. T9 Hirschberg's method used in a case of esotropia. The left corneal reflex is near the limbus and the angle is approximately equal to 40°. (From Kanski 2007, with permission of Butterworth-Heinemann)

the card with both hands. The eye that the patient uses to view the letter is the dominant eye. This is easily detected by having the patient occlude each eye in turn and when the dominant eye is covered the spotlight can no longer be seen through the hole. *Syn.* Dolman's test.
See **dominance, ocular; manoptoscope.**

hole in the hand t. A binocular vision test in which a distant object is viewed through a tube with one eye, while a hand is held at a distance of some 20 to 30 cm before the other eye. Subjects who see the object through an apparent hole in the hand have binocular vision, whereas seeing either the object through the tube only or the hand only indicates an absence of binocular vision. *Syn.* hole in the hand illusion.

Holmgren's t. *See* **test, wool.**

Howard–Dolman t. A test for measuring stereoscopic visual acuity consisting of two black vertical rods on a white background, viewed through an aperture from a distance of 6 m. By means of a double cord pulley arrangement, the subject manipulates one of the rods until it appears in the same plane as the fixed rod. The distance between the two rods is then measured, and calculations must be made to arrive at the stereoscopic acuity. *See* **acuity, stereoscopic visual; test, three-needle; test, two-dimensional.**

Humphriss immediate contrast t. *See* **method, Humphriss.**

infinity balance t. *See* **test, Turville infinity balance.**

Irvine's prism displacement t. *See* **test, four-prism dioptre base-out.**

inside-out t. for soft contact lenses Method of checking whether a soft contact lens is inverted before insertion. The lens is balanced on the forefinger and its profile is examined. If it is inside-out, the edge will be slightly turned out. Another method consists in gently pinching the lens: if it curls, it is the right way up; if the edges are turned out, it is inverted. A lens placed on the eye inside-out is uncomfortable.

Ishihara t. *See* **plates, pseudoisochromatic.**

Jackson crossed cylinder t. *See* **test for astigmatism, cross-cylinder.**

Jones 1 t. A test designed to evaluate the tear drainage system. Fluorescein dye is instilled into the conjunctival sac. Over a period of 5 minutes at 1-minute intervals, a cotton-tipped applicator is placed under the anaesthetized inferior nasal turbinate (a prominence on the inside wall of the nose). Absence of dye suggests a blockage somewhere in the passage, the nasolacrimal duct being the most common site. Jones 2 test may then be performed. *Syn.* fluorescein instillation test; primary Jones test. *See* **dilation and irrigation.**

Jones 2 t. After Jones 1 test, fluorescein is washed out and physiological saline is injected into the anaesthetized lower canaliculus. If the fluid recovered from the nose is fluorescein-stained, the test is positive indicating a partial obstruction in the nasolacrimal duct, otherwise there is a blockage in the punctum, canaliculus or common canaliculus or a defective pumping mechanism of the tears.
See **lacrimal apparatus; test, dye dilution.**

Krimsky's t. Method used to determine the objective angle of strabismus. The examiner's own eye is placed directly above a small penlight source fixated by the subject and observes the position of the corneal reflexes. Prisms are placed in front of the deviating eye until the examiner finds the prism power that makes the corneal reflex appear to occupy the same relative position as that in the fixating eye. *Syn.* prism reflex test. *See* **test, Bruckner's; test, Hirschberg's.**

Lang t. *See* **stereotest, Lang.**

lantern t. An occupational colour vision test used mainly to evaluate recognition of aviation and maritime signals. There are several such tests (e.g. Cam lantern, Edridge–Green lantern, Giles–Archer lantern, Holmes–Wright lantern, Farnsworth lantern or Falant). The latter two show colours in pairs, of which there are nine, and the observer's task is to name the colours.

Lea-Hyvarinen acuity t. A test chart designed to measure the visual acuity of young children. Each line is composed of four symbols, a square, a circle, house and heart (or apple), which are easy to recognize. The progression between the lines is in equal logarithmic steps and the spacing between the symbols is equal to the width of the symbols. There are charts for near vision and for distance vision testing. *Syn.* LEA acuity test. *See* **Glasgow acuity cards; test, Cardiff acuity.**

light-stress t. *See* **test, photostress.**

logMAR crowded t. *See* **Glasgow acuity cards.**

Maddox rod t. 1. *See* **Maddox rod.** 2. A test for measuring cyclophoria in which a Maddox rod is placed in front of one eye with the subject viewing a spot of light. If the rod is placed horizontally, the subject sees a vertical streak. If it does not appear vertical, it indicates the presence of incyclo- or excyclophoria and, by rotating the rod in a trial frame, the amount of cyclophoria can be evaluated. The test can also be performed with one Maddox rod in front of each eye, with axes parallel, while the subject views a spot of light through a 10 to 15 Δ prism in front of one eye (to displace one image relative to the other). The subject will then see two streaks. If they appear parallel, there is no cyclophoria. If not, one of the Maddox rods is rotated slowly until the subject reports that the two streaks are parallel. The angle of rotation as determined with a protractor scale indicates the amount of cyclophoria. The test can also be used to assess whether elevating or depressing extraocular muscles are underacting or overacting. The muscle most commonly affected is the superior oblique muscle of which the primary action is intorsion. *Syn.* double Maddox rod test. *See* **cyclophoria; cyclotorsion; test, double-prism.**

Maddox wing t. *See* **Maddox wing.**

Mars t. *See* **chart, Pelli-Robson.**

Mallett t. *See* **Mallett fixation disparity unit.**

manoptoscope t. *See* **manoptoscope.**

Melbourne Edge t. A contrast sensitivity assessment using a chart in which the subject must detect an edge. It consists of 20 circular patches of decreasing contrast. Each circle is divided by an edge that can be oriented in four different orientations (vertical, horizontal, 45°

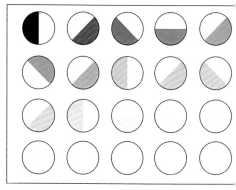

Fig T10 Melbourne Edge Test. (Courtesy of the National Vision Research Institute, Melbourne, Australia)

left, 45° right). The subject is asked to report the direction of the edge until it is no longer visible, which indicates the lowest contrast that can be detected (i.e. the peak of the contrast sensitivity function). The test is useful with low-vision patients and young children as it is independent of the resolution of letters or symbols. It can also facilitate diagnosis of visual cortex dysfunction because edge detection is mediated in the visual cortex (Fig. T10). *See* **contour; function, contrast sensitivity; sensitivity, contrast.**

motility t. A test aimed at investigating the integrity of the extraocular muscles and their innervation. The most common method is to have the patient fixate a penlight, which is moved in eight meridians while keeping the head still: up, up and to the right, right, down and to the right, down, down and to the left, left, up and to the left, following a star pattern. The test can be done either binocularly or monocularly. Such movements will test the action of all six extraocular muscles of both eyes. If, for example, the penlight is moved up and to the right of the patient, any limitation in movement indicates a fault in either the right superior rectus or the left inferior oblique muscle (Fig. T11).

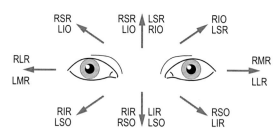

Fig. T11 Diagnostic positions of gaze indicating the muscles which have maximum power to move the eyes in the direction of the arrows (RIO, LIO, right and left inferior oblique; RIR, LIR, right and left inferior rectus; RLR, LLR, right and left lateral rectus; RMR, LMR, right and left medial rectus; RSO, LSO, right and left superior oblique; RSR, LSR, right and left superior rectus).

See movement, pursuit; muscle, yoke; pattern, alphabet; position, cardinal p's. of gaze; test, broad H; test, red glass.

neutral density filter t. A test designed to differentiate between functional and organic amblyopia by measuring visual acuity, with or without a neutral density filter. If acuity is greatly reduced when looking through the filter, the amblyopia is organic (e.g. glaucoma, central retinal lesions), but if the acuity is unaffected or even slightly improved, the amblyopia is functional. The validity of this test has been questioned. *Syn.* Ammann's test; dark filter test.
See amblyopia.

New Aniseikonia t. A test designed to measure aniseikonia. It consists of a booklet with pairs of half-moons, one green and the other red, and of different sizes. The patient wears red and green filters and is asked to point to the set of half-moons that appear to have identical vertical diameters. If the sizes are actually equal, the patient has no vertical aniseikonia; if the sizes are actually unequal, the patient has vertical aniseikonia of a percentage amount indicated next to the target. The booklet is rotated to a horizontal position to measure the horizontal aniseikonia.

non-invasive break-up time t. (NIBUT) A test that does not require any interference with the eye used for assessing the stability of the precorneal tear film. The patient's head rests on a chin rest at the centre of a hemispherical bowl of 20-cm radius, which is attached at the apex to a binocular microscope. A grid of white lines on a matte black background is inscribed on the inner surface of the bowl, and the image of this grid pattern projected onto the open eye is observed. The subject fixates a hole in the centre of the grid pattern and refrains from blinking. The time taken for the appearance of the first randomly distributed distortion or discontinuity of some of the reflected grid lines is a measure of the precorneal tear film break-up. The values for normal subjects vary between 5 and 200 seconds with a mean of around 40 seconds. The instrument used to measure NIBUT is often referred to as a toposcope.
See Tearscope plus; test, break-up time.

Norn's t. A test used for assessing tear secretion. It consists of instilling one drop of a mixture of 1% fluorescein and 1% rose bengal into the lower conjunctival sac. After 5 minutes, a slit-lamp examination is made of the colour of the stain in the central portion of the tear meniscus along the lower lid. The colour may be compared either with known dilutions of the mixture in capillary tubes or simply classified into five colours: intense red, pale red, intense orange, weak orange and yellow. In normal eyes, the colour is yellow or weak orange, whereas in a dry eye, it is red. *Syn.* tear dilution test.
See eye, dry; keratoconjunctivitis sicca; test, break-up time; test, non-invasive break-up time; test, phenol red cotton thread; test, Schirmer's.

t. object *See* test type.

ocular ferning t. A test designed for the assessment of ocular mucus. Conjunctival scrapings are placed on a glass slide, left to dry and examined under the microscope for the presence or absence of arborization (fern-like pattern). Normal eyes show ferning whereas in patients with cicatrizing conjunctivitis, such as ocular pemphigoid or Stevens–Johnson syndrome, ferning of the mucus is reduced or absent.
See pemphigoid, cicatricial.

optokinetic nystagmus t. (OKN) A test for eliciting OKN. The subject sits in front of a rotating drum covered with uniform black and white vertical stripes parallel to the axis of rotation (this apparatus is called an **optokinetoscope** or **optokinetic drum**). When the eyes respond with a slow movement in the same direction as the drum lasting about 0.2 s, and a fast phase in the reverse direction of about 0.1 s, the OKN has been elicited and this fact provides evidence of vision. As finer and finer black and white stripes are used, this reflex response will cease to be elicited for a particular spatial frequency of the stripes corresponding to the **objective visual acuity** of the subject. The test may also facilitate locating the site of a lesion in the optic radiations which has caused a homonymous hemianopia. If the lesion is in the parietal lobe, the OKN is asymmetric, being irregular when the drum is rotated towards the side of the lesion and regular when rotated in the other direction; and if the lesion is in the occipital lobe, the OKN will be symmetrical when the drum is rotated in either direction (Fig. T12).
See malingering; nystagmus.

Parks three-step t. An objective test for determining which extraocular muscle is paretic in a patient with hypertropia or hypotropia. A three-step procedure is used: (1) to determine the type of hypertropia (right or left); (2) to determine the magnitude of the hypertropia (e.g. with prisms and cover test) when the patient fixates to the

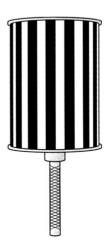

Fig. T12 Optokinetic drum.

right and to the left; and (3) to determine the magnitude of the hypertropia when the head is tilted towards each shoulder. Each step in this procedure reduces the number of possible muscles involved until it points to only one muscle of one eye. *Example*: paresis of the left superior oblique. Step (1), a left hypertropia points to a paresis of one of the following four muscles: left superior oblique, left inferior rectus, right inferior oblique or right superior rectus. Step (2), a hypertropia of the left eye increases when fixating to the right points to a paresis of either the left superior oblique or the right superior rectus. Step (3), a hypertropia of the left eye which increases when the head tilts to the left, points to a paresis of the left superior oblique. *Syn*. Parks-Bielschowsky three-step test. *See* muscle, cyclovertical; test, Bielschowsky's head tilt; test, forced duction.

Pelli-Robson t. *See* chart, Pelli-Robson.

Pepper t. A test used for assessing reading performance in low-vision patients. It emphasizes the visual rather than the cognitive component of reading. Thus, each chart consists of unrelated letters and words rather than continuous text. Each row contains either separate letters (at the top of the chart) or separate words (of increasing length in the lower portion of the chart), all of the same size. Missing the first or last half of the word indicates the position of the scotoma relative to the fixation point. The rows at the top of the chart are triple-line spaced, double-line spaced in the middle and single-line spaced at the bottom, thus requiring more and more exacting saccadic eye movements. There are five charts, each of different sized print. A reading rate, such as the number of correct units read per minute, can be determined with this test. *Syn*. Pepper Visual Skills for Reading Test (VSRT).

phenol red cotton thread t. A test used for measuring tear secretion. It is accomplished by using a special cotton thread, impregnated with phenol red dye. The thread is inserted under the lower eyelid for 15 seconds, and both eyes are closed. The absorption of tears is determined by the length of thread that has turned from red to yellow (due to the pH of tears). The average length varies between 3 and 48 mm, and less than 9 mm is usually indicative of a dry eye. This test is much quicker and much less uncomfortable than Schirmer's test and has good reliability. However, questions have been raised as to whether it is the actual secretion rate that is being measured. Several **cotton thread tests** exist to measure tear secretion using different cottons of different lengths and diameters, and some are used without phenol red dye.
See tear secretion; test, Norn's; test, Schirmer's.

phi phenomenon t. of Verhoeff *See* movement, phi.

photostress t. A test designed to differentiate the cause of a reduced visual acuity in one eye, between a lesion in the optic nerve and a disease in the fundus of the eye. For 10 seconds, a bright light is directed into the eye with the best acuity, while the defective eye is covered. The light is then removed and the patient is instructed to read the line just above the best visual acuity line for that eye. The time taken until the patient can just read that line is recorded. The same procedure is then repeated with the defective eye. If the recovery time is about the same in both eyes, the cause of the reduced visual acuity is an optic nerve lesion (e.g. retrobulbar optic neuritis); if the recovery time is much longer for the defective eye, the cause is in the fundus (e.g. retinal oedema, retinopathy, age-related macular degeneration). The latter is attributed to a delay in the regeneration of visual pigments after being bleached with a bright light. The recovery time to be able to read the line takes longer in old people than in young ones. *Syn*. light-stress test.

pinhole t. *See* disc, pinhole.

plus 1.00 D blur t. A test used to verify a patient's spherical correction or to determine whether a person is hyperopic. It consists of placing a +1.00 D lens in front of the eye; visual acuity should be reduced from 6/6 (20/20 or 0.00 LogMAR) to about 6/18 (20/60 or 0.48 LogMAR), which reduces visual acuity by about four Snellen lines. If the patient can still read smaller letters than 6/18, the spherical prescription is incorrect or the patient is hyperopic. This result could also be due to a much smaller pupil than average. This test is most helpful with young children as it helps relax accommodation. It also leads to best visual acuity because the best lens can be obtained by either decreasing the plus sphere or increasing the minus sphere lens. *Syn*. blur back test; maximum plus to maximum visual acuity technique.
See best vision sphere; hyperopia, absolute; method, fogging.

prism adaptation t. A prognostic test in cases of esotropia (convergent strabismus), indicating whether surgical intervention is favourable or not. Prior to the intervention, the patient has to wear a BO prism of an amount larger than the angle of deviation for an hour or more. An increase in the angle of deviation is an unfavourable prognosis and no increase or a decrease is considered favourable.

prism cover t. *See* test, cover.

prism dissociation t. *See* test, diplopia.

prism reflex t. *See* test, Krimsky's.

prognostic t. A test performed to predict the likely outcome of an intervention or the course of a condition. *Examples*: pinhole test; blue field entoptoscope; prism adaptation test.
See disc, pinhole; entoptoscope, blue field.

prone position t. *See* test, provocative.

provocative t. A test performed to reproduce signs of a suspected disease in order to help in the diagnosis of that disease. A common provocative test for open-angle glaucoma is the **water-drinking test** in which a fasting patient has to drink one quart of water (or about 1 litre in a 70 kg adult) within five minutes. The intraocular pressure (IOP) is measured before the water is taken and then at 15-minute intervals. An increase of 8 mmHg or more in 45 minutes is considered positive. Two common provocative tests for angle-closure glaucoma are: (1) The **dark room test** in which the patient is kept in a dark room for 1 hour and the IOP is measured before and after the test. An increase of 8 mmHg or more is generally considered positive. (2) The **prone position test** in which the patient lies in the prone position for 1 hour and if the IOP increases by 8 mmHg or more compared with the value before the test, the result is considered positive. In open-angle glaucoma, provocative tests have been found to be positive in less than half of the patients but that figure is higher in angle-closure glaucoma.

Purkinje tree t. *See* **angioscotoma.**

push-up t. **1.** *See* **method, push-up. 2.** A procedure used to ensure adequate lens movement of a soft contact lens. The lens is gently pushed upward by pressing on the patient's lower eyelid; it should move easily and return quickly to its original location.

random-dot E t. *See* **stereogram, random-dot.**

Raubitschek t. *See* **chart, Raubitschek.**

red glass t. A test for determining diplopia or suppression in which a bright target (e.g. a white light) is fixated while a red filter is held in front of one eye to interrupt fusion. The patient with diplopia will see a red light and a white light. The amount of deviation can be estimated by using a prism of an amount such that it eliminates the double image. The operation can be repeated in all the diagnostic positions of gaze to help identify a paretic extraocular muscle as the distance between the two images increases in the field of action of the paretic muscle. If only one light is seen it indicates suppression of one retinal image. *Syn.* red filter test.

See **action, primary; test, diplopia; test, motility**.

Scheiner's t. A test performed to measure the monocular near point of accommodation. It consists of using a Scheiner's disc in front of the eye, which observes a small target such as a thin black line. The target is moved towards the eye until it is no longer seen single. That point represents the near point of accommodation.

See **experiment, Scheiner's; method, push-up.**

Schirmer's t. A test used for measuring tear secretion. It is accomplished by using a 35 × 5 mm strip of filter paper (e.g. Whatman No. 41). The filter strip is folded so that one end, about 5 mm long, is inserted at the mid-portion (or lateral portion) of the lower eyelid of a patient seated in a dimly lit room. Tear secretion is considered normal if 10 mm or more of the paper from the point of the fold becomes wet in a four-minute period. More than 25 mm of wetting would indicate excessive tear secretion. Without any additional stimulation of any kind the test, called **Schirmer's test 1**, measures mostly the basal tear production, but because the filter paper tends to irritate the conjunctiva, reflex tear secretion is measured as well. **Schirmer's test 2** is aimed at measuring mainly basic tear secretion. It is carried out with the filter paper inserted inside the lower lid of an

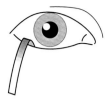

Fig. T13 Schirmer's test.

eye with topical anaesthesia. The amount of tear production is measured after five minutes. A value of more than 8 mm is considered to be normal and less than 8 mm may indicate a deficiency of basic tear secretion (Fig. T13).

See **alacrima; keratoconjunctivitis sicca; tear secretion; test, Norn's; test, phenol red cotton thread.**

screen t. *See* **test, cover.**

Seidel's t. A test performed to detect leaking of aqueous humour through a corneal wound by noticing the dilution of fluorescein which has been applied to the eye over the area of concern. The test is positive if there is a luminous green flow of aqueous seen through the slit-lamp under cobalt blue illumination.

sessile drop t. Measurement of the contact angle by observation of the formation of a drop of liquid on a solid surface. The image of the droplet may be photographed or projected.

See **angle, contact.**

shadow t. **1.** A test performed to give an approximate evaluation of the depth of the anterior chamber. It is carried out by placing a penlight on the temporal side of the eye at the level of the pupil and directing the beam of light horizontally towards the inner side of the eye. If the iris lies in a flat plane, which usually indicates a deep anterior chamber, the entire iris will be illuminated. If the iris is directed anteriorly, which usually indicates a narrow anterior chamber, the iris on the temporal side of the eye will be illuminated but the iris on the nasal side will be shadowed to varying degrees depending on the narrowness of the anterior chamber (Fig. T14). *Syn.* oblique illumination shadow test. **2.** *See* **retinoscopy. 3.** A test for the homogeneity of a lens (both material

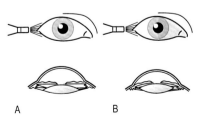

A   B

Fig. T14 Two different widths of the angle of the anterior chamber. A, open angle associated with a deep anterior chamber; B, narrow angle associated with a narrow anterior chamber. Only the iris on the temporal side is illuminated, as shown in the upper diagram.

and surface quality) in which the light from a small intense source of light passes through the lens and falls on a screen. Any defects will show as shadows.
See **angle of the anterior chamber; method, van Herick, Shaffer and Schwartz; method, Smith's.**
Sheridan–Gardiner t. A visual acuity test consisting of a large card (called the key card) which is held by the patient who is asked to point to the letter on that key card that is the same as the letter shown on the distance (or near) chart. The test consists of several cards with single letters of various sizes. It is most useful for testing children and illiterates.
simple penlight glare t. *See* **glare, disability.**
Simultan t. *See* **Simultantest.**
stereotest t. *See* **stereotest, Frisby; stereotest, Lang; stereogram, random-dot; vectogram.**
swinging flashlight t. *See* **pupil, Marcus Gunn.**
t. target *See* **test type.**
tear t. *See* **cytology, impression; dilation and irrigation; rose bengal; test, basic secretion; test, break-up time; test, Jones 1; test, non-invasive break-up time; test, ocular ferning; test, phenol red cotton thread; test, Schirmer's.**
tear dilution t. *See* **test, dye dilution; test, Norn's.**
Thorington t. A test designed to measure heterophoria at near and at distance. It consists of a horizontal row of letters on one side of a light source and a horizontal row of numbers on the other side of that source. A Maddox rod, orientated horizontally, is placed in front of one eye and the patient who is fixating the light source is asked to report through which letter or number the vertical streak appears to pass or to which it is closest. At 6 m, the number of letters must be placed 6 cm apart to represent 1 Δ steps. If the Maddox rod is in front of the right eye, the numbers on the right side of the source and the letters on the left, each number represents 1 Δ of esophoria and each letter represents 1 Δ of exophoria. The Thorington test can also be used at near. At 40 cm, for example, the separation of the letters and numbers must be 0.4 cm to represent 1 Δ. It can also be placed vertically with the Maddox rod orientated vertically to measure vertical heterophoria.
three-dimensional t. *See* **test, two-dimensional.**
three-needle t. A test for measuring stereoscopic visual acuity consisting of three fine rods placed vertically, two of them being fixed in the same plane, while the third one is movable in between. The subject views them through an aperture. The centre rod is placed in various positions backward and forward until the subject judges whether it is nearer or farther than the others (Fig. T15).
See **stereopsis; test, Howard–Dolman.**
three-step t. *See* **Parks's three-step.**
Titmus stereo t. *See* **vectogram.**
traction t. *See* **test, forced duction.**
Turville infinity balance t. A test for balancing the accommodative state of the eyes. It can also

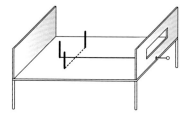

Fig. T15 Three-needle test.

be used for detecting suppression, vertical and horizontal associated phorias and (with a target composed of two horizontal lines) aniseikonia in the vertical meridian. It consists of a 3 cm-wide vertical septum placed in the centre of a mirror on which is reflected a reversed illuminated chart. Thus the patient can only see the right side of the chart with the right eye, and the left side with the left eye, which allows for simultaneous comparison of the chart seen by both eyes, while still retaining fusion for peripheral objects near the border of the chart. If the chart is projected onto a screen, the septum is placed halfway between patient and screen. The test is carried out after the conventional refractive procedures. *Syn.* infinity balance test.
See **balance, binocular; prism, aligning; suppression; test, balancing.**
two-dimensional t. A test for stereopsis consisting of two-dimensional objects as test material such as targets, cards, etc. as used in a stereoscope or a major amblyoscope (e.g. random-test stereogram, Titmus stereotest). Other tests for stereopsis are **three-dimensional** (3-D), the Howard–Dolman test being the most well known. Two-dimensional tests (2-D) are the most commonly used in clinical practice.
See **stereogram, random-dot; stereoscope; stereotest; test, Howard–Dolman; vectogram.**
t. type Any letter, figure or character used for vision testing. The term test object (*Syn.* test target) is a more general term, which encompasses any pattern or object (e.g. checkerboard, grating).
See **chart; grating; Jaeger test type; König bars; Landolt ring; optotype; pattern, checkerboard.**
Verhoeff phi phenomenon t. *See* **movement, phi.**
t-test *See* **Student's t-test.**
t. of Visual Analysis Skills *See* **test, developmental and perceptual screening.**
water-drinking t. *See* **test, provocative.**
Welland's t. *See* **test, bar reading.**
wool t. A test used for assessing colour vision deficiencies. It consists of a set of wool strands, which are to be matched with loose wool strands of the same colour. The best-known of these is the Holmgren's test. *Syn.* colour wool test.
Worth's four dot t. A test used for determining the presence of binocular vision. It consists of four illuminated discs: two green, one red and one white on a black background. The test is

viewed at any distance by a subject wearing red and green filters such that one eye sees the red and the white discs, while the other eye sees the two green discs and the white disc. Subjects are asked to report how many dots they see: four dots indicates normal binocular vision; two dots, both red, indicates suppression of the image in the eye wearing the green filter; three dots, all green, indicates suppression of the image in the eye wearing the red filter; and five dots, two red and three green, indicates diplopia. *Syn.* four-dot test. *See* **suppression; test, FRIEND; vision, Worth's classification of binocular.**

tetracaine hydrochloride (amethocaine hydrochloride) A topical corneal anaesthetic, commonly used in 0.25% to 1% solution. It may be used to carry out tonometry, to remove a foreign body, etc.

tetrachromatic theory *See* **theory, Hering's of colour vision.**

tetracycline *See* **antibiotic.**

textural gradient One of the monocular cues of depth perception produced by the change in the appearance of the grain of the structure of a surface, giving the impression that the thin small details must be farther away than the thick large ones (Fig. T16).
See **perception, depth.**

thalamus A pair of ovoid masses of grey substance located above the cerebral peduncles that serves as a relay station for sensory stimuli to the cerebral cortex. It contains the lateral geniculate body, which is a continuation of the pulvinar and which is situated at the posterior end of the thalamus.
See **geniculate body, lateral.**

theory An explanation of the manner in which a phenomenon occurs, has occurred or will occur.
   biological-statistical t. Theory of the development of refractive errors, based on the way in which the refractive components of the eye combine. It postulates a high correlation between the normally distributed refractive components to produce emmetropia. A breakdown of this correlation leads to ametropia. This theory depends essentially on hereditary factors.
   See **gene-environment interaction; myopia control; myopia, physiological; theory, emmetropization; theory, use-abuse.**
   corpuscular t. *See* **theory, Newton's.**
   duplicity t. The theory that vision is mediated by two independent photoreceptor systems in the retina: diurnal or photopic vision through the cones when the eyes see details and colours, and nocturnal or scotopic vision through the rods when the eyes see at very low levels of luminance. It can be illustrated when establishing a dark adaptation curve (sensitivity as a function of time), which is preceded by a bright preadaptation stimulus. The curve typically has two branches: an initial increase in sensitivity (i.e. lower light threshold) followed by a plateau, due to cone adaptation; then another increase in sensitivity followed by a plateau due to rod adaptation.
   See **interval, photochromatic; Purkinje shift; sensitivity, spectral; theory, two visual systems; vision, photopic; vision, scotopic.**
   emission t. *See* **theory, Newton's.**
   emmetropization t. A theory that explains the phenomenon of emmetropization on a biofeedback mechanism, involving cortical and subcortical control of the various components of the eye that contributes to its refractive power.
   See **emmetropization.**
   empiricist t. Theory that certain aspects of behaviour, perception, development of ametropia, etc. depend on environmental experience and learning, and are not inherited.
   See **empiricism; theory, nativist.**
   Fincham's t. Theory of accommodation which attributes the increased convexity of the front surface of the crystalline lens, when accommodating, to the elasticity of the capsule and to the fact that it is thinner in the pupillary area than near the periphery of the lens.
   See **capsule; theory, Helmholtz's of accommodation.**
   first order t. *See* **theory, gaussian.**
   gaussian t. The theory that, for tracing paraxial rays through an optical system, that system can be considered as having six cardinal planes: two principal planes, two nodal planes and two focal planes. The mathematical analysis can be carried out by the paraxial equation. *Syn.* first order theory; paraxial theory.
   See **Newton's formula; optics, paraxial; paraxial equation, fundamental; ray, paraxial.**
   Helmholtz's t. of accommodation The theory that in accommodation the ciliary muscle contracts, relaxing the tension on the zonule of Zinn while the shape of the crystalline lens changes, resulting in increased convexity, especially of the anterior surface. Fincham's theory complements that of Helmholtz.
   See **accommodation; theory, Fincham's; Zinn, zonule of.**
   Helmholtz's t. of colour vision *See* **theory, Young–Helmholtz.**
   Hering's t. of colour vision Theory that colour vision results from the action of three independent mechanisms, each of which is made up of a mutually antagonistic pair of colour sensations: red-green, yellow-blue and white-black. The latter pair is supposed to be responsible for the brightness aspect of the sensation, whereas the former two would be responsible for the coloured

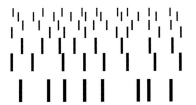

Fig. T16 An example of textural gradient.

Table T1 Main characteristics of the photopic and scotopic visual system

	Photopic vision	Scotopic vision
type of vision	diurnal (above 10 cd/m^2)	nocturnal (below 10^{-3} cd/m^2)
photoreceptor	cones	rods
max. receptor density	fovea	20° from fovea
photopigment(s) (and max. absorption)	long-wave sensitive (560 to 580 nm)	rhodopsin (507 nm)
	middle-wave sensitive (530 to 545 nm)	
	short-wave sensitive (420 to 440 nm)	
colour vision	present	absent
light sensitivity	low	high
dark adaptation:		
time to cone threshold	about 10 min	
time to rod threshold (about 3 log units below)		about 35 min
max. spectral sensitivity	555 nm	507 nm
spatial resolution (visual acuity)	excellent	poor
spatial summation	poor	excellent
temporal resolution (critical fusion frequency)	excellent	poor
temporal summation	poor	excellent
Stiles–Crawford effect	present	absent

aspect of the sensation. *Syn*. opponent-process theory; tetrachromatic theory.
See cell, colour-opponent; theory, Young–Helmholtz.

Huygen's t. *See* theory, wave.

lattice t. *See* theory, Maurice's.

Luneburg's t. A theory which hypothesizes that the geometry of the visual space can be described by a variable non-euclidean hyperbolic metric.

Maurice's t. Theory that explains the transparency of the stroma of the cornea. It states that the stromal fibrils, which have a refractive index of about 1.55 in the dry state, are so arranged as to behave as a series of diffraction gratings permitting transmission through the liquid ground substance (refractive index 1.34). The fibrils are the grating elements that are arranged in a hexagonal lattice pattern of equal spacing and with the fibril interval being less than the wavelength of light. The diffraction gratings eliminate scattered light by destructive interference, except for the normally incident light rays. Light beams that are not normal to the cornea are also transmitted to the oblique lattice plane. However, recent work has demonstrated inconsistencies in lattice space and there is some modification to the original postulate of this theory. *Syn*. lattice theory.

nativist t. Theory that certain aspects of behaviour, perception, development of ametropia, etc. are inherited and independent of environmental experience.
See gene-environment interaction; nativism; theory, empiricist.

Newton's t. The theory that light consists of minute particles radiated from a light source at a very high velocity. *Syn*. corpuscular theory; emission theory.
See theory, quantum; theory, wave.

opponent-colour t. *See* theory, Hering's of colour vision.

paraxial t. *See* theory, gaussian.

Planck's t. *See* theory, quantum.

quantum t. Theory that radiant energy consists of intermittent and spasmodic, minute indivisible amounts called quanta (or photons). This is a somewhat modern version of the theory originally proposed by Newton. *Syn*. Planck's theory.
See photon; theory, Newton's; theory, wave.

three-component t. *See* theory, Young–Helmholtz.

trichromatic t. *See* theory, Young–Helmholtz.

two visual systems t. The theory that there are two distinct modes of processing visual information: one pertaining to the identification ('what' system) and the other to localization ('where' system) of visual stimuli. The identification mode is concerned with resolution and pattern vision, and is associated with the foveal and parafoveal regions of the retina. It is subserved by primary cortical mechanisms. The localization mode is concerned with motion and orientation and is subserved by midbrain visual structures (Table T1).
See system, magnocellular visual; system, parvocellular visual; theory, duplicity.

use-abuse t. Theory that attributes the onset of myopia to an adaptation to the use or misuse of the eyes in prolonged close work with the concomitant lag of accommodation and hyperopic defocus. Environmental factors would be the main cause of myopia.
See myopia control; theory, biological-statistical.

wave t. Theory that light is propagated as continuous waves. This theory was quantified by the Maxwell equations. The wave theory of light can satisfactorily account for the observed

facts of reflection, refraction, interference, diffraction and polarization. However, the interchange of energy between radiation and matter, absorption and the photoelectric effect are explained by the quantum theory. Both the wave and quantum theories of light were combined by the concept of quantum mechanics, and light is now considered to consist of quanta travelling in a manner that can be described by a waveform. *Syn.* Huygens' theory.
See photon; theory, quantum; wavelength.

Young–Helmholtz t. The theory that colour vision is due to a combination of the responses of three independent types of retinal receptors whose maximum sensitivities are situated in the blue, green and red regions of the visible spectrum. This theory has been shown to be correct, except that the pigment in the third receptor has a maximum sensitivity in the yellow and not in the red region of the spectrum. Hering's theory of colour vision, which explains phenomena at a level higher than that of the cone receptors, complements this theory. *Syn.* Helmholtz's theory of colour vision; three components theory; trichromatic theory.
See pigment, visual; theory, Hering's of colour vision.

theoretical eye *See* eye, reduced; eye, schematic.

therapeutic soft contact lens *See* lens, therapeutic soft contact.

thimerosal *See* antiseptic.

third-degree fusion *See* stereopsis; vision, Worth's classification of binocular.

third cranial nerve *See* nerve, oculomotor.

third nerve paralysis *See* palsy, third nerve.

Thorington test *See* test, Thorington.

Thorpe four-mirror fundus lens *See* slit-lamp.

three and nine o'clock staining *See* staining, 3 and 9 o'clock.

three-dimensional Adjective pertaining to depth perception or the illusion of depth (e.g. a perspective drawing).

three-needle test *See* test, three-needle.

threshold The value of a stimulus that just produces a response. *Syn.* limen.
　absolute t. Minimum luminance of a source that will produce a sensation of light. It varies with the state of dark adaptation, the retinal area stimulated, the wavelength of light, etc. The lowest level of luminance visible is typically around 10^{-6} cd/mm^2. It has been estimated that the absolute threshold results from a single photon absorbed by each of several different rods. *Syn.* light threshold.
　See interval, photochromatic; photon; vision scotopic.
　contrast t. *See* threshold, difference.
　corneal touch t. *See* corneal touch threshold.
　t. determination in visual field analysis *See* algorithm, Swedish Interactive Thresholding.
　difference t. The smallest difference between two stimuli presented simultaneously that gives

rise to a perceived difference in sensation. The difference may be related to brightness, but also to colour and specifically to either saturation (while hue is kept constant) or hue (while saturation is kept constant). The difference threshold of luminance is equal to about 1% in photopic vision. *Syn.* contrast threshold (if the difference is one of luminance); increment threshold; just noticeable difference (jnd).
　See sensitivity, contrast; law, Weber's.
　increment t. *See* threshold, difference.
　light t. *See* threshold, absolute.
　movement t. 1. The minimum motion of an object that can be perceived. 2. The speed at which an object moving between two points just appears to be moving.
　See hyperacuity; phenomenon, phi.
　resolution t. *See* resolution, limit of.
　stereo-t. *See* acuity, stereoscopic visual.

Thygeson's superficial punctate keratitis *See* keratitis, Thygeson's superficial punctate.

thymoxamine (moxisylyte) *See* alpha-adrenergic antagonist.

thyroid eye disease *See* disease, Graves'.

thyrotoxicosis *See* disease, Graves'.

tight junction Refers to cells in which their membranes are fused rather than separated by a small extracellular space. The movement of substances through that space is restricted. *Example*: squamous cells of the corneal epithelium bound to each other by linking protein strands. *Syn.* zonulae occludentes.
　See blood-brain barrier.

tight lens syndrome *See* contact lens acute red eye.

tilt after-effect; *See* after-effect, tilt.

tilt, head *See* head posture, abnormal; head tilt; test, Bielschowsky's head tilt.

tilted optic disc *See* disc, tilted optic.

timolol maleate *See* adrenergic receptors; beta-blocker.

tinted lens *See* lens, tinted.

tissue A basic anatomical and physiological component of the living organism, consisting of a collection of similar cells and their intercellular substances. *Examples*: connective tissue, epithelial tissue, muscular tissue, nervous tissue.

Titmus stereo test *See* vectogram.

TNO test *See* stereogram, random-dot.

'tobacco dust' *See* retinal detachment, rhegmatogenous; sign, Shafer's.

tobramycin *See* antibiotic.

tomograph, confocal scanning laser *See* glaucoma detection; ophthalmoscope, confocal scanning laser.

tomography A radiographic technique for making a detailed X-ray image of a selected plane section of the body while blurring out the images of other planes. The data can be manipulated to represent three-dimensional images of structures.

computed t. (CT) A radiographic method of viewing a three-dimensional image of a layer of body structures, which is constructed by a computer from a series of plane cross-sectional X-ray images made along an axis. The images indicate the X-ray absorption (called attenuation) of tissues (e.g. bones with the highest density attenuate most, lungs attenuate least and blood vessels are in between). The X-rays are received by numerous gas or solid-state detectors, and computers are used to store, process and manipulate the information received from these detectors. The method yields far better differentiation of tissues than conventional radiography thus providing more precise diagnostic information. Usage includes the detection of orbital fractures, orbital cellulitis, intraorbital calcification, cerebral haemorrhage and orbital tumours. *Syn.* computerized axial tomography (CAT); CAT scan; CT scan. *See* **glaucoma detection; magnetic resonance imaging; radiology.**

confocal scanning laser t. *See* **ophthalmoscope, confocal scanning laser.**

optical coherence t. (OCT) A non-invasive, optical diagnostic imaging technique which enables in vivo cross-sectional tomographic visualization of internal microstructure in biological systems. OCT is analogous to ultrasound imaging except that it uses light (near-infrared) rather than sound, thus achieving approximately 1 to 100× higher image resolution. This is accomplished by using polychromatic (broad bandwidth) or tunable light sources in combination with interferometric techniques to detect depth resolved reflectivity profiles, due to subtle refractive index changes. Several adjacent one-dimensional optical A-scans are combined into two- or three-dimensional tomograms for quantitative analysis of the optic nerve head topography, peripapillary fibre layer thickness, macular retinal thickness, as well as corneal visualization. Quantitative results are compared with an age-matched normative database. Cross-section of the retinal layers is represented in colour with red for highly reflective structures, green-yellow intermediate and blue-black for low reflectivity. OCT can be used for early diagnosis of retinal diseases (e.g. cystoid macular oedema, central serous retinopathy, retinal detachments, macular hole), better understanding of retinal pathogenesis, monitoring of nerve fibre layer thickness and optic nerve head changes in glaucomatous eyes, as well as corneal thickness changes following refractive surgery. Most recent developments enable several 10 thousand measurements per second, allowing three-dimensional retinal images nearly free of motion artifact. In combination with improved resolution, this technique has the potential to perform non-invasive optical biopsy of the human retina, i.e. visualization of intraretinal morphology in retinal pathologies approaching the level achieved with histopathology.

See **glaucoma detection; interference.**

positron emission t. (PET) A neuroimaging technique in which a positron-emitting isotope (e.g. carbon-11, nitrogen-13, oxygen-15 and fluorine-18) incorporated into a metabolically active molecule (e.g. fluorodeoxyglucose) is injected intravenously and used as radioactive tracers to generate images of regional cerebral blood flow and glucose consumption contained in the tracers and thus, indirectly brain function. The emitted positron collides with an electron, giving rise to two photons, which strike detectors placed around the head. Tomographic images can be used to construct a three-dimensional image of the relative concentration of the tracer within the brain. PET has been used to study normal and abnormal brain function and to assess tumours, stroke, cortical lesions and also mapping of the visual cortex. *See* **magnetic resonance imaging, fMRI; neuroimaging, functional.**

tone, colour Term often used in colorimetry, photography and industry to indicate hue. *See* **hue.**

tone, muscle *See* **tonus.**

tonic accommodation *See* **accommodation, resting state of.**

tonic convergence *See* **vergence, tonic.**

tonic pupil *See* **pupil, Adie's.**

tonic vergence *See* **vergence, tonic.**

tonicity *See* **solution, hypertonic; solution, hypotonic; solution, isotonic.**

tonography Technique used for measuring the facility of outflow of aqueous humour from the eye under the continuous pressure exerted by the weight of a tonometer over a given period of time. The instrument usually employed for tonography is an electronically recording Schiötz tonometer. In this technique, the pressure is continuously recorded over a 4-minute period and the outflow is deduced by utilizing a specifically designed diagram, called a nomogram (which is a graphical representation of one, or more, mathematical relationships whereby the desired value may be found without calculation by placing a straight edge across the diagram). The results of tonography can indicate the presence of established glaucoma, although the technique is not very reliable for borderline cases.

tonometer An instrument for estimating intraocular pressure. It measures either the degree of corneal deformation produced by a known force or the force needed to produce a given degree of corneal deformation. *See* **glaucoma detection; manometer; pressure, intraocular; rigidity, ocular; Tonopen.**

air-puff t. *See* **tonometer, non-contact.**

applanation t. A tonometer in which the intraocular pressure is estimated by the force required to flatten a constant corneal area as, for example, in the **Perkins,** (Fig. T17) the **Goldmann** (Fig. T18) and the **Proview** tonometers in which the probe is pressed on the closed nasal

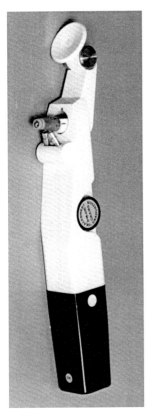

Fig. T17 Perkins tonometer.

eyelid until the patient sees a phosphene. The Goldmann tonometer (Figs. T18 and T19) is used in conjunction with a slit-lamp and provides an accurate reading with which all other tonometers are usually compared. The Perkins tonometer is a hand-held instrument.
See **law, Imbert–Fick; Tonopen.**
electronic t. Any tonometer with an electronic readout. These instruments act swiftly, the procedure usually being completed within a fraction of a second.
Goldmann t. *See* **tonometer, applanation.**
impression t. A tonometer in which the intraocular pressure is estimated by the degree of indentation of the cornea. The excursion of the plunger of the tonometer is read from a calibrated scale and converted into values of the intraocular pressure, often using appropriate tables. An older type of such instrument was that of **Schiötz**, which is rarely used nowadays. Modern instruments include the **Ocular blood flow analyser** in which a probe tip covered with a membrane is applied and deformed by the cornea while air at a constant pressure pushes against the membrane. The rate of air flow that escapes from the probe is measured and converted to a reading of intraocular pressure. *Syn.* indentation tonometer.

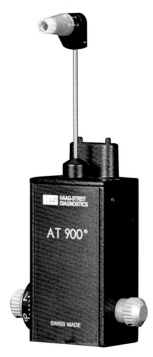

Fig. T18 Goldmann applanation tonometer. The instrument is mounted on a slit-lamp and the applanated corneal surface is observed monocularly through one eyepiece of the microscope. (Image from Haag-Streit AG, Koeniz, Switzerland, www.haag-streit.com)

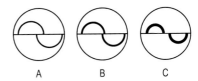

Fig. T19 Fluorescein pattern seen when the head of the Goldmann applanation tonometer rests against the anterior corneal surface. A, the dial reading is greater than the IOP; B, the dial reading is equal to the IOP and the applanated corneal area has a diameter of 3.06 mm; C, the dial reading is less than the IOP.

See **rigidity, ocular.**
indentation t. *See* **tonometer, impression.**
Mackay–Marg t. An electronic tonometer in which a plunger in the centre of a flat footplate which applanates the cornea protrudes by a very small amount (5 mm). The intraocular pressure is related to the counter force required to resist displacement of this plunger when the cornea is flattened by the footplate. The result is read by interpretation of a graph on a strip chart.
See **Tonopen.**
Maklakov's t. *See* **tonometer, applanation.**

non-contact t. A tonometer that does not require any contact to be made between the tonometer and the eye. Hence no anaesthesia is required with this instrument. It consists of sending a puff of air towards the cornea of sufficient strength to flatten a predetermined area of cornea. The time taken from the onset of the puff of air to the applanation of the cornea (which is monitored optically) is recorded electronically and is proportional to the intraocular pressure. A digital readout of pressure, in mmHg, appears within about 15 ms after the measurement is initiated. The principle is applied in the hand-held **Pulsair** non-contact tonometer and in the **Reichert Non-Contact** tonometer. *Syn.* air-puff tonometer; pneumatic tonometer.

Perkins t. *See* **tonometer, applanation.**

Pulsair noncontact t. *See* **tonometer, non-contact.**

rebound t. A hand-held, compact, portable tonometer. It incorporates its own battery supply and digital readout. A pair of coils coaxial to a probe shaft is used; a solenoid coil propels a lightweight magnetized probe against the cornea and it bounces back. A sensing coil detects several motion parameters from the voltage that the moving probe induces. They are recorded and analyzed. The intraocular pressure is related to the duration of the corneal impact, the shorter the duration, the higher the pressure. The probe is disposable and its tip is covered with a round plastic cover to minimize corneal damage. The results correlate well with the Goldmann tonometer, although with slightly higher readings.

Reichert Non-Contact t. *See* **tonometer, non-contact.**

Schiötz t. *See* **tonometer, impression.**

Tonomat t. *See* **tonometer, applanation.**

tonometry Measurement of intraocular pressure (IOP) with a tonometer. All existing tonometers only provide an estimate of the IOP, but a true measure can only be obtained with a manometer. *See* **manometer; pressure, intraocular; tonometer.**

Tonopen A hand-held, compact, portable applanation tonometer based on the same principle as the Mackay–Marg tonometer with a 1.5-mm transducer tip. It is a very small instrument, 18 cm long by 2 cm in width, weighing 56 g. It incorporates its own battery power supply and liquid crystal digital readout and provides both intraocular pressure readout and an indicator of the reliability of the instrument. The results correlate well with the Goldmann tonometer, although it slightly overestimates low IOPs and underestimates high IOPs. It can take measurements in an eye with an irregular or oedematous cornea or through a soft contact lens and in a variety of clinical settings (Fig. T20). *See* **tonometer, applanation.**

tonus A state of partial contraction present in a muscle in its passive state as, for example, when the eye is in the physiological position of rest. *Syn.* muscle tone.

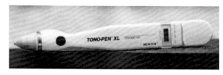

Fig. T20 Tonopen.

See **accommodation, open-loop; accommodation, resting state of; vergence, tonic.**

topical Adjective usually referring to medication applied directly to the eye. *See* **systemic.**

Topogometer An older device attached to a keratometer that allowed a measurement of the curvature of the cornea off the visual axis. It has been replaced by modern methods of measuring corneal topography such as videokeratography. *See* **corneal topography; videokeratoscope.**

topography, corneal *See* **corneal topography.**

Toposcope 1. An instrument for measuring the curvature of the surfaces of a contact lens, based on moiré fringes. A bar pattern is reflected from the lens surface, and the reflected image is viewed with a microscope that has a second bar pattern in the eyepiece. The two bar patterns superimposing each other at slightly different orientations create the **moiré patterns**. The magnification of the microscope is changed until the fringes are parallel to the central index line seen in the field, and a dial monitoring this change in magnification indicates the radius of curvature in millimetres. **2.** *See* **test, non-invasive break-up time.** *See* **optic zone radius, back; radiuscope.**

toric lens *See* **lens, toric.**

toroidal surface *See* **lens, toric.**

torsion Rotation of an eye around its fixation axis. If the upper pole of the vertical meridian of the cornea appears to rotate inward, it is called **intorsion** (also called **incyclotorsion**), and outward, **extorsion** (also called **excyclotorsion**). If the eye rotates to the right it may be called **dextrotorsion** and if it rotates to the left it may be called **laevotorsion**. It may occur as a result of a head tilt, extraocular muscle weakness or rotation of the eye to a tertiary position. *Syn.* cycloduction; cyclorotation; cyclotorsion (it is often regarded as synonym); torsional movement. *See* **cyclotorsion; law, Donder's; muscle, cyclovertical; position, tertiary; hemianopia, incongruous.**

torticollis, ocular Head tilting usually accompanied by a twisting of the neck adopted to minimize the effect of a palsy of one or more of the vertically acting extraocular muscles (most often the superior oblique). *See* **spasmus nutans.**

tortoiseshell Material used in the manufacture of spectacle frames. It is obtained from the shell plates of the hawksbill turtle. *See* **spectacle frame, plastic; spectacles.**

total astigmatism; diameter; reflection *See* under the nouns.

toughened glass *See* glass, safety.

tourmaline A mineral crystal or boron silicate compounded with elements of aluminium, iron, magnesium or potassium which polarizes light by absorbing the ordinary ray and transmitting the extraordinary ray.
See birefringence; light, polarized; polarizer.

toxic amblyopia *See* amblyopia, toxic.

toxocariasis A rare infestation caused *Toxocara Canis* or *Toxocara Catis*, which are common parasites of dogs and cats. The condition affects children and adults. It is caught by ingestion of soil or food contaminated with ova from animal faeces. After ingestion, the larvae hatch within the stomach and circulation and may affect the liver, lung, eye (**ocular toxocariasis**) or brain and cause fatigue and breathing difficulties. Ocular manifestations which are typically unilateral include chronic endophthalmitis with leukocoria, anterior uveitis, vitritis, fundus granuloma and vitreoretinal traction which may lead to retinal detachment. Management includes steroid and occasionally vitrectomy.

toxoplasmosis An infectious disease caused by the protozoan *Toxoplasma gondii*, of which the cat is a definitive host and livestock and humans are intermediate hosts. It occurs either as a congenital or as an acquired type. The ocular features in the congenital type include cataract, microphthalmos and optic atrophy; in the acquired type vitritis, anterior uveitis with elevated intraocular pressure, retinochoroiditis and with symptoms of floaters, blurring and photophobia. The main treatment is to attempt eradicating the parasite. The condition tends to recur, but if the immune system is not compromised, it is self-limiting.
See uveitis.

trabecula A supporting structure consisting of bands of connective tissue, usually collagenous, providing support in various organs.

trabecular meshwork Meshwork of connective tissue located at the angle of the anterior chamber of the eye and containing endothelium-lined spaces (the **intertrabecular spaces**) through which passes the aqueous humour to Schlemm's canal. It is usually divided into two parts: the **corneoscleral meshwork** which is in contact with the cornea and the sclera and opens into Schlemm's canal and the **uveal meshwork** which faces the anterior chamber.
See glaucoma, phacolytic; gonioscopy; iris, plateau; line, of Schwalbe; syndrome, pigment dispersion.

trabeculectomy A type of filtration surgery aimed at lowering the intraocular pressure by excising a small portion of the sclera and peripheral iris to create a passage allowing aqueous humour to flow from the anterior chamber out of the eye into the subconjunctival space. The hole is protected by a scleral flap, which is sutured back at the end of the procedure to reduce the risk of overfiltration and hypotony. The procedure is ended with injection of steroid and antibiotic drugs, which are then used as eyedrops for a period of time.
See cyclodialysis; filtration surgery; mitomycin C; sclerectomy.

trabeculoplasty, laser A procedure aimed at improving the outflow of aqueous humour in open-angle glaucoma by producing a series of laser burns (usually with an argon laser) to the trabecular meshwork.

trabeculotomy A surgical procedure aimed at lowering intraocular pressure by unblocking the entry of Schlemm's canal to ease the outflow of aqueous humour. This procedure is used principally in congenital glaucoma especially when goniotomy has failed.
See glaucoma, congenital.

trachoma A chronic, bilateral, contagious conjunctivitis caused by the serotypes A, Ba and C of *Chlamydia trachomatis*. The conjunctivitis results in conjunctival scarring (**Arlt's line**) and may lead to entropion and trichiasis and dry eyes. Follicles at the limbus may leave some sharply defined depressions (**Herbert's pits**). There is also keratitis with corneal infiltrates, pannus and vascularization. As the disease progresses there is trichiasis, corneal ulceration and opacification, which may result in blindness. Trachoma is one of the main causes of blindness in the world. It is a disease most commonly encountered in hot regions of the globe where hygienic conditions are poor. Treatment includes a course of antibiotics such as tetracycline or erythromycin and surgical correction of entropion and trichiasis may be necessary. *Syn.* egyptian conjunctivitis; granular conjunctivitis.

tract 1. A bundle of nerve fibres (e.g. the optic tracts). **2.** A system of organs serving the same function, e.g. the respiratory tract.
geniculocalcarine t. *See* radiations, optic.
optic t's. Two cylindrical bands of nerve fibres carrying visual impulses along the visual pathway of which they form a part. They run outward and backward from the posterolateral angle of the optic chiasma, then sweep laterally, encircling the hypothalamus posteriorly on their way to the lateral geniculate bodies. A few fibres leave the tracts for the superior colliculi, and some of these fibres end in the pretectal olivary nuclei and are involved in the pupillary light reflex. Lesions in the tracts result in binocular visual field defects and abnormal pupillary response in some circumstances.
See brachium; hemianopia, incongruous; pathway, visual; reflex, hemianopic pupillary.

tractional retinal detachment *See* retinal detachment, tractional.

training, visual Methods aimed at improving visual abilities, e.g. visual perception, spatial localization, heterophoria, hand/eye coordination, etc. to achieve optimal visual performance and comfort. These techniques represent an enlargement of the practice of orthoptics. *Syn.* vision therapy.

transcleral illumination *See* transillumination.

transduction Generally, the conversion of one form of energy into another. *Example*: the transformation of light energy into receptor potentials in the photoreceptors of the retina (also called **phototransduction**). The absorption of light by the pigments of the photoreceptors triggers a cascade of biochemical events that results in the breaking off of *opsin* and the photoisomerization of 11-*cis* retinal (retinaldehyde) into all-*trans retinal* (R → R*) ending in a decrease in cGMP (cyclic guanosine monophosphate), which leads to a closure of the ion channels and consequently to a change in resting potential from around −40 mV in the dark to around −70 mV in light, that is a hyperpolarization of the cells. *See* depolarization; hyperpolarization; isomerization; potential, receptor; pigment, visual; rhodopsin.

transillumination 1. The shining of light through a translucent membrane. This is principally used to better visualize ocular tumours, cysts or haemorrhages within the eye. It is accomplished by directing a narrow intense beam of light on the side of the eye. *Example*: If a tumour is present in the eye, some light will not be reflected and the pupil will appear partially or completely black, instead of bright red as when the healthy eye is thus illuminated. *Syn*. transcleral illumination. *See* meibography. **2.** *See* illumination, retro-.

transition of a scleral contact lens The zone between the optic (corneal) and haptic (scleral) portions. *See* blending; lens, scleral contact.

translocation *See* chromosome; mutation.

translucent Pertains to a medium or substance that transmits light but diffuses or scatters it on the way so that objects cannot be seen through it, e.g. paraffin wax, tracing paper, cloth, smoke, fog, ground glass, etc. *See* transparent.

transmission 1. The passage of radiations through a medium or a substance. Transmission can be either diffuse (light is scattered in all directions) or regular (i.e. without diffusion). *See* absorption; translucent; transmittance; transparent. **2.** The passage of a nerve impulse from one neuron to another across a synapse (nerve transmission). *See* neurotransmitter; synapse. **3.** The passage of infection or disease from one person to another.

transmission curve A graph in which the transmission of an optical medium is plotted against the wavelength. *See* lens, tinted.

transmittance A measure of transmission expressed as the ratio of the intensity of the transmitted light I' to the intensity of the incident light I, for a specified wavelength, i.e.

$$T = I'/I.$$

It is usually given as a percentage, i.e.

$$T = I'/I \times 100.$$

Syn. total transmittance. *See* absorption; density, optical.

transparent Pertains to a medium or a substance that transmits light without scattering and with little absorption, so that objects can be seen through it. Optical lenses, prisms, etc. are made of such material. *See* opaque; translucent.

transplant, corneal *See* keratoplasty.

transport, active A process by which particles (e.g. ions, molecules) are transported across cell membranes, against, in almost all instances, the concentration gradient. It requires energy, which is provided by the metabolism of carbohydrates, proteins or lipids and cellular energy, which is obtained from splitting adenosine triphosphate (ATP). *Example*: The sodium potassium pump that keeps sodium ions out of a cell and potassium ions in. When active transport results in a compound being released, it is termed 'secretion'. This process is one of the mechanisms (consequent to ultrafiltration) by which aqueous humour is produced in the ciliary body. *See* potential, action; ultrafiltration.

transposition 1. The act of converting the prescription of an ophthalmic lens from a sphere with minus cylinder form to a sphere with plus cylinder form or vice versa. It is done by (1) adding the sphere, (2) changing the sign of the cylinder and (3) rotating the axis by 90 degrees. *Example*: −3 D sphere, −2 D cylinder axis, 180° transposes to −5 D sphere, +2 D cylinder axis 90°. **2.** A surgical procedure used to correct muscle paralysis. In this procedure, adjacent muscles are transferred (transposed) to the paralysed muscle, allowing for partial movement in the field of action of the paretic muscle. There are various procedures: one in which parts of the recti muscles are sutured together (the superior and inferior recti are disinserted and joined to the lateral rectus) to correct lateral rectus palsy and improve abduction (**Hummelsheim's procedure** or with several variations, **Jensen's procedure** being one); another in which the lateral and medial recti muscles are disinserted and attached adjacent to either the superior or inferior rectus, to improve elevation or depression, respectively (**Knapp's procedure**) and another is to split the anterior fibres of the superior oblique, which is palsied and insert them anteriorly and laterally to reduce excyclotorsion (**Harado-Ito procedure**). *See* action, primary; focimeter; palsy, sixth nerve; palsy, third nerve; strabismus surgery.

Trantas' dots *See* conjunctivitis, vernal.

trauma to the eye Injury to the eye which may occur as a result of blunt (most common) or sharp objects, a chemical substance or a penetrating

foreign body. All tissues of the eye may be affected: eyelids (e.g. laceration), cornea (e.g. abrasion), conjunctiva, lens (e.g. cataract), retina (e.g. retinal dialysis), orbit (e.g. fracture) and can cause visual impairment from moderate to sight-threatening, visual field defects, diplopia and pain.
See **cataract; chalcosis; chemical burn; choroidal rupture; commotion retinae; corneal abrasion; disease, Berlin's; endophthalmitis; haematoma; haemorrhage, suprachoroidal; hyphaemia; iridodialysis; lens, prolapse of the; lid laceration; luxation of the lens; mydriasis, traumatic; neuropathy, optic; orbital fracture; retinal detachment, tractional; retinal dialysis; ring, Vossius'; siderosis; syndrome, shaken baby; vitreous detachment.**

travoprost *See* prostaglandin analogues.

Treacher Collins syndrome *See* syndrome, Treacher Collins.

tremors *See* movement, fixation.

trephine A surgical instrument with a circular cutting edge used to cut out a disc of tissue (e.g. a disc of cornea in keratoplasty).

triad, near *See* reflex, near.

trial case A case containing pairs of positive and negative spherical lenses, plano cylinders, thin prisms as well as discs, pinhole discs, etc. used in refraction with a trial frame. The contents of the case are referred to as a **trial set**.

trial frame Spectacle frame with variable adjustments for interpupillary distance, side length, etc. in which each lens rim is fitted with a number of cells into which trial lenses can be placed when testing vision (Fig. T21).
See **phoropter; Simultantest.**

trial lens *See* lens, trial.

trial lens clip *See* clipover.

trial, randomized controlled (RCT) An experimental design used for testing the effectiveness of a new medication or a new therapeutic procedure. Individuals are assigned randomly to a treatment (experimental therapy) or experimental group and to a control group (placebo or standard therapy) and the outcomes are compared. All confounding factors are matched between the two groups except the factor being investigated, which is present only in the treatment or experimental group. The trial is strengthened by 'blinding' or masking (single-blind, double-blind or triple-blind

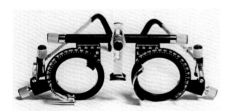

Fig. T21 Trial frame.

study) and cross-over design. RCT is the most accepted scientific method of determining the benefit of a drug or a therapeutic procedure. It represents the best evidence available, which is integrated into the final decision about the management of a condition by healthcare practitioners in what is called **evidence-based healthcare**.
Syn. randomized clinical trial.
See **sampling; significance; study.**

trial set A number of objects used to measure the refraction of the eye. It includes a trial case with various lenses, prisms, pinhole discs, Maddox rod, etc., and a trial frame.

triamcinolone *See* antiinflammatory drug; chalazion; retinopathy, diabetic.

triangle, colour *See* chromaticity diagram.

triangulation, amplitude of *See* convergence, amplitude of.

triangulation, angle of *See* angle of convergence.

tricarboxylic acid cycle *See* cycle, Krebs.

trichiasis A condition in which the eyelashes, due to entropion, blepharitis or injury, are directed toward the globe and cause irritation of the cornea and conjunctiva. Temporary relief may be achieved with epilation, but permanent treatment consists of cryotherapy or laser ablation or in severe cases surgical excision and replacement with a mucous membrane (Fig. T22).
See **distichiasis; epilation; lens, therapeutic soft contact; pemphigoid, cicatricial; pseudotrichiasis; trachoma.**

trichromatic theory *See* theory, Young–Helmholtz.

trichromatism Colour vision characterized by the fact that any perceived hues can be matched by three independent primaries (e.g. red, green and blue). *Syn.* trichromacy; trichromatic vision.

trichromatism, anomalous A form of defective colour vision in which three primary colours are required for colour matching, but the proportion of each primary is not the same as those required by a normal trichromat. There are three types of anomalous trichromatism: deuteranomaly, protanomaly and tritanomaly. *Syn.* anomalous trichromacy; anomalous trichromatic vision.
See **colour, primary; colour vision, defective.**

trifield lens *See* field, visual f. expander.

trifluridine; trifluorothymidine *See* antiviral agents.

trigeminal ganglion *See* ganglion, gasserian.

trigeminal nerve *See* nerve, trigeminal.

trimethoprim *See* antibiotic.

triophthalmos A double-faced fetus with three eyes. This occurs when the eyes on the joined sides of conjoined twins have combined to form a single one.

triplet Lens system composed of three lenses as, for example, a convex crown glass lens cemented between two concave flint lenses. The aim of such

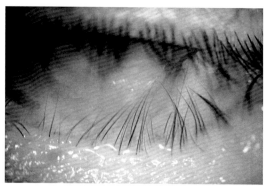

Fig. T22 Trichiasis. (From Kanski 2003, with permission of Butterworth-Heinemann)

a system is to minimize aberrations. It is used in optical instruments (Fig. T23).
See **doublet; eyepiece, orthoscopic; lens, achromatizing.**

triplopia Condition in which a subject sees three images of a single object. This condition may be the result of crystalline lens sclerosis, multiple pupils, etc.
See **diplopia; polyopia.**

trisomy *See* **chromosome.**

trisomy 13 *See* **syndrome, Patau's.**

trisomy 18 syndrome *See* **syndrome, Edwards'.**

trisomy 21 syndrome *See* **syndrome, Down's.**

tritan A person who has either tritanopia or tritanomaly.

tritanomal A person who has tritanomaly.

tritanomaly A type of anomalous trichromatism in which an abnormally high proportion of blue is needed when mixing blue and green to match a standard blue-green stimulus. This condition is exceedingly rare: it is estimated at about one person in a million. *Syn.* tritanomalous trichromatism; tritanomalous vision.
See **anomaloscope; colour vision, defective; plates, pseudoisochromatic.**

tritanope A person who has tritanopia.

tritanopia A rare type of dichromatism in which blue and yellow are confused. The tritanope only sees two colours: reds on the long-wave side, and greens or bluish greens on the other side of his neutral point, which is situated around 570 nm. Tritanopia occurs more often as an acquired type as a result of retinal disease or detachment, glaucoma, diabetes, retinitis pigmentosa, etc. Congenital tritanopia is very rare; it is estimated at about five males and three females in 100 000. *Syn.* blue blindness; blue-yellow blindness.
See **colour vision, defective; dichromatism; plates, pseudoisochromatic; test, Farnsworth-Munsell 100 Hue.**

trochlea *See* **fossa, trochlear; muscle, superior oblique.**

trochlear nerve *See* **nerve, trochlear.**

trochlear paralysis *See* **palsy, fourth nerve.**

troland Unit of retinal illuminance equal to that produced when the luminance L of the observed object is one candela per square metre seen through a pupil p having an area of one square millimetre i.e. $T = L \times p$. *Syn.* photon (obsolete).
See **retinal illuminance.**

tropia *See* **strabismus.**

tropicamide *See* acetylcholine; cycloplegia; mydriatic.

Troxler's phenomenon *See* phenomenon, Troxler's.

true image *See* **image, true.**

true negative A result to a test that does not detect a condition when the condition is absent.
See **false negative; specificity.**

true positive A result to a test that detects a condition when it is actually present,
See **false positive; sensitivity.**

truncation Removal of the peripheral part of a contact lens. The truncation is often undertaken at the base of a prism ballast lens.
See **ballast.**

trypan blue A blue dye used in cataract surgery; it is applied directly onto the anterior lens capsule, which it stains, thereby aiding its visualization and facilitating its removal. It is also used in eye banks to evaluate the quality of the endothelium

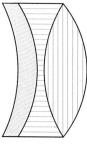

Fig. T23 Triplet.

of human donor corneas as it stains the nuclei of damaged or dead cells.
See phacoemulsification.

Tscherning ellipse *See* ellipse, Tscherning.

t-test *See* Student's t-test.

tubercle, lacrimal *See* lacrimal tubercle.

tubercle, lateral orbital A small elevation on the orbital surface of the zygomatic bone just behind and within the orbital margin, about 11 mm below the suture of the zygomatic and frontal bones. It serves as an attachment for the check ligament of the lateral rectus muscle, the lateral palpebral ligament, the suspensory ligament of Lockwood and the levator palpebrae superioris muscle. *Syn.* Whitnall's tubercle.
See ligament of Lockwood; ligament, palpebral.

tubercle, Whitnall's *See* tubercle, lateral orbital.

tuberculosis Chronic infection caused by the microorganism *Mycobacterium tuberculosis*, which causes primarily a pulmonary disease but also of various ocular tissues.
See disease, Eales'; keratitis, interstitial; neuropathy, optic; uveitis, bacterial.

tuberous sclerosis *See* sclerosis, tuberous.

tuck procedure *See* procedure, tuck.

tumbling E chart *See* chart, E.

tungsten-halogen lamp *See* lamp, halogen.

tunica vasculosa lentis *See* artery, hyaloid.

tunnel vision *See* vision, tunnel.

Turcot's syndrome *See* syndrome, Turcot's.

turgescence The swelling of a tissue, usually as a result of water accumulation.

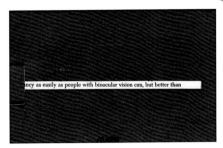

ncy as easily as people with binocular vision can, but better than

Fig. T24 Typoscope.

See deturgescence.

Turk's disease *See* syndrome, Duane's.

Turner's syndrome *See* syndrome, Turner's.

Turville infinity balance test *See* test, Turville infinity balance.

twitch, eyelid *See* myokymia.

twilight vision *See* vision, mesopic.

two visual systems theory *See* theory, two visual systems.

Tyndall effect *See* effect, Tyndall.

typoscope A reading shield made of black material in which there is a rectangular aperture allowing one or more lines of print to be seen. It reduces extraneous light reflected from the surface of the paper and assists in staying on the correct line (Fig. T24). It can be helpful for people with low vision who have, for example, media involvement. Recent models embody built-in lighting to provide even and controlled illumination. *Syn.* reading slit.

U

UGH syndrome *See* syndrome, UGH.

Uhthoff's symptom Temporary blurring of vision occurring when there is an increase in body temperature (e.g. during or following exercise) in patients with multiple sclerosis, optic neuritis and other optic neuropathies. The symptom may also occur as a result of emotional stress, menstruation, increased illumination or a hot bath. Uhthoff's symptom is sometimes considered to be a prognostic indicator of multiple sclerosis in patients with idiopathic optic neuritis. *Syn.* Uhthoff's phenomenon; Uhthoff's sign; Uhthoff's syndrome.

ulcer A localized lesion of the skin or of a mucous layer in which the superficial epithelium is destroyed and deeper tissues are exposed.
See abscess.
corneal u. A superficial loss of corneal tissue resulting from an infection that has led to necrosis. It may be caused by a bacterium (e.g. *Pseudomonas aeruginosa, Streptococcus pneumoniae*), by a virus (e.g. herpesvirus) or by a fungus (e.g. *Candida, Aspergillus, Penicillium*). It causes pain and usually reduced visual acuity, especially if the ulcer occurs in the centre of the cornea. Corneal ulcers usually look dirty grey or white and are

opaque areas of various sizes and a mucopurulent discharge may be present. If induced by contact lenses, especially extended wear lenses, patients must cease wearing their lenses immediately and the appropriate therapy instituted: antibacterial, antifungal or antiviral agent.
See **corneal facet; keratitis, herpes simplex; keratitis, hypopyon; keratitis, rosacea; keratitis, ulcerative; keratocele; keratomycosis; leukoma.**

dendritic u. *See* **keratitis, herpes simplex.**

von Hippel's internal u. A depression noted in the posterior surface of the cornea. This lesion resembles posterior lenticonus, except that it is thought to be due to an infection or inflammation. The lesion can be differentiated from Peter's anomaly by the presence of endothelium and Descemet's membrane in the former. Due to its posterior location, the lesion does not usually disturb visual function.
See **Peter's anomaly.**

marginal corneal u. Benign condition due to a hypersensitivity reaction to bacterial conjunctivitis, particularly staphylococcal blepharoconjunctivitis. It is characterized by infiltration of the peripheral cornea by white cells and by ocular irritation. The condition is usually self-limiting but painful. Treatment includes frequent cleaning of the eyelid margin with a cotton-tipped applicator or face cloth or cotton ball with baby shampoo, warm compresses, antibiotic ointment and occasionally topical corticosteroids.

Mooren's u. A rare, autoimmune, superficial ulcer of the cornea of unknown origin. It starts near the limbus as an overhanging advancing edge, which in severe cases spreads over the entire cornea and may even invade the sclera. The patient complains of pain, photophobia and blurred vision. There are two types: a self-limiting form, usually unilateral, affecting old people, and a progressive form, bilateral, affecting young people. The condition is difficult to treat and this may include topical and systemic steroids, immunosuppressants, or conjunctival excision.
See **keratitis, peripheral ulcerative.**

serpiginous u. *See* **keratitis, hypopyon.**

shield u. A localized corneal ulcer noted in severe cases of vernal conjunctivitis. The lesion is usually oval or pentagonal resembling a warrior's shield. It is located in the upper portion of the cornea as a result of irritation from the large papillae on the palpebral surface of the overlying eyelid.

ulcerative keratitis *See* **keratitis, ulcerative.**

ultrafiltration This is one of the mechanisms that produce aqueous humour from blood plasma in the ciliary epithelium of the ciliary processes. This mechanism takes advantage of the natural pressure gradient between the capillary vascular pressure and intraocular aqueous pressure, to drive fluid into the eye. Ultrafiltration is one of three physiological processes that create aqueous fluid, the others being active transport and diffusion (osmosis).
See **aqueous humour; ciliary body; diffusion; osmosis; transport, active.**

ultrasonography A technique utilizing high-frequency ultrasound waves (greater than 4 MHz, but high frequency of 20 MHz is also used, particularly for B-scan) emitted by a transducer placed near the eye. The silicone probe, which rests on the eye, is separated from the transducer by a water column to segregate the noise from the transducer. The ultrasound wave is reflected back when it encounters a change in density of the medium through which it is passing. The reflected vibration is called an echo. Echoes from the interfaces between the various media of the eye are converted into an electrical potential by a piezoelectrical crystal and can be displayed as deflections or spikes on a cathode-ray oscilloscope.

There are two basic techniques used for examination: a contact system (often referred to as **applanation**) described above in which the probe is in contact with cornea and an immersion system in which the transducer and the cornea are separated by a water bath. This latter method eliminates the risk of indentation of the cornea and underestimation of the anterior chamber depth and axial length. Two types of ultrasonographic measurements are used: (1) The time-amplitude or **A-scan** which measures the time or distance from the transducer to the interface and back. Thus echoes from surfaces deeper within the eye take longer to return to the transducer for conversion into electrical potential and so they appear further along the time base on the oscilloscope display. The A-scan is useful for the study of the biometric measurements, such as the axial length of the eye, the depth of the anterior chamber, the thickness of the lens, the distance between the back of the lens and the retina and the thickness of the cornea, as well as measurements of intraocular tumour size (e.g. choroidal melanoma) (Fig. U1). (2) The intensity-modulated or **B-scan** in which various scans are taken through the pupillary area and any change in acoustic impedance is shown as a dot on the oscilloscope screen, and these join up as the transducer moves across a meridian. The B-scan is useful to indicate the position of a retinal or vitreous detachment, or of an intraocular foreign body or a tumour, and for the examination of the orbit. The B-scan is especially useful in the examination of the posterior structures of the eye when opacities prevent ophthalmoscopic examination (e.g. cataract, corneal oedema). *Syn.* echography.
See **biometry of the eye; length of the eye, axial.**

ultraviolet (UV) Radiant energy of wavelengths smaller than those of the violet end of the visible spectrum and longer than about 1 nm. The wave band comprising radiations between 315 and 380 nm is referred to as **UV-A**. Excessive exposure to these radiations can cause cataract. The wave band comprising radiations between 280 and 315 nm is referred to as **UV-B**. Excessive exposure to all these radiations can cause photokeratitis and corneal opacity, while radiations between 295

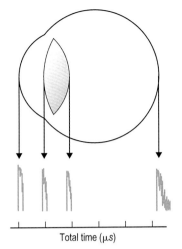

Fig. U1 Histogram of ultrasound reflections (or echoes) in the eye (A-scan). Echoes from the various boundaries are given against total time, i.e. the time interval from the cornea to the boundary and back to the cornea. The velocity of the ultrasound waves in the eye is approximately 1550 m/s (it is 1641 m/s in the lens and 1532 m/s in the humours). In this diagram, the total time between the cornea and the retina is 32 μs. The length is then equal to $32/2 \times 10^{-6} \times 1550 \times 10^3 = 24.80$ mm.

and 315 nm can cause cataract. The wave band comprising radiations between 200 and 280 nm is referred to as **UV-C**. Excessive exposure to these radiations can cause photokeratitis and corneal opacity (Table U1).
See blepharospasm; keratoconjunctivitis, actinic; laser, excimer; lens, absorptive; nanometre; pinguecula; wavelength.

umbo An area (0.15 to 0.20 mm) in the centre of the foveola. Stimulation of this area results in the highest visual acuity.

umbra The completely dark part of the shadow cast by an opaque object.
See penumbra.

unaided vision; visual acuity *See* acuity, unaided visual.

uncompensated heterophoria *See* heterophoria, uncompensated.

uncrossed diplopia *See* diplopia, homonymous.

undercorrected spherical aberration *See* aberration, spherical.

undercorrection A term applied to a corrective lens prescription of slightly lower power than required. It

has been prescribed in an unsuccessful attempt to slow the progression of myopia in children because it reduces the accommodative stimulus.
See defocus, myopic; myopia control.

undersampling Applied to the retina, a condition in which the density of photoreceptors is too low to be able to resolve the high spatial frequency of a visual target. *Example*: the limitation on visual acuity in the periphery of the retina where the photoreceptors are too far apart in the sampling distribution.
See aliasing; frequency, Nyquist.

unharmonious retinal correspondence *See* retinal correspondence, abnormal.

unilateral Pertaining to only one side.
See bilateral; contralateral; ipsilateral.

uniocular *See* monocular.

univariance A principle in which a light stimulus to an individual retinal receptor elicits the same response regardless of intensity and wavelength. For example, a cone receptor does not distinguish between a green or red patch and produces an identical response, which may be stronger or weaker. To distinguish colours from intensity, two or more adjacent cones need to be stimulated.

unoprostone isopropyl *See* prostaglandin analogues.

upbeat nystagmus *See* nystagmus.

upgaze Movement of the eyes upward with the head in the straight-ahead position.
See elevation of the eye.

urea *See* hyperosmotic agent.

use-abuse theory *See* theory, use-abuse.

Usher's syndrome *See* syndrome, Usher's.

uvea The vascular tunic of the eye, consisting of the choroid, ciliary body and the iris. The uvea contains most of the blood supply of the eye (Fig. U2). *Syn.* uveal tract; vascular tunic of the eye.
See melanoma, uveal; uveitis; vein, vortex.

uveal effusion syndrome *See* syndrome, uveal effusion.

Table U1 Divisions of the ultraviolet spectrum

UV-A (near)	380–315 nm
UV-B (middle)	315–280 nm
UV-C (far)	280–200 nm

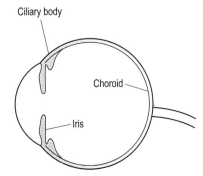

Fig. U2 The uvea.

uveal melanoma *See* melanoma, uveal.

uveal meshwork *See* meshwork, trabecular.

uveal tract *See* uvea.

uveitis Inflammation of the uvea. All three tissues of the uvea tend to be involved to some extent in the same inflammatory process because of their common blood supply. However, the most severe reaction may affect one tissue more than the others as in iritis, cyclitis or choroiditis or sometimes two tissues, e.g. iridocyclitis. When all the uveal structures including the surrounding structures (anterior chamber, vitreous and retina) are involved, the condition is called **panuveitis**. The symptoms also vary depending upon which part of the tract is affected. The cause may be idiopathic or due to an infection by bacteria (e.g. tuberculosis, syphilis), fungi, viruses (e.g. HIV, varicella zoster) or a parasite (e.g. toxoplasmosis), while others are associated with systemic conditions (e.g. juvenile idiopathic arthritis, sarcoidosis, lupus erythematosus, multiple sclerosis), *See* **arthritis, juvenile idiopathic; disease, Reiter's; hypopyon; ophthalmia, sympathetic; phthisis bulbi; syndrome, Behçet's; synchisis scintillans; syndrome, Vogt–Koyanagi–Harada; Table I6, p. 162**

acute anterior u. The most common form of uveitis in which the primary site of inflammation is the anterior chamber and it includes iritis, iridocyclitis and anterior cyclitis. It presents with pain, photophobia and lacrimation and some loss of vision because of exudation of cells (aqueous flare), protein-rich fluid and fibrin into either the anterior chamber or vitreous body, as well as ciliary injection, adhesion between the iris and lens (posterior synechia), miosis, hypopyon, keratic precipitates and iris nodules (Koeppe's and Busacca's). The condition is idiopathic in many cases but it can result from trauma, herpes simplex virus, varicella zoster virus or associated with ankylosing spondylitis, sarcoidosis, syphilis, Behçet's disease, Vogt–Koyanagi–Harada syndrome, tuberculosis (in which case there are usually granulomata on the iris and the condition is called **granulomatous uveitis**) or ankylosing spondylitis

and less commonly psoriasis, inflammatory bowel disease and Crohn's disease. Nearly half of the cases are human leukocyte antigen (HLA-B27) positive. **Chronic** anterior uveitis, which is less common than the acute type, is associated with juvenile idiopathic arthritis, Fuchs' heterochromic iridocyclitis and renal disease. Treatment includes topical corticosteroids and mydriatics to reduce the risk of posterior synechia and to relieve a spasm of the ciliary muscle (Fig. U3). *See* **arthritis, juvenile idiopathic; iridocyclitis; iridocyclitis, Fuchs' heterochromic; nodules, Busacca's; nodules, Koeppe's.**

bacterial u. Infection of the uvea by a microorganism, of which the most common are *Mycobacterium tuberculosis*, (tuberculosis) which typically causes a granulomatous anterior uveitis with posterior synechia and vitritis, retinal vasculitis and choroiditis; the spirochaetes *Treponema pallidum* (syphilis), which causes iris atrophy, chorioretinitis and pigmentary retinopathy; the spirochaetes *Borrelia burgdorfei* (Lyme disease), which is transmitted to humans by tick bites from rodents or deer and may cause anterior uveitis, anterior or posterior; and *Mycobacterium leprae* (leprosy, Hansen disease), which causes anterior uveitis, iris pearls at the pupil margin, iris atrophy, miosis and keratitis. Management includes drug combinations of an antituberculosis agent (e.g. pyrazinamide, ethambutol) and antibiotic, high dose penicillin with steroids for syphilis and antibiotic drugs for Lyme disease.

fungal u. Uveitis caused by a fungus such as *Aspergillus, Candida albicans, Cryptococcus neoformans* and *Histoplasma capsulatum*. It is often accompanied with other disorders (e.g. choroiditis, retinitis). It may have spread from other bodily tissues (e.g. skin, mouth, gastrointestinal tract) in patients who are intravenous drug addicts, patients with indwelling venous catheters, chronic pulmonary disease or patients who are immunosuppressed. *See* **endophthalmitis; syndrome, presumed ocular histoplasmosis.**

intermediate u. The primary site of this inflammation is the vitreous and it includes the pars plana zone (**pars planitis**) of the ciliary body, **posterior**

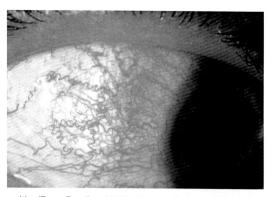

Fig. U3 Acute anterior uveitis. (From Bowling 2016, with permission of Elsevier)

cyclitis and hyalitis. The cause is unknown in most cases, but others are associated with systemic conditions such as multiple sclerosis, sarcoidosis or HIV infection. It affects around 10% of all cases of uveitis and is bilateral in about 80% of cases. Symptoms are floaters and, sometimes, blurred vision, and there may be anterior chamber cells and flare. Ophthalmoscopic examination may show vitreous condensation and gelatinous exudates ('**cotton balls**' or '**snowballs**'). Snowbanking, i.e. a whitish plaque or exudates involving the pars plana, often the inferior part of it, appears mainly in pars planitis. Intermediate uveitis may be associated with retinal vasculitis (i.e. inflammation of a retinal blood vessel). In a few cases the condition is self-limiting within a few months. However, in most cases the condition lasts several years and may lead to complications such as cystoid macular oedema, posterior subcapsular cataract, retinal detachment or cyclitic membrane formation. Treatment includes corticosteroids and in resistant cases immunosuppressive agents or surgery (e.g. cryotherapy).

phacoanaphylactic u. Granulomatous anterior uveitis caused by leakage of lens proteins into the aqueous humour. It may result from either a traumatic rupture of the lens capsule or to a degradation of lens proteins in cataracts. It may cause secondary glaucoma. *Syn*. phacogenic uveitis.

posterior u. The primary site of this type of uveitis is the retina or choroid and it includes choroiditis, retinochoroiditis and neuroretinitis. Symptoms include floaters and visual loss if the choroiditis involves the macular area. Ophthalmoscopically there is an accumulation of debris in the vitreous, and choroidal lesions appear as yellow-white areas of infiltrates surrounded by normal fundus. Retinitis is also present in most cases, as well as retinal vasculitis. Posterior uveitis may be idiopathic but it may be associated with the HIV virus, Behçet's disease, histoplasmosis, sarcoidosis, toxoplasmosis, syphilis, tuberculosis, Vogt–Koyanagi–Harada syndrome, sympathetic ophthalmia, etc. Management includes steroids and systemic immunosuppressive agents.

viral u. Uveitis caused by a virus. Common viruses are herpes simplex, which is usually associated with keratitis and may cause anterior uveitis with keratic precipitates, sectoral iris atrophy and reduced corneal sensation; **varicella zoster**, which may be associated with herpes zoster ophthalmicus, with anterior uveitis (granulomatous in some cases) and sectoral iris atrophy; **human T-cell lymphotrophic virus**, which causes leukaemia and may cause uveitis; **measles**, which may cause posterior uveitis and retinitis and in childhood, conjunctivitis and keratitis with subacute sclerosing panencephalitis as a late complication; **rubella**, which may cause anterior uveitis as well as pigmentary retinopathy; **cytomegalovirus** retinitis and iridocyclitis, which may occur in immunosuppressed individuals due to therapy (e.g. for HIV, although this has become less common because of more successful therapy, such as the Highly Active Antiretroviral Therapy (HAART)) and cause vision loss, floaters and retinal necrosis; **human immunodeficiency virus (HIV)**, which depletes CD4 T cells, which are essential to initiate an immune response to pathogens and consequently causes AIDS in about half of the infected cases.

See **blepharoconjunctivitis, herpes simplex; herpes zoster ophthalmicus; syndrome, acquired immunodeficiency.**

uveoscleral outflow; pathway *See* **pathway, uveoscleral.**

V

validity The extent to which a measurement correctly measures what it is supposed to measure or to which extent the findings of an investigation reflect the truth. In health sciences, validity is commonly assessed by determining the sensitivity and specificity factors and the limits of agreement of one instrument or procedure with another or with a standard reference.
See **reliability; sensitivity; specificity.**

value f *See* **f number.**

value, Munsell *See* **Munsell colour system.**

value, V- *See* **constringence.**

valve Any structure that regulates the flow of a liquid or gas through an orifice or passage in one direction and closes the aperture to backward flow.
v. of Hasner A fold of mucous membrane at the lower end of the nasolacrimal duct. If well developed, it generally prevents air from being blown back from the nose into the lacrimal sac. *Syn*. plica lacrimalis; valve of Bianchi.
See **lacrimal apparatus.**
v. of Krause A fold of mucous membrane at the junction of the lacrimal sac and the nasolacrimal duct. *Syn*. valve of Beraud.
See **lacrimal apparatus.**

v. of Rosenmuller A fold of mucous membrane found at the junction between the common canaliculus and the lacrimal sac. It is not strictly a valve because fluids can be blown back to emerge at the puncta. It is not always fully developed. *See* lacrimal apparatus.

van Herick, Shaffer and Schwartz method *See* method, van Herick, Shaffer and Schwartz.

vancomycin *See* antibiotic.

variance *See* standard deviation.

varicella-zoster virus *See* herpes zoster ophthalmicus; herpesvirus.

varifocal lens *See* lens, progressive.

vasa hyaloidea propria *See* artery, hyaloid.

vasculitis Inflammation of blood vessels. It may damage the lining of the vessels and cause obstruction to blood flow with consequent damage or necrosis of tissues supplied by the affected vessels.

vascularization *See* neovascularization; pannus.

vase, Rubin's *See* Rubin's vase.

vectogram A polarized stereogram consisting of two polarized images at right angles to each other. When viewed through polarizing filters, it presents one image to one eye and another image to the other eye. The Vectograph is a chart based on this principle in which almost one-half of a chart is seen by one eye and almost the other half by the other eye while some lines, letters or numbers are seen binocularly to lock fusion. The **Vectograph** is useful for balancing refraction and to detect suppression and fixation disparity. The **Titmus stereotest** (Fig. V1) consists of various vectograms, including one with a stereoscopic pattern representing a **housefly,** to establish whether the patient has gross stereopsis (it produces approximately 3000 seconds of arc of retinal disparity at 40 cm). Children are often tested by asking them to hold one of the wings of the fly, which they will do above the plate if it is seen stereoscopically. The other vectograms of the test provide finer tests for stereoscopic acuity.

See acuity, stereoscopic visual; disparity, retinal; stereogram, random-dot; suppression; test, balancing; test, two-dimensional.

VEGF (vascular endothelial growth factor) A major protein involved in regulating the differentiation and proliferation of vascular endothelial cells thus promoting the growth of new blood vessels (**angiogenesis**). VEGF is essential for normal embryonic development and contributes to the maintenance and repair of tissues. There are several VEGF proteins, depending on the number of amino acids that they contain (e.g. VEGF 121, VEGF 165, VEGF 189 and VEGF 206). However, under certain circumstances (e.g. higher than normal levels of VEGF as happens in hypoxia), it may participate in cancerous processes, inflammatory processes (e.g. rheumatoid arthritis) and ocular neovascularization as in exudative (wet) age-related macular degeneration and diabetic retinopathy. Anti-VEGF drugs are used to inhibit the action of VEGF.
See anti-VEGF drugs; opticin.

veil, Sattler's *See* Sattler's veil.

veiling glare *See* glare, veiling.

vein A tubular vessel that carries blood towards the heart.
See artery.
anterior ciliary v. One of many veins that drains the ciliary body, the deep and superficial plexuses, the anterior conjunctival veins and the episcleral veins to empty into the vortex veins.
anterior facial v. Vein branching from the angular vein at the side of the nose and running obliquely downward and backward across the face. It crosses the mandible and joins the posterior facial vein to form the common facial vein, which opens into the internal jugular. The anterior facial vein drains the part of the eyelids anterior to the tarsus.
aqueous v. One of several veins serving as exit channels for the aqueous humour, which it discharges from the canal of Schlemm into the episcleral, conjunctival and subconjunctival veins.

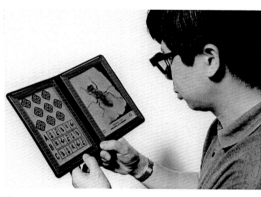

Fig. V1 Titmus stereotest.

central retinal v. A vein formed by the junction of the superior and inferior retinal veins at about the level of the lamina cribrosa on the temporal side of the central retinal artery. After a short course within the optic nerve, it empties into the cavernous sinus, the superior ophthalmic vein and sometimes into the inferior ophthalmic vein. *See* **artery, central retinal; retinal vein occlusion; venous pulsation.**
conjunctival v. One of many veins that drains the tarsal conjunctiva, the fornix and the major portion of the bulbar conjunctiva.
inferior ophthalmic v. Vein that commences as a plexus near the floor of the orbit, runs backward on the inferior rectus muscles and divides into two branches, one which runs to the pterygoid venous plexus and the other which joins the cavernous sinus, usually via the superior ophthalmic vein. The inferior ophthalmic vein receives tributaries from the lower and lateral ocular muscles, the conjunctiva, the lacrimal sac and the two inferior vortex veins.
palpebral v. One of the veins of the upper or lower eyelid that empties for the most part into the anterior facial vein as well as into the angular, supraorbital, superior and inferior ophthalmic, the lacrimal and the superficial temporal veins.
posterior ciliary v. *See* **vein, vortex.**
superior ophthalmic v. Vein that is formed near the root of the nose by a communication from the angular vein soon after it has been joined by the supraorbital vein. It passes into the orbit above the medial palpebral ligament, runs backward to the sphenoidal fissure where it usually meets the inferior ophthalmic vein and drains into the cavernous sinus. It has many tributaries: the inferior ophthalmic vein, the anterior and posterior ethmoidal veins, the muscular vein, the lacrimal vein, the central retinal vein, the anterior ciliary vein and two of the posterior ciliary veins (the superior ones).
vortex v. One of usually four (two superior and two inferior) veins which pierce the sclera obliquely on either side of the superior and inferior recti muscles, some 6 mm behind the equator of the globe. The two superior ones open into the superior ophthalmic vein and the two inferior open into the inferior ophthalmic vein. These veins drain the posterior uveal tract. *Syn.* posterior ciliary vein; vena vorticosa.
See **vein, anterior ciliary.**

velocity of light *See* **light, speed of.**

velonoskiascopy A subjective method of detecting ametropia in which a thin rod held near the eye is moved across the pupil while the subject fixates a distant light source. The rod casts a shadow on the retina if the eye is ametropic. This shadow will appear to move with the rod in myopia and opposite to the movement of the rod in hyperopia. By moving the rod across the pupil in different meridians, astigmatism can be explored. No shadow is seen in emmetropia.

vena vorticosa *See* **vein, vortex.**

venous-stasis retinopathy *See* **retinal vein occlusion.**

ventral Relating to either the front (anterior) or to the bottom in brain orientation.
See **dorsal; system, parvocellular visual.**

venous pulsation A normal expansion and contraction of veins, which is easily seen by ophthalmoscopy at the point of entry of the central retinal vein into the optic nerve. It is absent in papilloedema.

vergence 1. Denotes divergence of light travelling from, or convergence of light travelling from, or to an object or image. The object vergence at a refracting surface is equal to

$$L = -n/l$$

where n is the index of refraction of the first medium and l the distance between the object plane and the refracting surface in metres. The **image vergence** at a refracting surface is equal to

$$L' = n'/l'$$

where n' is the index of refraction of the second medium and l' the distance between the image plane and the refracting surface in metres. The unit of vergence is the dioptre. **2.** Disjunctive movements of the eyes such as convergence, divergence, cyclovergence, infravergence or supravergence.
See **distance, image; distance, object; duction; paraxial equation, fundamental; power, refractive.**
v. accommodation *See* **accommodation, convergence.**
accommodative v. *See* **convergence, accommodative.**
disparity v. *See* **fusion, motor.**
v. facility Ability of the eyes to make fusional vergence movements in a given period of time without changing accommodation. Clinically, this is measured by introducing a pair of large prisms (e.g. 12 Δ base-out) in front of a patient's eyes fixating a target until it appears single. The operation is repeated many times, and the results are commonly presented in cycles per minute (one cycle indicates that single vision was reported both with the prisms and after removing the prisms). The test can discriminate between symptomatic and asymptomatic patients with binocular vision difficulties.
See **convergence, fusional; fusion, motor; lens flippers.**
v. formula *See* **paraxial equation, fundamental.**
fusional v. *See* **convergence, relative.**
v. power *See* **power, refractive.**
proximal v. *See* **convergence, proximal.**
v. reflex *See* **reflex, vergence.**
relative v. *See* **convergence, relative.**
tonic v. Passive state of vergence of the eyes in the absence of a stimulus, i.e. when the eyes are in total darkness or when looking at a bright empty

field. This position is maintained by the tonus of the extraocular muscles. Only at death or when paralysed do the eyes return to their anatomical position of rest and tonic vergence disappears. *Syn.* dark vergence; tonic convergence.
See **accommodation, resting state of; position of rest, physiological; tonus.**
   vertical fusional v. Movement of the eyes upward until an object that was imaged on slightly disparate vertical parts of the retina falls on corresponding retinal points.

Verhoeff phi phenomenon test *See* **movement, phi.**

Verhoeff's circles Two black concentric circles designed for use with the duochrome test and as a target for the cross-cylinder method. The thickness and overall diameter of the inner ring are equivalent to a 6/6 (20/20) Snellen letter while the thickness and overall diameter of the outer ring are equivalent to a 6/15 (20/50) Snellen letter. *Syn.* Verhoeff's rings.
See **chart, Snellen; test for astigmatism, cross-cylinder; test, duochrome.**

Verhoeff's rings *See* **Verhoeff's circles.**

vernal catarrh; conjunctivitis *See* **conjunctivitis, vernal.**

vernier visual acuity *See* **acuity, vernier visual.**

version Conjugate movements of the two eyes in the same direction, such as **dextroversion**, both eyes rotate to the right; **laevoversion (levoversion)**, both eyes rotate to the left; **supraversion (sursumversion)**, both eyes rotate upward; **infraversion (deorsumversion)**, both eyes rotate downward: these versions bring the eyes into the **secondary positions of gaze.** Movements of the eyes up and to the right are called **dextroelevation**, up and to the left, **laevoelevation**, down and to the right, **dextrodepression** and down and to the left, **laevodepression**; these versions bring the eye into the **tertiary positions of gaze.** Version eye movements are performed by yoke muscles (Fig. V2). *Syn.* conjugate eye movements.

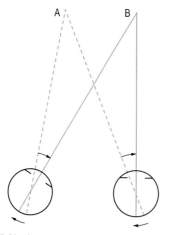

Fig. V2 Version movements of the eyes from A to B.

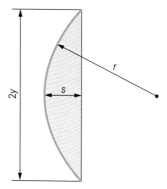

Fig. V3 Vertex depth (or sagittal depth) *s* of a spherical surface (*r*, radius of curvature; 2*y*, diameter of the surface).

   See **deviation, conjugate; muscle, yoke; positions of gaze, cardinal; test, motility.**

version prisms *See* **prisms, yoke.**

vertex The point where the optical axis intersects a reflecting or refracting surface. In a spectacle lens, the back vertex is the point of intersection of the optical axis with the surface nearest to the eye, the other being the front vertex. *Plural*: vertices.
   v. depth Distance between the posterior pole of a spectacle lens and the plane containing the posterior edge of the lens. The vertex depth *s* is given by the following formula

$$s = r - \sqrt{(r^2 - y^2)}$$

where *r* is the radius of curvature of the surface of the spectacle lens and *y* is the semidiameter at the edge of the surface (Fig. V3 and Table V1). *Syn.* sag.
See **clearance, apical; lens measure.**
   v. distance Distance along the line of sight between the apex of the cornea and the posterior surface of a spectacle lens. This distance normally varies between 11 mm and 15 mm.
See **clearance, apical; plane, spectacle.**
   v. focal length The linear distance separating the principal focal point (focus) of an optical system or lens from the front or back vertices. They are called the **front vertex focal length** (f_v) and the **back vertex focal length** (f'_v), respectively. In the case of a biconcave or biconvex lens, the front and back vertex focal lengths are equal. In the case of a positive meniscus lens, the back vertex focal length is shorter than the front vertex focal length and vice versa in the case of a negative meniscus lens.
See **power, back vertex; power, front vertex.**
   v. power *See* **power, back vertex; power, front vertex.**

vertexometer **1.** Synonym of focimeter. **2.** Synonym of distometer.
See **distometer; focimeter.**

vertical fusional vergence *See* **vergence, vertical fusional.**

Table V1 Vertex depths of various spherical surfaces. They also represent the centre thickness of a planoconvex lens with a front surface of radius of curvature r and diameter 2y, with an edge thickness of zero. Index of refraction of the lens 1.49.

Surface power (D)	Radius r (mm)	Lens diameter 2y (mm)			
		40	50	60	70
1	490	0.41	0.64	0.92	1.25
2	245	0.82	1.28	1.84	2.51
3	163.3	1.23	1.92	2.78	3.79
4	122.5	1.64	2.58	3.73	5.11
5	98	2.06	3.24	4.70	6.46
6	81.7	2.49	3.92	5.71	7.88
7	70	2.92	4.62	6.75	9.38
8	61.3	3.38	5.33	7.85	10.99
9	54.4	3.81	6.08	9.01	12.74
10	49	4.27	6.86	10.26	14.71
12	40.8	5.23	8.55	13.13	19.80
14	35	6.28	10.51	16.97	35.00
16	30.6	7.43	12.94	24.47	
18	27.2	8.75	16.45		
20	24.5	10.35			

vertigo The sensation of irregular movement in space of either oneself or of external objects. It can be experienced after vestibular stimulation.

vesicle 1. A small bladder or sac containing liquid. **2.** A small elevation on the skin containing fluid, usually serous fluid. **3.** Any structure that has the appearance of **1** or **2**.
optic v's. Hollow, spherical, neuroectodermal protrusions located one on each side of the forebrain. They are derived from the optic pits after closure of the embryonic neural tube. They subsequently invaginate to form the optic cup. The surface ectoderm overlying the optic vesicles invaginates to form the lens vesicle and eventually the crystalline lens. *Syn.* primary optic vesicle.
See **anophthalmia; cup, optic; ectoderm; pit, optic.**

vestibular nystagmus *See* **nystagmus.**

vestibulo-ocular reflex *See* **reflex, vestibulo-ocular.**

v gauge A device used to measure the total diameter of a rigid contact lens. It consists of a channel cut into a long rectangle of plastic or metal. The channel increases in width from 6.0 to 12.50 mm and a scale is printed beside it. The lens is placed with its concave surface down at the widest end of the channel and that end of the gauge is raised so that the lens slides down the channel until it stops. The diameter is then read from the scale where the lens touches the side of the channel. *Syn.* v-channel gauge.

vial A very small bottle. It may contain a soft contact lens, medicine or perfume.

vidarabine *See* **antiviral agents.**

videokeratoscope An electro-optical instrument for measuring the corneal topography. It produces a colour-coded three-dimensional map of the shape of the cornea and of the dioptric power of the different corneal regions. These instruments are computer-assisted, providing rapid online analysis of the image, and most of them are based on the corneal reflection of the Placido pattern or the Scheimpflug principle in which a series of slit-beam images are integrated (**scanning-slit videokeratoscope**). Topographic data are usually presented as a colour-coded map of the cornea showing regions of different power. These instruments are used to evaluate keratoconus, irregular corneal shape, and contact lens fitting; monitor the cornea after keratoplasty or refractive surgery, etc. There are many commercial models, some with scanning-slit technology which provides a map of the curvature and elevation of the anterior and posterior corneal surface.
See **corneal topography; keratoscope; photokeratoscope; Scheimpflug photography; Topogometer.**

Vieth–Müller circle *See* **horopter, Vieth–Müller.**

viewing angle *See* **angle, visual.**

viewing, eccentric Fixation in which the eye moves so as to place the image of an object outside the fovea. The object is perceived by the patient as looking 'past' it and not directly at it as in eccentric fixation. Eccentric viewing is often applied by people with low vision suffering from macular degeneration to improve reading a letter or a word by looking slightly above, below or to the side of it.
See **fixation, eccentric; vision, low.**

vignetting 1. A graduated reduction in retinal illuminance caused by light reaching the pupil at increasingly oblique angles. **2.** The difference in absorption between the two portions of photochromic fused bifocal lenses when the segment is not made of photochromic glass.
See **lens, photochromic; retinal illuminance.**

violet One of the hues of the visible spectrum evoked by stimulation of the retina by wavelengths shorter than 450 nm and somewhat longer than 380 nm.

virtual image; object *See* under the nouns.

virus A submicroscopic (20 to 600 nm in diameter) particle (called a virion), which typically contains a protein coat (called a capsid) surrounding genetic material in the form of a double or a single strand of RNA or DNA. Viruses replicate only within cells of living hosts. They can infect cells and are the cause of various diseases. This is accomplished by releasing the viral genetic material into the host cytoplasm if it is RNA or into the host nucleus if it is DNA, and thus inducing the production of new viral particles and newly infected cells. There are many viruses: DNA viruses as for example the adenovirus (some of which can cause epidemic conjunctivitis), herpesvirus and pox viruses, and RNA viruses as for example the picorna virus (e.g. hepatitis A), toga viruses (e.g. rubella), corona viruses (which can cause respiratory infection) and the retroviruses (e.g. HIV). *See* **antiviral agents; herpesvirus; gene therapy.**

viscocanalostomy A type of non-penetrating filtration surgery aimed at lowering intraocular pressure by dissecting a superficial scleral flap and excising a deeper partial-thickness scleral flap below, leaving a thin membrane consisting of trabeculum and Descemet's membrane, through which the aqueous humour diffuses. It then drains from the anterior chamber not through a scleral opening, but slowly into the subconjunctival space or through Schlemm's canal into which a high-density viscoelastic substance has been injected. The superficial flap is sutured in place at the end of the procedure. Intraocular pressure reduction is not usually as large as with trabeculectomy. *See* **filtration surgery.**

viscosity The property of a thick and sticky fluid to resistance to flow. For example, water has low viscosity whereas honey has high viscosity.

viscosity agents *See* **methylcellulose; wetting solution.**

visibility 1. The property of being visible to the eye. 2. The range of vision through different densities of atmosphere.

visible spectrum *See* **light; spectrum, visible.**

vision (V) 1. The appreciation of diversity in the external world, such as form, colour, position, etc. resulting from the stimulation of the retina by light. 2. *See* **acuity, unaided visual.**
achromatic v. *See* **achromatopsia.**
alternating v. *See* **lens, contact.**
ambient v. Vision mediated primarily by the peripheral retina and involved in spatial orientation and recognition of motion.
See **vision, focal.**
anomalous trichromatic v. *See* **trichromatism, anomalous.**
binocular v. Condition in which both eyes contribute towards producing a percept which may or may not be fused into a single impression.

See **fusion, sensory; monoblepsia; period, critical; test, bar reading; test, FRIEND; test, hole in the hand; test, Worth's four dot; vision, single binocular; vision, Worth's classification of binocular; zone of clear, single, binocular vision.**
binocular single v. *See* **vision, single binocular.**
blue v. *See* **chromatopsia.**
blurred v. Vision characterized by poor visual acuity or in which the edges of objects are indistinct. It may be due to uncorrected or poorly corrected ametropia or presbyopia, anomalies of the ocular media (e.g. cataract, corneal opacity, haemorrhage in the vitreous), amblyopia, excess lacrimation, spasm of accommodation, optic neuritis, angle-closure glaucoma, diabetes, multiple sclerosis, migraine, etc.
central v. Vision of objects formed on the foveola or the macula.
See **fusion, sensory.**
chromatic v. *See* **vision, colour.**
colour v. (CV) Vision in which the colour sense is experienced. It is mediated by three cone receptors, each with a different visual pigment. *Syn.* chromatic vision.
See **pigment, visual; theory, Hering's of colour vision; theory, Young–Helmholtz; trichromatism.**
daylight v. *See* **vision, photopic.**
defective colour v. *See* **colour vision, defective.**
deuteranomalous v. *See* **deuteranomaly.**
dichromatic v. *See* **dichromatism.**
distance v. Vision of objects situated either at infinity or more usually at some 5 or 6 m.
See **chart, Snellen; vision, near.**
diurnal v. *See* **vision, photopic.**
double v. *See* **diplopia.**
eccentric v. *See* **fixation, eccentric; vision, peripheral.**
entoptic v. *See* **image, entoptic.**
extrafoveal v. *See* **vision, peripheral.**
field of v. *See* **field, visual.**
focal v. Vision mediated by, primarily, the macular area of the retina and involved in the examination and identification of objects.
See **vision, ambient.**
green v. *See* **chromatopsia.**
gun barrel v. *See* **vision, tunnel.**
haploscopic v. Vision as obtained by looking in a haploscope.
indirect v. *See* **vision, peripheral.**
industrial v. The branch of optometry concerned with vision and perception by the individual at work, the evaluation of visual performance in a given occupation, the prescribing of protective ocular devices and the determination of the optimum environment (e.g. illumination) to accomplish a visual task efficiently.
intermediate v. Vision of objects situated beyond 40 cm from the eye but closer than, say, 1.5 m.
See **vision, distance, vision, near.**
island of v. *See* **island of vision.**
low v. Vision impairment even after correction by conventional lenses, resulting from either congenital anomalies or ocular diseases such as cataract, glaucoma, age-related macular degeneration,

pathological myopia, trachoma, onchocerciasis, etc. The correction and rehabilitation of patients with low vision is achieved by special aids called **low vision aids** (LVA), such as a telescopic lens, and appropriate counselling (e.g. about illumination and reading distance). The criteria that the health authorities normally use to classify a person as having partial sight take into consideration not only the corrected visual acuity but also the extent of visual field loss (generally less than 20°). *Syn.* partial sight; subnormal vision.

The **World Health Organization (WHO)** defines low vision as visual acuity less than 6/18 (20/60) and equal to or better than 3/60 (10/200) in the better eye with best correction.
See aids, low vision; blindness; bracketing; chart, Bailey–Lovie; chart, contrast sensitivity; clipover; deaf-blind; lamp, halogen; lens, cross-cylinder; lens, telescopic; magnification, apparent; magnification, relative distance; magnification, relative size; magnifier; rule, Kestenbaum's; spectacles, magnifying; spectacles, pinhole; telescope, galilean; test, Pepper; typoscope; viewing, eccentric.

mesopic v. Vision at intermediate levels between photopic and scotopic vision, and corresponding to luminances ranging from about 10^{-3} to 10 cd/m^2. Both cones and rods function in mesopic vision. *Syn.* twilight vision.

monochromatic v. Synonym of monochromatism. *See* monochromat.

monocular v. Vision of one eye only.

multiple v. *See* polyopia.

near v. (NV) Vision of objects situated 25 to 50 cm from either the eye or more commonly the spectacle plane.
See Jaeger test types; vision, distance.

night v.; nocturnal v. *See* vision, scotopic.

panoramic v. Vision of some animals whose eyes are located laterally so that the two visual fields overlap only slightly or are adjacent, thus providing vision over a much larger region of the environment than if the two lines of sight were aimed in the same direction.

peripheral v. Vision resulting from stimulation of the retina outside the fovea or macula. *Syn.* eccentric vision; extrafoveal vision; indirect vision.
See fusion, sensory; vision, central.

photopic v. Vision at high levels of luminance (above 5 cd/m^2) and resulting from the functioning of the cones. In this condition, the eye is most sensitive to light of wavelength 507 nm. *Syn.* daylight vision; diurnal vision; photopia.
See theory, duplicity; Table E1 p. 106; Table T1, p. 362; threshold, differential.

protanomalous v. *See* protanomaly.

red v. *See* chromatopsia.

v. science The scientific study of how the visual system contributes to an understanding of the environment by processing and interpreting the light stimulation to the eye. Various disciplines contribute to vision science including anatomy, biology, optics, optometry, physiology and psychology. *Syn.* visual science.

scotopic v. Vision at low levels of luminance, below about 10^{-3} cd/m^2 and resulting from the functioning of the rods. *Syn.* night vision; nocturnal vision; scotopia.
See theory, duplicity.

v. screener An instrument used to measure various visual functions rapidly and inexpensively. There are various models, but most are modified stereoscopes with an internally illuminated set of targets and an optical system or variable target positioning to simulate either a near or far testing distance. Most of these instruments measure visual acuity, heterophoria, fusion, stereopsis, colour vision and visual field.
See photorefraction.

simultaneous v. *See* lens, contact.

single binocular v. Condition in which both eyes contribute towards producing a single fused percept.
See fusion, sensory.

spatial v. *See* perception, depth.

stereoscopic v. *See* stereopsis.

stress, v. *See* syndrome, Meares–Irlen.

subnormal v. *See* vision, low.

telescopic v. *See* vision, tunnel.

v. therapy; v. training *See* training, visual.

tritanomalous v. *See* tritanomaly.

tunnel v. Vision limited to the central part of the visual field as though one were looking through a hollow tube. It may be a symptom of hysteria, malingering, the final stage of either open-angle glaucoma or retinitis pigmentosa, etc. *Syn.* gun barrel vision; telescopic vision.
See amblyopia, hysterical; field, visual f. expander.

twilight v. *See* vision, mesopic.

Worth's classification of binocular v. For the purpose of visual rehabilitation, binocular vision is often classified into three grades: (1) simultaneous binocular vision (first-degree fusion or superimposition); (2) fusion (sensory fusion or second-degree fusion or flat fusion); and (3) stereopsis (third-degree fusion).
See fusion, sensory; superimposition.

yellow v. *See* xanthopsia.

Vistech A clinical test designed to measure contrast sensitivity. It consists of a chart containing five horizontal rows, each with nine circular patches of sinusoidal gratings. The gratings are either vertical or 15° to the right or to the left. Each row has a different spatial frequency, starting from the top of the chart: 1.5, 3.0, 6.0, 12.0 and 18.0 cycles per degrees when viewed at a distance of 40 cm. The contrast level of each of the nine gratings decreases from 33% to 0% from left to right in approximately 0.25 log unit steps. The patient is asked to look along each row, identifying the orientation of the grating. The testing is carried out monocularly with optical correction, if any. The last grating of each row that is incorrectly identified is noted on an evaluation form, which is provided with the test. The end points of each of the five rows are connected to form a contrast sensitivity curve for each patient. It is then compared with

normal values indicated on the form. There is also a version for testing at distance. A new version of the Vistech called **Functional Acuity Contrast Test (FACT)** uses similar stimuli but with a constant step size of 0.15 log units. It provides better resolution when determining contrast sensitivity changes. *Syn.* Vision Contrast Test System (VCTS).
See **chart, contrast sensitivity; test, Arden grating.**

visual Relating to vision.

visual acuity; agnosia; agraphia *See* under the nouns.

Visual Analysis Skills Test *See* **test, developmental and perceptual screening.**

visual allesthesia; angle; area; association areas; axis; centre; cliff *See* under the nouns.

visual cortex *See* **area, visual.**

visual deprivation *See* **deprivation, visual.**

visual direction *See* **line of direction.**

visual display unit The visual image appearing on the screen of a cathode ray tube.
See **syndrome, computer vision.**

visual efficiency scale, Snell–Sterling *See* **Snell–Sterling visual efficiency scale.**

visual evoked cortical potential *See* **potential, visual evoked cortical.**

visual extinction *See* **phenomenon, extinction.**

visual fatigue; field *See* under the nouns.

visual field, binocular *See* **field, binocular visual.**

visual field expander *See* **field, visual f. expander.**

visual hallucination; illusion *See* under the nouns.

visual integration *See* **integration, visual.**

visual line of direction *See* **line of direction.**

visual neglect *See* **neglect, visual.**

visual optics; pathway; pigment; plane; point *See* under the nouns.

visual perseveration *See* **palinopsia.**

visual purple *See* **rhodopsin.**

visual search A perceptual task pursued to find a particular feature in a visual display or environment. One such occurrence is finding a given letter in a page of text.

visual science *See* **vision, science.**

visual system, magnocellular; parvocellular *See* **system, magnocellular; system, parvocellular.**

visual system, sustained *See* **system, parvocellular visual.**

visual system, transient *See* **system, magnocellular visual.**

visual training *See* **training, visual.**

visualization 1. The ability to form a mental image of an object not present in the field of view. 2.

Synonym for imagery. *Example*: visualizing the face of a person speaking on the radio.
See **imagery.**

visus Vision.

Visuscope A modified ophthalmoscope containing a small graticule target for the measurement of eccentric fixation. The examiner projects a shadow of the target on the patient's retina. The patient is asked to look at the centre of the target. The position of the foveal reflex relative to the centre of the graticule target indicates whether the patient has eccentric fixation and in which direction and by how much. A modified version is the **Euthyscope**, in which the graticule target consists of black spots rather than a star and concentric circles as in the Visuscope. The Euthyscope is used more for eccentric fixation therapy.
See **pleoptics.**

vitamin A deficiency A deficiency of vitamin A leads to interference with tissue nutrition and growth, atrophy of epithelial tissues, reduced resistance to infection of mucous membranes and various eye disorders including abnormal production and regeneration of rhodopsin resulting in night blindness, mucin deficiency due to goblet cell dysfunction and consequent xerophthalmia with Bitot's spots, conjunctival xerosis, and if longstanding corneal xerosis, corneal ulcerations and keratomalacia. Management includes a balanced diet and may require large vitamin A supplement with a topical antibiotic to prevent secondary infections.
See **carotene; hemeralopia; keratomalacia; photopigment; rhodopsin; xerophthalmia; xerosis.**

vitamin B deficiency *See* **homocystinuria; keratitis, punctate epithelial; neuropathy, nutritional optic.**

vitamin C and E *See* **macular degeneration, age-related.**

vitelliform macular dystrophy *See* **disease, Best's.**

vitiligo A disease of the skin characterized by areas of depigmentation of various sizes and shapes. In the eye, it can be seen in the choroid or iris. It is often associated with syphilis or tuberculosis and forms part of the **Vogt–Koyanagi–Harada syndrome**.
See **poliosis.**

vitrectomy Removal of the whole or a portion of the vitreous humour and replacement by saline or, more commonly, silicone oil or a gas (SF_6, C_2F_6 or C_3F_8), which serves as a tamponade agent. Indications for this surgical intervention include gaining access to a diseased retina, following retinal detachment, persistent vitreous opacities (usually as a result of unabsorbed haemorrhage), severe penetrating trauma, luxation of the lens, or removal of some foreign bodies which cannot be removed with a magnet. The intervention is usually performed through an opening in the pars plana of the ciliary body.
See **injection, intravitreal; retinopexy; tamponade.**

vitreoretinal degeneration *See* disease, Wagner's; syndrome, Stickler's.

vitreoretinopathy, familial exudative An autosomal dominant disorder involving chromosome 11q, although some cases may be X-linked. It is characterized by abrupt cessation of peripheral vessels at the equator, especially on the temporal side, resulting in vitreous degeneration, peripheral telangiectasia and fibrovascular proliferation. Complications include subretinal exudation and tractional retinal detachment. Possible treatments include photocoagulation or cryopexy.

vitreous base A dense broad band (3 to 4 mm wide) of vitreous attachment to the peripheral retina near the ora serrata. Collagen vitreous fibrils blend anteriorly with the basal lamina of the non-pigmented epithelium of the pars plana of the ciliary body and posteriorly with the internal limiting membrane of the retina.

vitreous body *See* vitreous humour.

vitreous chamber *See* chamber, vitreous.

vitreous detachment Separation of the vitreous body from the internal limiting membrane of the retina due to shrinkage from degenerative or inflammatory conditions, trauma, progressive myopia, old age, diabetes and in aphakic eyes in which the lens extraction was intracapsular. The most common cases are elderly individuals in whom the posterior part of the vitreous, which becomes liquefied (synchysis), detaches from the internal limiting membrane (called **posterior vitreous detachment**). Symptoms are flashes, floaters, myodesopia and photopsia because as the eye moves the vitreous body comes into contact with the retina and occasionally haemorrhage. The condition is sometimes associated with retinal tears and retinal detachment and then requires retinopexy.
See horseshoe tear; retinal break; retinopexy; ring, Weiss'; syneresis.

vitreous floaters *See* floaters.

vitreous haemorrhage *See* haemorrhage, preretinal; retinopathy, diabetic.

vitreous humour A transparent, colourless, gelatinous mass of a consistency somewhat firmer than egg white which fills the space between the crystalline lens, the ciliary body and the retina, and constitutes four-fifths of the volume of the eye. The vitreous is about 99% water; the remaining 1% includes hyaluronic acid, organic salts and soluble and insoluble proteins especially collagen (mainly type II). Its outer surface has a high collagen density, called the **cortex**, which merges with the ciliary epithelium and the internal limiting membrane of the retina. It is firmly attached to the retina (**vitreoretinal adhesion**) around the optic disc, to the lens at the ligament of Wieger and most firmly to the pars plana

of the ciliary body near the ora serrata in an area known as the **vitreous base**. In the elderly and in pathological conditions the vitreous is no longer in a gel state, tending to become fluid. *Syn.* vitreous body. *Note*: Most practitioners refer to this term as simply vitreous.
See artery, hyaloid; asteroid hyalosis; floaters; hyaloid remnant; synchisis scintillans; syndrome, Wagner's; vitreous base; vitreous detachment.

vitreous, persistent hyperplastic primary A congenital, abnormal, vitreous development characterized by a retrolental mass formed by remnants of the hyaloid system and tunica vasculosa lentis. The eye presents with leukocoria and there may also be cataract and congenital glaucoma. Treatment should begin as early in life as possible to avoid the risk of damage to the globe and amblyopia.
See artery, hyaloid; hyaloid remnant.

vitritis Inflammatory reaction of the vitreous as a result of a disease in the adjacent structures, such as the ciliary body, the choroid or the retina, which causes infiltration of cells into the vitreous sometimes causing fluffy 'cotton balls' or 'string of pearls' lesions. Patients complain of floaters and/or blurred vision. *Note*: also spelt vitreitis.
See endophthalmitis; hyalitis; uveitis, intermediate.

Vogt's striae *See* striae, Vogt's.

Vogt, palisades of *See* palisades of Vogt.

Vogt's white limbal girdle A white arc-like opacity in the cornea located concentric with the limbus in the 3 and 9 o'clock positions. Type 1 is a discontinuous band separated from the limbus by a clear zone. Type 2 is an unbroken band, made up mainly of hyaline deposits and is continuous with the sclera. This degeneration becomes more prevalent with age.

Volk lens *See* slit-lamp.

von Graefe's sign *See* disease, Graves'; sign, von Graefe's.

von Graefe's test *See* test, diplopia.

von Hippel's disease *See* disease, von Hippel's.

von Hippel–Lindau syndrome *See* syndrome, von Hippel–Lindau.

von Recklinghausen's disease *See* neurofibromatosis type 1.

vortex vein *See* vein, vortex.

V pattern *See* pattern, alphabet.

Vossius' ring *See* ring, Vossius'.

V syndrome *See* pattern, alphabet.

V-value *See* constringence.

W

wafer A very thin lens to be cemented on a larger lens to make a bifocal lens.

Wagner's disease *See* syndrome, Wagner's.

wall eye *See* eye, wall.

warpage, corneal *See* corneal warpage.

water content Water in a contact lens expressed as a percentage of the total mass of the lens in its hydrated state under equilibrium conditions with physiological saline solution containing 9 g/l sodium chloride at a temperature of 20 ± 0.5°C and with a stated pH value.

$$\text{Water content} = \frac{M - m}{M} \times 100$$

where M is the mass of hydrated lens and m is the mass of dry lens.
The **U.S. Food and Drug Administration (FDA)** has categorized hydrogel contact lenses into four groups according to their water content and their surface reactivity (referred to as ionic if it contains more than 0.2% ionic material and non-ionic otherwise). Group 1: water content less than 50% and non-ionic. Group 2: water content greater than 50% and non-ionic. Group 3: water content less than 50% and ionic. Group 4: water content greater than 50% and ionic.

water-drinking test *See* test, provocative.

waterfall after-effect; illusion *See* after-effect, waterfall.

watery eye *See* epiphora.

wave, alpha *See* alpha waves.

wave number *See* wavelength.

wave theory *See* theory, wave.

wavefront A virtual surface emanating from an object or an optical system, perpendicular throughout to a bundle of rays.
See aberration, wavefront.

wavelength Distance in the direction of propagation of a periodic wave between two successive points at the same position in the wave (e.g. the distance between two crests). *Symbol:* λ. *Note 1:* The wavelength in a medium is equal to the wavelength in vacuum divided by the refractive index of the medium. Unless otherwise stated, values of wavelength are generally those in air. The refractive index of standard air (15°C, 101 325 N/m²) lies between 1.00027 and 1.00029 for visible radiations. *Note 2:* The reciprocal of the wavelength is called the **wave number**. *Note 3:* The wavelength is longer for red light than for blue light. Wavelength λ is equal to

$$\lambda = c/v$$

where c is the velocity of light and v is the frequency of light. (Fig. W1)
See fluorescence; infrared; interferometer; light; phase; phenomenon, Bezold–Brücke; spectrum, electromagnetic; ultraviolet; theory, wave.

wavelength, complementary *See* colour, complementary.

wavelength discrimination Ability to distinguish one wavelength from another. It varies across the visible spectrum. This is determined by comparing one-half of a field illuminated with one wavelength against the other half illuminated with the same intensity wavelength which is then adjusted to a slightly different wavelength until it appears different in hue. The discrimination is best around 495 nm and 590 nm. Individuals with colour vision deficiency exhibit very different patterns than color normals.

wavelength, dominant (of a colour stimulus, not purple) Wavelength of a monochromatic light stimulus, that, when combined in suitable proportions with the specified achromatic light stimulus, yields a match with the colour stimulus considered. *Note:* When the dominant wavelength cannot be given (this applies to purples), its place is taken by the complementary wavelength (CIE). *See* chromaticity diagram; colour, complementary.

W cell *See* cell, W.

Weber's fraction; law *See* law, Weber's.

Weber's syndrome *See* syndrome, Weber's.

Weber–Fechner law *See* law, Weber's.

wedge, optical A filter in which the transmittance varies continuously along a path (straight or curved) on its surface. If the filter transmits all the wavelengths more or less equally, it is called a **neutral wedge**.
See phenomenon, Bielschowsky's.

weeping Excessive lacrimation.
See epiphora; lacrimal apparatus; lacrimation.

weeping reflex *See* reflex, lacrimal.

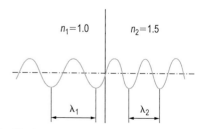

Fig. W1 Wavelength of light in air and in a medium of refractive index n_1 and n_2, respectively ($\lambda_2 = \lambda_1/n_2$).

Wegener's granulomatosis A systemic disease appearing in middle age with varying degrees of vasculitis, which principally affects the respiratory tract and the kidneys. Ocular manifestations include orbital congestion, proptosis, restrictive eye movements, peripheral ulcerative keratitis, dacryocystitis and pain. Management consists of corticosteroids and immunosuppressive agents and decompression of the orbital congestion, if severe.

Weill–Marchesani syndrome *See* syndrome, Weill–Marchesani.

Weiss' ring *See* ring, Weiss'.

Welland's test *See* test, bar reading.

Wernicke's disease *See* disease, Wernicke's.

Wernicke's hemianopic pupil; pupillary reaction; pupillary reflex; sign *See* reflex, hemianopic pupillary.

Wessley ring *See* ring, Wessley.

Wesson Fixation Disparity Card *See* disparity, retinal.

wettability *See* angle, contact.

wetting angle *See* angle, contact.

wetting solution A solution that (1) transforms a hydrophobic surface into a hydrophilic one; (2) acts as a lubricant; (3) helps to clean the surface or (4) helps to prevent contamination of the lens while being inserted. It is spread on both surfaces of a rigid contact lens prior to insertion. However, the effect of a wetting solution only lasts a short time because it is quickly removed by the tear layer. It is no longer available on its own. *See* enzyme; tears, artificial.

'what' system *See* system, parvocellular visual.

Wheatstone amblyopia *See* amblyoscope, Wheatstone.

'where' system *See* system, magnocellular visual.

white 1. An achromatic visual sensation of maximum lightness. **2.** A visual sensation evoked in the normal human eye by a mixture of different wavelengths of nearly the same characteristics as daylight as, for example, the light produced by illuminants C or D. *See* colour, achromatic; colour, complementary; light, white.

white body *See* body, white.

white dot syndromes *See* syndrome, white dot.

white pupil; pupillary reflex *See* leukocoria.

Whitnall's ligament *See* muscle, levator palpebrae superioris.

Whitnall's tubercle *See* tubercle, lateral orbital.

wide-angle lens *See* lens, wide-angle.

Wieger, ligament of *See* ligament of Wieger.

Wies' procedure *See* procedure, Wies'.

Wilbrand's knee That portion of the decussating optic nerve fibres from the inferior nasal retina which loop forward into the contralateral optic nerve for a distance of up to 3 mm from the anterior part of the optic chiasma and then pass backward into the optic tract. The existence of Wilbrand's knee in normal subjects has been questioned.
See scotoma, junction.

Willis, circle of *See* circle of Willis.

Wilson's disease *See* disease, Wilson's.

Wilson three-mirror fundus lens *See* slit-lamp.

wing cells *See* corneal epithelium.

wing, Maddox *See* Maddox wing.

wink The rapid voluntary closure and opening of one eye.
See blink.

with movement *See* movement, with; neutralization; retinoscope.

with the rule astigmatism *See* astigmatism, with the rule.

Wolfring, glands of *See* gland of Wolfring.

Wollaston ellipse *See* ellipse, Tscherning.

Wollaston lens *See* lens, Wollaston.

Wollaston polarizer; prism *See* prism, Wollaston.

Wood's light *See* light, Wood's.

word blindness *See* alexia.

working distance *See* distance, working.

Worth amblyoscope *See* amblyoscope, Worth.

Worth's classification of binocular vision *See* vision, Worth's classification of binocular.

Worth's four dot test *See* test, Worth's four dot.

Wundt's visual illusion *See* illusion, Wundt's visual.

X

xanthelasma A cutaneous deposition of lipid material that appears in the skin of the eyelids, most commonly near the inner canthi. It appears as a yellowish slightly elevated area. It is a benign and chronic condition that occurs primarily in the elderly. It may be associated with raised blood cholesterol, high-density lipoprotein and triglyceride levels, leading to heart disease or diabetes. *Syn.* xanthoma; xanthelasma palpebrarum; xanthoma palpebrarum. *See* corneal arcus; plaques, Hollenhorst's.

xanthogranuloma, juvenile (JXG) Benign proliferation of single or multiple small yellowish-brown papules or nodules, which may be found in the skin and the anterior uvea, especially in the iris. The condition mainly appears in young children, although it may occur in adults. The lesions consist of dermal infiltration by histiocytes, lymphocytes, eosinophils and Touton giant cells. The skin lesions increase in size and number but eventually regress spontaneously into an atrophic scar, otherwise they may need to be treated by excision or corticosteroid injection. Although the condition rarely affects the eye, when it occurs it is commonly associated with hyphaemia (in the anterior chamber), uveitis and secondary glaucoma with visual loss. Therapy includes topical and systemic corticosteroids. *Syn.* juvenile nevoxanthoendothelioma.

xanthoma *See* xanthelasma.

xanthopsia A condition in which all objects appear of a yellow colour. It may occur as a result of picric acid and santonin poisoning, or jaundice. *Syn.* yellow vision.
See chromatopsia.

***x*-axis** *See* axis, transverse.

X cell *See* cell, X.

X chromosome *See* chromosome.

X-Chrom lens *See* lens, X-Chrom.

xenograft A surgical graft of tissue transplanted from one species to another species. *Example*: a graft of pig tissue to a human.
See allograft.

xeroderma pigmentosum An autosomal recessive inherited disease in which there is progressive pigmentary degeneration of the skin, especially in sun-exposed areas. It results from a deficient enzyme used in the repair of DNA damaged by ultraviolet light. The condition begins in infancy and is characterized by the appearance of numerous pigmented spots resembling freckles and telangiectases. Eventually atrophic patches appear as well as wart-like excrescence and often squamous cell carcinoma. Patients are photophobic and the eyelids are frequently affected with atrophy and ectropion, which may be accompanied with conjunctival inflammation and corneal ulceration. Protection of the eyes and skin is essential as well as surgical removal of the carcinomatous tumours, but many patients eventually succumb to metastases.

xeroma *See* xerophthalmia.

xerophthalmia Extreme dryness of the conjunctiva and cornea due to a failure of the secretory activity of the mucin-secreting goblet cells of the conjunctiva. It is caused by vitamin A deficiency. The conjunctiva and cornea lose their lustre and become skin-like in appearance. The first sign is night blindness, followed by conjunctival xerosis with Bitot's spots and if long-standing corneal xerosis, corneal ulceration and possibly severe keratomalacia. Management includes ocular lubrication and systemic administration of vitamin A. *Syn.* xeroma; xerosis of the conjunctiva (if the cornea is not involved).
See keratoconjunctivitis sicca; keratomalacia; mucin; spot, Bitot's; vitamin A deficiency.

xerosis Excessive tissue dryness as may be found in the skin and the eye (e.g. conjunctival xerosis) most commonly as a result of vitamin A deficiency.
See spot, Bitot's; xerophthalmia.

X-linked inheritance *See* inheritance.

x pattern *See* pattern, alphabet.

xylometazoline *See* antihistamine.

Y

***y*-axis** *See* axis, anteroposterior.

YAG laser *See* laser, neodymium-YAG.

Y cell *See* cell, Y.

Y chromosome *See* chromosome.

yellow One of the hues of the visible spectrum evoked by stimulation of the retina by wavelengths situated in a narrow region between about 560 and 590 nm, i.e. between red and green. The complementary colours to yellow are blues.

yellow spot *See* macula lutea.

yellow vision *See* xanthopsia.

yoke muscles *See* muscle, yoke.

yoke prisms *See* prism, yoke.

Young's experiment *See* experiment, Young's.

Young's modulus of elasticity *See* modulus of elasticity.

Young's optometer *See* optometer, Young's.

Young–Helmholtz theory *See* theory, Young–Helmholtz.

Y pattern *See* pattern, alphabet.

y sutures of the lens *See* lens sutures.

z-axis *See* axis, vertical.

Zeis, glands of *See* gland, of Zeis.

Zeiss lens *See* lens, Zeiss.

Zellweger's syndrome *See* syndrome, Zellweger's.

Zernike polynomials *See* aberration, wavefront.

zero point *See* point, zero.

zinc A metallic element of which several salts are essential for growth. It can be found in many tissues of the body including the brain. Most ocular tissues such as the retina, choroid, Bruch's membrane and the retinal pigment epithelium contain zinc. Zinc deficiency is associated with age-related macular degeneration.
See **macular degeneration, age-related.**

zinc sulphate An astringent and antiseptic agent sometimes used topically in solution 0.2% or 0.25% to clear mucus from the outer surface of the eye (due to precipitating proteins), to give temporary relief of minor eye infections and to treat some types of bacterial conjunctivitis.

Zinn, annulus of *See* annulus of Zinn.

Zinn, circle of *See* circle of Zinn.

Zinn, zonule of A series of fibres passing from the ciliary body to the capsule of the lens at or near its equator, holding the lens in position and enabling the ciliary muscles to act upon it. The lens and zonule form a diaphragm that divides the eye into a small anterior area, which contains aqueous humour, and a larger posterior area, which contains vitreous humour. The zonule forms a ring that is roughly triangular in a meridional section. It is made up of fibres that are transparent and straight for the most part. The tension of these fibres varies with the state of contraction of the ciliary muscle and thus affects the convexity of the lens. The zonule of Zinn is made up of many non-cellular fibres, the fibrils of which consist of a cysteine-rich microfibrillar component of the elastic system, fibrillin. The fibres have been classified as follows: (1) The **hyaloid zonule (orbiculo-posterior capsular fibres)** which originate from the pars plana of the ciliary body and insert into the capsule just posterior to the equator at the edge of the patellar fossa. (2) The **anterior zonule (orbiculo-anterior capsular fibres** or **anterior zonular sheet)**, which originate from the pars plana of the ciliary body and insert into the capsule just anterior to the equator. These are the strongest and thickest of the zonular fibres. (3) The **posterior zonule (cilio-posterior capsular fibres** or **posterior zonular sheet)**, which originate from the pars plicata of the ciliary body and insert into the lens capsule posterior to the equator. These are the most numerous. (4) The **equatorial zonule (cilio-equatorial fibres)** which originate from the pars plicata of the ciliary body and insert into the lens capsule at the equator. *Syn.* suspensory apparatus of the lens; suspensory ligament; zonular fibres.
See **canal, Hannover's; canal of Petit; ciliary processes; Fig. C1, p. 47; ora serrata.**

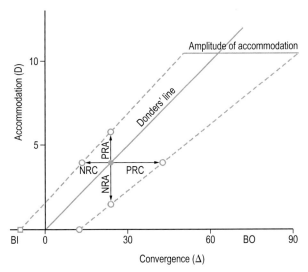

Fig. Z1 Zone of clear, single, binocular vision (NRC, negative relative convergence; PRC, positive relative convergence; NRA, negative relative accommodation; PRA, positive relative accommodation; BI, base-in prism; BO, base-out prism).

Zollner's visual illusion *See* illusion, Zollner's visual.

zone, ciliary *See* iris.

zone of comfort *See* criterion, Percival.

zone of the cornea, optical *See* optical zone of the cornea.

zone, optic *See* optic zone.

zone, papillary *See* iris.

zone, scleral *See* scleral zone.

zone of clear, single, binocular vision In Donders' diagram, it is the region determined by the extremes of accommodation and convergence that can be evoked while retaining a clear, single image. Clinically, this is determined by measuring the limits of negative and positive relative convergence by using base-in and base-out prisms to blur, or by measuring relative accommodation by binocularly adding concave or convex lenses, for various binocularly fixated distances (Fig. Z1). *See* **accommodation, relative amplitude of; convergence, relative; criterion, Percival;** criterion, Sheard; Donders' diagram; prism, rotary; vision, binocular.

zonula occludentes *See* tight junction.

zonular fibres *See* Zinn, zonule of.

zonule of Zinn *See* Zinn, zonule of.

zonulolysis Dissolution of the fibres of the zonule of Zinn by an enzyme so as to facilitate intracapsular extraction. The method is rarely used nowadays. The term may also refer to breakage of the zonule due to trauma. *Syn.* zonulysis.

zoom lens *See* lens, zoom.

zoster, herpes *See* herpes zoster; herpes zoster ophthalmicus.

zygomatic bone *See* orbit.

zygomatic foramen *See* Table O4, p. 245.

zygomatic nerve *See* nerve, zygomatic.

zygomycosis *See* phycomycosis.